Medical Ethics

A Clinical Textbook and Reference for the Health Care Professions

Edited by

Natalie Abrams

Michael D. Buckner

A Bradford Book

The MIT Press
Cambridge, Massachusetts, and London, England

Printed in the Unites States of America.

Library of Congress Cataloging in Publication Data:
Main entry under title:

Medical ethics.

  "A Bradford book."
  Includes bibliographical references and index.
  1. Medical ethics.   I. Abrams, Natalie.   II. Buckner,
Michael D.
R724.M2928   1982   174'.2   82-42556
ISBN 0-262-01068-2
ISBN 0-262-51024-3 (pbk.)

Design and Composition:
Horne Associates, Inc.

Jacket Design:
Irene Elios

To Robert, Jacqueline, Peter, and Alexander Abrams;
and Mallory Lennox

Acknowledgments

The idea for this reader emerged several years ago when our attempts to teach clinical ethics to medical students was frustrated by the primarily theoretical and abstract thrust of the available readers in bioethics. Our constant search for readings covering the practicalities of clinical practice convinced us of the need for such a text. The project became feasible with the large increase in research during the past seven years as increasing numbers of philosophers, sociologists, physicians, nurses, and health professionals turned their attention to issues in the ethics of clinical practice.

We would like to express our appreciation to those of our colleagues in medicine, nursing, and philosophy who during the past several years have provided support and encouragement for our work at New York University's School of Medicine. In particular, we would like to thank William Ruddick, Ph.D., who for the past few years has shared the task of teaching philosophy to medical students and helped lay the foundations for this text.

The text would not have been possible without the tireless editorial assistance of Carolyn Riehl, the administrative coordinator of our Philosophy and Medicine Program. In these tasks she was assisted by our secretary Rose Horowitz, by Lori Martin, and by the medical students Bernard Birnbaum and Karen Hopkins, who contributed cases to the text. Michael Brown and Peter Santogade, M.D., served as consultants for the collection and organization of case histories.

Finally, we would like to express our gratitude to Harry and Betty Stanton of the MIT Press/Bradford Books for their early and enthusiastic support of this project.

Much of the teaching and research that led to the development of this book was supported by grants from the National Endowment for the Humanities, Division of Education Programs; The New York Council for the Humanities; and the Office of Interdisciplinary Programs, Department of Health and Human Services.

New York City   N.A.
August 1982   M.D.B.

CONTENTS

II. CLINICAL IDEALS AND BEHAVIOR   *91*

PSYCHIATRIC ISSUES

PLACEBOS

ABORTION

General Introduction

During the past decade the discipline of bioethics has achieved a place in the curricula of nearly all university philosophy departments and most health profession schools, including medicine, nursing, dentistry, and allied health fields. Selected bioethical issues have influenced courses in related social science departments such as history, sociology, and anthropology. Most theology departments and divinity schools are concerned with the impact of these issues on the ministry. In response to their demand, there has been an attendant increase in anthologies and other texts on bioethics. Unfortunately, because most of these have been developed by college faculty for humanities courses, they do not meet the special needs of the professional schools in either content or format. Specifically, they are not focused upon the issues of most relevance to physicians and other health professionals in training, and the articles included are usually too abstract to benefit the professional in his or her actual practice.

Out of our experience in teaching medical, dental, and undergraduate students at New York University, we have developed a reader which we believe is well suited to the curricula present in most health profession schools. We assume that ethics develops from the need to make choices and commitments in the course of action. Thus, a basic reader in professional ethics must begin with concrete situations, cases, and issues. It should serve the student and teacher as a source book for developing the discussion of ethical issues. To this end, we have aimed at providing primary material on matters of greatest concern to health practitioners. We have selected items that best capture the working realities of health care and the moral dilemmas and choices that are forced upon the conscientious health practitioner. The text places priority upon providing the student with descriptions of medical situations and the choices to be faced in patient care, presentation of particular positions or decisions, and debate over the rationale and justification for various options.

An essential component in enabling the young professional to develop a moral consciousness about his or her work is to have a considered and well-articulated concept of professional identity. This requires discussion of a variety of issues not usually included in the standard bioethics reader, such as ideals and models of professional identity, the nature of professional training, and the fundamentals of professional service. Such an orientation leads to a set of readings quite different from the items usually included under the rubric "doctor-patient relationship." Much of the relevant work in this area has been developed by sociologists rather than "ethicists," although analyses developed by the latter are essential for the articulation of a moral professional code, or a "professional ethic." In this regard, we have included a unique set of readings in the second section, Clinical Ideals and Behavior.

The nature of medical work has been undergoing extensive change during the past several decades. There has been the development of new professions sharing the general goal of caring

for and curing sick people, the development of new methods of care, the extension of old
facilities such as hospitals in a manner resulting in their transformation, and a basic redefinition of the individual's commitment to the "life" of being a professional. This has led to a
perplexity concerning the norms appropriate to conduct between doctor and patient as
well as to a host of new questions concerning the authority relationship between "health professionals" and the obligations of professionals as employees of institutions. Selections to
cover each of these issues are also included in the section on clinical ideals and behavior. It is
hoped that students, e.g., medical students concerned about their status as young physicians,
will be able to devote some reflection to the ideals and norms that are possible as they enter
their professional careers. In addition to general discussions of roles, ideals, authority, communication, etc., we have provided selections concerned with the medical students' experiences and training.

Another aspect of the clinical orientation of the text has led us to avoid organizing selections under the topics "Paternalism" and "Truth Telling." Although these are favored themes
in the philosophical literature, they are only part of more general questions about the nature
of communication and the nature of authority in decision making in medical care. The young
physician knows that if lying is permissible in a particular situation, it is nonetheless a wrong
that requires special justification. But it is the nature of the justifications, and their ubiquitous presence in most aspects of communicating with patients, that is the matter of first concern. These concerns with communication are invariably integrated with efforts to teach
"interviewing" to preclinical students. The physician often overlooks the ethical aspects of
interviewing as a form of communication. Thus, we have included selections that attempt
to reveal the norms implicit in this form of communication.

Given the practical nature of medical science, the practicing professional, physician,
nurse, or health care student is concerned with individual patients and the application of
types of solutions to their problems rather than with developing taxonomies and abstract
systems of principles and analysis. Therefore, we have structured several major sections
of the third section, Issues in Clinical Ethics, around types of medical situations, and subdivisions around types of patient groups or diseases, including children, prisoners, the
elderly, and patients with Down's syndrome. We have devoted an entire subdivision to the
problems inherent in achieving the informed consent of the patient. Problems arise with
individuals in extremely debilitating and stressful conditions, and individuals who lack the
capacity either to be informed or to voluntarily commit any act. Also raised are basic objections to the notion that consent is impossible in certain situations, e.g., with infants or
the comatose, and arguments that the judiciary must become more involved in guardian
proceedings.

Consistent with this clinical focus, we have developed a section on Aggressiveness of
Patient Care, which covers the range of issues from terminating life-supporting technology to
the question of degree of therapeutic support for various kinds of patients. All medical students confront these difficult situations in their first clinical days and will live with them
throughout their entire professional careers, although perhaps never with the vividness and
stress present when they serve as residents. Our selections discuss newborns, critically injured,
and the elderly. The topic is approached from ethical, legal, and religious perspectives.

Two other sections of the text merit specific mention. The first is a section of more than
fifty cases in the Appendix. Although many of the readings contain extensive case histories,
the Appendix should prove valuable for class discussion. The cases there are intended as

supplements for all assignments. This is facilitated by a method of cross referencing employed in the text. First, in the introductions to each chapter and section, relevant cases are referenced by number. Second, each case is listed with a series of corresponding chapter heads for which assignment of that case would be relevant. Since many cases are relevant to several chapters, the listings are extensive. (See preface to cases.)

Appendix B consists of a number of codes, statutes, and regulations; and Appendix C includes highly edited presentations of the judicial opinions from major legal decisions concerned with biomedical issues discussed in the text. This legal material, supplemented with several sections reviewing case law concerned with "due care" and Supreme Court rulings, provides the text with a rich body of legal source material.

Although the dominant orientation of the text is clinical, the goal is to provide material which raises the most important ethical questions about the nature of medical practice. There are many selections which include an extensive discussion of the underlying concepts or implicit principles in the positions held by various partisans to a dispute. Even when this is not the case in a particular selection, it is expected that the discussion of a problematic clinical situation will lead the reader to an exploration of the concepts involved in the formulation of alternatives and in the choice to characterize the situation in a certain manner. The first section, Conceptual Foundations, provides a substantial body of selections on the basic concepts which serve to structure our understanding of the clinical issues. It includes items on such concepts as rights, informed consent, confidentiality, death, and personhood.

In conclusion, we would like to provide some suggestions concerning the use of the text. The first section, Conceptual Foundations, is meant to serve, as are the cases in the Appendix, as a source of correlative readings for assignments from the second and third sections. We believe that this text is particularly suitable for inclusion in one of the standard comprehensive courses in medical schools, e.g., an introduction to medicine or behavioral science. These courses are increasingly covering ethical issues and would improve in focus if students could be provided with a text which can lead them beyond the usual handouts. The text is also designed to be used in regular bioethics courses, and can be a second source text for faculty who teach such topics as interviewing, and doctor-patient communication, for which an understanding of the basis of criticism of medical practice, the patient's perspective, and the physician's view of ideal medical practice and health care is important.

The text can also be employed to advantage as a primary source book for humanities and social science courses which wish to follow the same approach to developing discussion of ethical issues as that advocated by the editors, viz., beginning with concrete issues and "practical concepts" and then moving to more extended abstract debates. It could best be supplemented for such courses with assigned readings from some of the more academic journals, e.g., *Ethics, Philosophy and Public Affairs,* and *Philosophy of Medicine,* or a special issues anthology, many of which are available. The sections of cases in the Appendix would be particularly valuable as a basis for student assignments and class discussion.

I. CONCEPTUAL FOUNDATIONS

The articles in this section have been selected for their succinct discussion of basic ideas involved in the clinical issues covered in this text. Unlike the selections in other sections, these do not present a contested position or survey the various ethical aspects of a problematic procedure or sphere of decision. Rather, they are intended to provide definitions and analyses of concepts which often structure debate in clinical ethics. As such they can be best read as the various clinical sections are studied.

We have attempted to provide readings on the philosophical concepts which are particularly relevant in the biomedical context. Although these are perhaps the most "philosophical" of the selections in this text, they are not the most abstract or discursive essays available on the concepts. Thus, for example, faced with the immense output of writing on the concept of "rights" in recent years, not to mention nearly classical review essays by such eminent writers as Hart, Feinberg, Dworkin, Flatham, and Melden, we have selected a clear, concise section of a text on medical ethics by Gregory Pence. A similar principle was followed in choosing Veatch's discussion of the concepts of death in which the motivating questions governing the relevance of these concepts to biomedical ethics are presented within the essay.

Several of these basic concepts are so fundamental to the organization of practice in health care that their primary discussion in the literature has been as if they belong to biomedical ethics. The concepts of informed consent, paternalism, and confidentiality are typical of these, although the development of philosophical work on the professions as such, including nursing, law, and business, has revealed the relevance of these notions for those fields as well. We have tried to present selections which illuminate a germinal notion; thus Clouser's discussion of "sanctity," Feinberg's treatment of "personhood," and Freidson's sociological account of the concept of a "profession" all present historically enlightened and commonsense accounts. Perhaps the most medically restricted account is Rachels' discussion of active/passive euthanasia.

One topic is presented, however, which extends beyond conceptual clarification and which engages an important debate, viz., the right to health care. The topic occurs here because of the generalized and abstract nature of the discussion. Once they are engaged in clinical practice, most health practitioners and physicians feel that the question of the general right to access, or what is termed the macroallocation issue, is an abstract issue. This is itself a stance that may be subjected to criticism. Nonetheless, it is true that the debate occurs more often on a "policy level" and quickly involves general issues concerning social justice and the nature of the state. The two selections by Telfer and Sade nicely establish the question and can be coordinated with our section on Delivery of Care, in which allocation issues are discussed. Also of interest are the selections by Pellegrino and Fried under Institutional Responsibility, which address the question of the level of responsibility for policy decision. (See cases 1, 2, 3, 4, 8–11, 12, 13, 14–18, 19, 20, 21–23, 24–28, 29–31, 32, 33, 34, 35, 36, 37, 38–43, 44–48, 49–51, 53, 54, 55, 56, 57, 59, 60, 62, 63, 64, 65, 66, 67, 68, 69, 71, 73.)

Informed Consent

1.

The Principle of Autonomy
Tom L. Beauchamp   James F. Childress

The Functions of Informed Consent

In recent years virtually all medical and research codes of ethics have held that physicians must obtain the informed consent of patients before undertaking significant therapeutic or research procedures. While these consent measures have largely been designed to protect the autonomy of patients and subjects, they also serve other functions. Alexander Capron has helpfully identified several important functions: [1]

1. The promotion of individual autonomy
2. The protection of patients and subjects
3. The avoidance of fraud and duress
4. The encouragement of self-scrutiny by medical professionals
5. The promotion of rational decisions
6. The involvement of the public (in promoting autonomy as a general social value and in controlling biomedical research

The Justification of Informed Consent

The *functions* of informed consent mentioned by Capron can also be reconstructed as formal *justifications* of the requirement that informed consent be obtained. Thus, one justification of the requirement is that of protecting patients and subjects by preventing harm to them—a justification based on the principle of nonmaleficence. This justification is especially appropriate for legal requirements governing consent. Nonetheless, this justification in terms of the principle of nonmaleficence is not fundamental to moral justifications of first-party consent. While a person's own decision may *indirectly* function to prevent harm, he may also autonomously choose a greater risk than others would choose for him. The principle of autonomy justifies allowing a person this option of greater risk.

Another important justification for informed consent is based on the principle of utility: informed consent will maximally protect and benefit *everyone* in society, including health professionals, patients, and the institutions of medical practice and research themselves. Rules of consent serve to protect and benefit patients and professionals, to allay public fears (especially about research), to encourage self-scrutiny by phy-

Source: Tom L. Beauchamp and James F. Childress, *Principles of Biomedical Ethics,* p. 63, Oxford University Press, 1979.

sicians and investigators, and to maintain relations of trust. This justification is closely related to Capron's fourth and sixth functions.

Even though both the justification based on utility and the justification based on non-maleficence are appropriate for some consent requirements, neither is the primary justification of informed consent. Both the historical roots and the primary justification of informed consent are located in the principle of autonomy—not in the principles of nonmaleficence or utility. There is a moral duty to seek a valid consent *because* the consenting party is an autonomous person, with all the entitlements that status confers. By contrast, neither utility nor non-maleficence leads to this strong conclusion, for both would justify not seeking consent in some circumstances—utility when it would not maximize the social welfare and nonmaleficence when no apparent harm would result. When informed consent is justified by the principle of autonomy, it is introduced, as Robert Veatch puts it, "not to facilitate social benefits, but as a check against them,"[2] for persons have rights independent of such considerations as immediate social utility and risk to patients or subjects. However, by contrast to the justification for obtaining first-party consent, which is based on protecting autonomy, the justification for obtaining second-party consent derives largely and perhaps exclusively from the moral demand that subjects and patients be protected from harm—a demand derived from the principles of nonmaleficence and beneficence.

The Elements of Informed Consent

Whether first parties or second parties are in question, it is generally agreed that informed consent must be solicited whenever a procedure is intrusive, whenever significant risks might be run to persons, and whenever the purposes of the procedure might be questionable. But there is controversy concerning the elements that constitute informed consent. Accordingly, each of the following four elements and the issues each raises will now be discussed:

Information elements:

  1. Disclosure of information

  2. Comprehension of information

Consent elements:

  3. Voluntary consent

  4. Competence to consent

Each of these four components should be understood as a necessary condition of valid informed consent. However, this broad generalization will have to be qualified and refined as each of the elements is studied. We begin with the last of the four elements in the above list.

Competence

Competence to consent could perhaps be more appropriately described as a *presupposition* of informed consent than as an *element* of informed consent. Logically, competence is a precondition of acting voluntarily and apprehending information. It is fundamental in biomedical contexts, because certain physical and mental defects can result in a situation where patients and subjects are not—in psychological fact or in law—able to give informed consent. Obviously many conditions external to an agent may inhibit voluntary action, but many internal conditions may also limit voluntary consent. It is usually the latter that give rise to questions about competence. For example, minors commonly are not capable of responsible actions, while the mentally disabled and the comatose present even more troublesome cases.

The concept of competence is a multidimensional one. Competence and incompetence are often assessed by diverse and even inconsistent theories of comprehension, rationality, freedom, physiological state, etc., and judgments of incompetence often apply to a limited range of decision making, not to all decisions made by a person. Some persons who are legally incompetent may be competent to conduct most of their personal affairs, and vice versa. The same person's ability to make decisions may vary over time, and the person may at a single time be competent to make certain practical decisions but incompetent to make others. For example, a person judged incompetent to drive an automobile may not be incompetent to decide to participate in medical research, or may be able to handle simple affairs easily, while faltering before complex ones. Accordingly, the notions of *limited* competence and *intermittent* competence are useful, because they require a statement of the precise decisions a person can make, while avoiding the false dichotomy of "either competent or incompetent." Use of these notions would preserve maximum autonomy, justifying intervention only in those areas where a person clearly is of questionable competence.

Two cases illustrate the difficulties often encountered in attempting to judge competence. In one case a sixty-eight-year-old man with kidney disease and multiple additional problems also develops intermittent psychotic behavior. The psychiatric diagnosis is that of chronic psychotic organic brain syndrome resulting from cerebral arteriosclerosis. Nonetheless, two psychiatrists declare the patient competent to make fundamental decisions affecting his treatment, based on behavioral and psychiatric indications. Because the patient exhibits what his attending physician regards as erratic and irrational behavior, the psychiatrists' declaration of competence is reluctantly accepted by the physician and by certain members of the family. In this difficult case the patient's behavior is perhaps best understood in terms of limited and intermittent competence. In the second case, a man who generally exhibits normal behavior patterns is involuntarily committed to a mental institution because of certain bizarre actions that follow from his unique and unorthodox religious beliefs. Because the man's religious beliefs lead to serious self-destructive behavior (pulling out an eye and cutting off a hand), he is judged incompetent, despite his generally competent behavior and despite the fact that his peculiar actions follow "reasonably" from his—many would say, equally peculiar—religious beliefs. While this puzzling case probably cannot be understood in terms of intermit-

tent competence, it may be that the notion of limited competence again applies.

Perhaps the major question in recent years about competence centers on *standards* for its determination. Conventional standards isolate various abilities to comprehend information and to reason about the consequences of one's actions. In particular, a person is said to be incompetent unless both capable of processing a certain amount of information and capable of choosing both ends and the means to those ends. The most promising headway toward a useful definition has come through criminal and civil law. Courts have disagreed on which of the following three properties is most crucial to a determination of competency:[3] (1) capacity to reach a decision based on *rational reasons,* (2) the reaching of a *reasonable result* through a decision, or (3) the *capacity to make a decision* at all. Without attempting to distinguish all the arguments and possible reasons for adopting any one of these three standards, it seems reasonable to combine them as follows: a person is competent if and only if that person can make decisions based on rational reasons. In biomedical contexts this standard entails that a person must be able to understand a therapy or research procedure, must be able to weigh its risks and benefits, and must be able to make a decision in the light of such knowledge and through such abilities, even if the person chooses not to utilize the information.

A further problem is that the term "competence" often functions to hide a significant value judgment about another person. A person who appears to others to be irrational or unreasonable might be declared incompetent in order that "treatment" may be provided. Such a declaration readily hides a value judgment about what a rational person ought to consent to do, presented in the guise of an empirical determination of incompetence. It is thus seldom a simple *empirical* question as to whether a person is or is not competent. If precise criteria were available for making such determinations, the gray area would vanish. But since such criteria are not available, *moral* judgments about what to do with possibly incompetent persons cannot be avoided.

Disclosure of Information

Most medical and research codes specify conditions under which a person can be said to have sufficient information on the basis of which he or she could make an informed choice. Commonly mentioned as necessary items of disclosure are contemplated procedures, alternative available procedures, anticipated risks and benefits, and a statement offering the person an opportunity to ask further questions and to withdraw at any time (in the case of research). Several writers on the subject of informed consent have proposed additional or supplementary conditions—for example, statements of the purpose of the procedure, the uncertain risks involved, persons in charge, and, if research is involved, how subjects were selected. Such lists could be indefinitely expanded, but many possible inclusions are not applicable to all areas of medical research and practice. Expansive lists of conditions are sometimes appropriate, while in other contexts they would waste precious time and might even prove to be damaging to patients or subjects. Accordingly, it is more important to determine which primary moral standards should govern the disclosure of information. We shall concentrate on this topic.

Standards of disclosure. One major question is how the distinction is to be drawn between adequately informed consent, on the one hand, and partially informed or even uninformed consent, on the other hand. Three general standards of disclosure have emerged in legal and ethical writings on informed consent: (1) what is operative in the biomedical professions, (2) what the reasonable person would want to know, and (3) what individual patients or subjects of research want to know. In the past there has been a strong reliance on (1). For example, it was only recently reported that

The view accepted by the majority of American jurisdictions bases the duty to disclose on a community standard; it requires only such disclosures of risks as is consistent with the practice of the local medical community. Expert medical testimony is required to show a breach of local medical standards.[4]

This standard was devised under the conviction that the doctor's proper role is that of acting in the patient's best medical interest. The obligation to disclose information is in effect subservient to a medical judgment of what is in the patient's best interest. Medical care standards, rather than patient's rights, are thus considered the operative guidelines governing proper disclosure. For this reason many have come to think—rightly, in our view—that this standard strips away too much autonomy from patients.

Lately this standard has been declining in significance, even in the courts, for two primary reasons. First, the amount of material information a person needs to make a decision is not a technical medical judgment, and is perhaps better within the comprehension of an average juror than an average physician. Second, medical custom often expresses the values and goals of the medical profession, but information provided to patients and subjects should be as free as possible of the values and goals of medical professionals, especially those doing research. The latter are more likely than most to believe in the scientific merit and social worth of their procedures; and they may well see risks and benefits in a quite different perspective than would others.

The reasonable person standard (2) now seems the prevalent criterion, and certainly it is an improvement over (1). But before the standard of the reasonable person can be accepted as the operational standard of disclosure for both research and practice, we need to know more precisely what it involves, including its relation, if any, to (3). The best present resource for an answer to this question is case law, which has gradually assembled a set of considerations that explicate the concept of a reasonable person, such as the following:

1. All material information necessary for a decision must be given, as judged by persons who would compose a jury rather than by expert testimony or by a medical body. [5]

2. Known risks of significant bodily harm and death must be disclosed. [6]

3. The reasonable person is a composite or ideal of reasonable persons in society, and the individual subject is not in question. The latter standard might be too subjective and would require too much guesswork by physicians. [7]

4. Standards of disclosure in medicine are not different from those of other professions where there is a similar fiduciary relationship. [8]

Although somewhat amorphous and open-ended, these legal criteria are useful for purposes of generalizing into moral contexts. However, even this claim is paradoxical. As Judge Robinson noted in *Canterbury v. Spence,* medical duties to disclose, as set forth in the law, are themselves ultimately based on moral considerations of autonomy. The judge calls these considerations "the patient's right of self-decision" and "the patient's prerogative to decide." [9] Their point is that duties of disclosure are *at their root* moral rather than legal or medical ones, and these moral duties inform both law and medicine as to the appropriate standards. What has been said, then, about general moral standards based on autonomy and present case law might be focused into the following minimum standard of disclosure: the patient or subject should be provided with information that a reasonable person in the patient's or subject's circumstances would find relevant and could reasonably be expected to assimilate. In this way the moral requirement to respect autonomy is translated into a consent standard.

Nonetheless, there are special problems about the development of more specific standards and about how the reasonable person standard can actually be employed in the disclosure of information in some areas of biomedical research and practice. One such

problem has been suggested on the basis of recent empirical research that attempts to discover whether information disclosed to patients is actually used by these patients in reaching their decisions. For example, data collected in a study by Ruth Faden indicate, among other things, that though 93 percent of the patients surveyed believe they benefited from the information disclosed, only 12 percent actually used the information disclosed as the basis of their decision to consent. [10] This study, involving family-planning patients, reaches conclusions similar to those of an earlier study by Fellner and Marshall of persons consenting to be kidney donors. [11] In both studies data indicate that patients make their decisions largely prior to and independent of the actual process of disclosing information. These data do not in any way show that patient decisions were *uninformed* or that disclosed information was *irrelevant,* for the patients may have only believed that the additional information was not such as to shake their prior commitment to a particular course of action. For example, a kidney donor could very reasonably decide that the eventual death of his brother far outweighs any information disclosed by a physician. Nonetheless, the above empirical findings do throw into open question what should count as facts that are material to the decision-making process for actual *individual* patients, as contrasted to *average reasonable* patients.

Based on the above considerations, we suggest that the average reasonable-person standard presently operative in law should be supplemented by a standard which takes account of the independent informational needs of actual reasonable persons in the process of making a difficult decision. Yet an entirely subjective standard—(3) above—seems inappropriate, because patients often do not know what information would be relevant for their deliberations. Perhaps the best solution is a compromise standard, combining (2) and (3): whatever a reasonable person would judge material to the decision-making process should be disclosed, and, in addition, any remaining information material to an individual patient should be offered through a process of asking a patient what else he or she wishes to know and providing truthful answers to any questions asked. Autonomy is not adequately protected unless some more rigorous criterion of this general description is adopted. If subjects fail to have an adequate idea, given their own concerns and needs, of what they are deciding, then there is no *informed* consent, even if they do possess all the information a disembodied "reasonable person" would possess. And since the protection of autonomy is the central justification of informed consent requirements in morals and the law, this modified, more stringent version of the reasonable-person standard seems morally required.

Comprehension of Information

Just as a sufficient quantity of information is needed for a consent to be informed, so adequate comprehension of the information by subjects or patients is a necessary condition of a valid informed consent. Without sufficient comprehension a person cannot use the information in making decisions—should he or she elect to use the information. Many conditions other than mere lack of sufficient information can limit comprehension. Irrationality and immaturity can do so, for example. But even if there were no problems about competence, problems about adequate comprehension would remain, for information may be presented in a distorted way or in unsuitable circumstances so that communication of the information fails to occur.

It is sometimes argued that a patient or subject cannot comprehend enough information to give informed consent. Franz Ingelfinger argues, for example, that "the chances are remote that the subject really understands what he has consented to,"[12] and Robert Mulford similarly argues that "the subject is ordinarily not qualified to evaluate the true risks and expected benefits."[13] This position is based on an inadequate view of so-called "full" disclosure. So long as one clings to the

ideal of complete disclosure of all possibly relevant knowledge, such claims about the limited capacity of subjects will be given credence. But if this ideal standard is replaced by an acceptable reasonable-person standard, there should no longer be any temptation to succumb to the Ingelfinger-Mulford form of pessimism. From the fact that we are never *fully* voluntary, fully informed, or fully autonomous persons, it does not follow that we are never *adequately* informed, free, and autonomous. A different lesson is to be learned: because comprehension is both limited and difficult, we should strive harder in biomedical and educational contexts to foster information and to avoid undue influence. Apprehending one's medical situation is not substantially different from apprehending one's financial situation when consulting with a CPA, or one's legal situation when consulting with a lawyer, or even one's marital situation when consulting with a marriage counselor. The shades of understanding are manifold, but various degrees of apprehension may nonetheless be adequate for an informed judgment.

Another problem is whether we ought to recognize waivers of informed consent. What are we to say about those idiosyncratic individuals who choose to have less information than would a "reasonable" person? Robert Veatch has argued that anyone who refuses to accept as much information as the reasonable person would accept cannot be said to have apprehended the relevant information and therefore cannot be said to have given an acceptable consent—at least not to involvement in research.[14] But is this view correct? Some persons do not want to know anything about what will be done. Indeed, some studies claim to show that over 60 percent of patients want to know virtually nothing about procedures or the risks of the procedures,[15] and other studies, as we have seen, indicate that only about 12 percent of patients use the information provided in reaching their decisions.[16]

There seem to be two major alternative ways of treating such persons. First, it might be maintained that when the reasonable-person standard is not being met, the contemplated procedure cannot be undertaken until sufficient information has been imparted, notwithstanding the person's autonomously expressed desire not to be informed. According to this approach, persons should not be coerced against their autonomous wishes into receiving undesired information. Second, a contrasting view is that when a patient or subject has been sufficiently informed to know whether or not further information is wished, and when the right to further information has been waived, no further information should be provided. In this second view, the person's informed waiver is itself sufficient to constitute *valid* consent to therapy or research, even if it is not an *informed* consent to that procedure.

Either alternative presents risks. On the one hand, forced information is a prima facie violation of autonomy, and many circumstances can be imagined in which information waivers would be justified. For example, if a deeply committed Jehovah's Witness were to inform a doctor that he wishes to have everything possible done for him, but does not want to *know* if transfusions or similar procedures would be employed, it is hard to imagine a moral argument to the conclusion that he must be told. On the other hand, to consider the second alternative, the fact must be faced that patients commonly have an inordinate trust in physicians, and the general recognition of waivers of consent in research and therapeutic settings could make patients more vulnerable to those who would use far too abbreviated consent procedures merely because they are convenient.

There probably cannot be any general theoretical solution to this problem of waivers. Each case of consent and the possibility of a waiver will have to be considered in its own complexity. There may, however, be a procedural way to resolve the problem. There could be rules against allowing waivers, but these rules could be considered as specifying prima facie duties which can be relaxed after special consideration by deliberative bodies, such as institutional review committees and

hospital ethics committees. Such rules would be developed to protect patients and subjects, but if protective bodies themselves were to find that the person's interest in a particular case was best protected by a waiver, they could allow the waiver. This procedural solution is not a mere avoidance of the problem. It would be easy to violate autonomy and to fail to live up to our responsibilities by inflexible rules which either permit or prohibit waivers. This procedural suggestion at least provides a flexible arrangement for meeting such problems.

A similar and related problem arises when patients or subjects reach their decisions on irrelevant grounds, even though they have been adequately informed. Such persons comprehend the relevant information but reach their decision based on emotional, irrational, or false views. For example, a person might falsely and irrationally believe that a doctor will not fill out his insurance forms unless he consents to a procedure the doctor has suggested; and he might persist in this belief even when informed of its falsity. Similarly, a sufficiently informed psychiatric patient capable of consent might consent to involvement in a nonpsychiatric, nontherapeutic research procedure under the false assumption that it is therapeutic. In these cases the adequate information that is both disclosed and apprehended plays no role in the decision to be involved in the research or to accept the therapy. The question then arises whether autonomous subjects should be coerced into giving up their false beliefs and irrational tendencies in order that they may decide on the basis of pertinent information alone.

In a general statement about the coercion of information, H. Tristram Engelhardt has argued that "One cannot try (nor should one) to force subjects who can be rational free agents to use that rationality and freedom to its fullest,"[17] because informed consent only entails that patients and subjects make their own free and rational assessments. Robert Veatch has similarly argued that where subjects specifically object to further information or persuasion, the information should not be imposed.[18] While these statements set forth commendable ideals, they do not imply that we should never coerce patients or subjects to further information. When a patient's or subject's autonomy is clearly limited by his own ignorance, as in the case of false belief, it may be legitimate to promote autonomy by attempting to impose the information. In this respect these cases resemble the waiver cases just discussed. In both, unsatisfactory apprehension leads to the problem, and as with the waiver cases, the best general solution is probably a procedural one.

It might be argued that these conclusions about apprehension hold for therapeutic settings but do not fit research settings where persons would be involved in nontherapeutic research. In the therapeutic environment the physician acts to the end of a patient's best interests, but in research settings the person is used as a means to the investigator's ends. Nonetheless, we believe this distinction between the two settings is largely irrelevant to the points made in this section about deficient apprehension. Factors such as the amount of risk involved and the person's identification with the purposes of research could make a decisive difference as to whether he should be involved, quite independent of whether it is a clinical or a research setting. Moreover, by participating in research, subjects might derive certain benefits which they could appreciate and which would be important to them, even though they consented on what the "reasonable person" would judge to be irrelevant grounds.

Voluntariness

Voluntariness connotes the ability to choose one's own goals, and to be able to choose among several goals if a wide choice is offered, without being unduly influenced or coerced to any of the alternatives by other persons or institutions. The mere *absence* of constraining influences may, however, not indicate that a subject is acting *freely*. On some occasions the person may have to be provided with the means to realize a chosen end, as well as given freedom of choice. For example, it makes no sense to say that a person is free to choose a nonvalidated therapy instead of a validated one, if only the validated one is actually made available. In contexts of informed consent, voluntariness is optimal when there is adequate disclosure, adequate comprehension, and a subject capable of choice who in fact chooses a specific action. However, the primary *meaning* of "voluntariness" is exercising choice about an action free of coercion or undue influence by another person.

How shall we understand the notions of coercion and undue influence? Coercion occurs when one person intentionally uses an actual threat of harm or forceful manipulation to influence another. The harm could be physical, psychological, economic, etc. By contrast, undue influence occurs whenever someone uses an excessive reward or irrationally persuasive technique to induce a person to a decision the person might otherwise not reach. If admission to a hospital of persons needing care were made contingent upon their enrollment in a research protocol that was unrelated to their illness, undue influence would have been exerted. But if the only temptation inviting enrollment in a nontherapeutic research project is time off from one's work at no extra pay for the duration of the experiment, no undue influence would have been exerted. Coercion and undue influence are points on a continuum, and it is probably not possible to locate these points precisely.

Mere influence or pressure to make a decision, however, contrasts sharply with coercion and undue influence. We almost always make decisions in a context of competing wants, needs, familial interests, legal obligations, persuasive arguments, etc. Many inducements will thus be pressures but not unduly influential ones—though no sharp boundary line can perhaps be drawn in some cases between pressure to decide and undue influence. For example, a person may be pressured by an office solicitor to make a blood donation. The solicitation would normally be acceptable, but could become unacceptable if salary or year-ending bonus considerations were brought into the picture as inducements. Consent to therapy and research may therefore be voluntary and valid even when some pressures play a significant role in the decision.

Many examples indicate how these distinctions can be brought to bear on practical contexts of informed consent. In one case hepatitis research was being done on mentally retarded children in New York. One allegation surrounding this case is that the parents were "coerced" into "volunteering" their children. Allegedly they were coerced —or, as some would prefer to say, unduly influenced—because there was a waiting list for admission to the school and parents were told that their children could be immediately admitted if they were "volunteered" for the hepatitis study. If this allegation of manipulative tactics were true, which is still in doubt, it would be a clear case of an unwarranted action. On the other hand, there is nothing about admission to institutions or about institutions themselves which makes unfair influence inevitable. Even in generally coercive environments, such as prisons, it is sometimes possible that informed consent to medical and research procedures can occur. It may be especially important to ensure that the right of autonomous determination is defended in such institutions, since there will be a natural presumption that voluntary action is impossible, e.g., in the case of research with prisoners. Yet in environments where many options are foreclosed, not all options need be so. There is no reason why prisoners could not validly consent to medical research—say, in the form of drug testing—if coercive tactics were not specifically involved, and if undue inducements, such as large amounts of money, were not allowed. Thus, a distinction ought to be drawn between generally coercive environments and individual acts of coercion. Informed consent may be valid in the former, but cannot be in the latter.

NOTES

1. "Informed Consent in Catastrophic Disease and Treatment," *University of Pennsylvania Law Review,* vol. 123, p. 364, December 1974.

2. Robert M. Veatch, "Three Theories of Informed Consent: Philosophical Foundations and Policy Implications," National Commission for the Protection of Human Subjects of Biomedical and Behavioral Research, *Appendix: Volume I. Belmont Report: Ethical Principles and Guidelines for the Protection of Human Subjects of Research* (Washington: DHEW Publication No. (OS) 78–0013, 1978).

3. We are indebted to Professor Donald Bersoff of the University of Maryland Law School for suggesting this tripartite approach.

4. "Informed Consent and the Dying Patient," *The Yale Law Journal,* vol. 83, p. 1637, 1974. Much the same point is made in *Canterbury v. Spence,* 464 Federal Reporter, 2nd Series, 772, where the standards operative in the biomedical professions are analyzed as of two types: (1) good medical practice standards, and (2) what a reasonable practitioner would disclose under the circumstances. See the excerpt from the case reprinted in Tom L. Beauchamp and LeRoy Walters, eds., *Contemporary Issues in Bioethics,* p. 143, Dickenson Publishing Co., Encino, Calif., 1978. (Hereafter this anthology is abbreviated B-W.)

5. Cf. *Wilkinson v. Vesey,* 110 R.I. 606, 626; 295 A.2d 676, 688 (1972).

6. Cf. *Cobbs v. Grant,* 8 Cal. 3d 229, 502 P.2d 1. 1979.

7. Cf. *Canterbury v. Spence,* 464 Federal Reporter, 2nd Series, 772, as reprinted in B-W, p. 144 (and also footnote 8). *Cobb v. Grant,* however, seems more subjective in that it appeals to "the patient's need" to know as a critical standard.

8. Cf. *Berkey v. Anderson,* 1 Cal. APP. 3d 790, 805; 82 Cal. Reporter 67, 78 (1969).

9. *Canterbury v. Spence,* in B-W, p. 144.

10. Ruth R. Faden, "Disclosure and Informed Consent: Does It Matter How We Tell It?" *Health Education Monographs,* vol. 5, p. 198, 1977; and Ruth R. Faden and Tom L. Beauchamp, "Informed Consent and Decision Making: The Impact of Disclosed Information," *Social Indicators Research,* 1979.

11. C. H. Fellner and J. R. Marshall, "Kidney Donors—The Myth of Informed Consent," *Ameri-*

can Journal of Psychiatry, vol. 126, p. 1245, 1970.

12. Franz J. Ingelfinger, "Informed (but Uneducated) Consent," as reprinted in B-W, pp. 434–435.

13. Robert D. Mulford, "Experimentation on Human Beings," *Stanford Law Review,* vol. 20, p. 106, November 1967.

14. Veatch, "Three Theories of Informed Consent."

15. Cf. Ralph J. Alfidi, "Controversy, Alternatives, and Decisions in Complying with the Legal 114, January 1975, as reprinted in B-W, p. 148.

16. Cf. the articles in footnote 10 above.

17. "Basic Ethical Principles in the Conduct of Biomedical and Behavioral Research Involving Human Subjects." National Commission for the Protection of Human Subjects of Biomedical and Behavioral Research, *Appendix: Vol. 1. Belmont Report,* 2 p. 8–22. (see footnote 2 above).

18. Veatch, "Three Theories of Informed Consent."

Paternalism

2.
The Justification of Paternalism
Bernard Gert   Charles M. Culver

In discussing the justification of paternalism, two features are essential: one is a clear account of paternalistic behavior; the other is a general theory about moral justification.[1] We think it is important to relate particular cases to a general theory of justification and to a general account of paternalistic behavior, for otherwise one does not get the full benefit of agreement on clear cases for application to cases that are not so clear.

The following is our definition of paternalistic behavior:[2]

A is acting paternalistically toward S if and only if A's behavior (correctly) indicates that *A believes that*

1. His action is for S's good.

2. He is qualified to act on S's behalf.

3. His action involves violating a moral rule (or will require him to do so) with regard to S.

4. S's good justifies him in acting on S's behalf independently of S's past, present, or immediately forthcoming (free, informed) consent.[3]

5. S believes (perhaps falsely) that he (S) generally knows what is for his own good.

From this account, it becomes clear that paternalistic behavior needs justification because it involves doing that which requires one to violate a moral rule; indeed, in almost all cases it involves an actual violation of a rule.[4] The definition also makes clear that one feature used in justifying a violation of a moral rule is not open to A when acting paternalistically, namely, the consent of S toward whom A is violating the rule. For if A has S's consent, A's behavior is no longer paternalistic. Thus, standard medical practice where one causes pain is not usually pa-

Source: *Ethics,* vol. 89, no. 2, January 1979, p. 199. Copyright 1979 by The University of Chicago.

An earlier version of this paper was read on October 17, 1976, at the Conference in Philosophy, Law, and Medicine, sponsored by Kalamazoo College and Western Michigan University. The material in this paper is the product of a faculty seminar at Dartmouth which included the following members of the Departments of Philosophy, Psychiatry, and Religion: Bernard Bergen, Ph.D.; K. Danner Clouser, Ph.D. (Department of Humanities, Hershey Medical School); Ronald Green, Ph.D.; James Moor, Ph.D.; Joel Rudinow, Ph.D.; Gary Tucker, M.D.; and Peter Whybrow, M.D.

ternalistic because the physician almost always has the consent of the patient for doing so.

Since in paternalistic behavior we do not have the consent of the person toward whom the moral rule is violated, the only way in which the violation can be justified is if we are thereby preventing significantly more evil to S by the violation than we are causing.[5] For if A believes that his violation of the moral rule with regard to S is justified only because of benefits that accrue to others, then A's behavior is not paternalistic. This is not to say that paternalistic behavior cannot benefit anyone other than S, but if it is to be justified paternalism, it must be justifiable solely by reference to S's good. Here we may run into a linguistic difficulty: Although we have talked of "S's good" and of "benefiting S," what is intended is the prevention or relief of S's suffering some evil, that is, death; pain; disability; or loss of freedom, opportunity, or pleasure. Unless we can accurately describe the benefit to S, or S's good, in terms of avoiding or relieving one of these evils, we are not justified in paternalistically violating the moral rule with regard to S. And even if we can describe S's good in these terms, this does not provide a sufficient condition for justifying our paternalistic behavior, only a necessary condition. It must also be true that the evils that would be prevented to S are so much greater than the evils, if any, that would be caused by the violation of the rule, that it would be irrational for S not to want to have the rule violated with regard to himself. But even this is not sufficient; to make it sufficient one must also be able to universally allow the violation of this rule in these circumstances, or in somewhat more technical terminology, be able to publicly advocate this kind of violation.

The following example illustrates many of the above points:

Mr. K is pacing back and forth on the roof of his five-story tenement and several times appears to be about to jump off.

When questioned by the police he sounds confused. When interviewed by Dr. T in the emergency room, Mr. K admits being afraid he might jump off the roof and says that he fears he might be losing his mind. He speaks of the depression he has been experiencing the past several months and begins weeping uncontrollably. He claims not to know the source of his despair but says he can stand it no longer. He adamantly refuses hospitalization but will not say why. Dr. T decides that he must commit Mr. K to the hospital for a 48-hour period for Mr. K's own protection.

According to our definition, this is a clear case of paternalistic behavior. Dr. T commits Mr. K to the hospital for what he believes is Mr. K's own good. Dr. T believes he is qualified to carry out such an act on Mr. K's behalf; he knows he is violating a moral rule with regard to Mr. K by depriving him of his freedom; he believes Mr. K's good justifies his acting without Mr. K's consent; and further, he views Mr. K as being someone who believes he generally knows what is for his own good.

Since this is an instance of paternalism, it requires justification as noted above. Dr. T could attempt to justify depriving Mr. K of his freedom without his consent by claiming that there was a very great likelihood that by so doing he was preventing the occurrence of a much greater evil: Mr. K's death (or serious injury through attempted self-destruction). Dr. T could further claim that in his professional experience the overwhelming majority of persons in Mr. K's condition who were in fact hospitalized did subsequently recover from their depression and acknowledge the irrational character of their suicidal desires.

Note that it need not be Dr. T's claim that self-inflicted death is an evil of such magnitude that paternalistic intervention to prevent it is always justified. Rather, he could claim that it is justified in Mr. K's case on several counts. First, Mr. K seems to have no reason for killing himself, and so his action seems irrational. Second, there is evidence that he suffers from a condition that is well known to be transient. Third, the violation of a moral rule (deprivation of freedom) which Dr. T has carried out results in Mr. K's suffering a much lesser evil than the evil (death) which Mr. K may perpetrate on himself.

But it is not sufficient justification for Dr. T merely to show that the evils prevented for Mr. K by his paternalistic action outweigh the evils caused to Mr. K; he must also be willing to publicly advocate the deprivation of Mr. K's freedom in these circumstances. That is, he must be willing to claim that all rational persons could agree with his judgment that in these circumstances Mr. K should be deprived of his freedom for a limited period of time. We believe that, accepting the case as described, not only could all rational persons agree, but also all rational persons would agree with Dr. T's judgment completely, and thus Dr. T's paternalistic behavior is strongly justified.

In contrast consider the following case:

Mrs. R, a twenty-nine-year-old mother, is hospitalized with symptoms of abdominal pain, weight loss, weakness, and swelling of the ankles. An extensive medical workup is inconclusive, and exploratory abdominal surgery is carried out which reveals a primary ovarian cancer with extensive spread to other abdominal organs. Her condition is judged to be too far advanced for surgical relief and her life expectancy is estimated to be at most a few months. Despite her oft-repeated request to be told "exactly where I stand and what I face," Dr. T tells both the patient and her husband that the diagnosis is still unclear but that he will see her weekly as an outpatient. At the time of discharge she is feeling somewhat better than at admission, and Dr. T hopes that the family will have a few happy days together before her condition worsens and they must be told the truth.

Dr. T's behavior is clearly paternalistic: He has deceived Mrs. R for what he believes to be her own good; he believes he is qualified to do so on her behalf; he believes the benefit to her justifies his violating the moral rule against deception, without her consent; and he views her as someone who believes she generally know what is for her own good.

Dr. T could attempt to justify his paternalistic act by claiming that the evil—psychological suffering—he hoped to prevent by his deception is significantly greater than the evil, if any, he caused by lying. While this might be true in this particular case, it is by no means certain. By his deception Dr. T is depriving Mrs. R and her family of the opportunity to make those plans that would enable her family to deal more adequately with her death. In the circumstances of this case as described, Mrs. R's desire to know the truth is a rational desire; in fact, there is no evidence of any irrational behavior or desires on the part of Mrs. R. This contrasts very sharply with Mr. K's desire to kill himself, which is clearly irrational. Furthermore, although we regard Mr. K's desire not to be deprived of freedom, considered in isolation, as a rational one, we would not consider it rational for one to choose a very high probability of death over a few days of freedom.

The Nature of Justification

We have already noted that in order to justify one's paternalistic behavior, it is necessary (not sufficient) that the evil prevented for S by the violation be so much greater than the evil, if any, caused to S by it, that it would be irrational for S not to choose having the rule violated with regard to himself. When this is not the case, as in Dr. T's deception of Mrs. R, then the paternalistic behavior cannot be justified. If it would not be irrational for S to choose suffering the evil rather than have the moral rule violated with regard to himself, then no rational person could universally allow the violation of the rule in these circumstances. This becomes clear when we specify what counts as "these circumstances." For us, specifying the circumstances is the same as specifying the kind of violation that one could publicly advocate. We hold that the only factors that are relevant in specifying a given kind of violation are: (1) the moral rule(s) which is (are) violated; (2) the probable amounts of evil caused, avoided, or prevented (relieved) by the violation (probable amount includes both the kind and severity of the evil and the probable length of time it will be suffered); and (3) the rational desires of the person(s) affected by the violation. Thus these factors alone determine the circumstances we must take into account when we determine the kind of violation. What is then needed is to determine whether to publicly advocate this kind of violation. This is done by deciding whether the evil prevented (relieved) or avoided by universally allowing this kind of violation outweighs the evil that would be caused by universally allowing it. If all rational persons would agree that the evil prevented by universally allowing the violation would be greater than the evil caused by universally allowing it, the violation is strongly justified; if none would, it is unjustified. If there is disagreement, we call it a weakly justified violation, and whether it should be allowed is a matter for decision.[6]

In order to make this point clearer let us use the case of Mrs. R to clarify some of the technical terminology we have used. Dr. T is deceiving Mrs. R. This requires moral justification. For us (as for almost all philosophers after Kant) morally justifying a violation of a moral rule requires that one be able to hold that everyone be allowed to violate the rule in the given circumstances. If one is violating a moral rule in circumstances where one would not allow others to violate it, one is not acting impartially. And it is universally agreed that morality requires impartiality. We believe that one should determine whether he would allow everyone to violate the moral rule in the given circumstances by seeing if he would publicly advocate this kind of violation. We regard determining the kind of violation as determining what counts as the relevant circumstances in which one is violating the rule. In the case under discussion, Dr. T is violating the rule against deception in the circumstances where there is

a high probability that he is preventing mental suffering for several weeks or months; there is an even higher probability that he is depriving a person of the opportunity to make the most appropriate plans for her future; and the person affected by the deception has a rational desire not to be deceived.[7]

Given this description of the kind of violation, determining whether one would publicly advocate it or not is the same as determining whether one would allow everyone to deceive in circumstances so described. The following may make the point even clearer. Suppose someone ranks unpleasant feelings for several weeks as a greater evil than the evil involved in the loss of some opportunity to plan for the future. Should he be allowed to deceive those who may have a different rational ranking, if his deception will result in their suffering what the deceiver regards as the lesser evil? Would any rational person hold that everyone be allowed to deceive in these circumstances; that is, would any rational person publicly advocate this kind of violation? We think that once the case is made clear enough, no rational person would publicly advocate such a violation. For it amounts to allowing deception in order to impose one's own ranking of evils on others who have an alternative rational ranking. Allowing deception in such circumstances would clearly have the most disastrous consequences on the trust one could put in the words of others, and thus allowing this kind of violation would have far worse consequences, on any rational ranking, than not allowing it. Thus no rational person would publicly advocate such a violation. On this analysis, Dr. T's deception was an unjustified paternalistic act.

We are not maintaining that all lying to patients is unjustified. But we think it is justified only when, if a person, acting rationally, were presented with the alternatives, he or she would always choose being lied to. The following is such a case.

Mrs. E is in extremely critical condition after an automobile accident which has taken the life of one of her four children and severely injured another. Dr. P believes that her very tenuous hold on life might be weakened by the shock of hearing of her children's conditions; so he decides to deceive her for a short period of time.

Anyone acting rationally who was presented with the option of being deceived for a short period of time or of greatly increasing his or her chance of dying would choose the former. Thus, if Mrs. E said that she wanted to know, knowing that the truth might kill her, we would not regard such a desire as a rational one. (We are excluding any other considerations such as religious beliefs or her desire to die because of such a loss.) In these circumstances, we have deception which significantly decreases the chance of death and causes no significant evil. Would a rational person publicly advocate this kind of violation? What would be the effect of universally allowing this kind of violation? As far as we can see, there would be no significant loss of trust, and whatever loss there might be would seem to be more than balanced by the number of lives that would be saved. Thus we hold that all rational persons would publicly advocate this kind of violation.

In discussing the justification of paternalism, it is very easy to fall into the error of supposing that all we need do is compare evils prevented with evils caused and always decide in favor of the lesser evil. It is this kind of view, a relatively straightforward negative utilitarianism, which seems to be held by many doctors and may account for much of their paternalistic behavior. If A holds this view, then A thinks that if he is preventing more evil for S than he is causing S, he is justified in violating a moral rule with regard to S.[8] Taking this kind of straightforward negative utilitarian view, one can easily understand why paternalistic acts of deception done in order to prevent or postpone mental suffering, as in the case of Mrs. R described above, are so common. Little if any evil seems to be caused, and mental suf-

fering is prevented, at least for a time; thus it seems as if such acts are morally justified. Paternalistic acts by which someone is deprived of freedom, as in commitment, are recognized to be more difficult to justify, for then we have a significant evil—the loss of freedom—which is certain and which has to be balanced against the evil we *hope* to prevent.

But negative utilitarianism is not an adequate ethical theory. We do not regard the foreseeable consequences of a particular act as the only morally relevant considerations; they are, of course, very significant, as they help determine the kind of act involved. But if an act is a violation of a moral rule, we must consider the hypothetical consequences of universally allowing this kind of violation. In a great many individual cases, balancing the evil that would be caused against the evils that would be prevented in universally allowing this kind of moral rule violation will lead to just the same moral judgment as if only the consequences of the particular act had been weighed. It is probably for this reason that some writers have taken the simpler balancing to be sufficient.

However, part of the standard philosophical literature against utilitarianism is comprised of examples in which it is inadequate to consider only the foreseeable consequences of a particular act. For example, consider a well-trained and very competent law student who did not study during the weeks preceding the state bar examinations he is now taking. He therefore cheats on them in order to decrease his chance of failing to qualify for the practice of law and thereby prevent the unpleasant feelings to himself and his parents which would accompany failure. His cheating has not caused harm to anyone (assume that the exam is not graded on a curve) and on a simple negative utilitarian view would therefore be morally justified. But we may hypothesize that if we allow cheating for the purpose of decreasing unpleasant feelings, then some individuals, who may believe themselves qualified when in fact they are not, will cheat and thereby pass. Thus we will destroy the value of these tests on which we in part rely to determine who is qualified for legal practice. The effect of less qualified people becoming lawyers is an increased risk of the population's suffering greater evils such as the deprivation of freedom, and this outweighs the suffering caused to those who fail to qualify.[9] Thus, by using this more complex balancing, we conclude that such acts of cheating are not morally justified.

The procedure used in the earlier examples may be applied to the cheating example as follows: The amount of evil caused directly by this particular act of cheating is believed to be nil; the evil avoided or prevented is unpleasant feelings for the person and his parents. There are supposedly no persons directly affected by this violation of the moral rule against cheating; so the rational desires of others need not enter the calculation. But imagine that anyone who thought that no harm would come of his cheating, and that he could prevent a few people having unpleasant feelings, was allowed to cheat. We believe that the hypothetical long-range evils associated with universally allowing this kind of violation so far outweigh the unpleasant feelings that would be prevented, that it would be irrational to universally allow this kind of violation. Thus it could not be publicly advocated.

Further Examples of the Justification Procedure

Paternalistic acts committed by physicians may involve the violation of a number of moral rules, but the three most common violations seem to be depriving of freedom, deceiving, and causing pain or suffering. We believe that in the case of all three violations there are both justified and unjustified paternalistic acts. We have given examples of depriving of freedom (Mr. K) and of deception (Mrs. E), which we have argued are justified, and an example of deception (Mrs. R), which we have argued is not. Let us consider two more cases of medical paternalism in order to review the various components of our account of

moral justification and to show how certain changes in these components can affect the final moral judgment reached.

Mr. C is a twenty-six-year-old single patient with a past history of intense participation in physical activities and sports, who has suffered severe third-degree burns over two-thirds of his body. Both of his eyes are blinded due to corneal damage. His body is badly disfigured and he is almost completely unable to move. For the past nine months he has undergone multiple surgical procedures (skin grafting, removal of his right eyeball, and amputation of the distal parts of the fingers on both hands). He has also required very painful daily bathings and bandage changings in order to prevent skin infections from developing over the burned areas of his body. The future he now looks forward to includes months or years of further painful treatment, many additional operations and a final existence as at least a moderately crippled and a mostly (or totally) blind person. From the day of his accident he has persistently stated that he does not want to live. He has been interviewed by a medical center psychiatrist and found to be bright, articulate, logical, and coherent. He is firm in his insistence that treatment be discontinued and that he be allowed to die. Nonetheless his physicians are continuing to treat him.[10]

According to our definition Mr. C's doctors are acting paternalistically: They believe that saving Mr. C's life justifies causing him great physical and psychological pain without his consent, they believe that they are qualified to act for Mr. C's good, and they believe that Mr. C believes he generally knows what is for his own good.

Mr. C's physicians could claim that they are acting as they are because they believe that the pain they are causing him by continuing treatment is a lesser evil than the death that would occur should they stop. This is certainly a rational ranking on their part. If Mr. C agreed, then the physicians would still be violating a moral rule but with Mr. C's consent, and thus no moral dilemma would exist. But Mr. C ranks the evils differently: he prefers death to months of daily pain, months or years of multiple surgical procedures, and a final existence as a deformed and crippled person. His ranking, like that of his physicians, is a rational one.

We would then say that the kind of violation being engaged in by the physicians involved their causing a great amount of pain by imposing their (rational) ranking of evils on a person whose own (rational) ranking is different. No rational person would publicly advocate this kind of violation because of the terrible consequences of living in a world where great pain could be inflicted on persons against their rational desires whenever some other person could do so by appealing to some different rational ranking of evils of his or her own. Thus when we universalize the kind of violation in which the physicians are engaged we conclude that their paternalistic act is unjustified. (Note that the form and conclusion to this analysis are similar to those in the case of deceiving the cancer patient.)

We have mentioned above that if Mr. C agreed with his physicians, no moral dilemma would exist. The case could also be varied in another way which would change our moral judgment. Suppose Mr. C had to undergo only one week of painful treatment and then had a high likelihood of resuming an essentially normal life. If he claimed to prefer death over one week of treatment, we would say that his ranking of evils was not rational. While we would sympathize with his loathing of his daily painful treatments, we would also expect that if forced to undergo them he would at some future time acknowledge that his present desires had been irrational. We would now describe the kind of violation being engaged in by the physicians as involving their causing a great amount of pain for a short time by imposing their rational ranking of evils on a person whose own ranking of evils is irrational.[11] A rational person would publicly advocate this kind of violation.

Thus universalizing this kind of violation, we conclude that the paternalistic intervention of the physicians would be justified.

All of the above cases have involved the balancing of great evils such as dying, deception about terminal illness, and the infliction of severe pain. The paternalistic interventions described have been obvious and often dramatic: commitment to a mental hospital or lying about whether a person's child was alive. The health care professionals making the decisions have all been physicians, and in most of the cases (though we have not mentioned this feature) the possibility of legal intervention has been present, in the form of suits for negligence or battery or injunctions to stop treatment. However, we believe that the vast majority of paternalistic interventions in medicine take place on a smaller scale. The following case illustrates what we consider to be a much more common kind of paternalism.

Mrs. W is a fifty-year-old patient in a rehabilitation ward who is recovering from the effects of a stroke. A major part of her treatment consists of daily visits to the physical therapy unit where she is given repetitive exercises to increase the strength and mobility of her partially paralyzed left arm and leg. She is initially cooperative with Mr. S, her physical therapist, but soon becomes bored with the monotony of the daily sessions and frustrated by her failure to adequately move her partially paralyzed limbs and by her very slow progress. She tells Mr. S she does not wish to attend the remaining three weeks of daily sessions. It is Mr. S's experience that if patients like Mrs. W stop the sessions early they do not receive the full therapeutic benefit possible and may suffer for the remainder of their lives from a significantly more disabled arm and leg than would be the case if they exercised now in this critical, early-poststroke period. Accordingly he first tries to persuade her to continue exercising. When that is not effective he becomes rather stern and scolds and chastises her for two days. She then relents and begins exercising again, but it is necessary for Mr. S to chastise her almost daily to obtain her continued participation over the ensuing three weeks.

Mr. S's scolding and chastising is paternalistic behavior by our account: He is causing Mrs. W psychological pain without her consent for what he believes is her own good. He further believes he is qualified to do so and also believes that Mrs. W believes she generally knows what is for her own good.

Mr. S could attempt to justify his action by claiming that the relatively minor amount of evil he is inflicting through chastising her into exercising is much less than the relatively greater evil Mrs. W may experience by being significantly more disabled than need be for the ensuing years of her life. Thus Mr. S could claim that Mrs. W's ranking of the relevant evils is irrational. We would describe the kind of violation being engaged in by Mr. S as his inflicting a mild degree of suffering on Mrs. W (through his chastising and her resumed exercising) by imposing his rational ranking of evils on Mrs. W, whose ranking is not rational. A rational person could publicly advocate this kind of violation, and we conclude that Mr. S's paternalistic behavior is justified.

Note that this case involves the balancing of evils which, while significant, are not of the intensity of our earlier cases. The amount of evil associated with the possibility of Mrs. W's needlessly greater lifelong disability seems just significant enough (and her balancing of the evils of three weeks of exercising versus lifelong disability seems just irrational enough) to justify causing her some mild to moderate degree of transient suffering without her consent.

However, there are some kinds of violations we would think not justified in Mrs. W's case. We would think it unjustified to inflict great physical pain on her to force her to exercise. The amount of evil associated with the possibility of her increased disability is simply not great enough so that one could publicly advocate that kind of violation.

Philosophically, the most interesting alternative to consider is the possibility of lying to her. Suppose Mr. S told her that unless she continued to exercise for three more weeks she would regress and never be able to walk again. Suppose further that he knew that in her case this was untrue, that in fact she was almost certainly going to be able to walk in any event, but that, as described above, physical therapy would very likely decrease her ultimate level of disability. If Mr. S did lie in this way, it might prove quite effective in quickly remotivating Mrs. W to exercise daily without the need for Mr. S to chastise her at all. In fact, such a deception might cause Mrs. W less total suffering than daily chastising would if she now perceived the exercising as something she wanted to do because through doing it she was staving off the possibility of a certain inability to walk. Thus, using a simple negative utilitarian method of calculation, it might seem that if chastisement were justifiable paternalism, lying would be even more strongly justifiable. But when we describe the kind of violation that Mr. S would commit by lying we see that this is not the case. It is true that Mrs. W's desire to discontinue physical therapy is, in the circumstances, one that we would regard as irrational. Thus we do not have lying in order to impose one person's rational ranking of the evils on another person's different rational ranking, but rather lying in order to substitute a rational ranking for an irrational one. Thus we must describe the kind of act as deception in order to prevent the possibility of a permanent (up to 20 to 30 years) though moderate amount of disability, and thereby causing a temporary (three weeks) mild physical discomfort (of physical therapy). Would a rational person allow lying in these circumstances; that is, would he publicly advocate this kind of violation of the rule against deception? We find this a difficult question to answer. Allowing lying in a situation where trust is extremely important (i.e., between a doctor, nurse, or therapist and a patient) in order to prevent evil significant enough that it is irrational not to avoid it (i.e., the possibility of permanent moderate disability) is an issue on which we think rational persons could disagree. The erosion of trust that would follow from universally allowing this kind of violation may have such significant evil consequences (e.g., legitimate warnings may come to be disregarded) that it is not clear that even preventing a significant number of persons from suffering permanent moderate disability is enough to counterbalance these consequences. Our conclusion in this circumstance is that rational persons would disagree; some would publicly advocate violation; some would not.

The conclusion of the preceding paragraph rests upon the assumption that lying is the only method whereby one can get Mrs. W to continue her treatment. However, if we have an alternative to lying, namely, the method of chastising and scolding, then we hold that all rational persons would publicly advocate using this method rather than lying. We have found, in informal testing, that when presented with these alternative methods of getting Mrs. W to continue treatment, everyone regarded chastising and scolding as morally preferable to lying, and that some regarded lying as completely morally unacceptable. If one uses a simple negative utilitarian theory, this result cannot be accounted for since in this particular case lying results in no more and almost certainly less overall suffering than chastising and scolding. However, if one applies the method of justification that we have been presenting, these moral intuitions are accounted for quite easily. For using *only* the relevant facts of the particular case—(1) the moral rules violated: causing pain (the unpleasantness caused by the scolding) versus deception (lying about consequences of stopping treatment); (2) the evil probably prevented: unpleasantness of treatment in both cases plus unpleasantness of scolding in the former case—as determining the kind of violation and then seeing whether one could publicly advocate this kind of violation, one will end up with the result that accords with the moral intuitions that one actually finds.

We believe the above case is typical of a multitude of everyday situations in medicine where doctors, nurses, and other health care workers act or are tempted to act paternalistically toward patients. Consider the problems presented by the patient with emphysema who continues to smoke, by the alcoholic with liver damage who refuses to enter any treatment program, or by the diabetic or hypertensive patient who exacerbates his or her disease by paying little heed to dietary precautions. Each of these patients is apt to stimulate paternalistic acts on the part of a variety of health care professionals (as well as the patient's own family members). We think it is an important task to determine, whenever possible, which kinds of paternalistic acts are justifiable and which are not.

NOTES

1. In this paper we intend to apply the general theory of moral justification contained in Bernard Gert, *The Moral Rules,* 2d ed., Harper Torchbooks, New York, 1975.

2. For a fuller account, see Bernard Gert and Charles M. Culver, "Paternalistic Behavior," *Philosophy and Public Affairs,* vol. 6, p. 45, fall 1976.

3. This feature has been slightly reworded from that presented in Gert and Culver. Also, James Rachels has pointed out that our earlier discussion of feature 2 suggested that being qualified required superior knowledge and that this is misleading. He correctly noted that one could believe oneself qualified not because of superior knowledge, but because of superior ability to act, e.g., when the subject of paternalism is suffering from a phobia.

4. It is not necessary that one explicitly hold some theory about what counts as a violation of a moral rule. All that is required is that one believes A is doing one of the following: killing; causing pain (physical or mental); disabling; depriving of freedom, opportunity, or pleasure; deceiving; breaking a promise; or cheating. All of these are universally regarded as requiring moral justification and hence are regarded by us as violations of moral rules.

5. See Gert, pp. xx–xxi, 98–100, 119, 126.

6. We think that following the procedure outlined in this paper will reduce the number of cases in which there is disagreement. In those cases of disagreement that remain we believe that some

type of decision-making body should be consulted whenever possible. This is an important practical matter that we do not discuss further here.

7. We realize the lack of precision of this description but we believe that often no greater precision is possible. This is one factor which makes coming to decisions sometimes difficult. See Aristotle, *Nicomachean Ethics*, 1.3.1094b.

8. Since it is only the evils caused and prevented with regard to S that are relevant, we are not involved in the kinds of interpersonal comparisons of utility that seem to present so many problems to utilitarian theorists.

9. It is this fallibility of persons, their inability to know all the consequences of their actions, which explains not only why no rational person would publicly advocate cheating simply on the grounds that no one would be hurt by it but also why moral rules are needed at all. We cannot consider the nature of a violation after we see how things actually turn out but must do so when the violation is being contemplated; then the fallibility of persons will play its proper role. See Gert, p. 126.

10. This case is adapted from Case 228, "A Demand to Die" in *Hastings Center Report,* vol. 5, p. 9, June 1975.

11. We realize that there will not be universal agreement on the rationality of all examples of the ranking of evils, but we think there will be agreement on many and thereby a portion of the initially unclear cases will become much clearer (see note 6 above).

Confidentiality

3.

The Rule of Confidentiality
Tom L. Beauchamp James F. Childress

Suppose the parents of a child suffering from a genetic disease insist that the physician not reveal this information to others in the family who may be at risk for having children with the same disease. Suppose, for example, that the child has Lesch-Nyhan syndrome, a disease involving uncontrollable self-mutilation. Because this disease is X-linked, the mother's sisters would be at risk. But the mother, let us suppose, dislikes her sisters, who live far away and never communicate. Furthermore, she feels the stigma of being a carrier of the disease and so wishes to conceal the information. In this case, her physician faces a conflict between his duty to respect the confidences of his patients and his general social responsibility. There is no way to avoid this conflict if his attempts to obtain the mother's permission to disclose this information should fail. The right and perhaps the duty to break therapeutic confidences under some circumstances indicate that the therapeutic role may sometimes have to yield to one's role as citizen and as protector of the interests of others.

There is widespread agreement, expressed in various ethical codes for health care professionals, that a rule of confidentiality should prevail in relationships with patients. The Hippocratic Oath urges secrecy regarding what "ought not to be spoken abroad" but does not limit secrecy to what is seen or heard in professional practice. The AMA Code holds that a "physician may not reveal the confidences entrusted to him in the course of medical attendance, or the deficiencies he may observe in the character of his patients, unless he is required to do so by law or unless it becomes necessary in order to protect the welfare of the individual or of the community" (Section 9). The World Medical Association International Code of Medical Ethics expressly holds that the physician owes his patient *"absolute secrecy on all [information] which has been confided to him or which he knows because of the confidence entrusted to him"* (emphasis added). Still, most codes and general theories hold that the rule of confidentiality is not absolute. In fact, it may be possible to specify several conditions under which confidentiality should not be main-

Source: Tom L. Beauchamp and James F. Childress, *Principles of Biomedical Ethics,* p. 209, Oxford University Press, New York, 1979.

tained—e.g., some more specific variants of the conditions listed in the AMA Code. Before we turn to those conditions for justified breaches of confidentiality, we need to inquire into the basis of the rule and the warrants that support it.

Although we may find a person who betrays secrets despicable, it is not clear that he violates a general moral principle or rule against telling secrets. In most instances, he betrays other people who entered into certain relationships with him and counted on him to respect their confidences. His actions are despicable because he betrays the *trust* of other persons. Trust is confidence in and reliance upon others to respect certain principles and rules in their interactions. It is the expectation that others will respect boundaries, which often (but not always) are moral ones. Some of the limits set by professional codes, for example, are more matters of custom than of morality. But the patient may rely upon the health care professional to respect these customs and may rightly believe that their implicit contract has been violated if the professional fails to live up to these customary standards. Assurance of confidentiality is also important because it enables people to seek help without the stigma that would result from public knowledge, because it encourages full disclosure that is essential for effective treatment, and because it is necessary for the maintenance of trust.

Another argument builds on the right of autonomy. One aspect of respecting autonomy is respect for a person's *privacy*. According to a landmark law review article in 1890 on the right of privacy, the individual has the right "of determining, ordinarily, to what extent his thoughts, sentiments, and emotions shall be communicated to others."[1] Whatever privacy includes, it involves personal control over information about oneself and over access to that information. Without such personal control, important human relationships such as love, friendship, and trust would be diminished. At stake are both the *amount* and the *kind* of information. As Charles Fried suggests,

while we might not mind if a person knows a general fact about us, we might feel that our privacy has been invaded if he knows the details.[2] Similarly, we might not object if a good friend knows the nature of our illness, but we might protest that he has invaded our privacy if he observes us actually suffering from that illness.

We grant others access to information about ourselves as a part of such relationships as love, friendship, and trust. We may also have specific reasons for granting this information to some persons: when we wish to be treated by a physician, a psychiatrist, or other health care professionals, we may have to share personal information. Less may be required for the physician than for the psychiatrist or psychologist. For successful treatment by the latter, we must expose our innermost thoughts, feelings, emotions, dreams, and fantasies. We grant these health care professionals access to information about ourselves for our own diagnostic and therapeutic benefit. In general, we should retain control over access to that information, authorizing access when appropriate. For example, we might authorize a physician to grant an insurance company or a prospective employer access to the information.

The harder questions, however, concern the stringency of the rule of confidentiality. Is it an absolute rule, as in the requirement of "absolute secrecy" in the International Code of Medical Ethics? Or should it be regarded merely as a rule asserting a prima facie duty?

Our view holds that the rule of confidentiality, which could be formulated as imposing duties on health care professionals or as creating rights for patients, states a prima facie duty. Anyone who thinks that a disclosure of confidential information is morally justified or even mandatory in some circumstances bears a burden of proof. While this approach requires a balancing of conflicting duties, it also establishes a structure of moral reasoning and justification. It is not enough to determine which act will respect the most duties or maximize the good, for the strong presumption against revealing confidences establishes the direction and burden of deliberation and justification.

Sometimes the health care professional has been viewed as having a "right" to violate confidences in some circumstances, but not as having a "duty" to do so. He is permitted, not obliged, according to this view. Nevertheless, there are clear legal duties to divulge confidential information when necessary to report contagious diseases, gunshot wounds, child abuse, etc. The AMA Code of 1957 holds that the physician should not violate the rule of confidentiality "unless he is required to do so by law or unless it becomes necessary in order to protect the welfare of the individual or of the community" (Section 9). Although some people interpret this statement as permitting but not requiring the physician to break confidences, we interpret it differently: one may not break a confidence except to fulfill another and more stringent duty—either a duty to obey the law, or a duty to protect the welfare of the patient or the community, e.g., a duty based on beneficence. There is no *right* to violate confidences in such cases unless there is also a *duty* to do so. The health care professional's breach of confidentiality thus cannot be justified unless it is necessary to meet a strong conflicting duty. This conclusion means that rules protecting confidences must sometimes give way to rules protecting other interests.

Before discussing duties that may justify violating the rule of confidentiality, we should note that some breaches of confidentiality are not violations of duties to the patient. For example, the company physician who informs his employers that an employee in a responsible position suffers from alcoholism may not actually violate a rule of confidentiality, for he may not be bound by this rule in the same way as a private physician. He could, for example, be under contract with the company and an employee's union to perform certain services, including the reporting of work-related information about patients. Nevertheless, both the company and the physician in such circumstances have the moral responsibility to

ensure that employee-patients actually understand at the outset that the traditional rule of confidentiality is not operative.

A distinction should be made between releasing information at the patient's *behest* and releasing it on the patient's *behalf without his consent.* Although the health care professional should generally release confidential information about a particular patient when the patient requests its release, the health care professional may encounter circumstances in which the patient refuses to authorize disclosures that would be in his best interest. When the patient authorizes disclosure of information—e.g., to his lawyer, to the court, to an insurance company, or to a family member—the health care professional does not violate the rule of confidentiality, which is designed to protect the patient's control over access to information about himself. Hereafter we shall be exclusively concerned with disclosures of confidential information without the patient's informed authorization.

What duties legitimately override the rule of confidentiality? While the AMA Code mentions both legal duties and actions necessary to protect patients or society, these two sets of conditions are not mutually exclusive. The law may lay down certain conditions for the protection of the individual and society or may simply allow general moral convictions to prevail. In either case, the law may not hold the health care professional accountable for a breach of confidentiality. Most instances of disclosing confidential information to protect *the patient* (rather than others) are not legally required. Some legal duties such as the requirement to report epileptic seizures to the division of motor vehicles may be paternalistic in some dimensions and utilitarian in others. Even the legal requirement to report child abuse is not paternalistic. The health care professional has a legal duty to report child abuse in order to protect the child, and he has a duty of confidentiality only to the child, not to the parents, even if they are also his patients. His fiduciary relationship is with the child, whose interests he must protect.

Legal duties to break confidentiality in order to protect *others* pose a conflict of obligations for the health care professional. On the one hand, he is obligated to protect his patient; on the other hand, he is legally obligated to act to protect the society, even if he thinks the law is silly or unjust. There also is a *moral* obligation to obey the law, at least in a relatively just system,[3] but it is only a strong prima facie duty, not absolute. Sometimes it may be necessary for the health care professional to violate the duty to obey the law in order to fulfill his responsibility to his patient. Sometimes he may justifiably reason that he cannot adequately treat his patient over time if he obeys the law—e.g., in complicated circumstances where there is a legal duty to report venereal disease.

Violations of the rule of confidentiality where there is no legal duty to disclose information raise additional issues. First, it is easier to justify violations of confidentiality on grounds of the prevention of harm to others than on grounds of paternalism, especially for competent adults. The duty to report child abuse would be strong even in the absence of a statute because of the child's dependence and vulnerability. However, where competent adults are involved, breaches of confidentiality to protect the patient from himself usually involve a violation of autonomy, and therefore are difficult to justify. Suppose that a physician has to decide whether to disclose to a thirty-year-old woman's parents that their daughter's marriage is in trouble and that this is the cause of a "nervous condition" which has resulted in her hospitalization. She has asked him not to say anything to her parents, but he is convinced that her parents, who are also his patients, would help her recover. The alleged benefit to the patient is not of sufficient magnitude or probability to warrant overriding autonomy and the rule of confidentiality in these circumstances. If the physician's efforts to convince the woman that she should tell her parents fail, he should maintain confidentiality even if he believes it is not in the patient's best interest.

Second, if the duty to prevent harms is more stringent than the duty to provide benefits, it is easier to justify violations of confidentiality in order to prevent harms to patients or others than to justify violations on grounds of benefit to patients. But a clear distinction cannot always be drawn between producing benefits and preventing harms; and the duty to prevent a trivial harm may not be stronger than the duty to produce a major benefit. The type of harms and benefits may also make a relevant difference. If psychiatrists have a duty to warn intended victims of violence, is the line to be drawn at threats to physical existence and integrity, e.g., murder and rape? Or do we extend it to include threats to property?

Third, how *probable* must the benefit or harm be before a breach of confidentiality is justified? Is a remote chance of substantial harm to many people sufficient?

Fourth, given the presumption against violating the rule of confidentiality and the significance of that rule, the health care professional should of course seek alternative and more acceptable ways of realizing a benefit or preventing a harm, short of disclosing confidential information (and violating other important moral principles and rules). Rarely is the breach of confidentiality justified if morally and legally acceptable alternatives exist. In one case, a physician had to determine whether to disclose a patient's homosexuality to his prospective wife, who was also the physician's patient. Although the physician chose to respect the rule of confidentiality, should he have tried to persuade the young man to tell his prospective wife? Or should he have discussed marriage and sexuality with the young woman so that she might have pressed her prospective fiance for more information? Since she was his patient, the physician had a stronger obligation to disclose information to her than he would have had if she had been a stranger, and this obligation makes his inaction less acceptable.[4]

Finally, most interesting cases of confidentiality involve uncertainty at the time the decision must be made. Uncertainty may occur on several different levels: basic information, diagnosis, prognosis, likelihood of an untoward event, etc. For example, suppose that the physician has to decide whether to inform the division of motor vehicles that his epileptic patient still suffers seizures, when this unconfirmed information came from a neighbor of the patient. In another case, a psychiatrist used hypnotic techniques to help a pilot recall suppressed information about his responsibility for the crash of a commercial plane. The information indicated that the pilot should not fly, at least temporarily. When the therapist was unable to convince the pilot that he should not fly until his problems were solved, what should he have done? How much certainty did he need for more vigorous action? Six months after returning to work, the pilot made an error of judgment that resulted in the crash of a transatlantic flight and the loss of many lives.[5] Suppose that a pilot of a commercial jet informs his physician that his forty-five-year-old mother was diagnosed as having Huntington's chorea. The physician has to determine whether to disclose to the airline this pilot's 50 percent risk of having the disease in the event the pilot fails to reveal it.[6] In these cases difficult matters of judgment are involved in determining the probability and magnitude of a harm (or benefit) that will justify the break of confidentiality. There can be no simple formula for deciding such cases independent of the individual risk benefit assessments themselves.

There is an important distinction between the probable effects of a disease (e.g., venereal disease) and the probable actions of an agent (e.g., a patient's threat to harm someone else). It may be easier to justify breaches of confidentiality to prevent a disease's negative effects than to prevent an agent's negative acts. Cases of doubt about whether an agent will do what he threatens to do may be harder to resolve than cases of doubt about the effects of a disease. The former cases, most of which emerge in psychiatric or psy-

chotherapeutic relations, require more room for patient autonomy, but they do not indicate that a patient should never be committed for suicidal or homicidal tendencies. The Assembly of District Branches and the Board of Trustees of the American Psychiatric Association in 1973 annotated the principles of medical ethics for psychiatry and held (with special reference to court-ordered disclosures of confidences): "When the psychiatrist is in doubt, the right of the patient to confidentiality and, by extension, to unimpaired treatment, should be given priority."[7] An annotated AMA code (1971) appealed to a version of the Golden Rule as a test of the physician's responsibility to report contagious diseases. This test could also apply to various doubtful cases: "the physician should act as he would desire another to act toward one of his own family in like circumstances" (Section 9).

NOTES

1. Samuel Warren and Louis Brandeis, "The Right of Privacy," *Harvard Law Review*, vol. 4, p. 193, 1890.

2. See Charles Fried, *An Anatomy of Values*, p. 141, Harvard University Press, Cambridge, Mass., 1970.

3. See James F. Childress, *Civil Disobedience and Political Obligation*, Yale University Press, New Haven, Conn., 1971; and John Rawls, *A Theory of Justice*, Chapter 6, Harvard University Press, Cambridge, Mass., 1971.

4. Harvey Kuschner, Daniel Callahan, Eric J. Cassell, and Robert M. Veatch, "The Homosexual Husband and Physician Confidentiality," *The Hastings Center Report*, vol. 7, p. 15, April 1977.

5. Bernard B. Raginsky, "Hypnotic Recall of Aircrash Cause," *The International Journal of Clinical and Experimental Hypnosis*, vol. 17, p. 1, 1969.

6. Aubrey Milunsky, *The Prevention of Genetic Disease and Mental Retardation*, p. 75, W. B. Saunders, Philadelphia, 1975.

7. "The Principles of Medical Ethics with Annotations Especially Applicable to Psychiatry," *American Journal of Psychiatry*, vol. 130, p. 1063, September 1973.

Definition of Death

4.

A Definition of Irreversible Coma
Report of the Ad Hoc Committee on Irreversible Coma

Our primary purpose is to define irreversible coma as a new criterion for death. There are two reasons why there is need for a definition: (1) Improvements in resuscitative and supportive measures have led to increased efforts to save those who are desperately injured. Sometimes these efforts have only partial success so that the result is an individual whose heart continues to beat but whose brain is irreversibly damaged. The burden is great on patients who suffer permanent loss of intellect, on their families, on the hospitals, and on those in need of hospital beds already occupied by these comatose patients. (2) Obsolete criteria for the definition of death can lead to controversy in obtaining organs for transplantation.

Irreversible coma has many causes, but *we are concerned here only with those comatose individuals who have no discernible central nervous system activity.* If the characteristics can be defined in satisfactory terms, translatable into action—and we believe this is possible—then several problems will either disappear or will become more readily soluble.

More than medical problems are present. There are moral, ethical, religious, and legal issues. Adequate definition here will prepare the way for better insight into all these matters as well as for better law than is currently applicable.

Characteristics of Irreversible Coma

An organ, brain or other, that no longer functions and has no possibility of functioning again is for all practical purposes dead. Our first problem is to determine the characteristics of a *permanently* nonfunctioning brain.

A patient in this state appears to be in deep coma. The condition can be satisfactorily diagnosed by points 1, 2, and 3 to follow. The electroencephalogram (point 4)

Source: Reprinted by permission of the author and the publisher from "A Definition of Irreversible Coma," a report of the Ad Hoc Committee of the Harvard Medical School, *Journal of the American Medical Association,* Vol. 205, No. 6 (August 1968), pp. 337–340. Copyright 1968, American Medical Association. The Ad Hoc Committee included Henry K. Beecher, M.D., chairman; Raymond D. Adams, M.D.; A. Clifford Barger, M.D.; William J. Curran, L.L.M., S.M.Hyg.; Derek Denny-Brown, M.D.; Dana L. Farnsworth, M.D.; Jordi Folch-Pi, M.D.; Everett I. Mendelsohn, Ph.D.; John P. Merrill, M.D.; Joseph Murray, M.D.; Ralph Potter, Th.D.; Robert Schwab, M.D.; and William Sweet, M.D.

provides confirmatory data, and when available it should be utilized. In situations where for one reason or another electroencephalographic monitoring is not available, the absence of cerebral function has to be determined by purely clinical signs, to be described, or by absence of circulation as judged by standstill of blood in the retinal vessels, or by absence of cardiac activity.

1. *Unreceptivity and unresponsitivity.* There is a total unawareness to externally applied stimuli and inner need and complete unresponsiveness—our definition of irreversible coma. Even the most intensely painful stimuli evoke no vocal or other response, not even a groan, withdrawal of a limb, or quickening of respiration.

2. *No movements or breathing.* Observations covering a period of at least 1 hour by physicians are adequate to satisfy the criteria of no spontaneous muscular movements or spontaneous respiration or response to stimuli such as pain, touch, sound, or light. After the patient is on a mechanical respirator, the total absence of spontaneous breathing may be established by turning off the respirator for 3 minutes and observing whether there is any effort on the part of the subject to breathe spontaneously. (The respirator may be turned off for this time provided that at the start of the trial period the patient's carbon dioxide tension is within the normal range, and provided also that the patient had been breathing room air for at least 10 minutes prior to the trial.)

3. *No reflexes.* Irreversible coma with abolition of central nervous system activity is evidenced in part by the absence of elicitable reflexes. The pupil will be fixed and dilated and will not respond to a direct source of bright light. Since the establishment of a fixed, dilated pupil is clear-cut in clinical practice, there should be no uncertainty as to its presence. Ocular movement (to head turning and to irrigation of the ears with ice water) and blinking are absent. There is no evidence of postural activity (decerebrate or other). Swallowing, yawning, vocalization are in abeyance. Corneal and pharyngeal reflexes are absent.

As a rule the stretch of tendon reflexes cannot be elicited; i.e., tapping the tendons of the biceps, triceps, and pronator muscles, quadriceps and gastrocnemius muscles with the reflex hammer elicits no contraction of the respective muscles. Plantar or noxious stimulation gives no response.

4. *Flat electroencephalogram.* Of great confirmatory value is the flat or isoelectric EEG. We must assume that the electrodes have been properly applied, that the apparatus is functioning normally, and that the personnel in charge is competent. We consider it prudent to have one channel of the apparatus used for an electrocardiogram. This channel will monitor the ECG so that, if it appears in the electroencephalographic leads because of high resistance, it can be readily identified. It also establishes the presence of the active heart in the absence of the EEG. We recommend that another channel be used for a noncephalic lead. This will pick up space-borne or vibration-borne artifacts and identify them. The simplest form of such a monitoring noncephalic electrode has two leads over the dorsum of the hand, preferably the right hand, so the ECG will be minimal or absent. Since one of the requirements of this state is that there be no muscle activity, these two dorsal hand electrodes will not be bothered by muscle artifact. The apparatus should be run at standard gains of 10 microvolts per millimeter (μv/mm), 50 μv/5 mm. Also it should be isoelectric at double this standard gain, which is 5 μv/5 mm or 25 μv/5 mm. At least 10 full minutes of recording is desirable, but twice that would be better.

It is also suggested that the gains at some point be opened to their full amplitude for a brief period (5 to 100 seconds) to see what is going on. Usually in an intensive care unit artifacts will dominate the picture, but these are readily identifiable. There should be no electroencephalographic response to noise or to pinch.

All of the above tests should be repeated at least 24 hours later with no change.

The validity of such data as indications of irreversible cerebral damage depends on the exclusion of two conditions: hypothermia [temperature below 90° F (32.2° C)] or central nervous system depressants, such as barbiturates.

Other Procedures

The patient's condition can be determined only by a physician. When the patient is hopelessly damaged as defined above, the family and all colleagues who have participated in major decisions concerning the patient, and all nurses involved, should be so informed. Death is to be declared and *then* the respirator turned off. The decision to do this and the responsibility for it are to be taken by the physician-in-charge, in consultation with one or more physicians who have been directly involved in the case. It is unsound and undesirable to force the family to make the decision.

5.

The Definition of Death: Ethical, Philosophical, and Policy Confusion
Robert M. Veatch

"Brain death" itself is a confusing term. It can have a noncontroversial meaning: the irreversible destruction of the brain tissue. It can also have a radically different meaning, one that is more philosophically and politically controversial. It can also mean "the death of the person as a whole as measured by the functioning of the brain." This ambiguity is the reason why I and many others would strongly recommend that the term "brain death" be abandoned.

The term reflects the ambiguity revealed in the Harvard report. Brain death can focus on technical, empirical criteria for the irreversible destruction of the brain. That was approximately the meaning of the term as used by the Harvard Committee. On the other hand, it can be used at a more conceptual level, as in arguments about whether the person as a whole should be considered dead when the brain has died.

The same linguistic point can be made about the term "cerebral death." It can mean the death of the cerebrum (leaving open the question of whether the person is dead when the cerebrum is dead) or it can mean the death of the person based on the destruction of the cerebrum. To make matters even more confusing "cerebral death" can be confused with "brain death." Sometimes, in spite of the obvious significant difference between the two, the terms are used interchangeably. This can lead to statements that the brain is dead when only cerebral activity has ceased. (No current law would permit pronouncement of death when only cerebral activity has ceased.) It can also lead to insistence on more rigorous criteria than necessary for measuring the prognosis of a person in irreversible coma or with irreversible loss of cerebral function.

The source of much of our confusion is the ambiguity of the term. We must keep separate three distinct questions. The empirical question is, "What are the best technical measures of the destruction of the brain?" The philosophical, conceptual question is, "What is it that is so essential to our concept of human life such that when it is lost we should treat the individual as dead?" The pol-

Source: Julius Korein (ed.), *Annals of the New York Academy of Sciences*, vol. 315, p. 307, 1978.

icy question is, "When should our laws and our courts regard a person as dead and when should a medical professional be authorized to pronounce a person dead?" Clearly no amount of biological, neurologic evidence will ever be decisive in deciding what it is an individual has lost when he has lost what is essential to our concept of humanness. The contribution to the discussion of the neurologists acting as neurologists should be empirical evidence of empirical predictors of the functioning of the brain and the likelihood of recovery of function once lost.

We should take pause when we realize that the Harvard report, which *de facto* was limited to this empirical, biological task, may have been wrong even at this level. It appears that the committee did not distinguish between criteria for irreversible coma, which it claimed to be identifying, and criteria for irreversible destruction of the brain, which would be relevant for any ethical or legal judgments based on the death of the whole brain. Whether the so-called Harvard criteria measure the destruction of the brain, or whether they measure irreversible coma, is a question that is primarily in the hands of those with appropriate neurologic skills. It appears, however, that the Harvard criteria may be precise measures of neither of these.

The important questions for those who are not specialists in those empirical disciplines are much more at the levels of concept and policy. At the conceptual level we ask, "What does it mean to be dead?" At the policy level we ask, "Under what circumstances should we call a person dead?"

Four Concepts of Death

Even if we know precisely the predictors of the destruction of the brain, it is still an open question whether we ought to call a person dead when his brain is destroyed. In general terms an entity is considered dead when there is a complete change in the status of that entity characterized by the irreversible loss of those characteristics that are essentially significant to it.[1]

Throughout history, in various times and cultures, many answers have been given to the question of what is essentially significant to the human. Four answers remain as plausible to large numbers of people. Each involves the irreversible loss of some essential characteristic.[2] The four essential characteristics are the presence of the soul, the flowing of "vital" body fluids, the capacity for bodily integration, and the capacity for consciousness and social interaction.

The irreversible loss of the soul. Probably more people in world history, and even more of those alive today, have believed that death means the irreversible loss of the soul than have held all the other concepts we shall consider. The link between the departure of the soul and death can be either analytical or synthetic. If the soul is simply *defined* as the element that departs at death, then we learn nothing about what holders of this concept of death thought death to be. It seems clear, however, that large numbers of people, including classical thinkers in Greek, some Christian, and most secular Western thought, until recently had a more synthetic notion of the relationship between the soul and death. The soul was the animating principle of thought and action in man and was identified with mental, emotional, and sometimes (but not always) with spiritual functions. It was nonmaterial, but nevertheless a metaphysical reality. It was important to nurture the soul and know its locus. Descartes, for instance, held that although the soul is united to all the portions of the body "there is yet . . . a certain part in which it exercises its functions more particularly than in all the others."[3] He was convinced that this was in the brain, "not the whole of the brain, but merely the most inward of all its parts, to wit, a certain very small gland which is situated in the middle of its substance," that is, the pineal body.

Although this view continues to be held by many people throughout the world, it is largely abandoned by most thinkers trained in the world view of Western science. It is beyond the pale of empirical scientific study and does not lend itself to the precision necessary for secular clinical and legal judgment. We shall abandon this concept, although some of its characteristics may be more plausible than other, more modern conceptions of what it means to be dead.

The irreversible stopping of the flow of "vital" body fluids. When modern man secularized his philosophical understanding of his nature, he had to find another, more biological formulation of what it meant to be dead. In answer to the question, "What is it about human life that its loss is so essential that the individual who loses it ought to be called dead?" modern man began to give answers focusing on the heart and lungs. We may try to deduce his concept of death from the empirical measures he made to determine whether an individual is dead. We could identify visual and tactile observations of respiration, pulse, and heart beat. More recently these have been made more sophisticated by the use of an electrocardiogram, but the tests are basically the same. They only tell us, however, that functions related to the heart and lung seem to be important.

If we ask what it is about the heart and lungs that is so important, it becomes clear that it is not their functioning per se that was thought essential. Consider the case of a patient whose lungs are permanently destroyed and who is maintained on a respirator or a blood oxygenator. Clearly he was and still is thought to be alive. Even the hypothetical person whose heart and lungs are permanently destroyed but who is maintained on a heart-lung machine would still be alive beyond any doubt. The critical function is not the heart and lung activity, but the flowing of the vital fluids—the blood and breath—that these organs normally produce.

The decisive problem with this concept of the essence of life is that it is not only simplistic, but biologically reductionistic. It makes no distinction between the human and the human's body. It is a vitalistic, animalistic notion of the human as essentially a biological species in which the biological functions of respiration and circulation are critical.

It is important to realize that there is no scientific or medical argument against that position. It is fundamentally not a scientific or medical question. If some individuals and some religious and philosophical schools of thought choose to answer the question "What is essential to the human's nature?" by pointing to respiration and circulation, no laboratory evidence will ever refute the stance. This position is, however, in conflict with the view of virtually every religious and philosophical group in human history. It can at least be said for the defenders of the idea that death occurs when the soul departs from the body, that they recognized that a human is more than his body and some of its lesser functions.

Irreversible loss of bodily integration. The new possibility of maintaining circulation and respiration in the absence of any brain activity has led many, but not all, to reexamine their concept of what it means to be dead. Henry Beecher, the chairman of the Harvard Committee, revealed his philosophical disdain for these functions when he considered the problem of hopelessly comatose patients. He asked, "Are these hopelessly comatose patients really still alive?" In answering his own question he contrasted the definition in *Black's Law Dictionary* to an alternative focusing on functions that are believed to relate to the activity of the brain. The functions he mentioned were "the individual's personality, his conscious life, his uniqueness, his capacity for remembering, judging, reasoning, acting, enjoying, worrying, and so on." He went on to argue that "We have proof that these and other functions reside in the brain, proof through studies of damage to the brain by surgery, or accident, or disease. . . . It seems clear that when the brain no longer functions, when it is destroyed, so also is the individual destroyed; he no longer exists as a person: he is dead."

Note that he says we have proof that these functions reside in the brain, but when he attempts to establish that these functions are the critical ones for deciding that a person should be treated as dead, he must shift to language such as "one believes" or "it seems clear." He is no longer in the realm of the scientific.

That he has shifted to the realm of metaphysics or ethics, however, does not necessarily mean that he is any less sure of himself. It is appropriate for him to say with confidence—with philosophical certainty—that the functions he has identified are more significant than the circulatory and respiratory functions.

The technical criteria that the Harvard Committee have identified imply that the integrative functions of the nervous system are implicitly the activities that defenders of a concept of death related to brain function see as man's essence. Spontaneous respiration, bodily reflexes, and response to stimuli are all integrative activities. Thus, according to this view, it makes sense to speak of the death of the person as a whole at the point when the person loses the ability to integrate his body as a whole.

It seems that this concept of death as the irreversible loss of bodily integrating capacity is philosophically preferable to the two previous concepts of death. It appeared that the battle was about over. Some who were raised prior to the asking of the more precise philosophical questions would continue romantically to hold onto the heart as the seat of the soul, the *sine qua non* of life. But it appeared that eventually all reasonable people would come to accept a concept of death that sees loss of integrating capacity as decisive. To be sure this could not be proven in any scientific empirical sense, but it was nevertheless taking on the character of a reasonably well-established philosophical certainty.

Then the neurologists began to differentiate cases more clearly and the philosophers began to ask their questions more carefully. Brierley and his colleagues reported two cases in which patients were apparently in irreversible coma—there was neurologic and histologic evidence that the cerebrum was destroyed—yet the patients breathed spontaneously and had intact lower brain centers. These were a challenge to the Harvard criteria as perfect predictors

of irreversible coma. The criteria may not ever classify someone in irreversible coma when he is not. That was the original fear. It appears, however, that they may be classifying some people as not in irreversible coma when they are. The criteria may predict something other than irreversible coma. They may predict destruction of the brain, or some third state in which more of the brain is destroyed than if the patient were only in irreversible coma. If so, the criteria may not be perfect predictors of either whole-brain or cerebral death.

This possibility is a real challenge. It is a challenge to what was thought to be a carefully derived empirical consensus. (Beecher said at one point, "It is clear that we have a definition of irreversible coma.") It is also a challenge at the philosophical or conceptual level. Is it really integrating capacity of the human body that is essential to his being treated as alive or is it something more specific, something residing in a more limited portion of the brain?

Irreversible loss of consciousness or capacity for special interaction. If one examines more closely the list of functions that Beecher takes as essential to being alive, it is clear that they are related to activities of the brain, but it is also clear that they do not relate to the brain as a whole. They are all what have sometimes been called the "higher brain functions": consciousness, remembering, judging, reasoning, enjoying, and the like. Neurologically we are left with the question, "Is it possible that all the essential functions could be irreversibly lost even though some of the brain cells remain alive?" Conceptually we must ask, "Is it really the integrating functions of the brain that are so essential or is it perhaps some other brain functions?"

We have found fault with the concept of death that focuses on the functions of respiration and circulation, in part because it is biologically reductionistic: it sees man as essentially animalistic. It abandons the earlier view that saw man as having both organic and nonorganic components—both body and soul. Yet everything that can be said in this regard against the concepts of death that focus on respiration and circulation can be said also against a concept that focuses on integrating capacity. Perhaps bodily integration is in some sense a more noble function than respiration and circulation, but it is still biologically reductionistic. If an individual who has irreversibly lost higher functions can still retain major integrating capacities because his lower brain centers are intact, such an individual would not meet the Harvard criteria; he would not have experienced death of the entire brain. It is still possible, however, that one could decide to call such an individual dead.

If the essential characteristic is not the vitalistic integrating capacity, then what is it? It could be capacity for consciousness— a capacity that seems to underlie most if not all of the higher functions that Beecher listed. That formulation takes cognizance of the mental capacities we have found lacking in the two previous concepts of what it means to die.

The Judeo-Christian tradition, however, has not seen man primarily as an isolated mentally functioning unit. Both Aristotle and the Judeo-Christian tradition have seen the human as essentially a political or social animal—one who has the capacity for social interaction with his fellow humans. Capacity for social interaction may then be the essential element whose loss constitutes death of the person as a whole. There is a danger that we may tend to evaluate social capacities qualitatively. The same risk exists, however, for the criteria of consciousness, integrating capacities, and even respiratory and circulatory function. Any capacities for social interaction must be a sign of life, no matter how rudimentary. In anatomic and physiologic perspective this may be identical to the capacity for consciousness. To have consciousness without capacity for some kind of social interaction seems impossible; to have social interaction without consciousness is equally implausible. So for questions of technical measurement of brain function, the distinction may not be important. It remains, however, crucial in

considerations of the human being's essential nature.

We have criticized concepts of death that identify loss of fluid-flow and integrating capacities as the essential characteristics. These concepts share the quality of being excessively biological; they are organically reductionistic. Yet reliance on capacities for consciousness or social interaction by themselves may err on the side of not giving enough of a place for the human body. The Judeo-Christian tradition that emphasizes man as a social animal still sees him as an animal. The body is an essential element. While avoiding the biological reductionism of other concepts of death, we should not slip into a Manichaeism that could accept the possibility of a living person free of his body. I doubt that the notion of disembodied consciousness will ever be more than a figment of the science fiction writer's imagination. Nevertheless, it is clear that a disembodied consciousness, conceivable, say, as a transferral of a memory to a magnetic tape equipped with sensory input and some kind of outputs, would not have all the necessary characteristics of humanhood. The body, the physical features, are necessary, if not sufficient, conditions.

The real question today is not the choice between heart and brain, but rather which part or parts of the nervous system are so essential to human function that their irreversible loss would constitute death of the person as a whole. Once one realizes that there are several brain functions that are potentially chosen as central, it is clear the philosophical debate is far from over. Reasonable people will disagree over whether a person should be pronounced dead when it is confirmed that only some portion of his brain is destroyed. The question becomes even more complex when one realizes that individual brain cells may live on after the most rudimentary brain functions have been lost. Thus, it makes little sense to hold out for the death of the entire brain in the sense of every cell's being dead. If one is going to hold to a concept of death based on brain function, it seems that at least some function above the cellular level ought to be present for a person to be considered alive. Yet if some functions—at least intracellular functions—are to be excluded when deciding which functions are significant, how does one go about deciding just which functions are necessary conditions for being considered alive? The ethical, philosophical, and theological issues remain crucial. Only when there is some degree of consensus, at least temporarily, on those issues can the more technical questions of measures of brain function and the more policy-oriented questions of when society should permit or require death to be pronounced be taken up in the context of the definition-of-death debate.

The Link between Conceptual and Technical Questions

Deciding the condition of certain body organs is important for many questions other than that of the pronouncement of death. But only after one has decided what it means to die can one begin to link technical measures of organ condition to the pronouncement of death. For some concepts of death, the technical measures follow quite easily. If the fluid flow through the body is crucial, the pulse, the heartbeat, the flowing of the breath through the nostrils become relatively straightforward tests.

If the loss of capacities for bodily integration is crucial, and one decides that the brain as a whole is the organ with decisive responsibilities for bodily integration, then tests to measure the irreversible destruction of the brain, or at least the irreversible loss of all brain function, become important.

Under these assumptions, if the Harvard criteria measure irreversible coma rather than complete destruction of the brain, the four technical measures would not be definitive in deciding to pronounce death. If, however, what they measure is closer to destruction of the whole brain, they are relevant in spite of the original decision to call them criteria for irreversible coma.

More recently attempts have been made

to determine the appropriate tests or criteria for measuring irreversible loss of consciousness, capacity for social interaction, or some other combination of higher brain functions. The EEG alone, for instance, may be a better test of loss of the critical functions. The bolus techniques may be, as well. There is no *prima facie* reason why brain-stem activities such as spontaneous respiration or reflexes would have to be absent in order to measure loss of higher brain function. If mental functions are necessary conditions for being alive, then we may have a problem quite analogous to the one that existed when the departure of the soul was the indicator of death: the processes may not be directly observable. Charron and others have argued that whatever our concept of death, the technical measures used must be of a publicly verifiable state. There is a major debate about whether mental processes can be reduced to physical states. Even if one makes the assumption that reduction of a complex mental process like consciousness to physical structures is possible, the physical structures may be so complex that no tests of their functioning are plausible. Certainly the electroencephalogram, which has been proposed as a measure of cerebral function, is at best a crude measure. The possibility that there could be electroencephalographic activity from some portions of perfused cortex, without the possibility of the person's ever regaining consciousness, suggests that much more precise technical measures would be required to avoid the possibility of classifying some individuals as alive when they are really dead according to concepts of death based on consciousness.

We must come to grips with the possibility, indeed the probability, that we shall never be able to make precise physiologic measures of the irreversible loss of mental processes. In this case we shall have to follow safer-course policies of using measures to declare death only in cases in which we are convinced that some necessary physical basis for life is missing, even if this means that some dead patients will be treated as

alive. But the fear of treating an occasional
dead patient as alive was the reason we
abandoned heart and lung measures. This
suggests that the arguments for moving
beyond heart and lung measures may be suspect, even if we are convinced at the level
of concept that a person should be considered
dead if he has lost integrating capacities or
capacity for consciousness and social interaction. Only when we are convinced that our
measures will not falsely consider someone
dead should the measures be used. It appears
that the Harvard criteria or similar tests of
entire brain function may have reached that
level of certainty if death is to be pronounced
when the entire brain is destroyed. (There
appears to be very little evidence, however,
to demonstrate that there really is destruction of the entire brain rather than certainty
that the patient will not recover any of the
functions being tested when the Harvard criteria are met.) We shall have to ask the technically competent people whether tests such
as the electroencephalogram alone provide
certainty that there will never be a recovery
of consciousness if we choose to use a concept of death based on loss of that function.

*The Link between Conceptual and Policy
Questions*

Just as the key technical questions for
purposes of pronouncing death are derived
from the philosophical decisions at the
conceptual level, so the policy questions will
also be derived from our philosophical conclusions about what it means to be dead.
Normally our public policy dealing with when
death should be pronounced should reflect
our philosophical stand. There may be
grounds for deviation, however. In a simpler
era, our policy that death "occurs precisely
when life ceases and does not occur until the
heart stops beating and respiration ends"
implied a policy that may not have been
based precisely on our understanding of
what it means to be dead.

Now we may be in a similar position regarding the choice between whole-brain-
oriented policies and policies that focus on
loss of consciousness and social interaction.

Even if we believe that a person should be
considered dead when he has lost the capacity for consciousness, we might favor legislation requiring pronouncement of death
when and only when the entire brain is destroyed. We might do this because we are
philosophically uncertain about the more
progressive concept of death or we may do
so for technical reasons. We may be convinced that there are no precise and accurate measures of the irreversible loss of
consciousness. Then a policy embodying
the concept should not be written into
law lest some neurologists might pronounce
death too quickly, attempting to use measures of loss of consciousness even if the
lower portions of the brain remained intact.
We might oppose writing such a policy into
law because we believe in principle that no
such measures can be devised. If, however,
we are convinced of the philosophical principles leading to the conclusion that a person is dead when he loses capacity for
consciousness, we should, in principle, be
willing to use tests of that capacity for pronouncement of death even if parts of the
brain remain viable. Thus, some tests might
be devised that measure the absence of a
necessary condition for consciousness even
if they do not measure the sufficient conditions.

There is another reason why our policy for
pronouncement of death may not correspond
precisely with our philosophical understanding of what it means to be dead. If the
conceptual issues are philosophical and theological in nature and not verifiable in a scientific sense, some difference of opinion will
likely remain in the society. Some laws would
permit (but not require) physicians to pronounce death when all brain functions (or the
relevant parts) are irreversibly destroyed.
This is based, presumably, on a respect for
the conscience of the individual physician.
I see no basis for respecting that conscience
in this way, however. To grant to the physician the option of not pronouncing death
when socially accepted criteria are met is
to violate the rights and the autonomy of
others involved and the dignity of our memory of the patient who may have supported

the social consensus. Certainly a physician should have the right to withdraw from his obligation to pronounce death in a case where he is personally convinced, based on his own religious or philosophical positions, that the patient is still alive. He cannot, however, use those personal values to continue treating a corpse as alive or a living person as a corpse.

Our traditional pluralistic solution to the problem of individual variation on questions of philosophy and theology is to grant a limited right of conscientious objection. The case should be no different here. Thus a state could chose to write a law specifying that a person should be considered dead if there is complete absence of brain function; and it might also recognize the plight of the Orthodox Jew or Bible-belt Baptist who had felt very strongly that he should be considered alive if his brain was destroyed but his heart continued to beat. This is not to say that such persons would really be alive or dead based on personal choice. Rather they would be *treated* as dead or alive on this basis. The only policy solution is to select the most plausible concept of death and adopt it as policy for purposes of pronouncement of death, but then allow limited conscientious objection for individuals who have strong objections to that concept of death. The individual might be permitted to write a document specifying that the consensus definition of death should not be used in his case, but some other definition selected from a number of options. The law might require pronouncement of death when there is irreversible loss of the function of the entire brain or the cerebrum, the capacity for consciousness, or some other specified function. It could permit an individual to execute a document specifying in his case that the older heart and lung criteria be used. In cases in which the individual has not executed such a document, we might follow the precedent of the Uniform Anatomical Gift Act and permit family members to exercise their judgment about what the patient would have wanted unless there is evidence of the patient's wishes to the contrary. The safer

course might be to retain the older heart-lung-oriented concept of death in cases in which the patient or his family do not express wishes to the contrary. That may, however, be sufficiently implausible as a social consensus that we should take the somewhat riskier course and adopt one of the other concepts of death, again permitting individual selection of some other concept of death. In any case, if individual discretion is permitted, it would have to be limited by the bounds of reasonableness to avoid having family members deciding that a patient with heart, lung, and brain function was dead or that a patient with none of these functions was alive.

Once we realize that the basic issues are philosophical and theological in nature—that the critical question is what is it that is so essential to the human's nature that its loss constitutes death—it makes sense to recognize the individual and cultural variations in the answers to that question. No technical information alone can ever answer the conceptual and policy questions (although it may well tell us the state of particular portions of the body). The confusions that exist among the technical, philosophical, and policy questions will require our devoting careful attention not only to the basic question of what is essential to the human's nature, but also to its implications for technical and policy matters.

NOTES

1. For a fuller development of the argument see my book *Death, Dying, and The Biological Revolution,* Yale University Press, New Haven, Conn., 1977.

2. Because the loss is irreversible, all the current talk about out-of-body and life-after-death experiences are really a confusion. It would be better to talk about apparent afterlife experiences while living, but with certain vital functions temporarily suspended. Certainly if death is the irreversible loss of function, then individuals who are still alive are not, and never have been, dead.

3. René Descartes, "The Passions of the Soul," in *The Philosophical Works of Descartes,* Cambridge University Press, Cambridge, England, 1911.

Active and Passive Euthanasia

6.

Active and Passive Euthanasia
James Rachels

The distinction between active and passive euthanasia is thought to be crucial for medical ethics. The idea is that it is permissible, at least in some cases, to withhold treatment and allow a patient to die, but it is never permissible to take any direct action designed to kill the patient. This doctrine seems to be accepted by most doctors, and it is endorsed in a statement adopted by the House of Delegates of the American Medical Association on December 4, 1973:

> The intentional termination of the life of one human being by another—mercy killing—is contrary to that for which the medical profession stands and is contrary to the policy of the American Medical Association.

> The cessation of the employment of extraordinary means to prolong the life of the body when there is irrefutable evidence that biological death is imminent is the decision of the patient and/or his immediate family. The advice and judgment of the physician should be freely available to the patient and/or his immediate family.

However, a strong case can be made against this doctrine. In what follows I will set out some of the relevant arguments, and urge doctors to reconsider their views on this matter.

To begin with a familiar type of situation, a patient who is dying of incurable cancer of the throat is in terrible pain, which can no longer be satisfactorily alleviated. He is certain to die within a few days, even if present treatment is continued, but he does not want to go on living for those days, since the pain is unbearable. So he asks the doctor for an end to it, and his family joins in the request.

Suppose the doctor agrees to withhold treatment, as the conventional doctrine says he may. The justification for his doing so is that the patient is in terrible agony, and since he is going to die anyway, it would be wrong to prolong his suffering needlessly. But now notice this. If one simply withholds treatment, it may take the patient longer to die, and so he may suffer more than he would if more direct action were taken and a lethal injection given. This fact provides strong reason for thinking that, once the initial decision not to prolong his agony has been made, active euthanasia is actually

Source: *The New England Journal of Medicine*, vol. 292, no. 2, January 9, 1975, p. 78.

preferable to passive euthanasia, rather than the reverse. To say otherwise is to endorse the option that leads to more suffering rather than less, and is contrary to the humanitarian impulse that prompts the decision not to prolong his life in the first place.

Part of my point is that the process of being "allowed to die" can be relatively slow and painful, whereas being given a lethal injection is relatively quick and painless. Let me give a different sort of example. In the United States about one in 600 babies is born with Down's syndrome. Most of these babies are otherwise healthy—that is, with only the usual pediatric care, they will proceed to an otherwise normal infancy. Some, however, are born with congenital defects such as intestinal obstructions that require operations if they are to live. Sometimes, the parents and the doctor will decide not to operate, and let the infant die. Anthony Shaw describes what happens then:

> When surgery is denied [the doctor] must try to keep the infant from suffering while natural forces sap the baby's life away. As a surgeon whose natural inclination is to use the scalpel to fight off death, standing by and watching a salvageable baby die is the most emotionally exhausting experience I know. It is easy at a conference, in a theoretical discussion, to decide that such infants should be allowed to die. It is altogether different to stand by in the nursery and watch as dehydration and infection wither a tiny being over hours and days. This is a terrible ordeal for me and the hospital staff—much more so than for the parents who never set foot in the nursery.[1]

I can understand why some people are opposed to all euthanasia, and insist that such infants must be allowed to live. I think I can also understand why other people favor destroying these babies quickly and painlessly. But why should anyone favor letting "dehydration and infection wither a tiny being over hours and days?" The doctrine that says that a baby may be allowed to dehydrate and wither, but may not be given an injection that would end its life without

suffering, seems so patently cruel as to require no further refutation. The strong language is not intended to offend, but only to put the point in the clearest possible way.

My second argument is that the conventional doctrine leads to decisions concerning life and death made on irrelevant grounds.

Consider again the case of the infants with Down's syndrome who need operations for congenital defects unrelated to the syndrome to live. Sometimes, there is no operation, and the baby dies, but when there is no such defect, the baby lives on. Now, an operation such as that to remove an intestinal obstruction is not prohibitively difficult. The reason why such operations are not performed in these cases is, clearly, that the child has Down's syndrome and the parents and the doctor judge that because of that fact it is better for the child to die.

But notice that this situation is absurd, no matter what view one takes of the lives and potentials of such babies. If the life of such an infant is worth preserving, what does it matter if it needs a simple operation? Or, if one thinks it better that such a baby should not live on, what difference does it make that it happens to have an unobstructed intestinal tract? In either case, the matter of life and death is being decided on irrelevant grounds. It is the Down's syndrome, and not the intestines, that is the issue. The matter should be decided, if at all, on that basis, and not be allowed to depend on the essentially irrelevant question of whether the intestinal tract is blocked.

What makes this situation possible, of course, is the idea that when there is an intestinal blockage, one can "let the baby die," but when there is no such defect there is nothing that can be done, for one must not "kill" it. The fact that this idea leads to such results as deciding life or death on irrelevant grounds is another good reason why the doctrine should be rejected.

One reason why so many people think that there is an important moral difference between active and passive euthanasia is that they think killing someone is morally worse than letting someone die. But is it? Is killing, in itself, worse than letting die? To investigate this issue, two cases may be considered that are exactly alike except that one involves killing whereas the other involves letting someone die. Then, it can be asked whether this difference makes any difference to the moral assessments. It is important that the cases be exactly alike, except for this one difference, since otherwise one cannot be confident that it is this difference and not some other that accounts for any variation in the assessments of the two cases. So, let us consider this pair of cases:

In the first, Smith stands to gain a large inheritance if anything should happen to his six-year-old cousin. One evening while the child is taking his bath, Smith sneaks into the bathroom and drowns the child, and then arranges things so that it will look like an accident.

In the second, Jones also stands to gain if anything should happen to his six-year-old cousin. Like Smith, Jones sneaks in planning to drown the child in his bath. However, just as he enters the bathroom Jones sees the child slip and hit his head, and fall face down in the water. Jones is delighted; he stands by, ready to push the child's head back under if it is necessary, but it is not necessary. With only a little thrashing about, the child drowns all by himself, "accidentally," as Jones watches and does nothing.

Now Smith killed the child, whereas Jones "merely" let the child die. That is the only difference between them. Did either man behave better, from a moral point of view? If the difference between killing and letting die were in itself a morally important matter, one should say that Jones's behavior was less reprehensible than Smith's. But does one really want to say that? I think not. In the first place, both men acted from the same motive, personal gain, and both had exactly the same end in view when they acted. It may be inferred from Smith's conduct that he is a bad man, although that judgment may be withdrawn or modified if certain further facts are learned about him—for example, that he is mentally deranged. But would not the very same thing be inferred about Jones from his conduct? And

would not the same further considerations also be relevant to any modification of this judgment? Moreover, suppose Jones pleaded, in his own defense, "After all, I didn't do anything except just stand there and watch the child drown. I didn't kill him; I only let him die." Again, if letting die were in itself less bad than killing, this defense should have at least some weight. But it does not. Such a "defense" can only be regarded as a grotesque perversion of moral reasoning. Morally speaking, it is no defense at all.

Now it may be pointed out, quite properly, that the cases of euthanasia with which doctors are concerned are not like this at all. They do not involve personal gain or the destruction of normal healthy children. Doctors are concerned only with cases in which the patient's life is of no further use to him, or in which the patient's life has become or will soon become a terrible burden. However, the point is the same in these cases: the bare difference between killing and letting die does not, in itself, make a moral difference. If a doctor lets a patient die, for humane reasons, he is in the same moral position as if he had given the patient a lethal injection for humane reasons. If his decision was wrong—if, for example, the patient's illness was in fact curable—the decision would be equally regrettable no matter which method was used to carry it out. And if the doctor's decision was the right one, the method used is not in itself important.

The AMA policy statement isolates the crucial issue very well; the crucial issue is "the intentional termination of the life of one human being by another." But after identifying this issue, and forbidding "mercy killing," the statement goes on to deny that the cessation of treatment is the intentional termination of a life. This is where the mistake comes in, for what is the cessation of treatment, in these circumstances, if it is not "the intentional termination of the life of one human being by another?" Of course it is exactly that, and if it were not, there would be no point to it.

Many people will find this judgment hard

to accept. One reason, I think, is that it is very easy to conflate the question of whether killing is, in itself, worse than letting die, with the very different question of whether most actual cases of killing are more reprehensible than most actual cases of letting die. Most actual cases of killing are clearly terrible (think, for example, of all the murders reported in the newspapers), and one hears of such cases every day. On the other hand, one hardly ever hears of a case of letting die, except for the actions of doctors who are motivated by humanitarian reasons. So one learns to think of killing in a much worse light than of letting die. But this does not mean that there is something about killing that makes it in itself worse than letting die, for it is not the bare difference between killing and letting die that makes the difference in these cases. Rather, the other factors—the murderer's motive of personal gain, for example, contrasted with the doctor's humanitarian motivation—account for different reactions to the different cases.

I have argued that killing is not in itself any worse than letting die; if my contention is right, it follows that active euthanasia is not any worse than passive euthanasia. What arguments can be given on the other side? The most common, I believe, is the following:

The important difference between active and passive euthanasia is that, in passive euthanasia, the doctor does not do anything to bring about the patient's death. The doctor does nothing, and the patient dies of whatever ills already afflict him. In active euthanasia, however, the doctor does something to bring about the patient's death: he kills him. The doctor who gives the patient with cancer a lethal injection has himself caused his patient's death; whereas if he merely ceases treatment, the cancer is the cause of the death.

A number of points need to be made here. The first is that it is not exactly correct to say that in passive euthanasia the doctor does nothing, for he does do one thing that is very important: he lets the patient die. "Letting someone die" is certainly different, in

some respects, from other types of action—mainly in that it is a kind of action that one may perform by way of not performing certain other actions. For example, one may let a patient die by way of not giving medication, just as one may insult someone by way of not shaking his hand. But for any purpose of moral assessment, it is a type of action nonetheless. The decision to let a patient die is subject to moral appraisal in the same way that a decision to kill him would be subject to moral appraisal: it may be assessed as wise or unwise, compassionate or sadistic, right or wrong. If a doctor deliberately let a patient die who was suffering from a routinely curable illness, the doctor would certainly be to blame for what he had done, just as he would be to blame if he had needlessly killed the patient. Charges against him would then be appropriate. If so, it would be no defense at all for him to insist that he didn't "do anything." He would have done something very serious indeed, for he let his patient die.

Fixing the cause of death may be very important from a legal point of view, for it may determine whether criminal charges are brought against the doctor. But I do not think that this notion can be used to show a moral difference between active and passive euthanasia. The reason why it is considered bad to be the cause of someone's death is that death is regarded as a great evil—and so it is. However, if it had been decided that euthanasia—even passive euthanasia—is desirable in a given case, it has also been decided that in this instance death is no greater an evil than the patient's continued existence. And if this is true, the usual reason for not wanting to be the cause of someone's death simply does not apply.

Finally, doctors may think that all of this is only of academic interest—the sort of thing that philosophers may worry about but that has no practical bearing on their own work. After all, doctors must be concerned about the legal consequences of what they do, and active euthanasia is clearly forbidden by the law. But even so, doctors should also be concerned with the fact that the law is forcing upon them a moral doctrine that may well be indefensible, and has a considerable effect on their practices. Of course, most doctors are not now in the position of being coerced in this matter, for they do not regard themselves as merely going along with what the law requires. Rather, in statements such as the AMA policy statement that I have quoted, they are endorsing this doctrine as a central point of medical ethics. In that statement, active euthanasia is condemned not merely as illegal but as "contrary to that for which the medical profession stands," whereas passive euthanasia is approved. However, the preceding considerations suggest that there is really no moral difference between the two, considered in themselves (there may be important moral differences in some cases in their *consequences,* but, as I pointed out, these differences may make active euthanasia, and not passive euthanasia, the morally preferable option). So, whereas doctors may have to discriminate between active and passive euthanasia to satisfy the law, they should not do any more than that. In particular, they should not give the distinction any added authority and weight by writing it into official statements of medical ethics.

NOTE

1. A. Shaw, "Doctor, Do We Have a Choice?" *The New York Times Magazine,* Jan. 30, 1972, p. 54.

7.

Killing and Giving Up   Lawrence C. Becker

Traditional medical ethics, reiterated recently in an AMA resolution,[1] have held that the intentional killing of a patient is impermissible but that under certain conditions, letting a patient die is permissible. James Rachels has argued that the distinction between killing and letting die in this range of cases is morally irrelevant.[2] I think Rachels' analysis is correct as far as it goes. (And it goes a long way toward clearing the air of confusions on this topic. In particular, he accurately points out that the supposed difference between killing-as-doing-something and letting-die-as-doing-nothing is a bogus issue. So is the characterization of active euthanasia as intentional, and passive euthanasia as somehow unintentional. Further, he correctly points out the tragic consequences of confusion on this issue.) His conclusion, however, is too strong. I agree that active euthanasia may sometimes be morally preferable to passive euthanasia. But I cannot agree that the killing/letting die distinction is, in itself, devoid of moral significance.

I think Rachels' argument ignores one issue of particular importance to medical ethics. That issue is the relation of killing to the character and personality traits which typify the good health care professional. I shall argue that the good health care professional must develop dispositions which (1) constitute character and personality traits deeply at variance with killing, but not similarly at variance with what may be called giving up efforts to save a life; and which (2) tend to be "unlearned" by (otherwise moral) acts intended to kill, but not by (otherwise moral) acts which constitute "giving up." Since the possession of these dispositions by health care professionals is morally significant, and since "giving up" is equivalent, in the cases which concern us here, to "letting die," I shall conclude that we have good reasons, in medical ethics, for insisting on the moral relevance of the killing/letting die distinction.

The good health care professional is committed to healing and/or to alleviating suffering. Very few, if any, are trained exclusively for the latter. Most are trained for, and professionally reinforced for, efforts to *improve the condition* of those who are ill, injured, or handicapped. Relieving pain is obviously an example of such an effort. Killing is not.[3]

Now the efforts needed to improve the condition of some patients are grueling in the extreme. They require not only large amounts of energy and concentration, but the ability to make and live with decisions based on very ambiguous evidence, and the discipline to stick with the effort even when there is no *clear* hope of success.

It is obvious that these abilities are necessary for the good health care professional. Medicine is not at bottom a theoretical activity, but a practical one, working with imperfect knowledge. This means that the results of a course of treatment will often be ambiguous not only prospectively but for a long time during treatment. It means that however ambiguous the evidence, decisions to treat or not to treat have to be made. And it means that damaging failures of nerve, of commitment, of the struggle to improve the patient's condition must not be allowed to occur.

It is equally clear that these abilities of the good health care professional are acquired, not inborn. The resultant personality and character traits often lead to a familiar range of vices: arrogance, precipitous decision making, inability to acknowledge one's errors, a tendency to depersonalize relationships with patients, and more to the point here: the translation of the commitment to improve the condition of one's patients into the pursuit of a craft for its own sake and the loss of the power to decide, rationally, when to *give up* efforts to heal, or to prolong life. That some health care professionals exhibit one or more of these vices is indisputable. But these vices are not necessary consequences of the dispositions requisite to the profession. In fact, they are mutations which *replace* the requisite dispositions and damage one's claim to the title "*good* health care professional."

In particular, it has frequently been argued that a physician who blindly and relentlessly pursues a hopeless course of heroic therapy on a helpless and unwilling patient has gone wrong *as a physician*. That is, that one of the traits necessary to being a good physician is missing: the ability to know when to give up. Defeat is often obvious, by any rational assessment, well before a patient dies. Exhortations to the effect that "where there is life there is hope" are merely that—exhortations. They function to help one avoid premature or irrational relaxation of effort.

Now I submit that it is "giving up" which is what ethicists who have made the killing/letting die distinction *for the medical context* have been trying (or should have been trying) to get at. Giving up is ceasing to administer health care—or, as in the case of giving last-resort doses of pain-killing drugs—administering health care without regard to its consequences for hastening death. Killing may sometimes be properly regarded as administering *aid*, but it is not administering *health care*. Giving up may amount to letting someone die, but it is very different from injecting a lethal dose of potassium chloride. Killing, as it figures in the problem under discussion, involves efforts to bring about death which go beyond giving up. Giving up may involve *acts* (turning off a respirator, witholding antibiotics). But those acts involve stopping, or refraining from administering, lifesaving health care. Killing, as used here, involves something more—such as the administration of a nontherapeutic poison.

Giving up is not inconsistent with the dispositions which are required in a good health care professional. Indeed, where giving up is unambiguously rational, it is required by them. But *killing* patients—as opposed to giving up on them—*is* inconsistent with those dispositions, even though killing may be, with respect to some patients, morally equivalent to or better than just letting them die.

Killing is inconsistent with the dispositions of good health care professionals because it is complicitous with the processes they are committed to combatting. It is an intervention to achieve the very thing they have been trained to prevent. Unlike killing, admitting defeat is not complicity. Giving up is not an intervention with anything but the hopeless effort to pursue lifesaving activities. Killing—in the sense relevant here —is much more than that.

It may be objected, I suppose, that this distinction rests on an arbitrary definition of medicine—one in which the notion of providing *health* care is emphasized to the exclusion of other concerns. It may be urged that what motivates the good health care professional is concern to relieve the patient's suffering—and, more generally, the desire to help people who are in distress. Thus, when the only way possible to help is to end the patient's life, and when killing is preferable to letting the patient die, killing is perfectly compatible with the dispositions of the good health care professional.

This is a superficially plausible objection, but its premise is just false. There are many ways of helping someone in distress, but the one of concern here is the one which (1) attends only to things which are in some sense health problems, and (2) attends to them by attempting to restore health. The controlling principle for the health care professional is *restoration* (of health), not merely *relief* (from the consequences of illness). The difference between these two controlling principles deserves emphasis. The restoration of health may involve subjecting the patient to even more suffering than that occasioned by the illness—and for a considerable length of time. To one engaged in the attempt to restore health, purely palliative measures are not aimed at.

It is not surprising, then, that health care professionals so often defend the moral relevance of the killing/letting die distinction. It may be a distinction without a difference as far as moral blameworthiness goes (when that is assessed only in terms of the motives of those involved, and the consequences to the patient). But it is surely not a distinction without a difference to the health care professional who is told, in some circumstances, to kill rather than to let die

—to kill rather than just give up. The difference is not merely that killing takes more— or a different sort of—moral courage. It is rather that killing runs against the core of the health care professional's deepest commitments and dispositions *qua* professional. *And especially in a professional context,* [4] it is difficult to subordinate those commitments and dispositions to the more general requirements of human conduct (which may occasionally entail the moral preferability of killing).

But *should* the health care professional subordinate them? Should he or she occasionally kill rather than just give up? One can certainly find cases in which it seems so. [5] And in these cases, *once a justifiable decision to give up has been made,* I agree that it would be wrong not to excuse a doctor or nurse who, out of common human sympathy, yielded to a patient's request to be killed. But to excuse an act is one thing. To justify that act—to advocate it as a matter of morally correct policy—is quite another. I think such acts should be excused, both morally and legally, for exactly the reasons Rachels sets out. They should be excused because as far as motives are concerned, and as far as consequences to the patient are concerned, there is no morally relevant distinction to be drawn. But I do not think that such acts can be fully *justified*—i.e., considered a proper part of health care policy, or a proper function of a health care professional.

I do not think they can be justified because they are so deeply at variance with the dispositions necessary in a health care professional, *and because by acting at variance with these dispositions* (and giving such acts the authorization of professional policy), the dispositions lose (some of) their controlling force. [6] It is unreasonable, it seems to me, to insist (as we all do) that health care professionals develop these necessary dispositions, and at the same time to insist that, in many cases, they ought *in their professional capacities* to do things so deeply at variance with them. This is unreasonable because it is self-defeating: acts at variance with the dispositions insisted upon damage those very dispositions.

I have made what might be called a *role-utilitarian*[7] argument: that if we want good health care professionals, we may insist that they learn when to give up, but it would be self-defeating to insist that they kill. The requirements of the *role* of a health care professional are compatible with learning when to give up on a patient, but not with learning when to kill a patient.

NOTES

1. In a statement endorsed by the House of Delegates of the American Medical Association in December, 1973.

2. James Rachels, "Active and Passive Euthanasia," *The New England Journal of Medicine*, vol. 292.2, p. 78, 1975.

3. Killing is not a therapy. However merciful it may be, however welcomed by the patient, it does not improve the patient's condition. It eliminates the patient. "Arguments" which claim, covertly or overtly, that positive euthanasia is merely an extension of the therapeutic mission are just misleading rhetoric.

4. Part of the difficulty here is surely the influence of the professional context. A physician out in a remote wilderness area, asked to kill a hopelessly injured companion who is in terrible pain, is in quite a different position from a physician in a modern hospital asked to administer a lethal poison.

5. Consider the physically helpless but rational patient, who is terminally ill but not suffering physically. Suppose that patient has exercised his or her legal right to have treatment stopped, and by refusing to eat, is using the only available means of bringing about a death earlier than the one expected from the disease. Suppose further that the patient asks to be given a lethal dose of barbituates.

6. There is ample evidence from psychology to support the behavior-modifying potency of acts at variance with an agent's character and personality traits.

7. I am indebted to W. K. Frankena for this piece of terminology.

Concept of a Profession

8.

The Formal Characteristics of a Profession
Eliot Freidson

What are the formal characteristics of the profession of medicine? In the most elementary sense, the profession is a group of people who perform a set of activities which provide them with the major source of their subsistence—activities which are called "work" rather than "leisure" and "vocation" rather than "avocation." Such activities are performed for compensation, not for their own sake. They are considered to be useful or productive, which is why those who perform them are compensated by others. When a number of people perform the same activity and develop common methods, which are passed on to new recruits and come to be conventional, we may say that workers have been organized into an occupational group, or an occupation. In the most general classification, a profession is an occupation.

However, a profession is usually taken to be a special kind of occupation, so that it is necessary to develop analytically useful distinctions between the profession and other occupations. I have argued that the most strategic distinction lies in legitimate, organized autonomy—that a profession is distinct from other occupations in that it has been given the right to control its own work. Some occupations, like circus jugglers and magicians, possess a de facto autonomy by virtue of the esoteric or isolated character of their work, but their autonomy is more accidental than not and is subject to change should public interest be aroused in it. Unlike other occupations, professions are *deliberately* granted autonomy, including the exclusive right to determine who can legitimately do its work and how the work should be done. Virtually all occupations struggle to obtain both rights, and some manage to seize them, but only the profession is *granted* the right to exercise them legitimately. And while no occupation can prevent employers, customers, clients, and other workers from evaluating its work, only the profession has the recognized right to declare such "outside" evaluation illegitimate and intolerable.

The Source of Professional Status

Obviously, an occupation does not "naturally" come by so unusual a condition as professional autonomy. The work of one group commonly overlaps, even competes, with that of other occupations. Given the

Source: Eliot Freidson, *Profession of Medicine*, p. 71, Harper & Row Publishers, Inc., New York, 1970.

ambiguity of much of reality, and given the role of taste and values in assessing it, it is unlikely that one occupation would be chosen spontaneously over others and granted the singular status of a profession by some kind of popular vote. Medicine was certainly not so chosen. A profession attains and maintains its position by virtue of the protection and patronage of some elite segment of society which has been persuaded that there is some special value in its work. Its position is thus secured by the political and economic influence of the elite which sponsors it—an influence that drives competing occupations out of the same area of work, that discourages others by virtue of the competitive advantages conferred on the chosen occupation, and that requires still others to be subordinated to the profession. As I have shown, the position of medicine was so established, from the rise of the university to our day.

If the source of the special position of the profession is granted, then it follows that professions are occupations unique to high civilizations, for there it is common to find not only full-time specialists but also elites with organized control over large populations.[1] Further, the work of the chosen occupation is unlikely to have been singled out if it did not represent or express some of the important beliefs or values of that elite—some of the established values and knowledge of the civilization. In the case of medieval medicine, it was its connection with the ancient learning that singled it out. Furthermore, since it is chosen by the elite, the work of the profession need have no necessary relationship to the beliefs or values of the average citizen. But once a profession is established in its protected position of autonomy, it is likely to have a dynamic of its own, developing new ideas or activities which may only vaguely reflect and which may even contradict those of the dominant elite. The work of the profession may thus eventually diverge from that expected by the elite. If a profession's work comes to have little relationship to the knowledge and values of its society, it may have difficulty surviving. The profession's privileged position is given by, not seized from, society, and it may be allowed to lapse or may even be taken away.[2] It is essential for survival that the dominant elite remain persuaded of the positive value, or at least the harmlessness, of the profession's work, so that it continues to protect it from encroachment.

Consulting and Scholarly Professions

Some kinds of work require for their performance the cooperation of laymen and require for their survival some degree of popularity with laymen: they are practicing or consulting occupations which must sustain a direct, continuous relationship with a lay clientele. Work involving a clientele has consequences for occupational organization which are markedly different from work which does not. In the former case the worker must contend with clients who are from *outside* the occupational community and who therefore may not be familiar or sympathetic with his occupation's ideas and practices. In the latter case the worker must contend on a daily basis only with his colleagues and other workers from *within* the occupational community. In the former case the survival of the occupation depends upon bridging the gap between worker and layman. Bridging the gap between worker and lay client is much more of a problem than bridging the gap between workers.

It is in the case of applied work, particularly work involving a broadly based lay clientele, that formal, legal controls are most likely to be imposed.[3] Only applied work is likely to have immediate consequences in human affairs, and some can be serious. When the public is considered too inexpert to be able to evaluate such work, those dominating society may feel that the public needs protection from unqualified or unscrupulous workers. Having been persuaded that one occupation is most qualified by virtue of its formal training and the moral fiber of its members, the state may exclude all others and give the chosen occupation a legal monopoly that may help bridge the gap between it and laymen, if only by restricting the layman's choice. The outcome is support of the profession by licensure or some other formal device of protecting some workers and excluding other. Licensing is much less likely to occur on behalf of the scholar or the scientist, for they are devoted to exploring intellectual systems primarily for the eyes of their colleagues. Nonetheless, in the case of the consulting or practicing professions such a legally exclusive right to work will not assure survival because the work cannot be performed, license or not, without being in some way positively attractive to a lay clientele.

Unlike science and scholarship, which create and elaborate the formal knowledge of a civilization, practicing professions have the task of applying that knowledge to everyday life. Practicing professions are the links between a civilization and its daily life and as such must, unlike science and scholarship, be in some sense joined to everyday life and the average man. Some of this linkage can be politically sustained—as when the legal order permits only one occupation to provide a given service to those seeking it—but some seems to depend upon the attractiveness of the work itself to the average man, upon the direct connection of the work with what the layman considers to be desirable and appropriate. In the case of medicine I have argued that improvement in the pragmatic results of practice, as well as mass education which brought the average man's ideas, knowledge, and norms closer to that of the profession, led to its becoming a successful consulting profession where before it was primarily an officially supported scholarly or scientific profession with a small practice among the elite.

But even if my interpretation of the historical development of the status of medicine is open to question, I hope that my taxonomic point is at once clear and persuasive. The structural differences between scholarly, learned, or scientific "professions" and practicing or consulting "professions" are of much greater consequence to the way each is established and maintained, and to the daily problems of work on the part of their members, than are their similarities. While,

in common usage, research scientists and physicians share the name "profession" and some common knowledge, these similarities have few consequences of significance.

Profession and Paraprofession

Just as the analysis of the development of medicine led to the observation of analytical differences between consulting and scholarly professions, so the analysis of the division of labor surrounding the formal organization of healing tasks led to the observation of structural differences in the position of various occupations in that division of labor. In the case of medicine, the division of labor is not simply a functional arrangement of specialists. Some occupations—dentistry, for example—are autonomous professions in their own right, even if they are not as prestigious as medicine.[4] Others, usually called "paramedical," are part of a division of labor organized into a hierarchy of authority, established and enforced by law, and swinging around the dominant authority and responsibility of the medical profession. Some of the occupations which are subordinate members of the medical division of labor, however, call themselves and are frequently called by others, "professions."

These paramedical occupations, of which nursing is perhaps the most prominent example, are clearly in a markedly different position than is medicine, for while it is legitimate for them to take orders from and be evaluated by physicians, it is not legitimate for them to give orders to and to evaluate physicians. Without such reciprocity we can hardly consider them the equals of physicians. And without the autonomy of physicians we can hardly believe it to be useful for them to be classified as the same type of occupation as the physician. They are specifically and generically occupations organized around a profession—paraprofessional occupations. This in itself makes a distinct species of occupation, particularly when people in such an occupation, given their proximity to a profession, are encouraged to take on professional attributes and to claim to be a profession. But whatever the claim, they do not stand in the same structural position as the profession on which they model themselves.

It might be noted that paraprofessional occupations usually seek professional status by creating many of the same institutions as those which possess professional status. They develop a formal standard curriculum of training, hopefully at a university. They create or find abstract theory to teach recruits. They write codes of ethics. They are prone to seek support for licensing or registration so as to be able to exercise some control over who is allowed to do their work. But what they persistently fail to attain is full autonomy in formulating their training and licensing standards and in actually performing their work. Their autonomy is only partial, being secondhand and limited by a dominant profession. This is the irreducible criterion which keeps such occupations paraprofessions in spite of their success at attaining many of the institutional attributes of professions. And the discriminatory power of full autonomy belies the value of using instead such institutional arrangements as training and licensing. That such arrangements are useful conditions for the development of an autonomous occupation is certain; that they are necessary conditions is moot; that they are sufficient conditions is plainly false.

The Formal Criteria of Profession

In analyzing the position of medicine and its associated occupations I have deliberately avoided adopting most of the criteria of profession used by many writers. Indeed, I have just explicitly denied the importance of training and licensing. This is not the place for a detailed examination and analysis of the many definitions which have been published before and after Cogan's review.[5] Furthermore, the parsimonious arrangement of those criteria by the most sophisticated and careful of recent analysts, William J. Goode, allows concentration on essentially

two "core characteristics" of professions, from which 10 other frequently cited characteristics are said to be derived.[6] These two core characteristics are "a prolonged specialized training in a body of abstract knowledge, and a collectivity or service orientation."[7] Among the "derived characteristics," which are presumably "caused" by the core characteristics, are five which refer to autonomy: "(1) The profession determines its own standards of education and training. . . . (3) Professional practice is often legally recognized by some form of licensure. (4) Licensing and admission boards are manned by members of the profession. (5) Most legislation concerned with the profession is shaped by that profession. . . . (7) The practitioner is relatively free of lay evaluation and control."[8] Obviously, in Goode's analysis, the core characteristics are critical criteria for professions insofar as they are said to be causal in producing professional autonomy as I have defined it, and many of the attributes others have specified. Let us look at them closely to see if this is so.

What precisely are the empirical referents of those core characteristics? In the first, training, are concealed at least three problems of specification—"prolonged," "specialized," "abstract." Since all training takes some time, how prolonged must training be to qualify? Since all training is somewhat specialized, how does one determine whether it is specialized enough to qualify? Since "abstract" is a relative rather than absolute term, how does one determine whether training is abstract or theoretical enough? It is difficult if not impossible to answer these questions with any reasonable degree of precision. Furthermore, I suggest that any answer one makes will fail to include all occupations clearly agreed to be professions or exclude all occupations clearly agreed not to be professions. Taking the three traditional professions of medicine, law, and the ministry, the range of variation in length of training (particularly in the ministry), the degree of specialization, and the amount and type of theory and abstract knowledge (particularly in the case of law) is in each case sufficiently wide that many other occupations not recognized as professions would fall within it. Nursing, for example, which is specifically excluded from the professions by Goode on the basis of training, falls within the range manifested by the three established professions.

Significantly, however, Goode excludes nursing because he feels its training is no more than "a lower-level medical education," which implies more the lack of autonomy it is supposed to produce than the specific attributes of nurse training. That is, it is not what nurses learn or how long it takes, but the fact that the bulk of what they learn is ultimately specified by physicians which is important. The objective content and duration of training is considerably less critical than occupational *control* over training.

Thus, not training as such, but only the issue of autonomy and control over training granted the occupation by an elite or public persuaded of its importance seems to be able to distinguish clearly among occupations. Pharmacy and optometry, for example, have the same minimum period of training and probably the same degree of specialization and abstract knowledge (so far as one can specify proportion and quantity for such terms). However, in most states the trained optometrist may legally diagnose (e.g., do refractions) and prescribe (order, make, and fit corrective lenses), while the trained pharmacist may not; the optometrist is clearly moving much closer to professional autonomy while the pharmacist is firmly subordinated to medicine.[9] It does not seem to be the actual content of training that explains or produces the differences. As I suggested in my analysis of the medical division of labor, the possibilities for functional autonomy and the relation of the work of an occupation to that of dominant professions seem critical. And the process determining the outcome is essentially political and social rather than technical in character—a process in which power and persuasive rhetoric are of greater importance than the objective character of knowledge, training, and work.

Consonant with the political character of the process, I might point out that the leaders of all aspiring occupations, including nursing, pharmacy, and optometry, insist that their occupations do provide prolonged training in a set of special skills, including training in theory or abstract knowledge which is generic to their field. And they can point to required courses in theory to buttress their assertions. These are institutional facts whose truth cannot be denied, but their meaning is suspect because the content and length of training of an occupation, including abstract knowledge or theory, is frequently a product of the deliberate action of those who are trying to show that their occupation is a profession and should therefore be given autonomy.[10] If there is no systematic body of theory, it is created for the purpose of being able to say there is. The nature of an occupation's training, therefore, can constitute part of an ideology, a deliberate rhetoric in a political process of lobbying, public relations, and other forms of persuasion to attain a desirable end—full control over its work.

Problematic as training is as a criterion, it has the virtue of empirical substance. The characteristics of an occupation's training refer to the formal rules and regulations embodied in the laws, regulations, and resolutions connected with political institutions, occupational associations, and educational organizations. The second "core characteristic" specified by Goode, however, and very commonly cited in other definitions, is much more problematic. The "collectivity or service orientation" usually refers to the orientation of the *individual* members of an occupation rather than to organizations. But clearly, the attitudes of individuals constitute an entirely different kind of criterion than the attributes of occupational institutions. Unlike the latter, which can be determined empirically by the examination of legislation, administrative regulations, and other formal documents including prescribed curricula, the attitudes of individuals must be determined by the direct study of individuals.

The actual existence of professional training institutions, the number of years and the nature of the courses required for a degree, and the nature of examinations required for a license are certainly established as facts. But curiously enough, there appears to be no reliable information which actually demonstrates that a service orientation is in fact strong and widespread among professionals. Even when one is quite willing to stretch the points of the scanty and inelastic data available, the blunt fact is that discussions of professions assume or assert *by definition* and without supporting empirical evidence that "service orientation" is especially common among professionals. I do not deny the reality of a service orientation as such (though it would be good to demonstrate it empirically) so much as I deny its distinct, exclusive, or predominant possession by professional occupations.

But a service orientation need not be considered to be an attribute of individual workers. On a different level of abstraction it can be considered to be an *institutional* attribute of an occupation. As a formal characteristic of an occupation, it is a claim about the membership as a body. The claim, of course, is also made by paraprofessions and by many other kinds of occupational organizations including trade unions and trade associations. As a property of occupational institutions, it too, like training, can be deliberately created so as to attempt to persuade politically important figures of the virtues of the occupation. *The profession's service orientation is a public imputation it has successfully won in a process by which its leaders have persuaded society to grant and support its autonomy.* Such imputation does not mean that its members more commonly or more intensely subscribe to a service orientation than members of other occupations.

Formal Institutions and Professional Performance

I have been arguing that the only truly important and uniform criterion for distinguishing professions from other occupations is the fact of autonomy—a position

of legitimate control over work. That autonomy is not absolute, depending for its existence upon the toleration and even protection by the state and not necessarily including all zones of occupational activity. The single zone of activity in which autonomy *must* exist in order for professional status to exist is in the content of the work itself. Autonomy is the critical outcome of the interaction between political and economic power and occupational representation, interaction sometimes facilitated by educational institutions and other devices which successfully persuade the state that the occupation's work is reliable and valuable.

Furthermore, I have argued that there is no stable institutional attribute which inevitably leads to such a position of autonomy. In one way or another, through a process of political negotiation and persuasion, society is led to believe that it is desirable to grant an occupation the professional status of self-regulative autonomy. The occupation's training institutions, code of ethics, and work are attributes which frequently figure prominently in the process of persuasion but are not individually or in concert, invariably, or even mostly, persuasive as *objectively determinable attributes.* It may be true that the public and/or a strategic elite always come to believe that the training, ethics, and work of the occupation they favor have some exclusive qualities, but this is a consequence of the process of persuasion rather than of the attributes themselves, and the attributes may not be said to be either "causes" of professional status or objectively unique to professions.[11]

NOTES

1. For an important attempt to conceptualize "the patterned distribution and control of knowledge in a society," see Burkart Holzner, *Reality Construction in Society,* Schenkman Publishing Co., Cambridge, 1968.

2. It can be argued that *as an occupation* the ministry has lost its professional position, particularly in countries where there is no state religion. In the United States the occupation controls ordination in individual churches but neither en-

trance into the occupation as such nor access to the legal privileges of the occupation (e.g., to perform a marriage ceremony). It is as if doctors could control entrance into and work in particular hospitals but not the development of competing hospitals or entrance into the occupation by those working at such hospitals.

3. See Holzner, op. cit., for the distinction between specialized knowledge and ideological knowledge.

4. Cf. Basil J. Sherlock, "The Second Profession: Parallel Mobilities of the Dental Profession and Its Recruits," *Journal of Health and Social Behavior,* vol. 10, p. 41, 1969.

5. Morris I. Cogan, "Toward a Definition of Profession," *Harvard Educational Review,* vol. 23, p. 33, 1953.

6. William J. Goode, "Encroachment, Charlatanism, and the Emerging Profession: Psychology, Medicine, and Sociology," *American Sociological Review,* vol. 25, p. 902, 1960.

7. Ibid., p. 903.

8. Ibid., p. 903.

9. Cf. Norman R. Denzin and C. J. Mettlin, "Incomplete Professionalization: The Case of Pharmacy," *Social Forces,* vol. 46, p. 375, 1968.

10. A number of attempts have been made to outline the natural history of occupations aspiring to professional status. See, for example, Everett C. Hughes, *Men and Their Work,* The Free Press of Glencoe, New York, 1958; Theodore Caplow, *The Sociology of Work,* University of Minnesota Press, Minneapolis, 1954; Harold L. Wilensky, "The Professionalization of Everyone?" *American Journal of Sociology,* vol. 70, p. 137, 1964. See also Corinne Lathrop Gilb, *Hidden Hierarchies, The Professions and Government,* Harper & Row, New York, 1966, for a number of comments on the way political status is developed by professions.

11. It may be noted that this argument is similar to, and in any case indebted to, that in Howard S. Becker, "The Nature of a Profession," National Society for the Study of Education, *Education for the Professions,* p. 24, National Society for the Study of Education, Chicago, 1962.

Rights

9.
Ethical Options in Medicine
Gregory Pence

Kinds of Rights

There are many different kinds of rights. Legal rights are very important, because the power of law and government backs them up. In the United States, the broadest legal rights are those conferred by the Constitution and the Bill of Rights. Legal rights can also be created by legislative vote, such as by new federal laws affecting the elderly and handicapped. Some legal rights can also be created by decisions of judges, the President, and administrators in their areas of jurisdiction. In the 1960s, Lyndon Johnson, by an administrative order, gave women equal rights in federal agencies, and federal judge Frank Johnson in Alabama, by judicial decision, gave new rights to mental patients. Similarly, administrators of the Department of Health, Education, and Welfare (HEW), adopted guidelines (applicable to large institutions receiving federal grants) giving new institutional rights to prisoners, the mentally infirm, children, and the handicapped. Rights granted by HEW are not legal rights, since an institution may refuse federal funds and decline to conform to HEW guidelines without breaking any laws. Another example of institutional rights are those the American Hospital Association adopted in its Patient's Bill of Rights. Compliance with these rights by member hospitals is entirely voluntary, and no legal rights of patients are violated by noncompliance. Similarly, other institutions like businesses and universities grant to members institutional rights that lack legal force.

Many people claim rights specified neither by existing law nor by institutional regulations. These are general *moral* rights. They are claimed to form the foundation for legal and institutional rights. In other words, most legal rights are understood as moral rights that happen to be enforced by law. Moral rights are seen as prior to, or independent of, legal and institutional rights. As one writer says, "Moral rights . . . form a genus divisible into various species of rights having little in common except that they are not (necessarily) legal or institutional."[1]

We will understand an essential problem about the right to medical care if we examine the principle of the reciprocity of rights and duties. The basic idea is that X's rights

Source: Gregory Pence, *Medical Options in Medicine*, Medical Economics Book Co., New Jersey, 1980.

are related to Y's duties to allow X to exercise his rights. Jones can't exercise his right to free speech unless others have duties to allow him to speak. Rights and duties are logically interdependent; they are two sides of the same coin. No rights exist without corresponding duties. A right must create an allegiance and respect in other people so it can be exercised.

A human right is held to be a very special kind of moral right. It's a right not just for Americans; the scope of these human rights is over all of humanity. Second, human rights are claimed to be the most fundamental and basic of all moral rights, so that any human right should overrule any conflicting, lesser right. According to this definition, if rights to equal medical care were human rights and not merely political, they would overrule conflicting political rights—for example, the rights of physicians to live and work where they choose.

Let's use a famous example: the UN Declaration of Human Rights. This document holds that "everyone, as a member of society . . . has the right to work . . . to protection against unemployment . . . to just and favorable renumeration . . . to rest and leisure . . . to periodic holidays with pay . . . to food, clothing, housing, and *medical care*"[2] (my emphasis). If these are indeed human rights, well-off Americans and Western Europeans have duties to provide food and medical care to the poor of the world. Having duties is stronger than philanthropy or charity. Not to fulfill these duties is to violate human rights.

Negative and Positive Rights

Traditional Western political theory has asserted a difference between acting and omitting regarding rights, but it's questionable whether this distinction can be logically upheld. Let's first see what's entailed. *Negative* rights are like the traditional rights of the Constitution and the Bill of Rights; they forbid others from interfering in an individual's life. John Locke claimed three famous rights as the natural rights of man:

life, liberty, and property.[3] *Positive* rights are rights to benefits, usually from governments. The rights to medical care and housing in the UN Declaration of Human Rights are positive rights. Negative rights are rights to be free from interference; positive rights require others to bestow benefits.

A right to work can be either a negative right forbidding interference in one's attempt to get employment or a positive claim to a job. A right to medical care negatively considered forbids interference by others and the state in matters between physicians and patients. As a positive right, it guarantees treatment to patients when they need it. No one violates a patient's negative right to medical care if he's not given treatment for Hodgkin's disease and is allowed to die. If medical care is a positive right, then not to treat this patient constitutes a violation of his rights.

We seem to be heading to the conclusion that either people don't have as many rights as they think or their rights are customarily violated. Much of the following discussion depends on what I call the *acting-omitting principle.*

We reject any morally significant distinction between acting and omitting with regard to euthanasia and lying. It's important to realize that in every case of this principle, there are always two choices, not one. If one accepts passive euthanasia for reasons X, Y, and Z, the principle forces one to accept active euthanasia for reasons X, Y, and Z. If one rejects euthanasia for all cases because of X, one must reject passive euthanasia in all cases because of X. If cases of passive euthanasia are justified only because of relieving suffering then cases of active euthanasia are similarly justified. The principle itself is logical and neutral; it favors neither active nor passive euthanasia.

Similarly, one must either reject lying by omission for patients' good if one totally rejects direct lying for similar reasons, or one must accept direct lying for patients' good if one already accepts omitting key information for patients' good. The principle, in short, forces us to look at the moral reasons for discontinuing life supports or lying, not the label on the act.

Applying this principle to rights to medical care, we reach similar conclusions. Either negative rights to medical care entail positive rights, or if people lack positive rights they also lack negative rights. For example, Jones can be harmed just as much by ignoring his positive right to be taken from the car accident by ambulance to the hospital as by interfering with his negative right to enter it on his own ability. Put in social terms, if society doesn't care whether babies are born with maximal possible health (positive rights to preventive care, genetic screening, and the like), then why should it care later whether anyone interferes with the now-grown baby's desire to obtain health (negative right)?

Many more practical examples could be brought forth showing that deliberately omitting can be as harmful—or as good—in many cases as deliberately acting. Yet when this thesis is applied to rights, we go directly against the mainstream of Western political theory. It's important to gain more insight on such an important point, for if it's true, many of us are in a certain ignorance. Therefore, we now consider a brief history of rights, after which we will be able to understand much more about rights to medical care.

A Brief History of Human Rights

This title is misleading, for we will not discuss human rights until relatively late on the historical scene, mainly because that's when they emerged. What we will really discuss are the antecedents of modern human rights.[4]

What we today call human rights were a century ago called natural rights, and such natural rights derived from natural law theory. Human rights can no more be understood apart from natural law theory than surgery can be understood apart from internal medicine. So we must go back in history and understand the beginnings of natural law.

Ancient Jewish religion held that Jews must obey laws commanded by Yahweh. These rules were laws in a sense different from laws of today, because they were backed not only by secular power but also by religious sanctions. Right ways of living were not only morally and religiously right (these two were the same) but also in concert with how Jews understood the natural workings of the universe. Jesus and Mohammed also emphasized that the law of God grounded religious life, ordinary morality, and political authority. At this time, the concept of natural rights is non-existent.

In the first and second centuries A.D., Stoics like Epictetus and Marcus Aurelius accepted a notion of natural law in which previously external commands of God became internal ordering causes of the physical universe. Beyond holding that everyone possessed a divine spark and hence were equal in some sense, natural law of the Stoics held little specific content. The important point is that the previous conception of law, which wouldn't make sense without a divine lawgiver, now becomes assimilated to physical regularities of matter, so that it would later be possible to speak of natural laws of matter without necessarily implying the existence of a God.

Thomas Aquinas (1225–1274), the great synthesizer of Christianity and Aristotelianism, preserved this ambiguity in natural law while distinguishing natural law from divine law. The latter is the higher law and based on revelation. Natural law, based merely on reason, is subordinate to divine law but overrules secular laws of civil societies. Two points are crucial here for modern rights: first, that civil laws violating natural laws are unjust and need not be obeyed; second, that natural law expresses the rational good of man written into the inner *telos* of things. It follows that if men have rights, they have them by reason of nature.

Up until this point, we haven't seen the interplay of three notions we take for granted: the individual, the state, and rights. These three ideas in their modern configuration are interdependent; that is, each makes sense only when the other two are present and as defined in conjunction with the other two. In essence, rights come to individuals as limiting conditions on the powers of the modern state. They define those areas in which individuals are free from state interference in their private lives.

However, we are getting ahead of the story. It was not until the time of Martin Luther and the Protestant Reformation in the 16th century that the modern notions of the individual and the state began to emerge. Luther helped, for he taught that individuals needn't go through priest or pope to reach God, but could pray, confess, and read the Bible on their own.

In the 17th century, Newton and Descartes continue natural law while science begins to emerge. Newton discovers the laws of universal gravitation, but he believes the hidden "attraction" of gravitation is divinely caused, and he thinks his work translating the bible is more important than his physics. Descartes bifurcates the universe into physical and mental realms and in essence gives us two sets of natural laws—one of science and one of the moral life.

By the Enlightenment of the 18th century, the theism of Luther and Newton is hard for many scientists to accept. Nevertheless, men retain belief in a natural moral law that is discoverable by reason and parallels such laws in science. Since universal laws are discoverable in science without belief in God, it seemed that similar laws could be discovered in morality.

Meanwhile, the modern nation state was asserting itself against the old kingships— against the divine rights of kings to rule. With the French and American revolutions, rights were claimed which stated what governments and kings could not do to individuals. Previously, John Locke had used natural law to claim natural rights for Englishmen of property. In doing so, he provided the theoretical justification for the Glorious Revolution that he and his protector, Lord Shaftesbury, ushered in. When the fathers of the American Revolution claimed rights (and only for males with property), they

were essentially stating what George III of England and Parliament were not to do to them. We then see how rights are claimed for individuals *against* the powers of the state.

Meanwhile, laissez-faire capitalism rises in the 18th century, emphasizing economic rights of individual entrepreneurs. Individual rights of noninterference were originally related to the "invisible hand" theory of the market: If the state doesn't interfere other than by establishing a framework for competition, individual competition and effort naturally bring forth economic growth. It's thus very natural that the most discussed right in politics was the right to property.

Kant, in the same period, claimed all men possessed equal natural rights because they possessed equal moral worth. For Kant, the seat of moral rights and freedom was a "noumenal" self, which is hidden and unverifiable.

Kant and many of his fellows of the Enlightenment held that people have natural rights because of their inherent rationality and moral worth, as revealed in the inherent rationality of the natural moral law. What is wrong with this view?

Marx in the 19th century immediately saw two problems. First, rights claimed against the state were always for men of property, not ordinary workers. For Marx, rights were bulwarks of a conservative, bourgeois status quo. Second, even if rights to life, liberty, and property covered everyone, these rights had no value without economic means to use them. A right to a fair trial means nothing if one can't afford a lawyer, and a right to travel means little if one hasn't got the fare.

Jeremy Bentham said rights were nonsense and natural rights were "nonsense on stilts." Bentham correctly perceived that individual rights of property and noninterference primarily benefited rich industrialists and landed gentry, not the great masses. Hence his denial of rights and emphasis on the utilitarian greatest good for the greatest number was a progressive theory in the late 18th and early 19th centuries.

A problem arises with the 20th century movement for equal rights. These claims were successful for women and minorities because all reasons for differential treatment were arbitrary and unjustified. Whatever justified natural rights for white males—rationality, moral worth, and the like—clearly isn't absent in some women and blacks, so that one could justifiably exclude all women and blacks. However, whatever criterion is chosen—whatever natural property, such as intelligence, is emphasized—as the basis for equal rights, it varies in degree among individuals. Yet human rights are supposed to be invariable and equal. Obviously, no natural endowment unequally distributed among people can justify equal rights.

Given this problem of finding a natural ground for natural rights, it's understandable that modern thinking about rights is conceptually incoherent. We find modern thinkers attempting the impossible task of holding that humans have equal rights while denying that humans equally share anything that can serve as the basis for the equality. At best, people assert an equal moral worth.

Many say the wisest policy is to balance conflicting rights against each other by "weighing" reasons. This makes sense if four people divide a pie even if John found it first. However, when 16 more people come along and want their interests also "weighed" in the scales, John becomes angry. Balancing conflicting rights makes sense only if there is a criterion that can limit rights and can be used to distinguish justified claims about rights from unjustified claims. But such a criterion is exactly what doesn't seem to exist.

The problem here isn't that what people claim as their rights aren't morally good. The problem is that much of the talk about rights is conceptually muddled. Rights stem from natural law theory, which in turn stems from a time when everyone believed in God. We inherit rights from a past tradition, a static homogeneous culture, and attempt to apply them to the modern, changing heterogeneous world. This is why there's more and more recourse to the courtroom to solve moral problems. Rights talk puts people into adversarial relationships appropriate to the courtroom and, since rights talk cannot itself solve conflicts, it inevitably must lead there.

The Right to Medical Care

Our historical sketch discussed only negative rights of noninterference and problems in justifying them. Once positive rights to benefits enter, the problems become altogether insoluble. Consider first the egalitarian who claims that rights to life and liberty are worthwhile only if there is an equal right to medical care. The positive right to medical care is a means of implementing negative rights of liberty and life. Consider second that to implement an equal right to medical care, physician's liberties must be violated. Moreover, the rights of both physicians and patients to choose each other may be curtailed.

The above conflict is an example of an important truth in political analysis: the incompatibility of maximum individual liberty with maximum social equality. This principle—which we call the incompatibility principle—is often ignored in political discussions. Suppose an egalitarian revolution divided equally everything that can be divided. Would individuals then have the liberty to make unequal trades? If not, they have little liberty. Jones may like Smith's car so much that he is willing to exchange them, even though others would consider it a poor trade. This small example at once defeats naive and vague ideas about a communist utopia of perfect equality. Whatever the goods equally distributed, governmental power must continue to enforce equality or clever individuals will pile up unequal wealth by trades.

Second, suppose—as is likely to happen—that any equal social right to medical care will be enforced, administered, and financed by government. Suppose Thomas is sick in a rural area and needs continuous home care but doesn't need to be in a hospital. To get him such care, government requires physician

Smith, in order to keep his medical license, to make rural home visits once every two weeks. Smith hates this idea because he'd rather practice cardiology; so his treatment of Thomas is not always the best. Other physicians are equally resentful and also don't always have their hearts in their jobs. Therefore, more and more administrators are appointed to check on physicians. These administrators have antagonistic, adversarial relationships with physicians, making physicians more hostile, suspicious, and resentful than before.

To pay for the extra care, salaries of new administrators, and a new bureaucracy, taxes increase—especially taxes of people like physicians. Among the first rights claimed early in the history of the United States was the right to spend money as one chose (there was no income tax). One may thus consider taxes as indirect infringements on liberty—as do libertarians in their political theory.

It's easy to imagine the decrease in liberty among physicians: less freedom to work and live where they choose, less freedom to order any procedure (some would be authorized, some not), and less freedom to make money. On the other hand, if well designed, the system could increase equality in medical care. The overall point, of course, is that maximum liberty and maximum equality are not good bedfellows; instead, they are quarreling lovers in unhappy tension with each other—one having the upper hand in one context, the other in the next.

Nor is this the end of problems about rights to medical care. Burdens of satisfying this right fall unfairly and unequally on members of health professions, even if everyone finances it. Rights to liberty and life depend merely on the noninterference of others. Positive rights to medical care depend on health professionals to satisfy them.

Individual Responsibility for Health

One kind of argument about rights to medical care needs special mention. Both sides

of this argument assume that life-style and environment greatly affect long-term health. The individualist side argues that people are most responsible for where they live and their life-styles, and hence are responsible for later sickness. The social-egalitarian side argues that people are generally not responsible for their environment or life-styles, and hence are not responsible for later sickness. Individualists argue that equal rights to medical care make healthy people pay for the unhealthy habits of others. Even Ivan Illich, a critic of Western medicine, argues that insistence upon such rights fosters the myth that medicine can bail out an unhealthy life and hence undermines the recognition of personal reponsibility for health.[5] Egalitarians, on the other hand, argue that whether a person has the money, time, and knowledge to lead a healthy life-style depends on factors largely outside his control.

The evidence that life-style significantly affects health is enormous.[6] Mormons in Utah—who tend not to smoke, drink, divorce, who sleep and eat regularly, and who don't carry guns—live much longer than neighboring Nevadans from Las Vegas and Reno, even though the states match for almost all other variables. Fuchs, who did this study, emphasizes that we are responsible for our health and that medicine can't really do much for those who continue to abuse their bodies.

We can agree that first, once one has a stroke or cancer, medicine can do little, and second, that life-style affects whether we'll have such problems. Nevertheless, we are still left with the problem of whether people can choose their health life-style. Fuchs is undoubtedly right about Mormons and Nevadans, but how many Mormons really chose to be Mormons living in Utah, and more important, how many chose to be so because it would make them healthier? Yet only if someone chose in some sense to lead this life-style for health reasons could he be said to be responsible for its outcome. Otherwise, a Mormon in Utah living to 90 rather than the normal 70 seems no more or less responsible for his health than someone dying at 55 rather than the normal 45 in Harlem.

Factors that increase health and longevity are the health virtues—excellences and personal traits disposing one to activities that promote peak physical condition. People are as responsible for these health virtues as they are for the practical or moral virtues. In other words, responsibility lies neither totally with the individual nor totally with his community. The truth lies somewhere in between, varies with different cases, and probably can be determined only with *phronesis* and more knowledge than we usually have about an individual's life. Just as we can't expect a good person to be trained in the virtues in an evil society, so we can't expect people in unhealthy environments to be trained to healthy habits. On the other hand, people raised with the best health habits, who have the knowledge and wealth to be healthy, and yet who nevertheless continue very unhealthy habits are especially responsible for their ill health.

Overall, we can't make blanket generalizations about whether people are indeed responsible for their health life-styles. This is partially an individual matter, partially not, and it varies in degree from case to case. Therefore, whether people have rights to medical care must be decided—at least for the foreseeable future—independently of whether one believes them responsible for their health.

Individualism and Rights

So far, the argument seems to favor individualists who champion negative rights of noninterference but vociferously deny positive rights. However, the reason rights to medical care are suspect is not simply that as positive rights they conflict with others' negative rights; the problem, instead, is that the whole tradition of rights is confused.

Let's take two examples. Robert M. Sade, in a famous article in the *New England Journal of Medicine*, denies a positive right

to medical care because it would conflict with physicians' negative rights to liberty and property.[7] Sade combines a Lockean appeal to natural rights with an appeal to the laissez-faire economics of Adam Smith. The problems we have been discussing are illustrated by Sade's comparison of physicians to bakers and rights to medical care to rights to eat. Assuming it's obviously wrong to force bakers to bake so people can eat, Sade argues that physicians shouldn't be forced to provide medical care. In essence, Sade assumes that if rights of others require positive acts on our part, then others have no such rights. It doesn't matter whether we are bakers or physicians.

Sade rejects positive rights because they decrease the power of negative rights. With equal logic one could reject negative rights because they preclude positive rights. Radical egalitarians do just this, and if enough people suffer, radical egalitarianism increases in appeal. Sade wants to bake his bread and eat it, too: Bakers should bake while starving masses stare inside, and yet bakers should, in the face of this starvation, still expect social protection of their right to profits.

Thomas Szasz also rejects positive rights to medical care in favor of negative individual rights.[8] Szasz argues not about property and freedom to work but about bureaucracy and freedom. Szasz predicts that if physicians work for the state, they will become agents of the state, not of the patient. When patients are assigned to physicians, patients lose traditional rights; physicians in turn create not a system of healing but a system to buttress conventional authority.

Several criticisms can be made of Szasz's position. First, medicine *already* buttresses conventional authority—the issue here is of degree. Second, Szasz's slippery slope assumes that state-paid physicians couldn't be insulated from political pressures as are Federal judges. Third, it's not the proper role of medicine to defend the political freedom of patients. Lawyers, judges, congressmen, and local legislators are available for that purpose. Fourth and most important, Szasz assumes a basis for negative rights in personal freedom, which he finds positive rights don't have. But of course, one is no more grounded in human nature than the other.

Both Sade and Szasz champion negative rights and assume a picture of the state common in idealization of the 18th century—idealizations that stress natural rights from natural law, laissez-faire economics, and incentives to bold individuals to explore lands thought to hold unlimited resources. These idealizations never applied *de facto* to most people of the 18th century and only doubtfully apply to the modern world of "mixed" capitalism, government support of research and medical education, and national concern for minorities, the poor, and the sick.

Second, negative rights were originally limitations on state powers and protected wealthy and politically strong individuals. Over centuries, rights became instruments of equality and benefits to the common person. As such, the new rights came with the new welfare state. The goal of this state—better called the "trustee" state—is not protection of original negative rights that established its authority, but the good of *all* of its citizens.

Negative rights were originally connected to the classic conception of the state, whereas new positive rights are connected to the modern trustee conception of the state. Both kinds of rights and conceptions of the state are often assumed simultaneously today. This is one reason that rights are so muddled. It's also a reason why the appeals of Sade and Szasz can draw only half-hearted support, and then mainly from conservatives and nonegalitarians. Sade and Szasz believe benefits of private property and individual liberty outweigh evils of poverty and unequal medical care; radical egalitarians perceive the slant of the scales going the other way.

Perhaps the problems are insoluble, given our limited theoretical tools. The general problem is how negative rights can coexist with positive rights. The specific problem is how a right to medical care might be just. Whether our view is general or specific, the best solutions to these problems inevitably end with some uneasy compromise between conflicting rights. As we have seen, one reason for this inevitable tension is a conflict between how rights are defined in contrast to the state. Perhaps we need to scrap the entire traditional triad (rights, state, individualism) and recreate a new triad (virtues, decentralized government, and social good). At least, we may need to *add* this second triad onto the first, for a balancing of rights can never accomplish tasks that can be done only by the virtues.

Rights and Virtues

We seem to be left in a mess about rights: We can find no universally shared natural foundation in all people upon which to base equal moral rights, and our conception of the state and its relation to rights is either fuzzy or bordering on incoherent. Ideally, we should abandon rights, define what goals we think society should promote and what behavior must be prohibited, and then define the virtues as character excellences as means to these goals.

However, even if we can't do this now, we needn't give in to cynicism or pessimism. We can be like consequentialists and see rights as they see morality—as rules of conduct that produce more good than bad consequences. The virtues are like rights then in that their exercise creates more good (defined as the promotion of worthwhile social goals) than bad.

What creates the greatest good depends on many things. In general, changing moral rules in midstream creates havoc, resentment, and bitterness; so conservatives are right in their observation that traditional systems, even if arbitrary, are better than rapid changes toward untried rules. On the other hand, those things that create the greatest good change from century to century, from society to society. American life-styles may not promote such a good in the Middle East or Africa, even if they do in America.

Once we accept this insight from utilitarianism, we needn't worry about finding some universally shared natural basis to justify rights. Moreover, we can explain why rights to inherit property may have been justified at one time—to increase capital formation needed for large-scale industries, bringing about cheap goods—but are less justified, if at all, now. We can explain why rights to life once meant that Lesch-Nyhan babies or cancer patients had to be treated to the very end, regardless of anyone's wishes, but needn't always be so treated today. Moreover, we can explain why some old rules about liberty may no longer be justified but some new ones may be needed (for example, about privacy and equal rights under the law).

Seen in this way, the question then becomes whether a proposed right to medical care would create the greatest good—given a definition of greatest good and given maximal factual knowledge. We shall make a case that most proposals cannot be so justified. Before doing so, it's important to point out that rights can't do the whole job, even when we consider them in a utilitarian framework.

The theme of this book is the need for the practical virtues as traits of character. One way to put this theme is that just as certain minimal rights of noninterference are justified as rules that increase the general good, so fostering the virtues as intrinsic excellences fosters this good. In cases of both rights and virtues, the salutary effect of their existence can be achieved only if paradoxically people value these things for themselves.

Behind the idea of a right to equal medical care is a praiseworthy moral feeling that has always motivated charity hospitals: People suffering in sickness need help and care. It's compassionate, kind, and benevolent to help them, even if they have in some sense brought their conditions on themselves—for example, by smoking cigarettes. It's important that poor sick people have medical care—not as their right enforced by bureaucratic government, but as a reflection of ourselves and our kind of society. We judge societies by how they treat their most unfortunate members. The highest motive for treating the sick is not that one's conscience is pricked by the claims of others. Nor should one be forced to do it by guilt or govern-

ment regulation. The highest motive is effected when, pained by suffering and having the power to stop it, one simply does. It doesn't matter if people ordinarily aren't moved to help. We aren't describing ordinary moral people, their beliefs or intuitions. We are discussing the highest form of moral excellence.

The poor and sick should be given some kind of care, because to give such care reflects the best ideals of how we want physicians, citizens, and society to be. The questions are how much care should be given and in what way. Will nationalized health systems and new bureaucracies work? It would seem not.

Our two best examples of nationally financed health programs are the Veterans Administration hospitals and the 1973 legislation that put treatment, including dialysis, for all end-stage renal disease patients, regardless of age, under Medicare coverage. Past experiences with these programs show that once they are running, they are almost impossible to change or shut down—no matter how costly or inefficient they are. The most important reason for this situation is that powerful lobbies prevent cost-effective changes. For example, hospital dialysis is more expensive than home dialysis (though generally patient out-of-pocket expenses are less than with home dialysis, because Medicare picks up more of the cost for institutional dialysis), cannot be easily adjusted to the patients' work schedules, and is bad for patient self-respect because it makes them overly dependent on the institution. But strong lobbies have successfully prevented any incentives to get dialysis patients on home treatment. Similarly, powerful lobbies have resisted attempts to make VA hospitals more efficient. Everyone wants less government spending, just so the cuts aren't close to home. Cut costs, but don't take away our local post office!

Increased bureaucratization from new medical rights is only one problem. Another problem is that United States citizens want contradictory goals. They want to have the best medical care available, but they don't want to pay for it.

We need some peculiarly American medical system to serve rural areas and inner cities. It's likely that sweeping changes to systems of other countries will not work here without modification. We have the problem of reconciling equality in medical care with the individual liberties of physicians. How can we justify forcing physicians to work and live where they don't want to be?

As it's put here, in the language of conflicting rights, the problem is insoluble. But the general goal of equalizing the distribution of medical care is not insoluble, although it won't be solved by coercive measures. Just as we won't get more organ donations by suing our relatives or by government decree, so we won't get more rural care by legal-financial coercion of physcians. As B.F. Skinner has discovered, punishment of any kind makes the one punished temporarily stop the undesirable behavior, but he will hate the punisher. Moreover, when the punishment is removed, the old behavior will recur since the original want hasn't been changed. The problem is why physicians don't want to go to the inner city and rural areas. The question can be put differently by asking why physicians don't have more of the practical virtues. It's not enough to rationalize by describing lack of good schools for their children, bad working conditions, and the like. It wouldn't be compassionate or courageous to serve if these things weren't true.

The distribution of medical care and the practice of virtues by physicians are matters that should be solved, at least partially, within medicine. Physicians won't want to serve the poor until systems of medical education emphasize the virtues of serving over the virtues of research. Medicine contains conflicting sets of virtues—one set of excellences about research and scientific skill, the other set about caring and kindness. Lately, the first set seems to have been emphasized—especially in medical education—over the second. The answer about helping the poor won't come until we wrestle with conflicting priorities within medicine.

Another part of the answer must come not from medicine but from society. Caring for the suffering need not mean nationalized health care. Just as Swedish systems will not work in the United States, so systems for Detroit may not work in Omaha. Some areas may emphasize state government, others local civic and religious institutions. Some areas may not care and will be judged accordingly.

Szasz correctly signals the dangers of government taking over medical care. Also, if this should happen, opportunities for compassion and caring will decrease. Charity means less when people receive public assistance and food stamps. There's a physician I know of who treats patients eligible for Medicaid and who doesn't bill Medicaid. These are 10 percent of his patients. He believes that a good physician treats some of the poor because it's charitable and compassionate to do so. Some of his younger colleagues may find this silly and stupid. The younger physicians were educated in the sixties and seventies when rights were emphasized, the physician in another time that emphasized virtues of character. This example illustrates the problem of rights and the advantages of virtues.

NOTES

1. Joel Feinberg, *Social Philosophy*, Prentice-Hall, Englewood Cliffs, N.J., p. 84, 1973.

2. UNESCO, *Human Rights: A Symposium*, Allan Wingate, New York, 1949.

3. John Locke, *Two Treatises of Government*, ed. Peter Laslett, Cambridge: At the University Press, 1963.

4. In preparing this account, I have relied on Alasdair MacIntyre's *A Short History of Ethics*, Macmillan, New York, 1966.

5. Ivan Illich, *Medical Nemesis*, Pantheon, New York, 1976.

6. Victor Fuchs, *Who Shall Live? Health Economics and Social Choice*, Basic Books, New York, 1977.

8. Robert M. Sade, "Medical Care as a Right: A Refutation," *New England Journal of Medicine*, vol. 285, p. 11, 1971.

9. Thomas Szasz, "The Right to Health," *Georgetown Law Journal*, vol. 57, p. 734, 1969.

Concept of a Person

10.

The Criterion of Common Sense Personhood
Joel Feinberg

A criterion of personhood in the descriptive sense would be a specification of those characteristics that are common and peculiar to commonsense persons and in virtue of which they are such persons. They are necessary conditions for commonsense personhood in the sense that no being who lacks any one of them can be a person. They are sufficient conditions in the sense that any being who possesses all of them is a person, whatever he or she may be like in other respects. How shall we formulate this criterion? If this question simply raises a matter of fixed linguistic convention, one might expect it to be easy enough to state the defining characteristics of personhood straight off. Surprisingly, the question is not quite that simple, and no mere dictionary is likely to give us a wholly satisfactory answer. What we must do is to think of the characteristics that come at least implicitly to mind when we hear or use such words as "person," "people," and the personal pronouns. We might best proceed by considering three different classes of cases: clear examples of beings whose personhood cannot be doubted,

clear examples of beings whose nonpersonhood cannot be doubted, and actual or hypothetical examples of beings whose status is not initially clear. We probably will not be able to come up with a definitive list of characteristics if only because the word "person" may be somewhat loose, but we should be able to achieve a criterion that is precise enough to permit a definite classification of fetuses.

Undoubted Commonsense Persons

Who are undoubted persons? Consider first your parents, siblings, or friends. What is it about them that makes you so certain that they are persons? "Well, they look like persons," you might say; "They have human faces and bodies." But so do irreversibly comatose human vegetables, and we are, to put it mildly, not so certain that they are persons. "Well then, they are males and females and thus appropriately referred to by our personal pronouns, all of which have gender. We can't refer to any of them by use of the impersonal pronoun 'it', because they

Source: Joel Feinberg, "Abortion," in Tom Regan (ed.), *Matters of Life and Death,* p. 188, Random House, New York, 1980.

have sex; so perhaps being gendered is the test of personhood." Such a reply has superficial plausibility, but is the idea of a "sexless person" logically contradictory? Perhaps any genetically human person will be predominately one sex or the other, but must the same be true of "intelligent beings in outer space," or spirits, gods, and devils?

Let's start again. "What makes me certain that my parents, siblings, and friends are people is that they give evidence of being conscious of the world and of themselves; they have inner emotional lives, just like me; they can understand things and reason about them, make plans, and act; they can communicate with me, argue, negotiate, express themselves, make agreements, honor commitments, and stand in relationships of mutual trust; they have tastes and values of their own; they can be frustrated or fulfilled, pleased or hurt." Now we clearly have the beginnings, at least, of a definitive list of person-making characteristics. In the commonsense way of thinking, persons are those beings who are conscious, have a concept and awareness of themselves, are capable of experiencing emotions, can reason and acquire understanding, can plan ahead, can act on their plans, and can feel pleasure and pain.

Undoubted Nonpersons

What of the objects that clearly are not persons? Rocks have none of the above characteristics; neither do flowers and trees; neither (presumably) do snails and earthworms. But perhaps we are wrong about that. Maybe rocks, plants, and lower animals are congeries of lower-level spirits with inner lives and experiences of their own, as primitive men and mystics have often maintained. Very well, that is possible. But if they do have these characteristics, contrary to all appearance, then it would seem natural to think of them as persons too, "contrary to all appearance." In raising the question of their possession of these characteristics at all, we seem to be raising by the same token the question of their commonsense

personhood. Mere rocks are quite certainly not crowds of silent spirits, but if, contrary to fact, they are such spirits, then we must think of them as real people, quite peculiarly embodied.

Hard Cases

Now, what about the hard cases? Is God, as traditionally conceived, a kind of nonhuman—or better, superhuman—person? Theologians are divided about this, of course, but most ordinary believers think of Him (note the personal pronoun) as conscious of self and world, capable of love and anger, eminently rational, having plans for the world, acting (if only through His creation), capable of communicating with humans, of issuing commands and making covenants, and of being pleased or disappointed in the use to which humans put their free will. To the extent that one believes that God has these various attributes, to that extent does one believe in a *personal* God. If one believes only in a God who is an unknown and unknowable First Cause of the world, or an obscure but powerful force sustaining the world, or the ultimate energy in the cosmos, then, it seems fair to say, one believes in an *impersonal* deity.

Now we come to the ultimate thought experiment. Suppose that you are a space explorer whose rocket ship has landed on a planet in a distant galaxy. The planet is inhabited by some very strange objects, so unlike anything you have previously encountered that at first you don't even know whether to classify them as animal, vegetable, mineral, or "none of the above." They are composed of a gelatinous sort of substance much like mucus except that it is held together by no visible membranes or skin, and it continually changes its shape from one sort of amorphous glob to another, sometimes breaking into smaller globs and then coming together again. The objects have no appendages, no joints, no heads or faces. They float mysteriously above the surface of the planet and move about in complex patterns while emitting eerie sounds resembling nothing so much as electronic music. The first thing you will wish to know about these strange objects is whether they are extraterrestrial *people* to be respected, greeted, and traded and negotiated with, or mere things or inferior animals to be chopped up, boiled, and used for food and clothing.

Almost certainly the first thing you would do is try to communicate with them by making approaches, gesturing by hand, voice, or radio signals. You might also study the patterns in their movements and sound emissions to see whether they have any of the characteristics of a language. If the beings respond even in a primitive way to early gestures, one might suspect at least that they are beings who are capable of perception and who can be *aware* of movements and sounds. If some sort of actual communication then follows, you can attribute to them at least the mentality of chimpanzees. If negotiations then follow and agreements are reached, then you can be sure that they are rational beings, and if you learn to interpret signs of worry, distress, anger, alarm, or friendliness, then you can be quite confident that they are indeed people, no matter how inhuman they are in biological respects.

A Working Criterion of Commonsense Personhood

Suppose then that we agree that our rough list captures well the traits that are generally characteristic of commonsense persons. Suppose further (what is not quite as evident) that each trait on the list is necessary for commonsense personhood, that no one trait is by itself sufficient, but that the whole *collection* of traits is sufficient to confer commonsense personhood on any being that possesses it. Suppose, that is, that consciousness is necessary (no permanently unconscious being can be a person), but that it is not enough. The conscious being must also have a concept of a self and a certain amount of self-awareness. But although each of these last traits is necessary, they are still not enough even in conjunction, since a self-aware, conscious being who was totally incapable of learning or reasoning would not be a person. Hence rationality is also necessary, though not by itself sufficient. And so on through our complete list of person-making characteristics, each one of which, let us suppose, is a necessary condition, and all of which are jointly a sufficient condition of being a person in the commonsense, descriptive sense of "person." Let us call our set of characteristics *c*. Now at least we can pose the most important and controversial question about the status of the fetus: What is the relation, if any, between having *c* and being a person in the normative (moral) sense, that is, a being who possesses, among other things, a right to life?

It bears repeating at the outset of our discussion of this most important question that formulating criteria of personhood in the purely moral sense is not a scientific question to be settled by empirical evidence, not simply a question of word usage, not simply a matter to be settled by commonsense thought experiments. It is instead an essentially controversial question about the possession of moral rights that cannot be answered in these ways. That is not to say that rational methods of investigation and discussion are not available to us, but only that the methods of reasoning about morals do not often provide conclusive proofs and demonstrations. What rational methods can achieve for us, even if they fall short of producing universal agreement, is to list the various options open to us, and the strong and weak points of each of them. Every position has its embarrassments, that is, places where it appears to conflict logically with moral and commonsense convictions that even its proponents can be presumed to share. To point out these embarrassments for a given position is not necessarily to refute it but rather to measure the costs of holding it to the coherence of one's larger set of beliefs generally. Similarly, each position has its own peculiar advantages, respects in which it coheres uniquely well with deeply entrenched convictions that even its opponents might be expected to share. I shall try in the ensuing discussion to state and illustrate as vividly as I can the advantages and difficulties in all the major positions. Then I shall weigh the cases for and against the various alternatives. For those who disagree with my conclusion, the discussion will serve at least to locate the crucial issues in the controversy over the status of the fetus.

A proposed criterion for moral personhood is a statement of a characteristic (or set of characteristics) that its advocate deems both necessary and (jointly) sufficient for being a person in the moral sense. Such characteristics are not thought of as mere indexes, signs, or "litmus tests" of moral personhood, but as more basic traits that actually confer moral personhood on whoever possesses them. All and only those beings having these characteristics have basic moral rights, in particular the right to full and equal protection against homicide. Thus, fetuses must be thought of as having this right if they satisfy a proposed criterion of personhood. The main types of criteria of moral personhood proposed by philosophers can be grouped under one or another of five different headings, which we shall examine in turn. Four of the five proposed criteria refer to possession of c (the traits we have listed as conferring *commonsense* personhood). One of these four specifies actual possession of c; the other three refer to either actual or potential possession of c. The remaining criterion, which we shall consider briefly first, makes no mention of c at all.

The species criterion. "All and only members of the biological species *Homo sapiens*, 'whoever is conceived by human beings,' are moral persons and thus are entitled to full and equal protection by the moral rule against homicide." The major advantage of this view (at least for some) is that it gives powerful support to those who would extend the protection of the rule against homicide to the fetus from the moment of conception. If this cri-

terion is correct, it is not simply because of utilitarian reasons (such that it would usefully increase respect for life in the community) that we must not abort human zygotes and embryos, but rather because we owe it to these minute entities themselves not to kill them, for as members of the human species they are already possessed of a full right to life equal in strength to that of any adult person.

The species criterion soon encounters serious difficulties. Against the view that membership in the species *Homo sapiens* is a *necessary* condition of membership in the class of moral persons, we have the possibility of there being moral persons from other planets who belong to other biological species. Moreover, some human beings—in particular, those who are irreversibly comatose "vegetables"—*are* human beings but doubtfully qualify as moral persons, a fact that casts serious doubt on the view that membership in the species *Homo sapiens* is a *sufficient* condition of being a moral person.

The species criterion might be defended against these objections if some persuasive reason could be given why moral personhood is a unique feature of all and only human beings. Aside from an arbitrary claim that this is "just obvious," a position that Singer argues amounts to a pernicious prejudice against nonhuman animals comparable with racism and sexism, the only possible way to defend this claim to uniqueness is by means of some *theological* argument: *All* human beings (including human fetuses) and *only* human beings (thereby excluding all nonhuman animals and possible beings from other planets) are moral persons *because God has made this so.* Now, if one already believes on faith that God had made it true that all and only humans are moral persons, then of course one has quite conclusive reason for believing that all and only humans are moral persons. But if we leave faith aside and confine our attention to reasons, then we shall have to ask what grounds there are for supposing that "God has made this so," and any reason we might have for doubting that it *is* so would count equally as a reason against supposing that God made it so. A good reason for doubting that 7 + 5 = 13 is an equally good reason for doubting that God made it to be the case that 7 + 5 = 13; a good reason for doubting that cruelty is morally right is, if anything, a better reason for denying that God made it to be the case that cruelty is right.

The modified species criterion. "All and only members of species generally characterized by *c,* whether the species is *Homo sapiens* or another, and whether or not the particular individual in question happens to possess *c,* are moral persons entitled to full and equal protection by the moral rule against homicide." This modification is designed to take the sting out of the first objection (above) to the unmodified species criterion. If there are other species or categories of moral persons in the universe, it concedes, then they too have moral rights. Indeed, if there are such, then *all* of their members are moral persons possessed of such rights, even those individuals who happen themselves to lack *c* because they are not yet fully developed or because they have been irreparably damaged.

The major difficulty for the modified species criterion is that it requires further explanation why *c* should determine moral personhood when applied to *classes* of creatures rather than to individual cases. Why is a permanently unconscious but living body of a human or an extragalactic person (or for that matter, a chimpanzee, if we should decide that that species as a whole is characterized by *c*) a moral person when it lacks as an individual the characteristics that determine moral personhood? Just because opposable thumbs are a characteristic of *Homo sapiens,* it does not follow that this or that particular *Homo sapiens* has opposable thumbs. There appears to be no reason for regarding right-possession any differently, in this regard, from thumb-possession.

The strict potentiality criterion. "All and only those creatures who either actually or potentially possess *c* (that is, who either have *c* now or would come to have *c* in the natural course of events) are moral persons now, fully protected by the rule against homicide." This criterion also permits one to draw the line of moral personhood in the human species right at the moment of conception, which will be counted by some as an advantage. It also has the undeniable advantage of immunity from one charge of arbitrariness since it will extend moral personhood to all beings in *any* species or category who possess *c,* either actually or potentially. It may also cohere with our psychological attitudes, since it can explain why it is that many people, at least, think of unformed or unpretty fetuses as precious. Zygotes and embryos in particular are treasured not for what they are but for what they are biologically "programmed" to become in the fullness of time: real people fully possessed of *c.*

The difficulties of this criterion are of two general kinds, those deriving from the obscurity of the concept of "potentiality," which perhaps can be overcome, and the more serious difficulties of answering the charge that merely potential possession of any set of qualifications for a moral status does not logically ensure actual possession of that status. Consider just one of the problems raised by the concept of potentiality itself. How, it might be asked, can a mere zygote be a potential person, whereas a mere spermatozoon or a mere unfertilized ovum is not? If the spermatozoon and ovum we are talking about are precisely those that will combine in a few seconds to form a human zygote, why are they not potential zygotes, and thus potential people, *now?* The defender of the potentiality criterion will reply that it is only at the moment of conception that any being comes into existence with exactly the same chromosomal makeup as the human being that will later emerge from the womb, and it is *that* chromosomal combination that forms the potential person, not anything that exists before it comes together. The reply is probably a cogent one, but uncertainties

about the concept of potentiality might
make us hesitate, at first, to accept it, for
we might be tempted to think of both
the germ cell (spermatozoon or ovum) and
the zygote as potentially a particular person, while holding that the differences between their potentials, though large and
significant to be sure, are nevertheless differences in degree rather than kind. It
would be well to resist that temptation,
however, for it could lead us to the view
that some of the entities and processes
that combined still earlier to form a given
spermatozoon were themselves potentially
that spermatozoon and hence potentially
the person that spermatozoon eventually
became, and so on. At the end of that
road is the proposition that everything is
potentially everything else, and thus the
destruction of all utility in the concept of
potentiality. It is better to hold this particular line at the zygote.

The remaining difficulty for the strict
potentiality criterion is much more serious.
It is a logical error, some have charged, to
deduce *actual* rights from merely *potential*
(but not yet actual) qualification for those
rights. What follows from potential qualification, it is said, is potential, not actual,
rights; what entails actual rights is actual,
not potential, qualification. As the Australian
philosopher Stanley Benn puts it, "A potential president of the United States is not
on that account Commander-in-Chief [of
the U.S. Army and Navy]." This simple point
can be called "the logical point about potentiality." Taken on its own terms, I don't
see how it can be answered as an objection
to the strict potentiality criterion. It is still
open to an antiabortionist to argue that
merely potential commonsense personhood
is a ground for *duties* we may have toward
the potential person. But he cannot argue
that it is the ground for the potential person's *rights* without committing a logical
error.

*The modified or gradualist potentiality
criterion.* "Potential possession of c confers
not a right, but only a claim, to life, but
that claim keeps growing stronger, requiring
ever stronger reasons to override it, until

the point when c is actually possessed, by
which time it has become a full right to
life." This modification of the potentiality
criterion has one distinct and important
advantage. It coheres with the widely shared
feeling that the moral seriousness of abortion increases with the age of the fetus. It is
extremely difficult to believe on other than
very specific theological grounds that a zygote
one day after conception is the sort of being that can have any rights at all, much less
the whole armory of "human rights" including "the right to life." But it is equally
difficult for a great many people to believe
that a full-term fetus one day before birth
does not have a right to life. Moreover, it is
very difficult to find one point in the continuous development of the fetus before
which it is utterly without rights and after
which it has exactly the same rights as
any adult human being. Some rights in post-
natal human life can be acquired instantly
or suddenly; the rights of citizenship, for example, come into existence at a precise
moment in the naturalization proceedings
after an oath has been administered and a
judicial pronouncement formally produced
and certified. Similarly, the rights of husbands and wives come into existence at just
that moment when an authorized person
utters the words "I hereby pronounce you
husband and wife." But the rights of the
fetus cannot possibly jump in this fashion
from nonbeing to being at some precise
moment in pregnancy. The alternative is to
think of them as growing steadily and gradually throughout the entire nine-month
period until they are virtually "mature" at
parturition. There is, in short, a kind of
growth in "moral weight" that proceeds in
parallel fashion with the physical growth
and development of the fetus.

An "immature right" on this view is not
to be thought of simply as no right at all,
as if in morals a miss were as good as a mile.
A better characterization of the unfinished
right would be a "weak right," a claim with
some moral force proportional to its degree
of development, but not yet as much force as
a fully matured right. The key word in this
account is "claim." Elsewhere I have given an

account of the difference between having a right (which I defined as a "valid claim") and having a claim that is not, or not quite, valid. What would the latter be like?

One might accumulate just enough evidence to argue with relevance and cogency that one has a right . . . although one's case might not be overwhelmingly conclusive. The argument might be strong enough to entitle one to a hearing and fair consideration. When one is in this position, it might be said that one "has a claim" that deserves to be weighed carefully. Nevertheless the balance of reasons may turn out to militate against recognition of the claim, so that the claim is not a valid claim or right.

Now there are various ways in which a claim can fail to be a right. There are many examples, particularly from the law, where *all* the claims to some property, including some that are relevantly made and worthy of respect, are rejected, simply because none of them is deemed strong enough to qualify as a right. In such cases, a miss truly is as good as a mile. But in other cases, an acknowledged claim of (say) medium strength will be strong enough to be a right *unless* a stronger claim appears on the scene to override it. For these conflict situations, card games provide a useful analogy. In poker, three-of-a-kind is good enough to win the pot unless one of the other players "makes claim" to the pot with a higher hand, say a flush or a full house. The player who claims the pot with three-of-a-kind "has a claim" to the pot that is overriden by the stronger claim of the player with the full house. The strongest claim presented will, by that fact, constitute a right to take the money. The player who withdrew with a four-flush had "no claim at all," but even that person's hand might have established a right to the pot if no stronger claim were in conflict with it.

The analogy applies to the abortion situation in the following way. The game has at least two players, the mother and the fetus, though more can play, and sometimes the father and/or the doctor are involved too.

For the first few weeks of its life, the fetus (zygote, embryo) has hardly any claim to life at all, and virtually any reason of the mother's for aborting it will be strong enough to override a claim made in the fetus's behalf. At any stage in the game, any reason the mother might have for aborting will constitute a claim, but as the fetus matures, its claims grow stronger, requiring ever-stronger claims to override them. After three months or so, the fact that an abortion would be "convenient" for the mother will not be a strong enough claim, and the fetus' claim to life will defeat it. In that case, the fetus can be said to have a valid claim or right to life in the same sense that the poker player's full house gives him or her a right to the pot: It is a right in the sense that it is the strongest of the conflicting claims, not in the sense that it is stronger than any conflicting claim that could conceivably come up. By the time the fetus has become a neonate (a newborn child), however, it has a "right to life" of the same kind all people have, and no mere conflicting claim can override it. (Perhaps more accurately, only claims that other human persons make in self-defense to their own lives can ever have an equal strength.)

The modified potentiality criterion has the attractiveness characteristic of compromise theories when fierce ideological quarrels rage between partisans of more extreme views. It shares one fatal flaw, however, with the strict potentiality criterion: Despite its greater flexibility, it cannot evade "the logical point about potentiality." A highly developed fetus is much closer to being a commonsense person with all the developed traits that qualify it for moral personhood than is the mere zygote. But being almost qualified for rights is not the same thing as being partially qualified for rights; nor is it the same thing as being qualified for partial rights, quasi-rights, or weak rights. The advanced fetus is closer to being a person than is the zygote, just as a dog is closer to personhood than a jellyfish, but that is not the same thing as being "more of a person." In 1930, when he was six years old, Jimmy Carter didn't know it, but he was a potential president of the United States. That gave him no claim *then,* not even a very weak claim, to give commands to the U.S. Army and Navy. Franklin D. Roosevelt in 1930 was only two years away from the presidency; so he was a potential president in a much stronger way (the potentiality was much less remote) than was young Jimmy. Nevertheless, he was not actually president, and he had no more of a claim to the prerogatives of the office than did Carter. The analogy to fetuses in different stages of development is of course imperfect. But in both cases it would seem to be invalid to infer the existence of a "weak version of a right" from an "almost qualification" for the full right. In summary, the modified potentiality criterion, insofar as it permits the potential possession of *c* to be a *sufficient condition* for the actual possession of claims, and in some cases of rights, is seriously flawed in the same manner as the strict potentiality criterion.

The actual-possession criterion. "At any given time *t,* all and only those creatures who actually possess *c* are moral persons at *t,* whatever species or category they may happen to belong to." This simple and straightforward criterion has a number of conspicuous advantages. We should consider it with respect even before examination of its difficulties if only because the difficulties of its major rivals are so severe. Moreover, it has a certain tidy symmetry about it, since it makes the overlap between commonsense personhood and moral personhood complete—a total correspondence with no loose ends left over in either direction. There can be no actual commonsense persons who are not actual moral persons, nor can there be any actual moral persons who are not actual commonsense persons. Moral personhood is not established simply by species membership, associations, or potentialities. Instead, it is conferred by the same characteristics (*c*) that lead us to recognize personhood wherever we find it. It is no accident, no mere coincidence, that we use the moral term "person" for those beings, and only those beings, who have *c.* The characteristics

that confer commonsense personhood are not arbitrary bases for rights and duties, such as race, sex, or species membership; rather they are the traits that make sense out of rights and duties and without which those moral attributes would have no point or function. It is because people are conscious; have a sense of their personal identities; have plans, goals, and projects; experience emotions; are liable to pains, anxieties, and frustrations; can reason and bargain, and so on—it is because of these attributes that people have values and interests, desires and expectations of their own, including a stake in their own futures, and a personal well-being of a sort we cannot ascribe to unconscious or nonrational beings. Because of their developed capacities they can assume duties and responsibilities and can have and make claims on one another. Only because of their sense of self, their life plans, their value hierarchies, and their stakes in their own futures, can they be ascribed fundamental rights. There is nothing arbitrary about these linkages.

Despite these impressive advantages, the actual-possession criterion must face a serious difficulty, namely, that it implies that small infants (neonates) are not moral persons. There is very little moral reason, after all, to attribute *c* more to neonates than to advanced fetuses still *in utero.* Perhaps during the first few days after birth the infant is conscious and able to feel pain, but it is unlikely that it has a concept of its self or of its future life, that it has plans and goals, that it can think consecutively, and the like. In fact, the whole complex of traits that make up *c* is not *obviously* present until the second year of childhood. And that would seem to imply, according to the criterion we are considering, that the deliberate destruction of babies in their first year is no violation of their rights. And *that* might seem to entail that there is nothing wrong with infanticide (the deliberate killing of infants). But infanticide *is* wrong. Therefore, critics of the actual-possession criterion have argued that we ought to reject this criterion.

Sanctity of Life

11.

The Sanctity of Life: An Analysis of a Concept

K. Danner Clouser

My task is to analyze a concept—the concept of "the sanctity of life."[1] One would like to know more precisely what it means, when it should be used, what it commits us to, whether it can be defended. What makes sense must be sorted out from what does not. My main hope is to stimulate thinking about this issue. To that end I want my analysis to remain more on the suggestive and broad level than on the narrow and definitive.

I will first make some general observations about the concept—its ordinary connotations and its immediate muddles. Then I will try out other possible interpretations of its meaning and logic. The fallout from that effort will then constitute my main claims about the concept. Anticlimactically, I will consider two counterexamples.

It is always helpful to know from the start what an author will be concluding; knowing the end product, one can be far more alert to the author's mistakes as they occur. Hence: I find the sanctity of life concept to be impossibly vague and to be a concept that is inaccurate and misleading, whose positive points can be better handled by other well-established concepts.

Connotations of Religious Origin

The first thing that must be said about this concept is that it is clearly religious in origin. It is found more explicitly in Eastern religions (Hinduism in particular). But it also appears throughout our Judeo-Christian traditions. There its theological status may not be clear, but in a variety of ways it surfaces. Basically it bespeaks life to be God's creation, over which we have no authority; life is a gift-in-trust from God, and we are pledged to practice good stewardship of it; it is for our use, but it is only on loan.

Much work could be done on explicating the religious conception of life's sanctity: its origin, its basis, its meaning. But that is *not* the focus of this article. Such an approach would be far too limiting, given my concern with ethics; that is, it would be appropriate only to those who accept the religious view-

Source: *Annals of Internal Medicine,* vol. 78, no. 1, January 1973, p. 119. Earlier versions of this paper were given at Coe College and at the Medical College of the University of Florida, Gainesville, Fla., as part of their Publix Lecture Series in the History and Philosophy of Medicine. Supported in part by The National Endowment for the Humanities grant EO-4579-71-197.

point. But in ethics we must seek that to which all rational men could agree. Our world is too pluralistic to derive its rules from a limited set of metaphysical commitments to which only a smaller subset of persons subscribe.

This is by no means to disparage the religious; it is only to say that these are not the commitments around which we could expect or require all men to rally. Generally, religious requirements are more stringent than what could be expected of all rational men. They go beyond the reasonable obligation, beyond the call of duty; they require you to go the second mile. Generally, religious practices will be in accord with, but more stringent than, whatever we find binding on all men.

Although "sanctity," after all, is a religious concept, refusing to discuss the religious meanings of "sanctity of life" does not cut us off from meaningful discussion of the concept, simply because the concept has been taken over by the world at large. It is used by the religious and the nonreligious, and in both cases with "religious" fervor. It it used and appealed to by almost everybody, and those who use it seem to think that all their fellow men should agree, at least in principle. It is this ordinary secular use that we shall look at more closely, insofar as it relates to human life in particular.

General Connotations and Related Muddles

Treasuring of life. In the very general sense, it would seem that the concept means the treasuring of all human life, no matter what. It is being used to argue that wherever there is human life, nothing can count against it; life can never be taken. It thus is posed as a conclusive reason instead of just a reason to be weighed with other reasons and arguments; that is, it is feigned to be conclusive rather than being simply one point among many to be considered. Furthermore, the connotations are that this concept applies to *all* human life, including fetal life and comatose life. "Sanc-

tity of life" is often appealed to as though it settles the abortion question as well as the question of the artificial support of unconscious life. In effect, this proposition says that where there is life, it would be inconsistent with "the sanctity of life" for us to interfere.

Surely, on closer examination we would find that this is simply not a defensible use of the sanctity of life concept. "Sanctity of life" should not be interpreted as defining what is human life and what is not, although it frequently is. One could say, with consistency, that he accepted both "sanctity of life" and abortion, because he did not happen to believe fetal life was human life. In short, "sanctity of life" leaves the definition of human life undetermined. It just does not say.

So it seems a mistake to think that "the sanctity of life" is a conclusive judgment, rule, or principle that, if accepted, solves the problem, leaving nothing more at issue. Rather, it is just one consideration among many that enter the argument. For example, there are times when we have believed it was justified to commit suicide, to put to death, to withhold lifesaving therapy, or to kill. In short, "sanctity of life" is not the decisive consideration; it is not a conclusive argument. At best, it is one consideration among many, and it is at times outweighed by these other considerations.

Quality of life. It is unclear whether "sanctity of life" means that life must be protected at all costs or whether it means that the *quality* of life must be protected at all costs (even if it requires the sacrifice of other life). The argument based on the quality of life is used for permitting abortion, for allowing badly deformed infants to die, for determining government medical priorities as to where money will go (say, to the elderly rather than to the young). This is frequently thought to be in opposition to the "sanctity of life" argument. Yet its proponents could claim the "sanctity of life" as their basis, contending that human life is so very special that it should not be degraded, that there are some forms and conditions of life not worth living. Thus the ambiguity of the "sanctity of life" argument allows it to be used against itself.

We have glanced superficially at some ordinary connotations of the concept. We have seen, surrounding it, ambiguities, contradictions, and a general lack of clear direction; at least we have seen enough to realize that it is not as clear, decisive, and helpful as many seem to believe. Now we must try even harder to find its meaning.

Its Meaning: Some Possibilities

A property of life? At least on the surface, in speaking of the "sanctity of life" it would seem we were attributing some property to human life. It would seem to be an attribute that comes into being and exists with each individual life, something that attaches to each life. (To define "individual life" would require a separate entourage of metaphysical distinctions, claims, and maneuvers.)

But our ordinary criteria for a property's existence are not fulfilled in this case. Our senses do not detect any such attribute, nor can we be led by an expert to "sense" some more mysterious and illusive property that might inhere in or hover about life. There is the possibility of a "derived" property, that is, a property that, although unperceived, "must" exist within the phenomenon of life because it happens to follow from some theory about life. It could be derived, for example, from the religious sense of sanctity. That is, it might follow from certain other propositions that are held—such as "God created life," "man is God's creation," "man is God's steward," and so on. But this is not our present point of focus. There is no universally accepted theory—if any at all—that entails a property called "sanctity."

There is another reason for believing sanctity is not some sort of property that adheres to life. If it were a "good," a treasured something or other, there surely would be a feeling of obligation to create as much human life as possible. Yet none of us feels the obligation to reproduce without ceasing!

This realization gives us an important clue: "sanctity of life" does not seem to be telling us to *do* something (create as much life as possible); it seems more to be telling us what *not* to do (do not take life). This point will be elaborated later.

A feeling? Of course, all this is not to say that we do not have special *feelings* about life—all the way from treasuring it to feeling a deep sense of mystery about it. We may experience awe at being alive. This is important to the ordinary concept of sanctity, as I shall show later; but it could hardly be the meaning of sanctity. That is, it simply would not do the work generally presumed to be done by appealing to the sanctity of life principle.

For one, "sanctity" seems more objective than simply feelings we have about life, however deep. It suggests something to be acknowledged, rather than a description of things felt. For another, neither command nor obligation follows from the fact that we feel a certain way about life. For example, the fact that we may sense the mysteriousness of existence does not imply anything about how we should treat life—our own or others. If we sometimes find life exhilarating it does not follow that we must "protect life at all costs" or "never allow a life to cease." On the other hand, it may very well be why we value life and establish certain rules for its protection.

A value? A right? One way of locating more precisely the ordinary meaning of "sanctity" would be to substitute some possible synonyms, and "listen" to the result. "The value of life" or "the importance of life" obviously do not have the same ring as "sanctity of life." For example, "because life is important, abortion cannot be legalized" or "we cannot allow respirators to be turned off because of the value of life." These phrases seem much weaker; they seem to be saying a lot less than is connotated by "the sanctity of life." The ring of "sanctity" has the strength of a quality-in-reality that attaches to a life principle; it sounds much more inviolable. There may be many reasons why the substitutions seem to have less force. Among them is that both "value" and "importance" sound too subjective; they sound more like something we impute to life than something it has in itself. They do not have the overtones of being facts that command acknowledgment. "Sanctity of life" seems to have this objective connotation, although, as was suggested earlier, this "inherent property" idea is hardly defensible.

The phrase "right to life" comes closer precisely because it suggests something somewhat more objective, something out there and given, and hence something to be acted in accord with. For example: "The fetus has a right to life"; "The comatose patient has a right to life." "Right to life" seems much closer to the thrust and intent of "sanctity of life." This is, at least partially, because both expressions imply an obligation binding on us, an obligation not to violate that particular life. This point will be elaborated later.

An overall life orientation? Perhaps we have been pressing too hard for a precise meaning. It may well be that the sanctity of life concept is simply not intended to be exact, to settle issues, to give direction. Rather, it might simply bespeak a very general orientation toward life, a kind of world view. As such we should not expect rigorous differentiations, decisive exclusions, and definitive direction. We should rather expect a pervading awareness, a gentle suasion, nudging our views and actions in one way or another. Widely diverse views and actions would be compatible with this world view, since the meaning (and hence criteria, implications, and applicability) would be so vague. Although this interpretation would concern the concept's use rather than its meaning, I have some sympathy with it. It is consistent with a point I think important, that "sanctity of life" is more something we pledge ourselves to, a commitment, than it is an objective property that demands acknowledgment.

Nevertheless, one particular aspect of this "world view" interpretation is very disconcerting. That is its indeterminateness; as

it stands it seems impossibly vague. It involves believing life has value, that it should be treated as important, that it should be preserved—all other things being equal. But, given this interpretation, it is not at all clear who would disagree. Is it even a helpful distinction? Does it separate anyone from anyone else? Wouldn't everyone—save wanton, whimsical killers—subscribe to this world view? As such, it hardly bears talking about, let alone appealing to for settling arguments.

Of course not everyone believes life is equally important; there would be widely discrepant ideas of what constitutes "adequate justification" for taking life. But that would be so even among those who were pledged to the sanctity of life world view. Surely nearly everyone agrees that life should be protected and not taken without a reason. And the sanctity of life world view is no more precise about life than that. What counts as a reason is not specified by the concept itself; so this world view is no more exacting about life than is the world at large.

What, precisely, does this sanctity of life world view come to? What would it mean to have this as one's general life orientation? If asked, a believer might respond with a variety of statements:

1. Life is precious.

2. I have respect for life.

3. Life should be caringly nurtured.

4. Life should not be taken without adequate justification.

5. Every living thing has a presumptive right to live.

All these in effect boil down to statements 4 and 5, and for our purposes statements 4 and 5 are equivalent. Feelings and attitudes about life ("precious," "respect") are really not to the point, except insofar as they affect one's behavior. What difference does "respect for life" make in one's actions? The most likely manifestation would be urging and practicing the principle that life not be taken except for very good reasons, and that is equivalent to 4, above. "Respect" would have to imply at least that, if it is to make any sense at all. Also, statement 3—caringly nurturing life—could be reduced to 4, or simply be deleted as a viable interpretation of "sanctity of life." That is, the sanctity of life principle is not ordinarily called on to justify or insist on humane treatment of individual lives (unless lack of such treatment is a threat to life itself). Usually it is cited only in decisions between life and death, not in a call for loving treatment.

If I have not gone astray in these reduction maneuvers, we are left with something like: urging and practicing that life not be taken without adequate reason. This is the heart of a world view committed to "sanctity of life." It means that life has a presumptive right to exist, and that the burden of proof sits on him who would take life, not on him who would preserve it. "Do not take life without adequate justification." This is at least more precise, but again almost everyone would agree because it leaves the crucial issue undetermined: namely, when is taking life justified? *That* is where all the disagreements are, and that is what is left undetermined by "sanctity of life."

Some Fallout from Our Inquiry

From our "world view" considerations, there are four significant results:

1. The concept now seems to be saying nothing more than "don't kill" or "don't deprive of life." And, as in all moral rules, it is a general prohibition to which there can be exceptions, but the exceptions must be justified.

2. Notice that it is now stated in the negative: "do not take life." It is now a prohibition. It is not making an ambiguous command like "treat life as sanctified" or "regard life as sanctified" or even the straight claims, "life is sanctified" or "life is precious." You do not have to figure out what "sanctity" is, or "precious" or "important" or "valuable"; the command is much more straightforward. *Whatever* human life life is, in any case, do not take it.

3. It follows that an important shift in the grounding of this admonition has also taken place. It does not depend on a quality or property called "sanctity"; it does not depend on the presence of this attribute which may or may not be there; it does not depend on people acknowledging the existence of this "property." It now depends more securely on our own self-interest and our concern for friends and family. That is, it is to the advantage of each of us that we honor this directive. We would be foolish not to urge everyone to do so; by advocating it, we enhance the safety of ourselves, our friends, and our family.[2] This is not to say that most of us would not act on it anyway, but, if we are looking for universal acceptance, this kind of self-interest is as strong a basis for it as we can hope to find.

4. The fourth advantage of this formulation is that it focuses the attention where the action really is, namely, on the *exceptions*. As with all moral rules, there is a general prohibition to which there can always be exceptions, provided the exceptions are justified. This puts the burden of proof on those who would disobey the moral rule. Then the interesting arena of debate becomes: What constitutes justifiable exceptions? This in an improvement over subscribing to "sanctity of life" principle, which seems to hide the fact of exceptions; "sanctity of life," when taken as the conclusive consideration rather than as one among many, obfuscates the vital role of exceptions and their justification. Consequently, the really crucial questions are much less apt to surface: What life is to be protected? What is human life? Is a fetus human life? Is allowing to die different from taking a life? Is extreme suffering a reason for allowing to die?

Just to sharpen this point a bit, compare being told "treat life as sanctified" and being told "do not take a life." Being told the first, it would never be clear where and if you transgressed it. *Whatever* you did—as long as you were remembering that life was precious—you might feel you were treating life as sacred. But under the admonition, "do not take life," anytime you were about to help die, let die, or turn off the respirator, you would immediately be forced to the real issue—what justifies it in this case? You are immediately pushed to give reasons, and you are thus in the arena where the real debate is: When and why is it justifiable to take a life? Proclaiming "sanctity of life" can keep one from ever directly facing up to these hard questions. In short, when you are transgressing the rule "do not kill," it is immediately apparent in a way that is not apparent when you are told "treat life as sanctified." In the former case the focus immediately shifts to where the issues really are. In the "sanctity" case, we bog down in the fat of ambiguity, imprecision, and hidden reasoning.

Summary

Before raising two niggling puzzles, I will summarize where we have been.

We began by noticing some of the misleading aspects of the "sanctity of life" concept, such as the assumption that it solved the question of what was and was not human life in those notorious borderline cases and the assumption that it was a conclusive consideration against which nothing could count.

We found muddles concerning exceptions. Even though we believe ourselves to accept the sanctity of life principle, we do tolerate many exceptions, even though we may see no reason for them.

We questioned the sense of regarding "sanctity as a property embedded in life itself or as a feeling about life. And, even if these views could somehow be defended, we still saw no way to derive what we *ought* to do from what is the case.

Our final foray into its territory considered the possibility that "sanctity of life" was a very general orientation toward life. This nonspecificity seemed to wash it out completely. But we learned some things in the process: that the command "don't kill" provides more precise guidance; that the "thou shalt not . . ." form of admonition is more helpful because the burden of justification is thereby placed on the transgressor (which, in turn, considerably sharpens the ingredient issues); and that a foundation is provided for advocating and defending the rule, namely, self-interest and concern for friends and family.

For most readers this is an appropriate stopping place. What follows is an attempt to deal with some of the related fine points.

Lingering Doubts

I do think that most of what is valuable, understandable, and defensible in the sanctity of life concept can be more clearly and helpfully handled by the moral rule, "do not take life." But after my reduction maneuvers are over there may be an irreducible remainder. I can find two instances not provided for here that may be accounted for by "sanctity of life." These issues are complicated; I can but sketch them here, but this will at least serve to initiate reflection on them.

One worry concerns future generations and our obligations to them. Intuitively, we may feel that we owe something, namely, continuation of the human race. Yet acting in accord with our moral rule, "Do not kill," would not necessarily guarantee future generations. And, for that matter, none of our moral rules (which essentially proscribe us from depriving others of life, pleasure, and freedom) or our moral ideals (which basically enjoin us to prevent suffering) would ensure the future of the human race. In fact, the moral ideal of preventing suffering might actually advise us *not* to perpetuate the race. Yet don't we feel a deep sense of obligation for continuing human life? Of course this may be caused by other than moral factors, but on the surface it seems to be a moral commitment. How do we account for this? Is this perhaps what sanctity of life really means? Is this the principle behind our felt commitment to create future generations? Life is precious; so keep it going.

Look at the "felt commitment" more closely. It seems more a commitment to keep the race going than simply to create life. That is, there is no obligation to create as much life as we can but only to see that human life continues—not this life, nor that life in particular, nor all the life possible—but life ordered and selected so as not to have undue suffering and to contribute to the progress of life. In short, we see even here that "sanctity of life" (if that's what we choose to call it in this instance) is not an unqualified commitment to the creating and survival of all life in any way, shape, or form. It is not all life that is precious, but only the continuation of *some* life rather than none.

We feel a commitment to preserve the life of the species, yet there seems to be no standard moral principle that underlies this felt commitment; we cannot reduce it to a more ultimate principle. So here is a plausible meaning for "sanctity of life," although it would be a struggle to restrict it to *just* that meaning; it would soon overflow this rigid boundary and assume some of its old misleading and indefensible senses.

Even in this case, however, the sanctity of life concept does not give wholesale endorsement to life but is quite compatible with modifying and restricting judgments about how much life, what quality of life, what qualifies as human life, and so forth. So this felt commitment is really a commitment to seeing that human life continues, but it leaves undecided the specific conditions under which it may continue.

It might be more helpful to speak of this as a commitment to *potentiality* rather than "sanctity" of life. Our obligation would be to realizing potential. This at least would tie it in with the deep-seated obligation we feel to actualize potential or at least preserve it, thus allowing it to develop. But, like "sanctity of life," this potentiality principle obvi-ously does not mean any and all potentiality should be realized. There must be other guidelines for what should be realized and what should not. Once again our attention is directed to the real concerns: which potentials should be allowed to develop, which not, and why. (Thus the stage is set for the whole cast of ethical problems involved in genetic engineering.)

The second puzzle has to do with the rational basis of ethics. Very roughly, it is this: the rational basis for urging us to follow the moral rules is that it is for our own good (and that of family and friends) if others follow these rules. It would be irrational of us not to advocate these rules; we run a risk of being hurt if we do not. But there *are* forms of life that could never represent any threat to us; they could not retaliate directly nor would we ever find ourselves in their situation. Hence why should we practice or urge morality with respect to them? There are not many such; a fetus would be one and perhaps a severely retarded child. Why should we urge concern toward these forms of life? We cannot be harmed by them, nor can we ever become them and hence eventually be harmed by attitudes and actions we have allowed and engendered. So why should we urge concern? The difficulty in answering this question is reflected in the moral ambiguity encompassing these cases. Why do some people respect life in these forms? The moral ideal of preventing suffering may account for some concern, but these lives *could* be snuffed out without anyone suffering pain or apprehension. So why protect them? Yet many of us feel a commitment to give these forms of life some protection. We might agree that there could be considerations that would *outweigh* their right to life, but there at least seems to be a felt obligation to grant them a prima facie right to life. This question is too complicated to pursue here. But, for the purpose of this discussion, have we raised a point that cannot be accounted for by the rational foundation of ethics? If so, then this may be the one place where the concept is finally applicable, because many feel it strongly in this case. Maybe it is here that there is a difference between those who espouse "sanctity of life" and those who do not. In the case of the fetus and the severely retarded child there seems to be, in some people, a deeply felt obligation to preserve the life. Yet it does not seem to be required on a rational ethical basis. So perhaps "sanctity" does stand by itself as a principle or commitment clear and distinct from others. Nevertheless, it is far more limited than is usually believed, with far less applicability than to the broad range of actions for which it is usually cited as the basic principle. Although I will not attempt it here, there might be a way to reduce even this small remainder. Such a move would at least have the advantage of conceptual economy, and it would place this felt obligation on firmer, more defensible ground than the sanctity of life concept, which is unclear, indefensible, and applicable only to this particular case. The reduction would show that for important, pragmatic reasons this felt obligation was an extension of the standard moral rule, "do not deprive of life," even though the beings in question are neither rational nor capable of retaliation, and we will never find ourselves in their place. It has to do with the importance of maintaining general respect for *all* human life by honoring it even in the borderline cases. That is, it might be argued that if we are to honor life in the clear-cut cases, we cannot allow disrespect to creep in on the borders. This would rid us of the need for the "sanctity" concept even in this limited, last-ditch stand. But I suggest it only as a possibility, the development of which I will spare you.

Conclusion

Many discussions within medical ethics appeal to and pivot on the sanctity of life concept. Yet the really critical issues are hidden by the hulking darkness of that concept. It has been my purpose to bring these submerged structural elements to the surface where they can be explicitly focused on and examined. To this end I discussed the meaning and use of this concept; my arguments were meant to be more suggestive than conclusive. My conclusion is this: the sanctity of life concept as it is generally used—not in its original religious sense—is only a slogan. It not only gives no clear guidance, but it can be positively misleading. There is no place for it in the formal structures of ethics, and what good emphases we can find within the concept are already taken care of by clearer, more defensible rules within ethics. Its best use as a slogan would be as a rhetorical reminder, urging us to weigh life heavily when it is balanced against other goods. And of course we are all for that on solid rational grounds.

There may be another benefit accruing from these reductionist efforts. By showing the secularized sanctity of life concept to be ineffectual, the way has been cleared for the religious meaning of that concept to be reinstated. Freed from the dilution of secular adaptation, this concept can more forcefully assume its pivotal role in the religious stance on these life and death issues.

NOTES

1. Although it might be worthwhile, I am not in this paper distinguishing between "the sanctity of life," "the concept of the sanctity of life," and "the sanctity of life principle." These will be used interchangeably, except where context makes it clearly not so.

2. For an excellent account linking "rationality" and "publicly advocating" in the justification of moral rules, see Bernard Gert, *The Moral Rules: A New Rational Foundation for Morality*, Harper and Row, Publishers, Inc., New York, 1970.

Right to Health Care

12.

Justice, Welfare, and Health Care
Elizabeth Telfer

I shall be examining some of the broad principles which are relevant to discussions as to the proper way to provide health care in the community. Such discussions have taken a very pointed turn in recent years, for example, in regard to the "pay beds" issue. The state of that practical issue is changing all the time; so I shall not attempt to relate what I say at all closely to the present state of play. Rather I hope to elucidate some of the background of ideas against which the protagonists in that debate pursue their argument.

In my discussion I shall assume the principle that the state is responsible for the health of the citizens, in the sense that it is bound, insofar as the community's resources permit, to see that it is possible for everyone who needs it to secure medical care. The detailed analysis of this principle, whether in terms of needs, rights, or justice, is a matter of controversy, but in broad outline the principle is entailed by any political philosophy which ascribes to a government the positive function of furthering the welfare

of its citizens; and such a political philosophy is readily accepted by all but extremists at the present time. Assuming this principle, then, I shall examine the various ways in which a government might try to implement its obligation to see that everyone gets the opportunity of health care. There are of course many possibilities here, but I think four broad types can be distinguished, which I shall call, respectively, laissez-faire, liberal humanitarian, liberal socialist, and pure socialist. I shall briefly describe each system, and then discuss the pros and cons of each.

Four Possible Systems of Health Care

The laissez-faire system leaves medical care entirely to private enterprise. Those who can afford it pay for their medical treatment on a business footing, either directly or through insurance schemes. The needy are looked after, if at all, by private charities. The government interferes only to the extent that it interferes in other commercial enter-

Source: *Journal of Medical Ethics,* vol. 2, no. 3, 1976, p. 107.

This paper owes much to the following: H.B. Acton, *The Morals of Markets,* Longman Group, London, 1971 (especially Chapters III and IV), and Brian Barry, *Political Argument* (Chapter VII), Routledge and Kegan Paul, London, 1965.

prises: that is to say, it enforces contracts, hears suits for damage, and tries to prevent fraud—perhaps in this case by insisting on qualifications of some kind for medical practitioners. The liberal humanitarian system is a modification of this. Those who can afford it pay for themselves, as before. But the needy are looked after not by private charity but by the state, using funds obtained by taxing the less needy. The liberal socialist scheme is what we have in Britain today. Everyone, or everyone who is able, has to contribute to a state scheme which provides for his medical care. But he may if he wishes pay also for private medicine. There can of course be systems between the liberal humanitarian and the liberal socialist, whereby everyone may belong to the state system but anyone may instead if he wishes opt out both of benefiting from it and also from all or part of his share of paying for it. Lastly there is pure socialism, which is what some now advocate: the complete abolition by law of non-state medicine.

I shall take it that the laissez-faire system is agreed to be inadequate; indeed, under such a system the state would in my view be abrogating its responsibilities toward the needy. It is true that the needy might be very well provided for if there were a strong enough tradition of charity of this kind. But it seems too haphazard a basis for such an important service. In any case, it might be said that the opportunity for health care is owed to everyone as a basic human right; if this is so, receiving it should not have to depend on people's goodwill, however forthcoming that goodwill is. Of course, replacing a laissez-faire system with one of the others might mean a loss of that worthwhile thing, exercise of the motive of charity. But there are some things which are so important that getting them done properly is more important than getting them done inadequately from the right motive. In any case, scope would remain on any scheme for the exercise of charity. We have today, for example, charities which support medical research, and which may feel justified in pursuing projects with a high risk of failure which those

bodies using taxpayers' extorted money feel unjustified in supporting.

I turn then to a consideration of the more plausible schemes. My strategy will be to mention first some of the advantages people have advanced in favor of liberal humanitarianism, and the criticisms made of it from a socialist point of view. Then I shall turn to the advantages and disadvantages of socialism, considering the liberal and pure versions together for the time being. Finally I shall touch on the vexed and topical question of liberal versus pure socialism.

The Liberal Humanitarian Scheme of Health Care

The first advantage attributed to the liberal humanitarian scheme is that it meets everyone's needs with minimum coercion: people are constrained only to the extent of paying taxes for the needy and not made to contribute to their own good, a practice which smacks of unwarranted interference. Second, it is said that resources are more usefully distributed: state aid can be concentrated on those who really need special help, and those who are paying for their own services will have an incentive not to squander them, as they do not have under a state scheme.

The third and fourth advantages of the liberal humanitarian scheme are what may be called moral, rather than merely medical. The third is the advantage of preserved incentive. People are encouraged to work harder if they can get what they need only by working, and discouraged if extra work brings no extra reward. Having an incentive to work hard is a double advantage: it benefits the community by increasing prosperity and it cultivates industriousness in the individual's character. The fourth advantage is similarly one of development of character: to have to decide for oneself how to manage such an important department of one's life develops a sense of responsibility and powers of decision.

In criticizing this system, the socialist can first point to the problem posed for the liberal humanitarian by those who are perfectly well able to provide for themselves, by means of private insurance, but neglect to do so. If they fall ill, even the liberal humanitarian will have to admit that the state must look after them; it is unfair that they should receive this benefit without paying for it, but one cannot leave a man to die because he has been improvident. The socialist can say that for him there is no problem, because everyone has to pay his way.

The second socialist criticism is a denial that the medical needs of the average man can in fact be met by a noncoercive liberal scheme, on the ground that the average man, not just the needy man, could not afford to pay for modern medicine individually, even if he had in his control all that part of his money which at present the state takes from him for general medical care. This assertion, if true, would be a knock-down argument against liberal humanitarianism. I shall not discuss it in detail, as it depends on economic rather than philosophical arguments. One point in its favor is that the distinction on which the liberal humanitarian scheme really rests, between being and not being too poor to buy necessities, does not apply to medical care even roughly, because one person's basic necessities in medical care may be vastly more expensive than another person's luxuries.

There may therefore be those who, although quite well off, will not be able to afford, or even necessarily afford the premiums to cover, what is medically necessary for them. At best, then, a scheme which really meets people's needs will require state subsidies not merely for the poorest but also for the illest; and this is already a departure from the basic liberal humanitarian scheme. Apart from this, the question whether a private system would be cheap enough for the consumer depends on such things as the way in which, and the scale on which, it is organized; the level of doctor's fees in such a system; and so on. I shall say a little on the latter question shortly.

The third criticism is that to have some people recipients of state aid when the majority are paying for themselves creates an unfortunately sharp division between haves and have-nots, the independent and the dependent, which is more blurred when all are in a state scheme. However strongly one might insist on the human right to medical care, those who are given it without paying, when others pay, will feel they are recipients of charity; and this feeling is damaging to self-esteem and embittering to those who cannot help their dependent position.

The fourth socialist criticism of liberal humanitarianism is the most important and the most baffling, since it combines many different strands. It can be expressed by saying that the scheme makes medical care a commercial matter, and this is unsuitable. But why might it be thought to be unsuitable? Medicine is not like love, which logically cannot be bought. People say here that it is wrong to "traffick in" or to "exploit" people's need. This description might, however, apply equally well to those who sell food, or any needed commodity, and no one suggests that they are immoral; a butcher or baker meets a need and in doing so meets his own needs too. There is, all the same, a difference in the medical case, which means that what may be called market safeguards do not protect the patient as well as they do the ordinary consumer. In general, the consumer is not actually suffering, as distinct from needy, and also he understands something of what he is buying; so he can "shop around" and look for cheap goods and services. But a patient will not want to wait and will not know how to judge; so he can very easily be exploited. Nor would an agreed "professional fee" system improve his position; on the contrary, if such fees were fixed at an over-high rate (as is perhaps the case with lawyers now) he would have no chance of finding the most favorable price for medical care.

The liberal humanitarian can agree with all these views but points out that they do not constitute a special difficulty for his scheme as opposed to a socialist one. Given the urgency with which medical care is needed, doctors can on a socialist scheme also blackmail the consumers (here society at large) to pay them too much, so that again everyone suffers. The patient, he will go on, is best safeguarded by a private system, which will at least leave some room for "shopping around"; apart from that he is protected by the compassion and goodwill of the majority of the profession.

Here, however, the socialist tends to retort that the market system implicit in the liberal humanitarian scheme is deficient precisely in that it leaves no room for compassion or goodwill. Those partaking in a market economy (he goes on) are in business to make a profit, and as large a one as possible, just as the consumer is trying to pay as little as possible: that is what the market is all about. Greed, then, rather than compassion, is the motive of the doctor in a liberal humanitarian scheme.

This socialist doctrine is, however, a muddle. It is true that what we may call a pure market transaction can be defined as one in which each party seeks to do as well as possible. But this is an artificial abstraction from actual practice, where what goes on might be a product of all kinds of forces; doctor and patient will both be governed by many nonmarket considerations in arriving at a fee. It is also true as a matter of fact that the doctor in commercial medicine must make enough to live on if he is to remain in business; so the bottom end of his scale is fixed. But there is no practical necessity for him to be a pure marketeer, trying to make the largest possible profit, and therefore no reason why his main motive should not be compassion just as much as if he had private means and worked for nothing. Nor does compassion for a person's sufferings entail refusal to take any money from him, any more than sympathy for a stranded motorist entails refusal to accept payment for a gallon of petrol. Of course, a doctor in a laissez-faire system has a problem if his patients are too poor to pay enough even to support him. But in a liberal humanitarian system such patients are subsidized by the state.

I think then that the claim that medicine should not be a commercial matter cannot be sustained in its crude form. But there is nevertheless a difficulty about commercial medicine which arises less obviously in a socialist system: considerations of cost, rather than of need, will obtrude too much into the doctor's medical thinking. Of course, the National Health Service doctor also is constantly being urged to economize. But if he thinks a certain expensive drug or treatment is needed for a patient, not merely useful or beneficial, he can go ahead. With a private patient, however, he will have to think all the time, "Can this patient afford it?" and this must be very inhibiting to the process of making a balanced decision on treatment.

The Socialist System of Health Care

The strengths of the socialist position will already have emerged to some extent through their criticisms of the liberal humanitarian: a socialist scheme can offer very large resources to any individual who needs expensive treatment, in a way which avoids both the stigma suffered by the involuntary noncontributor and the unfair advantages enjoyed by the negligent one. It is also said that a socialist scheme avoids the self-interested motivation of a commercial scheme. But as we have seen there is no need for doctors participating in a commercial scheme to do so out of self-interest. Moreover, there is no reason why doctors, and patients, should not be self-interested in a state scheme: patients wanting more than their share of attention, doctors wanting more and more money. No doubt the philosophy behind the socialist scheme is "from each according to his capacity, to each according to his need"—a kind of fraternal spirit. But there is nothing in the system to ensure that participants in fact see it this way. No doubt they can see their National Insurance contributions and taxes as benefiting the community rather than themselves; but then the liberal humanitarian can see his taxes in that way too.

It is also maintained in favor of a socialist system that it ensures equal treatment for equal needs. This unqualified claim is probably rather optimistic. On a socialist scheme influence, aggressiveness, and articulateness will to some extent win more attention and care than is fair, just as money may do on a commercial scheme. But to claim an advantage over liberal humanitarianism on grounds of equality the socialist has only to show that his scheme has more equal results than the liberal alternative; and this he can probably do. The question does arise, however, what importance is to be attached to achieving equality if everyone's basic needs are met; it might be maintained that above the level of basic needs the demands of equality are rather controversial. The real issue, then, is whether a socialist system meets people's needs more satisfactorily than its rivals. We have seen that where a large expenditure for one person is concerned this may be the case. But many would maintain that a socialist system is necessarily too wasteful of resources to be able to give a satisfactory routine service to all, on the grounds that the removal of any need to pay at the time encourages overextravagant use. How far this common charge is borne out in practice is a question for the sociologist rather than for the philosopher. But it should be noted that "unnecessary" calls upon the doctor's time are often due to ignorance rather than selfishness: an educated person does not think of calling in a doctor for a cold or flu or bleeding nose, not because he is too public-spirited, but because he himself knows what to do. It should therefore be possible for the socialist to lessen abuses without needing the deterrent of payment, by educating the public rather more than doctors at present seem to be willing to do.

I suggest then that the socialist might be able to escape the charge that his system is necessarily inefficient. But there are two other charges that are perhaps even more serious: that a socialist scheme is an unwarranted infringement of liberty, and that it undermines individual responsibility. The first charge is not so easy to maintain as some of those who make it seem to think. Obviously the scheme is a curtailment of liberty; but it would presumably be justified nevertheless if it promoted a great

common good that could be achieved in no other way. The issue of liberty, then, is partly the issue of whether the alternative liberal humanitarian system is economically viable. But even if it were, we must still ask whether the unhappiness of those who are stigmatized under it is a price worth paying for retaining greater freedom. And to this there is no easy answer.

The second criticism is that socialized medicine undermines individual responsibility for health. On a socialist system, it may be said, the state takes over that responsibility for health care which under a private system the individual possesses: the need to plan how his health care (and that of his family) is to be paid for, and to decide his priorities accordingly. Why is this said to be a bad thing? Many reasons are advanced. One is that the individual will come to think that all aspects of health care are now looked after by Them, and so cease to "take responsibility" for those things which on any system only he can provide: a sensible diet, adequate sleep, and so on. Whether this happens in fact is an empirical question; it seems to me likely that those people who do take this kind of responsibility for themselves are too individualistic to be affected one way or the other.

A second reason for criticizing the removal of responsibility is that it trivializes the individual's concern for his life: the more the important areas of life are taken over by the government, the more people see their main business in life as the contriving of amusements. Instead of thinking about health and education, they think about clothes and holidays. Now this is perhaps a tendentious description of the situation: if one were to say that state control of the utilities of life gives people more chance to cultivate their talents and develop their personal relationships, to think about things worthwhile in themselves rather than merely useful, the argument against state control would be less clear. But perhaps most people's capacity to achieve the aristocratic ideal of leisure, as opposed to mere amusements, is limited; if so, it might in general be true that too much socialism leads people to give trivial things undue importance in life.

The third and most important argument advanced against this kind of removal of responsibility is the claim that it saps character. On a liberal humanitarian scheme people have to make decisions and live with the results of them, whereas on a socialist scheme decisions are taken out of their hands. The argument is that a person who does not have to make decisions cannot express his individuality, because it is in making one's own choices, different from anyone else's, that individuality is both shown and fostered; and moreover he loses his autonomy, the capacity for self-determination which makes him a person in the full sense.

The socialist can reply that these considerations apply unqualifiedly only when every area of life is governed by the state; the nationalization of some aspects of life—such as education, housing, health— leaves plenty of scope for individual choice and decision. He might admit that there is even so a measure of deteriorization in character, but think it amply compensated for by the increased benefits; or he might take the line that there is no need to assume that people's characters suffer at all. But even if he is right in this latter claim about what actually happens, the liberal can object on moral grounds: even supposing that character remains intact in a socialist world, is it appropriate to treat adults as though they were like children, capable of deciding only unimportant matters? This is where the liberty and responsibility arguments coincide; liberty, it might be said, is liberty in the exercise of responsibility. Treating people properly involves respecting their liberty, or treating them as responsible creatures. But, as I said earlier, even the claims of liberty may have to bow to those of utility, or of humanity to those who would suffer under a libertarian scheme.

The Liberal Socialist Versus the Pure Socialist Systems of Health Care

I come now to the final section of my discussion: the issue of pure versus liberal socialism. At present our own system is a liberal version, which allows those who wish and are able to do so to buy extra services on a private basis. Many people now advocate that this should be forbidden by law, and pure socialized medicine imposed. The issue is very complex. In Great Britain the question is whether people should be allowed to supplement the services they can get under the National Health Service. But there is also the possibility of a system whereby people can opt out of the National Health Service altogether. I cannot go into the pros and cons of this latter system. Again, even in Great Britain there are two separate questions: whether private medicine in state hospitals should be forbidden, and whether private medicine should be forbidden altogether. I shall not be able to distinguish between these two positions with the exactness which they really require. A further complexity is that the degree of extra service which is available for private purchase varies very much. I shall assume that it consists only of earlier appointments and more leisurely consultations with general practitioners and specialists, freer choice of specialist, prompter hospital treatment for non-emergencies, and more privacy in hospital. Private treatment is not necessarily better in any respect other than these, and the degree to which it is better even in these will vary from place to place.

The usual argument concerns the right to private treatment. But I would suggest that for some people on some occasions private treatment may be not merely a right but a duty. Whatever the arguments against it, they can surely on occasion be morally outweighed, for those who can manage to afford private treatment, by obligations to others: the obligation to be restored to full health quickly and not be a drag on family or colleagues; the obligation to arrange a hospital stay at the least difficult time for family or colleagues; the obligation to continue working in hospital and to secure the privacy which makes this possible. The fact that not everyone can afford private medicine does not absolve those who can from this kind of duty. It would sometimes be true to say, contrary to the normal view, that a person who insisted on public medicine when he could afford private was being selfish and un-public-spirited.

Of course the usual defence of private medicine is in terms not of duties but of rights. People have a right, it is said, to spend their money on what they like: some, it is often added, spend their spare money on bingo or drinking; why should I not spend mine on health insurance? This is basically an appeal to liberty. The mention of those who spend their money on smoking or drinking is an attempt to add considerations of equality. It is salutary to be reminded that there are now a great many ordinary people who could afford private treatment if they gave it high priority. But there are still some who could not, and while this is so, a man cannot claim the right to buy private treatment merely on grounds of equality. What he has to say instead is, Why is it thought that people should be free to spend far more than the poorest can spend on every other kind of goods, but not on medical care?

One reply might be that people should not be free to spend unequally in any sphere: in other words, wealth should be redistributed equally. I have already refused to enter into discussion of this general question and suggested that what is uncontroversial and of paramount importance is the meeting of needs. But this is precisely why some people who are by no means egalitarians in general are against private medicine. The public system, they maintain, does not at present meet people's basic needs, especially their need of reasonably prompt treatment. The so-called extras which private medicine provides are on this view not mere luxuries but basic necessities, open to the rich but too expensive for the poor. Assertions that we are free to buy everything other than medical care are thus beside the point, insofar as there is no

other basic necessity beyond the reach of the poorest.

If this account is true, there are some medical necessities which can at present be got only by paying extra. But it does not follow that everyone's basic needs will more nearly be met if no one is allowed to pay extra. It is said that private patients use up a disproportionate amount of scarce resources; if they were done away with, queues would shorten and beds would multiply. But the extra services they receive are surely small in comparison with the extra money they pay; in other words, they are subsidizing the other patients. Without their money, resources would therefore be scarcer and queues longer, especially as some doctors would leave the profession, or the country, if there were no private patients. I suggest then that private medicine is one of those inequalities which are justified in that everyone, including the worst off, benefits from them.

The sensitive individual may still feel reluctant to avail himself of private medicine, even if he is convinced that the National Health Service can do with his money. I think this is to do with a sense of the fraternity of suffering: a wish not to cut oneself off from fellow-sufferers by having an easier time, even if one's easier time is of use to them. Such a feeling is certainly likable, just as is a person's reluctance to eat his Christmas dinner when he thinks of those who are starving. But if I am right about the value of the private patient's contributions, he should ignore his feelings on this matter.

I have reached few conclusions. As always in real-life issues, the philosophical aspect is too intertwined with the empirical, and the empirical too elusive in any case, to permit any dogmatism. What I have hoped to do is simply to bring out some of the principles at issue in any discussion of the rights and wrongs of socialized medicine.

13.

Medical Care as a Right: A Refutation
Robert M. Sade

The current debate on health care in the United States is of the first order of importance to the health professions, and of no less importance to the political future of the nation, for precedents are now being set that will be applied to the rest of American society in the future. In the enormous volume of verbiage that has poured forth, certain fundamental issues have been so often misrepresented that they have now become commonly accepted fallacies. This paper will be concerned with the most important of these misconceptions, that health care is a right, as well as a brief consideration of some of its corollary fallacies.

Rights—Morality and Politics

The concept of rights has its roots in the moral nature of man and its practical expression in the political system that he creates. Both morality and politics must be discussed before the relation between political rights and health care can be appreciated.

A "right" defines a freedom of action. For instance, a right to a material object is the uncoerced choice of the use to which that object will be put; a right to a specific action, such as free speech, is the freedom to engage in that activity without forceful repression. The moral foundation of the rights of man begins with the fact that he is a living creature: he has the right to his own life. All other rights are corollaries of this primary one; without the right to life, there can be no others, and the concept of rights itself becomes meaningless.

The freedom to live, however, does not automatically ensure life. For man, a specific course of action is required to sustain his life, a course of action that must be guided by reason and reality and has as its goal the creation or acquistion of material values, such as food and clothing, and intellectual values, such as self-esteem and integrity. His moral system is the means by which he is able to select the values that will support his life and achieve his happiness.

Man must maintain a rather delicate homeostasis in a highly demanding and threatening environment, but has at his disposal a unique and efficient mechanism for dealing with it: his mind. His mind is able to perceive, to identify percepts, to integrate them into concepts, and to use those concepts in choosing actions suitable to the maintenance of his life. The rational function of mind is volitional, however; a man must *choose* to think, to be aware, to evaluate, to make conscious decisions. The extent to which he is able to achieve his goals will be directly proportional to his commitment to reason in seeking them.

The right to life implies three corollaries: the right to select the values that one deems necessary to sustain one's own life; the right to exercise one's own judgment of the best course of action to achieve the chosen values; and the right to dispose of those values, once gained, in any way one chooses, without coercion by other men. The denial of any one of these corollaries severely compromises or destroys the right to life itself. A man who is not allowed to choose his own goals, is prevented from setting his own course in achieving those goals and is not free to dispose of the values he has earned, is no less than a slave to those who usurp those rights. The right to private property, therefore, is essential and indispensable to maintaining free men in a free society.

Thus, it is the nature of man as a living,

Source: *New England Journal of Medicine*, vol. 285, no. 23, p. 1288, Dec. 2, 1971.

thinking being that determines his rights—his "natural rights." The concept of natural rights was slow in dawning on human civilization. The first political expression of that concept had its beginnings in 17th and 18th century England through such exponents as John Locke and Edmund Burke, but came to its brilliant debut as a form of government after the American Revolution. Under the leadership of such men as Thomas Paine and Thomas Jefferson, the concept of man as a being sovereign unto himself, rather than a subdivision of the sovereignty of a king, emperor, or state, was incorporated into the formal structure of government for the first time. Protection of the lives and property of individual citizens was the salient characteristic of the Constitution of 1787. Ayn Rand has pointed out that the principle of protection of the individual against the coercive force of government made the United States the first moral society in history.

In a free society, man exercises his right to sustain his own life by producing economic values in the form of goods and services that he is, or should be, free to exchange with other men who are similarly free to trade with him or not. The economic values produced, however, are not given as gifts by nature but exist only by virtue of the thought and effort of individual men. Goods and services are thus owned as a consequence of the right to sustain life by one's own physical and mental effort.

If the chain of natural rights is interrupted, and the right to a loaf of bread, for example, is proclaimed as primary (avoiding the necessity of earning it), every man owns a loaf of bread, regardless of who produced it. Since ownership is the power of disposal,[1] every man may take his loaf from the baker and dispose of it as he wishes with or without the baker's permission. Another element has thus been introduced into the relation between men: the use of force. It is crucial to observe who has initiated the use of force: it is the man who demands unearned bread as a right, not the man who produced it. At the level of an unstructured society it is

clear who is moral and who immoral. The man who acted rationally by producing food to support his own life is moral. The man who expropriated the bread by force is immoral.

To protect this basic right to provide for the support of one's own life, men band together for their mutual protection and form governments. This is the only proper function of government: to provide for the defense of individuals against those who would take their lives or property by force. The state is the repository for retaliatory force in a just society wherein the only actions prohibited to individuals are those of physical harm or the threat of physical harm to other men. The closest that man has ever come to achieving this ideal of government was in this country after its War of Independence.

When a government ignores the progression of natural rights arising from the right to life, and agrees with a man, a group of men, or even a majority of its citizens, that every man has a right to a loaf of bread, it must protect that right by the passage of laws ensuring that everyone gets his loaf—in the process depriving the baker of the freedom to dispose of his own product. If the baker disobeys the law, asserting the priority of his right to support himself by his own rational disposition of the fruits of his mental and physical labor, he will be taken to court by force or threat of force where he will have more property forcibly taken from him (by fine) or have his liberty taken away (by incarceration). Now the initiator of violence is the government itself. The degree to which a government exercises its monopoly on the retaliatory use of force by asserting a claim to the lives and property of its citizens is the degree to which it has eroded its own legitimacy. It is a frequently overlooked fact that behind every law is a policeman's gun or a soldier's bayonet. When that gun and bayonet are used to initiate violence, to take property, or to restrict liberty by force, there are no longer any rights, for the lives of the citizens belong to the state. In a just society with a moral government, it is clear that the only "right" to the bread belongs to the baker, and that a claim by any other man to that right is unjustified and can be enforced only by violence or the threat of violence.

Rights—Politics and Medicine

The concept of medical care as the patient's right is immoral because it denies the most fundamental of all rights, that of a man to his own life and the freedom of action to support it. Medical care is neither a right nor a privilege: it is a service that is provided by doctors and others to people who wish to purchase it. It is the provision of this service that a doctor depends upon for his livelihood, and is his means of supporting his own life. If the right to health care belongs to the patient, he starts out owning the services of a doctor without the necessity of either earning them or receiving them as a gift from the only man who has the right to give them: the doctor himself. In the narrative above substitute "doctor" for "baker" and "medical service" for "bread." American medicine is now at the point in the story where the state has proclaimed the non-existent "right" to medical care as a fact of public policy, and has begun to pass the laws to enforce it. The doctor finds himself less and less his own master and more and more controlled by forces outside of his own judgment. . . .

Any doctor who is forced by law to join a group or a hospital he does not choose, or is prevented by law from prescribing a drug he thinks is best for his patient, or is compelled by law to make any decision he would not otherwise have made, is being forced to act against his own mind, which means forced to act against his own life. He is also being forced to violate his most fundamental professional commitment, that of using his own best judgment at all times for the greatest benefit of his patient. It is remarkable that this principle has never been identified by a public voice in the medical profession, and that the vast majority of doctors in this country are being led down the path to civil servitude, never

knowing that their feelings of uneasy foreboding have a profoundly moral origin, and never recognizing that the main issues at stake are not those being formulated in Washington, but are their own honor, integrity, and freedom, and their own survival as sovereign human beings.

Some Corollaries

The basic fallacy that health care is a right has led to several corollary fallacies, among them the following:

That health is primarily a community or social rather than an individual concern. [2] A simple calculation from American mortality statistics [3] quickly corrects that false concept: 67 percent of deaths in 1967 were due to diseases known to be caused or exacerbated by alcohol, tobacco smoking, or overeating, or were due to accidents. Each of those factors is either largely or wholly correctable by individual action. Although no statistics are available, it is likely that morbidity, with the exception of common respiratory infections, has a relation like that of mortality to personal habits and excesses.

That state medicine has worked better in other countries than free enterprise has worked here. There is no evidence to support that contention, other than anecdotal testimonials and the spurious citation of infant mortality and longevity statistics. There is, on the other hand, a good deal of evidence to the contrary. [4,5]

That the provision of medical care somehow lies outside the laws of supply and demand, and that government-controlled health care will be free care. In fact, no service or commodity lies outside the economic laws. Regarding health care, market demand, individual want, and medical need are entirely different things, and have a very complex relation with the cost and the total supply of available care, as recently discussed and clarified by Jeffers et al. [6] They point out that "'health is purchaseable', meaning that somebody has to pay for it, individually or collectively, at the expense of forgoing the current or future consumption of other things." The question is whether the decision of how to allocate the consumer's dollar should belong to the consumer or to the state. It has already been shown that the choice of how a doctor's services should be rendered belongs only to the doctor: in the same way the choice of whether to buy a doctor's service rather than some other commodity or service belongs to the consumer as a logical consequence of the right to his own life.

That opposition to national health legislation is tantamount to opposition to progress in health care. Progress is made by the free interaction of free minds developing new ideas in an atmosphere conducive to experimentation and trial. If group practice really is better than solo, we will find out because the success of groups will result in more groups (which has, in fact, been happening); if prepaid comprehensive care really is the best form of practice, it will succeed and the health industry will swell with new Kaiser-Permanente plans. But let one of these or any other form of practice become the law, and the system is in a straitjacket that will stifle progress. Progress requires freedom of action, and that is precisely what national health legislation aims at restricting.

That doctors should help design the legislation for a national health system, since they must live with and within whatever legislation is enacted. To accept this concept is to concede to the opposition its philosophic premises, and thus to lose the battle. The means by which nonproducers and hangers-on throughout history have been able to expropriate material and intellectual values from the producers has been identified only relatively recently: the sanction of the victim. Historically, few people have lost their freedom and their rights without some degree of complicity in the plunder. If the American medical profession accepts the concept of health care as the right of the patient, it will have earned the Kennedy-Griffiths bill by default. The alternative for any health professional is to withhold his sanction and make clear who is being victimized. Any physician can say to those who would shackle his judgment and control his profession: I do not recognize your right to my life and my mind, which belong to me and me alone; I will not participate in any legislated solution to any health problem.

In the face of the raw power that lies behind government programs, nonparticipation is the only way in which personal values can be maintained. And it is only with the attainment of the highest of those values—integrity, honesty, and self-esteem—that the physician can achieve his most important professional value, the absolute priority of the welfare of his patients.

The preceding discussion should not be interpreted as proposing that there are no problems in the delivery of medical care. Problems such as high cost, few doctors, low quantity of available care in economically depressed areas may be real, but it is naïve to believe that governmental solutions through coercive legislation can be anything but shortsighted and formulated on the basis of political expediency. The only long-range plan that can hope to provide for the day after tomorrow is a "nonsystem"—that is, a system that proscribes the imposition by force (legislation) of any one group's conception of the best forms of medical care. We must identify our problems and seek to solve them by experimentation and trial in an atmosphere of freedom from compulsion. Our sanction of anything less will mean the loss of our personal values, the death of our profession, and a heavy blow to political liberty.

NOTES

1. A. Rand, *Man's Rights, Capitalism: The Unknown Ideal,* p. 320, New American Library, Inc., New York, 1967.

2. J.S. Millis, "Wisdom? Health? Can Society Guarantee Them?" *New England Journal of Medicine,* vol. 283, p. 260, 1970.

3. Department of Health, Education, and Welfare, Public Health Service, *Vital Statistics of the United States 1967,* vol. II, Mortality, Part A, p. 1,

Government Printing Office, Washington, D.C., 1969.

4. H. Shoeck (ed.), *Financing Medical Care: An Appraisal of Foreign Programs*, Caxton Printers, Inc., Caldwell, Idaho, 1962.

5. M.J. Lynch and S.S. Raphael, *Medicine and the State*, Charles C Thomas, Springfield, Ill., 1963.

6. J.R. Jeffers, M.F. Bognanno, J.C. Bartlett, "On the Demand versus Need for Medical Services and the Concept of 'Shortage,'" *American Journal of Public Health,* vol. 61, p. 46, 1971.

II. CLINICAL IDEALS AND BEHAVIOR

This section presents a selection of readings unique in readers on biomedical ethics. It has been designed with the goal of providing an intensive view of the professional ideals and the pragmatic norms that govern the behavior of physicians and patients in a general sense, that is, independent of specific clinical situations. The articles range from insightful accounts of real behavior developed by sociologists, to normative presentations of ideals of professional conduct by physicians and philosophers. We have not included selections which primarily debate the adequacy of specific ideals or norms. The usual philosophical essays of analysis and reconstruction of a "debate" are absent. Instead it is expected that these selections will be read as primary material about which the course instructor can raise a variety of ethical questions. The point is to have the philosophical work done in the class by working upon these materials.

The section is composed of five parts. Each provides a different perspective on the norms, expectations, and commitments assumed by the participants in medical care situations. Although in one sense there is no medical care without both a physician and a patient (and usually a nurse, a hospital, etc.), in becoming a physician an individual becomes committed to a set of ideals that constitute his or her professional identity. These are discussed in the first part as "Ideals and Models of the Physician-Patient Relationship." Also included are accounts that model the relationship against a pattern of ideals. The next part on "Roles and Norms" has three subsections which review the notion of "authority" and then discuss the specific expectations and performances as exhibited by both doctors and patients. The part on "Professional-Patient Communication" scrutinizes communication as the fundamental general feature of the health care relationship, one that goes beyond technical medical interventions for caring and curing. The fourth part, "Institutional Responsibility," discusses questions generated by the institutional context of health care as it occurs in hospitals and prisons. The last part, "Professional Accountability," provides both extensive legal material on the responsibilities of physicians as developed in case law as well as discussions of the accountability of physicians to their patients when "advocacy" may be at issue.

Ideals and Models of the
Physician–Patient Relationship

The selections by Pellegrino and Szasz address the basic ideals governing the role of the physician in society. In his essay, Pellegrino carefully analyzes the identity of the physician as being based upon an elaboration of four fundamental concepts: "profession, patient, compassion, and consent." He provides a deft analysis of these notions during the course of which he rejects the popular term "client" as inappropriate for the doctor-patient relationship. By contrast Szasz focuses his discussion upon Plato's account of physicians and the nature of their relationship to patients and to the state. He reviews the general foundations of the duties of physicians with special attention to the paternalism inherent in the Platonic account. He concludes with a critique of the views that would hold experts and professionals as independent of other institutional allegiances and calls for a policy mandating the explicit declaration of other loyalties.

The selections by Freidson and Parson are sociological accounts of how the doctor-patient relationship is based upon implicit roles toward which people attempt to conform their behavior. Freidson's brief selection describes the highly individualistic character of the physician's role, and Parson's classic account provides the standard description of the patient's role as well as accounts of the medical situation and the physician's role. Although much discussed, selections from Parson's original work are usually absent from readers in medical ethics.

The section concludes with two articles which present the doctor-patient relationship as fundamentally an interpersonal one. Bayles reviews several models, including the agency, contract, friendship, paternalist, and fiduciary relationships. Unlike Pellegrino, he favors the use of the notion of "client." Fried argues for a version of a friendship model which he terms the good of "personal care." He concludes by discussing four fundamental rights that are generated by his account, viz., lucidity, autonomy, fidelity, and humanity. (See cases 7, 14, 18, 23, 25, 26, 27, *28*, 31, 44, 45, 47, 48, 49, *53, 65, 66, 67*, 69, *71*, 72, 74.)

14.

To Be a Physician   Edmund D. Pellegrino

Wheresoever manners and fashions are corrupted,
language is. It imitates the public riot.
—Ben Jonson

The world we perceive is the world we see through words
. . . hence the importance of teaching language
not so much as grammar as behaviour.
—Ashley Montagu

Authenticity is revealed ultimately in what we *are,* and this, in turn, by what we think it means to *be* a physician. Our being is revealed very often by what we take the words to mean which we use to justify our acts.

If we are to know something about what it is to *be* a physician, four words in common parlance are in need of rehabilitation: the words *profession, patient, compassion,* and *consent.* They are so ubiquitous in the speech of physician and patient that we all imagine we know what they mean. Yet language, as Jean Paul said, is "a cloud which everyone sees in a different shape." It is essential, therefore, for every physician to contemplate more closely the shape of the clouds these words make when he utters them.

Profession

The first word is *profession.* With the receipt of the M.D. degree, the student officially becomes a member of a profession. In sociological terms, the student joins a body of individuals sharing certain specific knowledge, rules of conduct, ideals, and entry requirements. Some are impressed with their entry into a privileged social group which

automatically entitles them to a certain respect, a wide discretionary space in decision making and considerable authority over others. The more crass may even rejoice in the license to charge fees for what only yesterday they did for nothing.

While each of these construals of the word has a certain truth, the original meaning is much more powerful, and specific, to being a physician. It comes from the Latin word *profiteri,* to declare aloud, to make a public avowal. It entered English in the thirteenth century, or thereabouts, to signify the act of public avowal and entry into a religious order. It was a public declaration of belief and an intent to practice certain ideals. In the sixteenth century, it included the public declaration of possession of certain skills to be placed in the service of others, as in the profession of medicine, law, or ministry. The word was visibly distorted in the nineteenth century when the language of an industrial society infected our parlance. A profession became simply a prestigious occupation. Instead of commitment, we began to talk of efficiency, productivity, utility—in Marxist as well as capitalist societies.

When a student consciously accepts his degree he makes a public avowal that he possesses competence to heal and that he will

Source: Edmund D. Pellegrino, *Humanism and the Physician,* University of Tennessee Press, Knoxville, 1979. This chapter is an amalgam of the following: "To Be a Physician," Convocation Address given at Texas A&M University in October 1977; and "Profession, Patient, Compassion, Consent: Meditations on Medical Philology," which was presented as the Commencement Address at the Hippocratic Oath Ceremony, University of California, Los Angeles, on June 3, 1977, and appeared in *Connecticut Medicine,* vol. 42, no. 3, p. 175, March 1978.

do so for the benefit of those who come to him. In that declaration, he binds himself publicly to competence as a moral obligation, not simply a legal one; he places the well-being of those he presumes to help above his own personal gain. If these two considerations do not shape every medical act and every encounter with the patient, the "pro-fession" becomes a lie: the physician is a fraud and his whole enterprise is undiluted hypocrisy.

These are strong words, but they derive ineluctably from the expectations engendered in others by the act of pro-fession—the personal and public voluntary acceptance of the obligations one is willing to assume in accepting a medical degree. This is the essence of the oaths—whether of Hippocrates, Maimonides, or any of the others—traditionally administered at graduations. These oaths are not meaningless condescensions to tradition but living witnesses to society of a personal commitment.

A few years ago, it was popular for medical graduates to refuse to take *any* oath. To their credit they took the oath seriously enough to resist when they could not agree with its content. I hope the more placid acquiescence of today is not evidence of moral lassitude or lack of the courage to dissent.

The physician remakes his pro-fession every time he dares to offer himself to a patient. The obligation is unavoidable. It leaves little room for incompetence, selfishness, or even legitimate personal concerns like fatigue, lack of time, or the demands of family. It is inconsistent with the prevalent bureaucratic ethos which buries individual acts in the faults of society, institutions, or, the "team." We must not be "auxiliary bureaucrats," the term Gabriel Marcel used for those in a mass society who excuse themselves as mere functionaries.

If our pro-fessions had, up to now, been authentic in the pristine sense, we would have less malpractice, governmental regulation, and consumerism to worry about. It is the actual or perceived failure to act in accordance with the full meaning of the word *pro-fession* which underlies much of the public disquietude with medicine today.

Patient

The next word to examine is *patient,* another badly tortured word whose original meaning has also been seriously attenuated. The Latin root is *patior-pati*—to suffer, to bear something. It was first used in its medical sense by Chaucer. A person becomes a patient when, in his perception of his own existence, he passes some point of tolerance for a symptom or a debility and seeks out another person who has professed to help. The patient bears and suffers something, and his expectation is that every act of the physician will be to relieve him of that burden and restore his lost wholeness—which is, incidentally, the meaning of the Anglo-Saxon word *heal.*

The patient therefore is a petitioner, a human in distress, and an especially vulnerable human. He enters a relationship of inequality. He is in pain, anxious, and lacking in the knowledge and skill necessary to heal himself or to make the decision about what is best for him. The person who has become a patient thus loses some of the most precious of human freedoms—freedom to move about as he wishes, to make his own decisions rationally, and freedom from the power of other persons. The patient bears, in a real sense, the burden of a wounded and afflicted humanity.

The patient is not a "client," a word appearing with distressing frequency in medical and medico-legal writing. *Client* is from the word *cliens* and has a lineage dating back to Roman times. The word referred to a plebeian and in the Middle Ages to a vassal under the protection of a patrician or lord. The client paid certain homage and performed services to the lord in return for this protection. Today, the client is a customer. It is alarming to see how the spirit of this word has come to pollute the relationship of physician and patient and how insensitive we have become to the original sense of what it means to be a patient.

Physicians all too frequently interpret the word "patient" to mean long-suffering or enduring trouble without discontent or complaint, a trait they ascribe to a "cooperative" patient. There are even a few physicians who see patients as their vassals, paternalistically protecting them in the distorted notion of their own moral authority, making decisions for rather than with the patient, and demanding compliant behavior from those they serve. We even talk, in a distorted way, of "educating" patients, meaning that they must conform to our notions of how to behave in illness.

Compassion

If we understand, and feel, the full meaning of the word *patient,* then we can also understand another word so often tortured on the rack of misuse—compassion. The word is simply a derivation of the same root, *patior,* which gives us the word "patient." It means, literally, to suffer with, to bear together, to share in another's distress, and to be moved by desire to relieve distress.

Compassion is not some facile combination of talents in public relations under the rubric of bedside manner; nor is it some mystical quality or charisma which radiates only from the gifted; nor again is it synonymous with mawkish or demeaning pity for the sick, or a saccharine piety and self-righteousness. These construals are all offensive to true compassion and an insult to the wounded humanity of the patient.

Compassion means to feel genuinely the existential situation of the person who is bearing the burden and who has undergone the insult of sickness to his whole being. We can never enter wholly into the state of being of another human, but we must strive with all our might to *feel* it to the fullest extent our sensibilities will allow. It is our failure to feel along with the patient that leads to the complaint we hear so often today of humiliation and being demeaned.

Consent

If we understand the full flavor of meanings of *profession, patient,* and *compassion,* then we can easily understand the last word so prevalent in current legal and moral dis-

course, *consent.* Here, the Latin root is *sentire,* a word which has two senses: one in the emotional and physical sense and the other in an intellectual sense. Therefore, *consent* is to *feel* together and to *know* something together.

Con-sent grows out of a human interaction between someone who seeks to know what to do and one who advises what should be done. It is not the mere satisfaction of some legal formality, a signature on a piece of paper duly witnessed. Con-sent demands, rather, that action be taken from the ground *between* patient and physician. Both must feel the action is the right one, and both must agree on the basis of knowledge that it is a rational choice as well.

Consent of this quality is morally indispensable if we only think of the vulnerable state of the patient and the inequality of the relationship with the physician. The obligation to obtain con-sent flows from the fact of being a pro-fessed healer, one who purports to repair wounded humanity. The physician must restore as much of the patient's lost freedom as possible. That means making available the knowledge—the alternatives and probabilities—necessary to a free and human decision to take one course as opposed to another, or to reject what the physician proposes.

But even these crucial four words express something which is still peripheral to the innermost center of humanistic medicine. Two more words must engage our reflections: *being* and *having,* and the difficult but crucial distinction between them.

Gabriel Marcel, the French philosopher, critic, and dramatist, said that "Everything really comes down to the distinction between what we *have,* and what we *are.*" This is not one of those meaningless messages so appealing to the minds of middle-aged moralists. Rather, it is a distillation of the dilemmas we face as persons and institutions in forming an authentic image of ourselves, one in which we and others can believe.

Without indulging in all the complex subtleties of Marcel's thought, what he seems to be saying is this: to *have* something is to hold ownership and control over a thing acquired from without. Whether it is a profession, an idea, an education, or a fortune, what we *have* is always external to our being; it can never enter into or define the infinitely greater mystery of what we are. No matter how impressive the things we *have,* they must not be our identity. If they are, then we lose the chance to *be* something. We lose the freedom of a personal choice and testimony. It is we who put our possessions to use and not our possessions that use us.

Physicians have a medical education, an M.D. degree, a set of skills, knowledge, prestige, titles. They *possess* many things by which they may mistakenly identify themselves and their profession. Many of the health professions—medicine included—confuse the possession of packets of knowledge, a white coat, or a technique with *being* a physician or healer.

Whatever else it may be, medicine comes fully into existence as medicine only in the moment of clinical truth, in the act of making a clinical decision. In this act, the physician chooses a right healing action, one that will restore health or contain established disease or prevent new disease. Among the many things that can be done, the focal point on which all medical activity converges is a choice of those that should be done for this person, at this time, and in this life situation. The right decision is the one that is *good* for this patient—not patients in general, nor what is good for physicians, for science, or even for society as a whole.

As soon as we introduce the word *right* with respect to action and *good* with respect to an end, we introduce morality—some system of strongly held beliefs against which behavior is to be judged as good or bad. Medicine is, therefore, at the root a moral enterprise because values enter into every decision. The physician's art and science are necessarily shaped by the special human relationship between a vulnerable person seeking to be healed and another professing to heal.

All health professionals participate to some degree in this central function of medicine. But it is the physician who stands closest to the point of convergence of the whole process, and thus he has the broadest moral responsibility. The closer we are to this moral center, the more we are physicians; the farther from it, or the narrower the range factors to be integrated, the less we are physicians, no matter how sophisticated our technical knowledge.

Whichever of the many conceptions of medicine one selects, one can be a physician only if one satisfies the essence of the medical act: to make a right choice that is "best" for this patient. Others may carry out the procedures required—and they need not be physicians at all—but what medicine uniquely *is,* is the capability morally to manage the clinical moment.

To *be* a physician is freely to commit oneself to the moral center of the relationship with the patient and to do so with one's whole person—that is the only condition for freedom, as Bergson so rightly observed. This is neither too harsh nor too simplistic a judgment. The malaise of medicine—the moral desuetude so many see in us and the bewilderment of our students about what we *are*—is rooted in our failure to sense the dimension of *being* a physician.

Without this dimension, even the idea of service can become degraded into mere performance of a function. Many of us function, but few serve. To transform functions into service we need what Marcel called attachment: "dedication to the intrinsic quality of what is done, its adaptation to the needs of the person served and personal accountability for its quality."

We cannot distinguish *having* from *being* without the capacity for critical self-examination. This is what the humanities—philosophy, history, literature at their best—have always taught the educated man. These studies are therefore tools of that intellectual and moral honesty which gives the lie to self-assurance and forces a constant reexamination of motives and values. There is no more effective antidote to the overweening pride that can so easily beset the physician.

15.
The Character of Physicians   Eliot Freidson

Any set of rules, prescriptive as well as proscriptive, is based on a set of assumptions about the persons involved—assumptions about their mental and physical capacities, their moral inclinations, their essential motivation to perform and conform, their capacity for change, and the like. The law, for example, is predicated upon an image of conscious, calculating, knowledgeable persons whose behavior may be influenced by the deterrence of known penalties for apprehension and conviction. In its treatment of offenses by those judged insane, juvenile, physically handicapped, or otherwise not normal persons, the law makes specific exceptions predicated on its assumptions about the character of these excepted persons. As in the law, so it is in the informal rules and regulations of a medical group. The physicians in the medical group seem to share a very special conception of themselves. They assume that the physicians are essentially ethical, conscientious, and competent, these qualities being organized into an individually expressed but stable pattern of behavior. From this follows the fundamental rule that one owes one's colleagues (and is owed by them) respect, trust, and protection unless overwhelming evidence points to the contrary.

The physician is seen as a person whose work behavior was laid down at some time in the past. Part of such behavior is an immutable function of personality. Such behavior cannot be changed in any significant way and can be only accepted and lived with.

Apparently this colleague of mine's behavior with respect to family doctors has quieted down. I haven't gotten as many complaints about him as I used to get the first year. And it is not for me to say what his problems are. I'm not a psychiatrist. I can guess that he hasn't really grown up yet. So this is a question of personality, which to me is something you live with.

Personality manifests itself in the way a physician manages his patients and also in such elements of work as the ostensibly technical matter of ordering laboratory tests.

As to those even who have been out of school for a long time who order a lot of tests, nothing can be done about them. You cannot change the individual. Some people want to have all kinds of tests, even if the chances of their revealing something are quite remote. And others are more apt to go without them.

Such elements of work style as the ordering of laboratory tests are also seen as a matter of taste, which relies on the idea that each individual exercises his free judgment and is essentially incomparable with any other in his choices. The pure individualism of the physicians, an individualism that is not a mere difference so much as an assertion of autonomy stemming from their work, is stressed.

Physicians are individualists basically in their work whether they work for a group or not. You are working as an individual with your patient, and this is your day-to-day work. Whatever your natural reactions are, whether you are on salary or in solo practice, you are still an individualist.

Source: Eliot Freidson, *Doctoring Together,* American Elsevier, New York, 1975.

16.

The Functional Setting of Medical Practice and the Cultural Tradition

Talcott Parsons

In the most general terms medical practice may be said to be oriented to coping with disturbances to the "health" of the individual, with "illness" or "sickness." Traditionally, the principal emphasis has been on "treatment" or "therapy," that is, on dealing with cases which have already developed a pathological state, and attempting to restore them to health or normality. Recently there has been increasing emphasis on "preventive medicine," that is, controlling the conditions which produce illness. For our purposes, however, the therapeutic functional context will present sufficient problems.

A little reflection will show immediately that the problem of health is intimately involved in the functional prerequisites of the social system as defined above. Certainly by almost any definition health is included in the functional needs of the individual member of the society so that from the point of view of functioning of the social system, too low a general level of health, too high an incidence of illness, is dysfunctional. This is in the first instance because illness incapacitates for the effective performance of social roles. It could of course be that this incidence was completely uncontrollable by social action, an independently given condition of social life. But insofar as it is controllable, through rational action or otherwise, it is clear that there is a functional interest of the society in its control, broadly in the minimization of illness.

All this would be true were illness purely a "natural phenomenon" in the sense that, like the vagaries of the weather, it was not, to our knowledge, reciprocally involved in the motivated interactions of human beings. In this case illness would be something which merely "happened to" people, which involved consequences which had to be dealt with and conditions which might or might not be controllable but was in no way an expression of motivated behavior.

This is in fact the case for a very important part of illness but, it has become increasingly clear, by no means for all. In a variety of ways motivational factors accessible to analysis in action terms are involved in the etiology of many illnesses, and conversely, though without exact correspondence, many conditions are open to therapeutic influence through motivational channels. To take the simplest kind of case, differential exposure, to injuries or to infection, is certainly motivated, and the role of unconscious wishes to be injured or to fall ill in such cases has been clearly demonstrated. Then there is the whole range of "psycho-somatic" illness about which knowledge has been rapidly accumulating in recent years. Finally, there is the field of "mental disease," the symptoms of which occur mainly on the behavioral level. At one time most medical opinion inclined to the "reduction" of *all* illness to a physiological and biological level in the sense both that etiology was always to be found on that level, and that only through such channels was effective therapy possible. This is certainly not the predominant medical view today. If it ever becomes possible to remove the hyphen from the term "psycho-somatic" and subsume all of "medical science" under a single conceptual scheme, it can be regarded as certain that it will not be the conceptual scheme of the biological science of the late nineteenth and early twentieth centuries. It is also

Source: Talcott Parsons, *The Social System,* The Free Press, New York, 1951.

certain that this conceptual scheme will prove applicable to a great deal of the range of social action in areas which extend well beyond what has conventionally been defined as the sphere of medical interests.

The fact that the relevance of illness is not confined to the nonmotivated purely situational aspect of social action greatly increases its significance for the social system. It becomes not merely an "external" danger to be "warded off" but an integral part of the social equilibrium itself. Illness may be treated as one mode of response to social pressures, among other things, as one way of evading social responsibilities. But it may also, as will appear, have some possible positive functional significance.

Summing up, we may say that illness is a state of disturbance in the "normal" functioning of the total human individual, including both the state of the organism as a biological system and of his personal and social adjustments. It is thus partly biologically and partly socially defined. Participation in the social system is always potentially relevant to the state of illness, to its etiology, and to the conditions of successful therapy, as well as to other things.

Medical practice as above defined is a "mechanism" in the social system for coping with the illnesses of its members. It involves a set of institutionalized roles which will be analyzed later. But this also involves a specialized relation to certain aspects of the general cultural tradition of modern society. Modern medical practice is organized about the application of scientific knowledge to the problems of illness and health, to the control of "disease." Science is of course a very special type of cultural phenomenon and a really highly developed scientific level in any field is rare among known cultures, with the modern West in a completely unique position. It may also be noted that scientific advance beyond the level to which the Greeks brought it is, in the medical field, a recent phenomenon, as a broad cultural stream not much more than a century old.

We have dealt at some length in Chapter VIII with science as a general feature of the cultural tradition, and with some of the conditions of its application to practical affairs. This need not be repeated here. We need only note a few points particularly relevant to the medical field. First, it should be quite clear that the treatment of illness as a problem for applied science must be considered problematical and not taken for granted as "common sense." The comparative evidence is overwhelming that illness, even a very large part of what to us is obviously somatic illness, has been interpreted in supernatural terms, and magical treatment has been considered to be the appropriate method of coping with it. In nonliterate societies there is an element of empirical lore which may be regarded as proto-scientific, with respect to the treatment of fractures for instance. But the prominence of magic in this field is overwhelmingly great.

This, however, is by no means confined to non-literate cultures. The examples of traditional China and our own Middle Ages will suffice. Where other features of the cultural tradition are not favorable to the traditionalized stereotyping which we think of as characteristic of magic in the full sense, we find a great deal, and sometimes predominance, of health "superstition" in the sense of pseudo rational or pseudo scientific beliefs and practices.

In the light of these considerations it is not surprising that in a society in which scientific medicine has come to be highly institutionalized, popular orientations toward the health problem are by no means confined to the scientific level. There is much popular health superstition, as evidenced by such things as the "patent medicines," for example the widely advertised "Dr. Pierce's Golden Medical Discovery," and many traditional "home remedies." Furthermore in the health field there is a considerable fringe of what are sometimes called "cults." Some religious denominations, of which Christian Science is perhaps the most conspicuous example, include a religious approach to health as an integral part of their general doctrine. Then there is a variety of groups which offer health treatments outside the medical profession and the professions auxiliary to it like dentistry and nursing. These are apt to include complex and bewildering mixtures of scientifically verifiable elements and various grades and varieties of pseudo-science.[1]

Finally the institutionalization of science is, as the analysis of Chapter VIII would lead us to expect, far from complete within the profession itself. There are many kinds of evidence of this, but for present purposes it is sufficient to cite the strong, often bitter resistance from within the profession itself to the acceptance of what have turned out to be critically important scientific advances in their own field. One of the classic cases is the opposition of the French Academy of Medicine to Pasteur, and for some time the complete failure to appreciate the importance of his discoveries. A closely related one is the opposition of the majority of the surgeons of the day to Lister's introduction of surgical asepsis. The conception of "laudable pus" is an excellent example of a medical "superstition."

It goes without saying that there is also an important involvement of expressive symbolism in medical practice. Rather, however, than attempting to review it at this point it will be better to call attention to certain aspects of it as we go along.

The Social Structure

The immediately relevant social structures consist in the patterning of the role of the medical practitioner himself and, though to common sense it may seem superfluous to analyze it, that of the "sick person" himself. There is also a range of important impingements of both roles on other aspects of the total structure of the social system which will have to be mentioned at the appropriate points.

The role of the medical practitioner belongs to the general class of "professional" roles, a subclass of the larger group of occupational roles. Caring for the sick is thus not an incidental activity of other roles—though, for example, mothers do a good deal of

it—but has become functionally specialized as a full-time "job." This, of course, is by no means true of all societies. As an occupational role it is institutionalized about the technical content of the function, which is given a high degree of primacy relative to other status determinants. It is thus inevitable both that incumbency of the role should be achieved and that performance criteria by standards of technical competence should be prominent. Selection for it and the context of its performance are to a high degree segregated from other bases of social status and solidarities. In common with the predominant patterns of occupational roles generally in our society it is therefore in addition to its incorporation of achievement values, universalistic, functionally specific, and affectively neutral. Unlike the role of the businessman, however, it is collectivity-oriented, not self-oriented.

The importance of this patterning is, in one context, strongly emphasized by its relation to the cultural tradition. One basis for the division of labor is the specialization of technical competence. The role of physician is far along the continuum of increasingly high levels of technical competence required for performance. Because of the complexity and subtlety of the knowledge and skill required and the consequent length and intensity of training, it is difficult to see how the functions could, under modern conditions, be ascribed to people occupying a prior status as one of their activities in that status, following the pattern by which, to a degree, responsibility for the health of her children is ascribed to the mother status. There is an intrinsic connection between achieved statuses and the requirements of high technical competence, as well as universalism and competence. In addition, of course, there is pressure in the society to assimilate the medical role to others of similar character in the total occupational system.

High technical competence also implies specificity of function. Such intensive devotion to expertness in matters of health and disease precludes comparable expertness in other fields. The physician is not, by virtue of his modern role, a generalized "wise man" or sage—though there is considerable folklore to that effect—but a specialist whose superiority to his fellows is confined to the specific sphere of his technical training and experience. For example, one does not expect the physician as such to have better judgment about foreign policy or tax legislation than any other comparably intelligent and well-educated citizen. There are, of course, elaborate subdivisions of specialization within the profession.

Affective neutrality is also involved in the physician's role as an applied scientist. The physician is expected to treat an objective problem in objective, scientifically justifiable terms. For example, whether he likes or dislikes the particular patient as a person is supposed to be irrelevant, as indeed it is to most purely objective problems of how to handle a particular disease.

With regard to the pattern variable, self vs. collectivity orientation, the physician's role clearly belongs to what, in our occupational system, is the "minority" group, strongly insisting on collectivity orientation. The "ideology" of the profession lays great emphasis on the obligation of the physician to put the "welfare of the patient" above his personal interests, and regard "commercialism" as the most serious and insidious evil with which it has to contend. The line, therefore, is drawn primarily vis-à-vis "business." The "profit motive" is supposed to be drastically excluded from the medical world. This attitude is, of course, shared with the other professions, but it is perhaps more pronounced in the medical case than in any single one except perhaps the clergy.

In terms of the relation of the physician's occupational role to the total instrumental complex there is an important distinction between two types of physicians: one of the "private practitioner," the other the one who works within the context of organization. The important thing about the former is that he must not only care for sick people in a technical sense, but must take responsibility for settlement of the terms of exchange with them because of his direct dependence on them for payment for his services, and must to a high degree also provide his own facilities for carrying on his function. It is a crucially important fact that expertness in caring for the sick does not imply any special competence one way or another in the settlement of terms of exchange. It may or may not be a good social policy to have costs of medical care, the means of payment for it, and so on settled by the members of the medical profession, as individuals or through organizations, but such a policy cannot be justified on the ground that their special training gives them as physicians a technical competence in these matters which others do not have.

An increasing proportion of medical practice is now taking place in the context of organization. To a large extent this is necessitated by the technological development of medicine itself, above all the need for technical facilities beyond the reach of the individual practitioner, and the fact that treating the same case often involves the complex cooperation of several different kinds of physicians as well as of auxiliary personnel. This greatly alters the relation of the physician to the rest of the instrumental complex. He tends to be relieved of much responsibility and hence necessarily of freedom, in relation to his patients other than in his technical role. Even if a hospital executive is a physician himself, he is not in the usual sense engaged in the "practice of medicine" in performing his functions any more than the president of the Miners' Union is engaged in mining coal.

As was noted, for common sense there may be some question of whether "being sick" constitutes a social role at all—isn't it simply a state of fact, a "condition"? Things are not quite so simple as this. The test is the existence of a set of institutionalized expectations and the corresponding sentiments and sanctions.

There seem to be four aspects of the institutionalized expectation system relative to the sick role. First is the exemption from normal social role responsibilities, which of course is relative to the nature and severity of the illness. This exemption requires legitimation by and to the various alters involved, and the physician often serves as a court of appeal as well as a direct legitimatizing agent. It is noteworthy that like all institutionalized patterns the legitimation of being sick enough to avoid obligations cannot be only a right of the sick person but is an obligation upon him. People are often resistant to admitting they are sick, and it is not uncommon for others to tell them that they *ought* to stay in bed. The word generally has a moral connotation. It goes almost without saying that this legitimation has the social function of protection against "malingering."

The second closely related aspect is the institutionalized definition that the sick person cannot be expected by "pulling himself together" to get well by an act of decision or will. In this sense also he is exempted from responsibility—he is in a condition that must "be taken care of." His "condition" must be changed, not merely his "attitude." Of course, the process of recovery may be spontaneous, but while the illness lasts he can't "help it." This element in the definition of the state of illness is obviously crucial as a bridge to the acceptance of "help."

The third element is the definition of the state of being ill as itself undesirable with its obligation to want to "get well." The first two elements of legitimation of the sick role thus are conditional in a highly important sense. It is a relative legitimation so long as he is in this unfortunate state which both he and alter hope he can get out of as expeditiously as possible.

Finally, the fourth closely related element is the obligation—in proportion to the severity of the condition, of course—to seek *technically competent* help, namely, in the most usual case, that of a physician and to *cooperate* with him in the process of trying to get well. It is here, of course, that the role of the sick person as patient becomes articulated with that of the physician in a complementary role structure.

It is evident from the above that the role of motivational factors in illness immensely broadens the scope and increases the importance of the institutionalized role aspect of being sick. For then the problem of social control becomes much more than one of ascertaining facts and drawing lines. The privileges and exemptions of the sick role may become objects of a "secondary gain" which the patient is positively motivated, usually unconsciously, to secure or to retain. The problem, therefore, of the balance of motivations to recover becomes of first importance. In general motivational balances of great functional significance to the social system are institutionally controlled, and it should therefore not be surprising that this is no exception.

A few further points may be made about the specific patterning of the sick role and its relation to social structure. It is, in the first place, a "contingent" role into which anyone, regardless of his status in other respects, may come. It is, furthermore, in the type case temporary. One may say that it is in a certain sense a "negatively achieved" role, through failure to "keep well," though, of course, positive motivations also operate, which by that very token must be motivations to deviance.

It is inherently universalistic, in that generalized objective criteria determine whether one is or is not sick, how sick, and with what kind of sickness; its focus is thus classificatory not relational. It is also functionally specific, confined to the sphere of health, and particular "complaints" and disabilities within that sphere. It is furthermore affectively neutral in orientation in that the expected behavior, "trying to get well," is focused on an objective problem, not on the cathectic significance of persons,[2] or orientations to an emotionally disturbing problem, though this may be instrumentally and otherwise involved.

The orientation of the sick role vis-à-vis the physician is also defined as collectively oriented. It is true that the patient has a very obvious self-interest in getting well in most cases, though this point may not always be so simple. But once he has called in a physician the attitude is clearly marked, that he has assumed the obligation to cooperate with that physician in what is regarded as a common task. The obverse of the physician's obligation to be guided by the welfare of the patient is the latter's obligation to "do his part" to the best of his ability. This point is clearly brought out, for example, in the attitudes of the profession toward what is called "shopping around." By that is meant the practice of a patient "checking" the advice of one physician against that of another without telling physician A that he intends to consult physician B, or if he comes back to A that he has done so or who B is. The medical view is that if the patient is not satisfied with the advice his physician gives him he may properly do one of two things. First he may request a consultation, even naming the physician he wishes called in, but in that case it is physician A, not the patient, who must call B in. The patient may not see B independently, and above all not without A's knowledge. The other proper recourse is to terminate the relation with A and become "B's patient." The notable fact here is that a pattern of behavior on the part not only of the physician but also of the patient is expected, which is in sharp contrast to perfectly legitimate behavior in a commercial relationship. If he is buying a car there is no objection to the customer's going to a number of dealers before making up his mind, and there is no obligation for him to inform any one dealer what others he is consulting, to say nothing of approaching the Chevrolet dealer only through the Ford dealer.

The doctor-patient relationship is thus focused on these pattern elements. The patient has a need for technical services because he doesn't—nor do his lay associates, family members, etc.—"know" what is the matter or what to do about it, nor does he control the necessary facilities. The physician is a technical expert who by special training and experience, and by an institutionally validated status, is quali-

fied to "help" the patient in a situation institutionally defined as legitimate in a relative sense but as needing help.

In this connection it should be noted that the burdens the physician asks his patients and their families to assume on his advice are often very severe. They include suffering— you "have to get worse before you can get better" as, for instance, in the case of a major surgical operation. They include the risk of death, permanent or lengthy disablement, severe financial costs, and various others. In terms of common sense it can always be said that the patient has the obvious interest in getting well and hence should be ready to accept any measures which may prove necessary. But there is always the question, implicit or explicit, "How do I know this will do any good?" The one thing certain seems to be that the layman's answer to this cannot, in the majority of severe and complex cases, i.e., the "strategic" ones, be based primarily on his own rational understanding of the factors involved and a fully rational weighing of them. The difference from the physician in this respect is often a matter of degree, but it is a crucially important difference of degree.

Finally, third, the situation of illness very generally presents the patient and those close to him with complex problems of emotional adjustment. It is, that is to say, a situation of strain. Even if there is no question of a "physic" factor in his condition, suffering, helplessness, disablement, and the risk of death, or sometimes its certainty, constitute fundamental disturbances of the expectations by which men live. They cannot in general be emotionally "accepted" without the accompaniments of strain with which we are familiar and hence without difficult adjustments unless the patient happens to find positive satisfactions in them, in which case there is also a social problem. The significance of this emotional factor is magnified and complicated insofar as defensive and adjustive mechanisms are deeply involved in the pathological condition itself.

For the normal person the direction of

these alterations is undesirable; they are frustrations. Therefore, it is to be expected that two types of reaction should be prominent, a kind of emotional "shock" at the beginning of illness, and anxiety about the future. In both cases there is reason to believe that most normal persons have an unrealistic bias in the direction of confidence that "everything will be all right"; that is, they are motivated to underestimate the chances of *their* falling ill, especially seriously ill (the minority of hypochondriacs is the obverse), and if they do they tend to overestimate the chances of a quick and complete recovery. Therefore, even the necessary degree of emotional acceptance of the reality is difficult. One very possible reaction is to attempt to deny illness or various aspects of it, to refuse to "give in" to it. Another may be exaggerated self-pity and whining, a complaining demand for more help than is necessary or feasible, especially for incessant personal attention. In any case this factor reinforces the others. It makes it doubly difficult for the patient to have an objective judgment about his situation and what is needed. Whether they pay explicit attention to it in any technical sense or not, what physicians do inevitably influences the emotional states of their patients, and often this may have a most important influence on the state of their cases.

These inherent frustrations of the technical expert acquire special significance because of the magnitude and character of the interests at stake. The patient and his family have the deepest emotional involvements in what the physician can and cannot do, and in the way his diagnosis and prognosis will define the situation for them. He himself, carrying as he does responsibility for the outcome, cannot help but be exposed to important emotional strains by these facts.

The absolute limits of the physician's control—which of course are relative to the state of medical science at the time and his own assimilation of it—are not the only source of frustration and strain. Within these limits there is a very important area of uncertainty. As in so many practical situations, some of the factors bearing on this one may be well understood, but others are not. The exact relation of the known to the unknown elements cannot be determined; the unknown may operate at any time to invalidate expectations built up on analysis of the known. Sometimes it may be known *that* certain factors operate significantly, but it is unpredictable whether, when, and how they will operate in the particular case. Sometimes virtually nothing is known of these factors, only that the best-laid plans mysteriously go wrong. In general, the line between the spontaneous forces tending to recovery—what used to be called the *vis medicatrix naturae*—and the effects of the physician's "intervention" is impossible to draw with precision in a very large proportion of cases.

The argument of the last few pages may be summed up in the proposition that one principal set of functional significances of the combination universalism, functional specificity, and affective neutrality is to enable the physician to "penetrate" sufficiently into the private affairs, or the "particular nexus" of his patients to perform his function. By defining his role in this way it is possible to overcome or minimize resistances which might well otherwise prove fatal to the possibility of doing the job at all.[3]

This importance is not, however, confined to the overcoming of potential resistances. It is also evident that these pattern elements are "for the protection of the physician" in a broader sense than in the case of the "nurse-chaperone," as she is sometimes actually called. The obverse functional danger to that of refusal to admit to the sphere of private affairs is that this admission should be too thorough, that the role of the doctor should be assimilated to that of other "significant persons" in the situation of the patient, that he really should become a personal intimate, a lover, a parent, or a personal enemy. All these roles are, it will be noted, defined in terms of the opposite combination of the values of the pattern variables being discussed from that which characterizes the professional pattern.

A good many instances were collected by the author in which physicians had been put in positions where there was a "pull" to assimilate their roles to patterns of this type, particularly that of a "personal friend" of the patient. There are various complicating factors, but in general it can be said that there was a marked tendency for the physician to feel uncomfortable. Asked why it was undesirable to allow the assimilation to take place, the usual answer ran in terms of the difficulty of maintaining "objectivity" and "good judgment" in relation to the job. There is every reason to believe that there was an element of correct insight in the testimony of these doctors, none of whom incidentally was a psychiatrist or psychiatrically trained. It is, however, difficult to judge how far this is a rational appraisal of the situation and how far a rationalization of other factors of which the respondent was not explicitly aware.

The enormous recent development of psychotherapy, and increase of our knowledge of the psychological aspects of human relations relative to it, calls attention to another most important aspect of this whole situation. Through the mechanisms of transference the patient, usually without knowing what he is doing, not only has certain resistances, but he actively attempts by projection to assimilate his physician to a pattern of particularistic personal relationship to himself. He attempts to elicit the reaction which is appropriate to his own need-dispositions. Though this is most conspicuous in psychiatric cases, as noted, there can be no doubt that it is also of the greatest importance throughout the field of doctor-patient relationships.

In the first place it is necessary for the physician to be protected against this emotional pressure, because for a variety of reasons inherent in his own situation it is not possible for him to "enter in" to the kind of relationship the patient, usually unconsciously, wants. Above all this functional specificity which permits the physician to confine the relationship to a certain content field, indeed enjoins it on him, and affective neutrality which permits him to avoid entering into reciprocities on the emotional level, serve to bring about this protection. The upshot is that he refuses to be "drawn in" and has institutional backing in his refusals of reciprocity.[4]

NOTES

1. An excellent and very detailed analysis of one of these border-line groups is given in the study by Walter I. Wardwell, *Social Strain and Social Adjustment in the Marginal Role of the Chiropractor,* unpublished Ph.D. dissertation, Harvard University, 1951.

2. This it will appear later is particularly important to the therapeutic process. It is not to be interpreted either that the cathectic significance of persons has no part in the etiology of illness or that cathexis of the physician as an object does not occur—but it is controlled.

3. It is interesting to note that the social or psychological research worker faces similar problems in his relations to people he wishes to interview or observe. The cognate features of his role have the same order of functional significance.

4. The fact that his role is collectively oriented, on the other hand, tends to draw him in and has to be counteracted by these other factors.

17.
Obligations to Clients   Michael Bayles

Securing the services of a professional, as difficult as that may sometimes be, is only a preliminary to the professional-client relationship. This chapter considers the ethical nature of the professional-client relationship and the obligations of professionals to clients that arise therefrom. In the compass of this chapter it is impossible to provide a complete and detailed analysis of these obligations, and important differences arise in applying these obligations to different professional situations. Therefore, the emphasis is on the standard or normal situation of a competent adult consumer. Modifications are needed for other situations, such as physicians treating small children and unconscious patients. On the basis of this analysis, a standard is offered to systematize obligations of professionals to clients and general obligations are then briefly developed.

The average client will probably have a physician's attendance during a fatal illness or injury, but most physician-patient contacts are for more mundane matters such as a bacterial infection or a broken bone. Only gross neglect by the patient or physician—for example, the failure of a patient to take any medicine at all or of a physician to ask whether the patient is allergic to penicillin before prescribing it—is apt to turn these matters into seriously life-threatening illnesses or injuries.

The central issue in the professional-client relationship is the allocation of responsibility and authority in decision making—who makes what decisions. The ethical models are in effect models of different distributions of authority and responsibility in decision making. One may view the professional-client relationship as one in which the client has most authority and responsibility in decision making, the professional being his employee; one in which the professional and client

are equals, either dealing at arm's length or at a more personal level; or as one in which the professional, in different degrees, has the primary role. Each of these conceptions has been suggested by some authors as the appropriate ethical model of the relationship. Each has some commonsense support.

Agency

According to this view, the client has most of the authority and responsibility for decisions; the professional is an expert acting at the direction of the client. The client hires a professional to protect or act for some interest; the professional provides services to achieve the client's goal—purchase of a house, removal of a gall bladder, design of a building. According to this conception, the professional acts not only for or in behalf of the client, but also acts under the direction of the client as in bureaucratic employer-employee relationships. This conception is especially plausible for lawyers. In filing a complaint or arguing for a client, a lawyer acts for and in behalf of the client. According to some people, a lawyer is merely a "mouthpiece" or "hired gun."

The agency model most clearly exemplifies what has been called the "ideology of advocacy." This ideology has two principles of conduct: (1) that the lawyer is neutral or detached from the client's purposes, and (2) that the lawyer is an aggressive partisan of the client working to advance the client's ends. This ideology is readily applicable to physicians, architects, and engineers. A physician, for example, should not evaluate the moral worth of patients but only work to advance their health.

The chief problem with the ideology of advocacy, where it does become an ideology, is that sometimes devotion to a client's inter-

Source: Michael Bayles, *Professional Ethics*, Wadsworth Publishing Co., Belmont, Calif., 1981.

ests is thought to justify any lawful action advancing the client's ends, no matter how detrimental the effect on others.

The agency view of the professional-client relationship is unduly narrow. A number of considerations indicate limits to a professional's proper devotion to a client's interests, and consequently to a client's authority in decision making.

1. As discussed in the next chapter, professionals have obligations to third persons that limit the extent to which they may act in behalf of client interests.

2. The agency view arises most often in the context of defending professionals, especially lawyers, from attribution of client sins. This focus is too narrow to sustain a general account of the professional-client relationship. It best pertains to an adversarial context in which two opposing parties confront one another. In counseling, a lawyer's advice "need not be confined to purely legal considerations. . . . It is often desirable for a lawyer to point out those factors which may lead to a decision that is morally just as well as legally permissible."

3. Professionals emphasize their independence of judgment. Unlike a soldier who is not expected to think for himself but to do things the army's way, professionals should exercise their training and skills to make objective judgments. The agency view ignores this feature.

4. Except in cases of dire need—medical emergencies, persons charged with crimes—professionals may accept or reject specific clients. With a few restrictions, they may also stop the relationship. Consequently, the agency view is too strong. Professionals must also be ethically free and responsible persons. For their own freedom and the protection of others, they should not abdicate authority and responsibility in decision making.

Contract

If a client ought not to be viewed as having most authority and responsibility, then perhaps the authority and responsibility should be shared equally. In law, a professional-client relationship is based on a contract, and the ethical concept of a just contract is of an agreement freely arrived at by bargaining between equals. If the relationship is a contractual one, there are mutual obligations and rights, "a true sharing of ethical authority and responsibility." As it recognizes the freedom of two equals to determine the conditions of their relationship, the contract model accords well with the liberal values of freedom and equality of opportunity.

However, no gain results from treating as equals people who are not relevantly equal in fact or from assuming a nonexistent freedom. The history of contracts of adhesion (the standard forms offered by monopolies or near monopolies such as airlines) indicates the injustice that can result from falsely assuming contracting parties have equal bargaining power. Many commentators have noted relevant inequalities between professionals and clients, especially in the medical context. First, a professional's knowledge far exceeds that of a client. A professional has the special knowledge produced by long training, knowledge a client could not have without comparable training. Second, a client is concerned about some basic value—personal health, legal status, or financial status—whereas a professional is not as concerned about the subject matter of their relationship. The client usually has more at stake. Third, a professional often has a freedom to enter the relationship that a client lacks. A professional is often able to obtain other clients more easily than a client can obtain another professional. Especially if a potential client has an acute illness or has just been charged with a crime, he or she is not free to shop around for another professional. From this point of view, the bargaining situation is more like that between an individual and a public utility.

Friendship

Instead of viewing the relationship as one between two free and equal persons dealing at arm's length, some authors suggest that the relationship is more personal. One does not relate to a professional as one does to a grocer or public utility. The personal element is most closely captured by viewing the relationship as one of pals or friends. According to this view, professional and client have a close relationship of mutual trust and cooperation; they are involved in a mutual venture, a partnership.

Perhaps the most sophisticated version of this conception is that proposed by Charles Fried. He is primarily concerned with the legal and medical professions. Fried seeks to justify professionals devoting special attention and care to clients and sometimes seeking ends and using means that they would not seek or use for themselves. Friends are permitted, even expected, to take each others' interests seriously and to give them more weight than they do those of other persons. Fried suggests that the attorney-client relationship is analogous to a one-way limited friendship in which the lawyer helps the client secure legal rights. The lawyer helps the client assert his autonomy or freedom within the bounds society permits. Others have suggested that the physician-patient relationship should similarly be viewed as a cooperative effort of friends or pals to deal with the patient's illness or injury.

The many dissimilarities between friendship and the professional-client relationship, however, destroy the analogy. First, as Fried recognizes, the professional-client relationship is chiefly in one direction; the professional has a concern for the client's interests but not vice versa. Second, friendship is usually between equals. Even in friendships between employer and employee, the employer's superiority in the office is changed to a position of equality in the bar for a drink. As the above discussion of the contract model indicates, professionals and clients are not equals. Third, the affective commitment of friendship is usually

lacking. Professionals accept clients for a fee, not out of concern for individuals. Thus, one commentator concludes that "Fried has described the classical notion, not of friendship, but of prostitution." As the factual assumptions of this model are incorrect and the analogy supporting it is weak, its ethical implications are unfounded.

The friendship analogy is not needed to justify a professional paying special attention to a client's interests. The role of a professional is to provide services to clients, and the acceptance of a client is sufficient to justify the special attention. A barber who accepts a customer pays special attention to a customer's hair over that of others who need a haircut more. One need not postulate the barber as friend to justify this attention. It is presupposed by any system of services for a fee.

Paternalism

Once one abandons models that assume the professional and client are equal and accepts the professional as to some extent in a superior position to the client, one faces the problem of the proper extent of professional authority and responsibility in decision making. Parents have knowledge and experience that children lack, and it is often ethically appropriate for them to exercise their judgment on behalf of their children. Similarly, as a professional has knowledge and experience a client lacks and is hired to further the client's interests, perhaps the relationship should be viewed as one of paternalism.

Paternalism is a difficult concept to analyze. A person's conduct is paternalistic to the extent his or her reasons are to do something to or in behalf of another person for that person's well-being. What is done can be any of a number of things, from removing an appendix to preventing the person from taking drugs. One can also have a paternalistic reason for acting in behalf of a person—for example, filing a counterclaim or asserting a legal defense. The key element of paternalism derives from the agent, X, acting regardless of the person's, Y's, consent to it. Y may be incapable of consent, as when a physician treats an unconscious patient in an emergency, or Y may never have been asked, or may have refused to consent to the act.

Conduct can be paternalistic even when Y in fact consents. For example, if X is prepared to do something to Y regardless of Y's consent, then X's reason is paternalistic even if Y does consent. Parents frequently manipulate a child into assenting to actions, although they were prepared to do them without the child's assent. The key element is that X would have done the action, if he could, even if Y had not consented. Such claims are difficult to establish, but this difficulty is a practical problem and does not affect the conceptual matter. In manufacturing consent, information can be withheld, false information provided, or more emphasis placed on some facts than on others. Professionals sometimes manufacture consent when action cannot legally be taken without client consent, such as accepting a settlement or performing an operation.

The concept of doing something to or in behalf of includes failure to do something. Suppose Y requests X to do something for him, but X refuses because she thinks it would be detrimental to Y's well-being; for example, a physician refuses to prescribe a tranquilizer for a patient. This also counts as doing something to or in behalf of a person without his consent; Y does not consent to the tranquilizers being withheld.

A voluminous literature exists concerning the justification of paternalism. The brief discussion here will outline only the major arguments. Paternalism requires justification because it involves doing something to or in behalf of another person regardless of that person's consent. It thus denies the freedom of people to make choices affecting their lives. They lack freedom as self-determination. The loss of control over their own lives, especially to professionals, is one reason for people's concern about professional ethics. Thus, paternalism is of central importance in professional ethics.

Three arguments are often offered to justify paternalism.

1. The agent has superior knowledge as to what is in a person's best interest.
2. The client is incapable of giving a fully free and informed consent. By "fully free" is meant without duress, psychological compulsion, or other emotional or psychological disturbance. By "informed" is meant with appreciation of the consequences of a course of conduct and its alternatives.
3. A person will later come to agree that the decision was correct. Although the person does not now consent, he will later. For example, an unconscious accident victim with a broken limb will agree that a physician was correct to set the bone.

To decide whether these justifications support viewing the professional-client relationship as paternalistic, it is useful to consider when reasonable people would allow others to make decisions for them. First, a person might not wish to bother making decisions because the differences involved are trivial. Second, decisions might require knowledge or expertise a person does not possess. Third, a person might allow others to make judgments if he or she is or will be mentally incompetent. Some people voluntarily enter mental hospitals.

The first of these reasons does not directly relate to the arguments for paternalism, but the second and third do relate to the first two arguments for paternalism. Reasonable persons would allow others to make decisions for them when they lack the capacity to make reasonable judgments. However, most clients do not have sufficiently impaired judgment to reasonably allow others to make important decisions for them. Moreover, even with individuals, the view is not plausible for the common legal and medical cases. A person who wants to purchase a house or make a will, or who has the flu or an infection, is rarely so distraught as to be unable to make reasonable decisions. Consequently, the argument from incapacity does not support adopting a paternalistic conception of the professional-client relationship for most cases, although it supports using that conception in special cases.

The first argument for paternalism, that from superior knowledge, fits with reasonable persons allowing others to make decisions when they lack knowledge. Moreover, clients go to professionals for their superior knowledge and skills; such knowledge and skill is a defining feature of a profession. However, many decisions require balancing legal or health concerns against other client interests. As many authors have noted, crucial professional decisions involve value choices. They are not simple choices of technical means to ends, and even choices of means have a value component. Professionals have not had training in value choices. Even if they had, they might not know a client's value scheme sufficiently to determine what is best for him when everything is considered.

Similarly, a physician can advise bed rest, but because of business interests a client can decide her overall interests are best promoted by continuing to work on certain matters. The client might especially need the income or be on the verge of completing a business deal that will earn a promotion. Physicians sometimes fail to realize that a patient's other concerns, even a vacation trip with the family, can precede health. They write and speak of the problem of patient noncompliance just as parents speak of noncompliance by children. Yet, one does not have everything when one has health.

Although a professional and client are not equals, sufficient client competence exists to undermine the paternalistic model as appropriate for their usual relationship. Clients can exercise judgment over many aspects of professional services. If they lack information to make decisions, professionals can provide it. Sometimes professionals argue that clients can never have the information they have. This is true, but not directly to the point.

Much of the information professionals have is irrelevant to decisions that significantly affect client values. The precise name of a disease and its manner of action are not relevant to deciding between two alternative drug therapies, but the fact that one drug reduces alertness is. To deny clients authority and responsibility by adopting the paternalistic model is to deny them the freedom to direct their own lives. Clients are not capable of determining the precise nature of their problem, or of knowing the alternative courses of action and predicting their consequences or carrying them out on their own. They need and want the technical expertise of a professional to do so. However, they are capable of making reasonable choices among options on the basis of their total values. They need professionals' information in order to make wise choices to accomplish their purposes.

Finally, when the professional-client relationship is conducted on the paternalistic model, client outcomes are not as good as when the client has a more active role.

Fiduciary

As a general characterization of what the professional-client relationship should be, one needs a concept in which the professional's superior knowledge is recognized, but the client retains a significant authority and responsibility in decision making. The law uses such a conception to characterize most professional-client relationships, namely, that of a fiduciary. In a fiduciary relationship, both parties are responsible and their judgments given consideration. Because one party is in a more advantageous position, he or she has special obligations to the other. The weaker party depends upon the stronger in ways in which the other does not and so must *trust* the stronger party.

In the fiduciary model, a client has more authority and responsibility in decision making than in the paternalistic model. A client's consent and judgment are required and he participates in the decision-making process, but the client depends on the professional for much of the information upon which he gives or withholds his consent. The term *consents* (the client consents) rather than *decides* (the client decides) indicates that it is the professional's role to propose courses of action. It is not the conception of two people contributing equally to the formulation of plans, whether or not dealing at arm's length. Rather, the professional supplies the ideas and information and the client agrees or not. For the process to work, the client must trust the professional to accurately analyze the problem, canvass the feasible alternatives, know as well as one can their likely consequences, fully convey this information to the client, perhaps make a recommendation, and work honestly and loyally for the client to effectuate chosen alternatives. In short, the client must rely on the professional to use his or her knowledge and ability in the client's interests. Because the client cannot check most of the work of the professional or the information supplied, the professional has special obligations to the client to ensure that the trust and reliance are justified.

This is not to suggest that the professional simply presents an overall recommendation for a client's acceptance or rejection. Rather, a client's interests can be affected by various aspects of a professional's work; so the client should be consulted at various times. The extent of appropriate client participation and decision making can be determined by advertence to the reasons for allowing others to make decisions for one. Professionals do not have expertise in a client's values or in making value choices. Their superior knowledge and expertise do not qualify them to make value choices significantly affecting a client's life plans or style. However, they

do have knowledge of technical matters. A patient will certainly let a physician determine the dosage of medicines. In short, client consent and involvement are not necessary when (1) the matter is chiefly a technical one or (2) the value effect is not significant.

The appropriate ethical conception of the professional-client relationship is one that allows clients as much freedom to determine how their life is affected as is reasonably warranted on the basis of their ability to make decisions. As clients have less knowledge about the subject matter for which the professional is engaged, the special obligations of the professional in the fiduciary model become more significant. The professional must assume more responsibility for formulating plans, presenting their advantages and disadvantages, and making recommendations. Because of the increased reliance on the professional, he or she must take special care to be worthy of client trust. Thus, although the fiduciary model is appropriate throughout the range of competent clients and services, a professional's responsibilities to the client increase as a client's knowledge and capacity to understand lessen.

Finally, some clients are not competent to make decisions. In this case, the paternalistic model becomes appropriate. These cases of an incompetent client will almost always be restricted to members of the legal and health professions. Even then it does not follow that the professional should make the decisions. If a client is incompetent, a legal guardian should be appointed to make decisions. When this is done, the professional has a fiduciary relationship to the guardian. Consequently, the appropriate occasions for professionals to adopt a paternalistic role are restricted to those in which a client is incompetent and a guardian has not yet been appointed.

18.

The Good of Personal Care Charles Fried

The traditional paradigm of the doctor-patient relation, the ideal of personal care, is just *the benefit of being treated with loyal devotion to one's own interests.* But is this a benefit to which one is entitled? Does one have a *right to personal care,* even at the cost of certain advantages to all? Certainly we must distribute benefits and burdens fairly, but the claim of a right to personal care can justify a waste of resources at best and at worst an unfair benefit to those who happen to be the recipients of this personal care. For it may well be that by pursuing a policy of personal care in respect to those presently before us we actually lessen our ability to help those unidentified persons who will need help later; we may actually worsen their situation. So we must ask whether, once fairness is assumed, there is anything to be said for the right and value of personal care? The first question to answer is whether there is any coherent sense to the notion of giving some preference, some intrinsic value to one's relation to the concrete person before one, otherwise than simply as a function of one's obligation to the group as a whole of which this person is a member.

The doctor's preference for his patient might be seen as a special case of the often noted (and deplored) phenomenon that the plight of identified persons in immediate danger calls forth a measure of effort and even heroism which would generally be unavailable to ward off perils of a similar or greater degree from a larger but unidentified (statistical) group where the measures involved are effective just because they prevent the peril from ever arising. Examples of this would be the heroic efforts to save the victims of mining accidents and the rela-tive lack of concern for measures of general safety that would have prevented the accidents from ever occurring. The familiar predilection for curative as opposed to preventive medicine is another example of this phenomenon.

In arguing for the obligation of personal care, I shall by implication at least be defending those attitudes, choices, and patterns of behavior that *favor the concrete, the immediate, the identified.* But can such preferences even be stated as part of a coherent set of moral principles? To begin with, a number of confusions should be put out of the way.

First, nothing about the optimization view entails that in every conceivable circumstance the impersonal, the preventive, the remote is the more efficient way of deploying our resources. Certainly a concern for overall, long-term efficiency makes such moves more eligible, but it may sometimes be that the best thing to do is to wait until the need arises in its most dramatic and palpable form and then to use all presently available means to meet it. Second, the uncertain promises and disasters of the future are not reason to prefer the immediate a priori; rather they are among the many factors that enter into our probability calculus as to the most efficient course of action overall. What we may not do is discount the future just because it is the future. Third, although I recognize that immediate, palpable need tends to call forth greater effort, still we must distinguish between realistically making use of this passion and justifying it as moral and rational on calmer reflection. Fourth, I reject utterly what may be called the symbolic value argument that justifies a preference for the immediate and palpable over the statistical as a way of

Source: Charles Fried, *Medical Experimentation: Personal Integrity and Social Policy,* American Elsevier Publishing Co., 1974.

teaching or symbolizing our concern for the individual. What, after all, is the value we are choosing to symbolize? Is it the value of human life? Then the question arises how exactly are we to conceive that value. Whether to do so in terms of unstinting devotion to the concrete case before us is just the issue to be resolved. Nor do I accept the notion that "we" understand the value of human life and happiness in terms of broader efficiency, but the only way in which "they" can be brought to do their part is to preach the primacy of the concrete. Among other things, by making this argument am I not letting the cat out of the bag, at least to those of "them" who get wind of our argument?

If personal care is to be established as a coherent concept, as a good in itself, no reliance can be placed on the preceding four arguments. At best those arguments show that some practices apparently illustrative of personal care might be referred to an optimizing approach after all. To rely on such arguments would make the good of personal care not an intrinsic good but a contingent good derived from an optimizing point of view and having no validity where optimization does not dictate such an answer. To establish the intrinsic value of personal care, I shall have to argue for the proposition that the relationship of assisting a person in need is an action and a relationship which have a special integrity of their own. They form a unit, a unit of value, and thus may one assert a coherent interest in personal care.

To begin with it should be noted at once that many important relationships other than that of doctor to patient make a similar claim as against principles that would require the individual to be judged by and subordinated to the interests of the larger group. For instance, the conduct of friends and family members illustrates familiar and indeed expected loyalty to the interests of one or a small and defined group of persons. It is not only in some emergency but regularly and pervasively that parents are expected to give a special care for the interest

of their own children, a care which greatly surpasses any possible claim that might be raised in behalf of a wider group of children or of the population at large. Similarly, the care and devotion that friends show each other can hardly be viewed as deriving wholly from the appreciation that it is just one's friends who stand in the greatest need of such attention. Indeed this narrower focus of our energies and concerns is best illustrated by the concern which we show for ourselves. I very much doubt that I—or very many of us—could justify the amount of time and resources lavished on our own concerns in terms of the proposition that this was, after all, the most efficient of all possible directions for such an expenditure. Although we recognize in varying degrees our obligation and inclination to do our best by our society, or nation, or humanity as a whole, this recognition is generally constrained by an assertion of a right to devote a certain amount of ourselves to ourselves, to our families, to our friends. These preferences may, to be sure, be shortsighted and selfish. That is the issue to be explored. That they exist can hardly be doubted.

In doing all that I can for a person in need, I also enter into a special and wholly different kind of relationship with that person from the relationship I enter into when I perform services to a large range of persons, some known, others unidentified. It is a relationship which, like that of friend to friend or of a person to himself, cannot be reduced to a special case of some larger general relation in which all men stand to each other. Rather human relationships and the action they entail must be analyzed discontinuously. Doing everything for a person, almost everything for a person, and only so much as some optimizing policy requires, are not simply points on a smooth continuum. Relieving a person in distress is a discrete human gesture like making love; one cannot remove aspects of the action one by one and still be left with the same thing. Since this argument is central to my thinking about values, relations, and rights, I must say more about it to make it plausible and to contrast it to the familiar modes of analysis which obscure what is crucial here.

Returning to the case before us, the issue may be drawn between two views of a valued relationship in which aid is rendered. Those who would disaggregate the relation would argue that the relation may be analyzed into (1) the material benefits conferred (as if these were themselves susceptible of analysis into atomic elements), and (2)—for those who insist that the personal quality of the relation is important—the benefits of friendship or sociability in the relation. And so these benefits must be committed to the view that if the material benefits were conferred outside of the relationship, say remotely by a stranger or even a machine, while the sociability or friendship were obtained from the known person, why this would be just as good. Indeed, they might go on to argue, this schism would probably be better, for it allows one to choose efficiently those who can best confer material benefits, while taking one's social pleasures where those are most likely to be found. After all, is it so clear that I should want to have, say, my doctor or a lifeguard as a friend; do I really want to enter into a *personal* relation with these persons?

Now it is precisely my assertion that we do indeed want to enter into personal relations in such cases. I do not assert—it would be absurd—that we want necessarily to enter into relations of friendship or love with them. But this shows that there are other kinds of personal relations than those of friends or lovers or relatives. The position that one might be indifferent between receiving crucial medical aid from a doctor and receiving it from a machine, while turning elsewhere for whatever "pleasures" of sociability are alleged to inhere in the doctor-patient relationship, is a position that, among other things, gravely misconceives the concept of sociability. The significance of personal relations cannot be precipitated out from the many other goods that are pursued in such relationships. It is not as if there

were the goods of productive labor, of teaching, of musical performance, of sexual gratification, of competition and challenge on one hand, and the good of sociability on the other. After all, what is this abstract good of sociability? I submit that to split off sociability from the significant encounters in which it occurs is like splitting off speed from running fast or driving fast. Sociability is, it might be said, an adverbial notion; it is a quality that certain interactions have. It is not something that it makes sense to think of split off from those interactions. And the more significant the interaction on other grounds, the greater the potentiality for significance in the personal relations in those interactions. But of course this means that there are many other significant personal relations than those that correspond to the ordinary notions of friendship or love—relations that are less open and pervasive, but as significant in their own right.

In the case of the doctor-patient relation the elements that combine to constitute the significance of that relation include:

• The importance and nature of the interests served by that relation. This suggests that not everything that now falls into that professional ambit necessarily has to. The identification of these interests and of what is distinct about them is discussed in the next chapter.

• The complex of intelligence, knowledge, and judgment that is needed to serve these interests. Particularly, as I shall argue, there is the fact that health has different significance for different persons, depending on their life plans and value systems, and the further fact that in some situations the doctor may need to help his patient not so much to realize his life plan as to realize that he must radically revise that plan.

• The expectations and confidence which tradition (maybe only mythology) relates to the role of the physician in our culture. This is not a circular argument: the fact of the expectations is not being used to account for the expectations. Rather my point is that the role of trusted personal adviser and helper is a distinctive and significant one, as a total role and not just for the discrete benefits conferred within it. In different times and cultures the precise outlines and kinds of functions included within this role may vary. Yet because of the significance of the role it is important that the commitments of that role be honored, even if the role might perhaps have been defined otherwise.

The intuitive notion is one of the integrity of a relationship, and therefore of conduct which meets the conception of that relationship. And so when a doctor does less than he is able for his patient, albeit in the name of the progress of medicine and the welfare of larger numbers of persons, this is disquieting because it does violence to the integrity of a relationship which the patient assumes he is in, and which doctors have traditionally stated they were in. The notion of the integrity of this relationship is, to be sure, a complex one. Even in its most extreme form, I would doubt that it carries with it the expectation that the doctor will do everything conceivable to further the interest of his patient. He will not, perhaps, endanger himself. He will not, perhaps, allow the claims of his patients to overwhelm his whole existence and all other relationships in which he might stand. But these qualifications themselves refer to structures of rights, relations, and expectations of the same form as his relation to the patient, of the same form as the relation of helper to helped. The best way to conceive of the system of these relationships is in terms of adjacent obligations, adjacent relationships. And the technique for resolving conflicts is not one of weighing up and balancing, but of drawing the boundary lines and the terms of the obligation.

The notion is one of doing unstintingly what it is that one does, though choosing with care the occasions on which one will do it. The notion of doing one's utmost in a system of adjacent relations can be contrasted to a notion in which the doctor conceives of himself as performing only one large-scale action, which is acting as the agent of the health care system to the population at large.

On this latter view his activity and his target is a population of persons, while in the former case his activity has as its object a sequence of discrete objects who are individual patients. And in that latter case, it is his responsibility not to exhaust his resources before he has attended to the totality of his object, which is the population at large, while in the former case if he has exhausted his resources (or himself) on a particular patient, then those with whom he has not entered into this relationship and to whom he is no longer available have no complaint.

How these integral actions and relations come about, what their contents are, in what their integrity consists, and the relationships between them are deep problems of psychology and ethics. I will not, because I cannot, offer a general theory for such problems here. At best in the course of this essay I will offer certain partial solutions to specific problems. Nevertheless it is important to give some sense of the notion of integrity in actions and relations, because it is that notion which captures the special dimension of the subject before us. And as a general concept it suggests an important criticism of the standard classical utilitarian view of ethics. On the utilitarian view, what a person does, the relationships he enters into, and the choices he makes are all made with an eye toward a distant global end, which is furthering the greatest good of the geatest number or some such optimizing goal. But, I am arguing here that the ethical life of human beings, the values they perceive and follow, inhere in the concrete actions they perform and the concrete relationships into which they enter. It is these which allow a man to live in the present and to give ultimate, intrinsic value to the things that he does. Traditionally the doctor has seen himself as a person who stands to his patients in a relation that is at least analogous to that of friend or lover. To be sure the relation is less intense and pervasive, but it is analogous because it has its own integrity, and it demands, at least within its more circumscribed ambit, complete and unstinting devotion. Moreover, being a relationship, its value is a value for *both* parties to it, doctor and patient, and both parties have rights that arise out of it. Although I have been focusing on the interests of patients in the ideal of personal care, it should be clear that this ideal implies an interest and a right on the part of the doctor as well to maintain the integrity of his activity, to work not as a tool or as the bureaucratic agent of a social system, but as one whose professional activity is a personal expression of his own nature, the relationships he enters into being freely chosen, the obligations freely assumed, not imposed.

The reciprocal of this relation may be better seen if we recall some of the other relationships that make this demand of integrity: friendship, love, family relationships, the relation to one's self are all examples I have mentioned. Nor are all such instances to be found in the realm of relations between persons. The relationship of an artist to his art or a scholar to truth has this quality. It is evident that the artist gives to his art an unstinting devotion which is analogous to the care a doctor gives his patient. And the relation between the artist's art and his other concerns, his concerns as a person, citizen, parent, and so on, are relations of adjacent demands, whose structure must be adjusted in some systematic way, rather than the relation of factors of supply whose price and productivity determine the optimum mix of products from the artist, as if from a business firm. There may not be many other professional relationships which have this quality; some think that the lawyer owes his client that degree of concern, and that the lawyer, like the doctor, is not to be viewed as a businessman selling a product or a bureaucrat allocating a scarce resource.

What the foregoing argument shows is that the concept of personal care is a pervasive one, which grows out of a relation that people can create only in the context of more or less direct contact, and that the actions and ends pursued in the context of such relations are qualitatively different from those pursued outside of them. Finally, we have seen that the distinct character of those relations, actions, and values gives rise to interests not only in those who benefit from them—in this case the patient—but in

the benefactor, here doctors, as well. For doctors, like others entering into relations of personal care, achieve in that relation the capacity to perform a distinct kind of service and to pursue a distinct kind of value. And the structure of these relations and values presupposes that they are deliberately entered into, chosen, assumed as obligations are assumed.

Personal Integrity

In most general terms, the goal of health care as it pertains to such fundamental human values relates to the maintenance of the integrity, of the coherence of the human person, with specific reference to the physical substrate of that integrity. The human person identifies himself with his body; he knows that he *is* his body, that his knowledge of and relation to the whole of the outside world depends on his body and its capacities, and that his ability to formulate and carry out his life plan depends also on his body and its capacities. The doctor's interventions are placed in a special category just because he intervenes at a special point in the system which is the person. In illness, the patient himself, not just some extraneous interest, is threatened. Compare the doctor to the garage mechanic. So long as the person's body and his health are regarded as an asset to be maintained and to be phased out when fully depreciated, the doctor is indeed only a serviceman charged with maintenance of a capital good. But a person's relationship to his body, to his health, is not his relation to his productive goods. Instead it is the person's relation to himself. Although a person may properly be conceived as allocating his life resource to best realize his plan and projects, underlying that conception is the conception of a person who has projects. The person comes logically and morally before the various ends he pursues. And so the doctor does not just help provide the means to get the person where he is going, he ministers to the person who has those ends.

The doctor stands in a special relation to his patient because he ministers to the basic unit which is the person, rather than to the attributes and creations which that person gathers around him in pursuit of his purposes. For the person is his body, and the body's health is the integrity of the person. Although I can appreciate that one would wish to avoid such philosophical depths (or shoals), there is no other way that one can have an adequate conception of what is the person's good, and in what his integrity consists.

The two most general aspects of the concept of personality are the ability truly and accurately to attain understanding of the outside world and the ability to formulate and realize the plan of one's life in relation to the outside world. The materials available to an autonomous person seeking to develop and realize his conception of good are his own natural capacities, the resources of the outside world, and the more or less free cooperation of other persons. It is in structuring and elaborating these resources that a person expresses himself and builds a life. Typically, one might say almost naturally, the supporting interaction of other autonomous persons is the highest and the richest resource available to a person. By conceiving of each other as both the instruments and the ends of their mutual strivings, men are capable of building a society of mutual respect and cooperation. This ideal good of what has been called social union gathers its significance from the fact that in such a social union each person's individual self-respect and sense of integrity are fostered and reinforced by the conditions of mutual cooperation in which the value and integrity of others is simultaneously affirmed.

Sickness and Death

While this conception of human good does involve striving, and creation involves the overcoming of obstacles, a person's conception of this good must also be realistic. It must accept and work with not only the potentialities but the limitations of the actual, concrete situation. And this is most important in respect to the factors of sickness and death. As death is seen as inevitable, it becomes not the ultimate evil and threat to the life plan and to personal integrity but rather an unavoidable constraint, an element in the total picture. The life one fashions, the good one realizes is bounded in time by the fact of mortality. It is no more worthwhile chafing at this fact than at any of the other natural limitations of man's situation. The fact of death is overcome not by seeming to annihilate that fact but by pursuing goods whose effects will outlive the person who pursues them. And, as has been seen in a number of great lives and in innumerable ordinary lives, by limiting life resources, death can give value and preciousness to the expenditure of those resources. Such a conception of death implies a corresponding conception of the doctor's role. Since he cannot remove the constraint of mortality, his function in this respect must be so far as possible to adjust the individual to the fact of this constraint and to loosen the constraint so that it is compatible with a reasonable and rich life plan. This would suggest that it is only one of the physician's duties to retard a premature death; it is as much his duty to help assure that when death does come it is a lucid event, somehow consistent with the life that preceded it. Death should not be an event which, at its approach, trivializes and belies the efforts of a whole lifetime to live fully in realistic contact with the external world of facts and persons.

The Function of Medical Care

It follows from this conception that the doctor's prime and basic function is not so much the prevention of death (which is not in his power) but the preservation of life capacities for the realization of a reasonable, realistic life plan. As in particular cases conflicts arise and decisions must be made between various capacities and between the risk of death and the impairment of various capacities, the doctor must see himself as the servant, not of life in the abstract, but of the life plans of his patients. And these will surely differ greatly among individuals and also differ relative to the stage of realization of the life plan in a particular case. When the doctor prepares himself to render service in general, and when society trains and equips the doctor to render such service, both must do so from some conception of what kinds of life plans persons actually have, what the capacities are that persons have for realizing them, and what the realistic, inevitable constraints must be.

On this view one of the most difficult and painful tasks of the doctor is in coping with the prospect of premature death and of disabling illness. It is these, rather than the fact of death, of course, which represent the true threats to realistically conceived life plans. Where there is a risk there must be a chance of loss or failure, and every life plan is to some extent a venture, to some extent a system of more or less calculated risks. The doctor helps to avert or minimize these failures. But where this is not possible he is implicated in a much more delicate process, which is the admission of and adjustment to defeat. A person who learns that he must die sooner than he might reasonably have expected or whose activities and capacities will be significantly curtailed by illness must reformulate to a greater or lesser extent his life plan, his conception of himself; he must change. It is a crucial function of the doctor to assist in this process by intervening so far as possible in the physical changes involved, by informing his patient about the realities of his new situation, and ultimately, by helping him to accept and adjust to these realities.

Cutting across these two related functions is a function of particular significance to the subject of this study. The ideal of human life to which the physician ministers is an ideal of a life fully, lucidly lived, a life whose major events and constraints are accepted and internalized into the structure that a free and thinking man creates of that life. And thus the experiences of illness, cure, and impending death must also be made into significant events having intrinsic value. Since the physician is deeply implicated in all of these events, however, and since he therefore encounters his patient at the *cruces* of his life, it is essential that this encounter be a social encounter out of whose human and social reality the most can be made. A dramatic but by now perhaps trite example of this point is the so-called natural childbirth movement. The physical event which radically alters the structure of the parents' life plan is there made into a significant event, an event which is lucidly lived, rather than a more or less extraneous occurrence to be gotten through or around somehow.

The intervention of the doctor, when he deals with serious illness, is replete with richer potentialities. For whenever human beings impinge upon each other, they may do so blindly, as it were, withholding some part of their human personality from that encounter and thus making themselves *pro tanto* mere inhuman instrumentalities of the other person's purposes, or the encounter may be a human and social encounter in which the full range of human capacities is implicated and complete human respect is shown. It might be, after all, that a patient will treat his doctor like some kind of medicine, like a more or less inanimate object used to arrive at an end. And a doctor might connive in such an instrumental relationship. But I take it to be the goal of a fully human life that important relationships be lived significantly and as human relationships. And this is why the model of the doctor as the supplier of a limited, instrumental service is a serious distortion.

Rights in Medical Care: Lucidity, Autonomy, Fidelity, Humanity

The rights implied by this identification of the fundamental concerns involved in medical care may be put under four heads: lucidity, autonomy, fidelity, and humanity. These four rubrics converge in the notion of the integrity of the relation of personal care.

Lucidity. The patient has a right to know

all relevant details about the situation he finds himself in. This follows from the significance of the situation of medical care for his understanding of what he is and what he might become. Thus lucidity is not just an instrumental benefit, contingently useful to the patient, to his doctor, or to some third persons in maximizing this or that set of goods. It is a constitutive good and therefore a right, since it is crucial to a fully human process of choosing one's good and to the process of choosing what kind of person one will be. To deny a patient an opportunity for lucidity is to treat him not as a person but as a means to an end. And even if the ends are the patient's own ends, to treat him as a means to them is to undermine his humanity insofar as humanity consists in choosing and being able to judge one's own ends, rather than being a machine which is used to serve ends, even one's own ends.

Further, an offense against lucidity denies the patient the opportunity to make out of the significant situation in which the patient encounters the doctor a human encounter, a human relation—that is one in which the parties to the relation may equally engage their major capacities, their capacities for intelligence, choice, and affection. Denial of lucidity is a sufficient condition for a relation of dominance, and that in itself is a violation of right.

Autonomy. A patient has a right to be free not only from fraud in the relation of medical care, but from force and violence as well. Thus if a patient, though fully informed, is subjected to a treatment against his will, this too violates his rights. Similarly if the doctor is forced to perform services against his will, this violates his autonomy. Admittedly, no more controversial philosophical notion exists than of this liberty. The intuitive notion is of liberty to dispose of one's self, that is of one's person, one's body, mind, and capacities according to a plan and a conception fully chosen for

one's self. The idea is one of being one's own man, and from that position entering into relations of friendship, love, generosity, and service. In the relation of medical care this means that both patient and doctor fully define their relation to each other, neither being imposed on as a resource at the command of the other.

Fidelity. Dealings among persons create expectations, reliance, and trust. Where each party acknowledges not only that his conduct causes expectations to arise in his counterpart, but acknowledges also that these expectations are justified, that is, he ratifies them, then deliberately to disappoint such expectations is a form of deceit. It is a form of deceit which is so clearly identified that it has its own name, faithlessness. Thus, lying is a form of faithlessness because the use of language not only generates expectations but acknowledges those expectations as justified. There is perhaps usually a conventional element to fidelity. The expectations one acknowledges are rarely specified in full in the particular encounter. Rather there is a more or less implicit incorporation by reference of a whole conventional system of expectations. This is the case in the relation of medical care, where the patient relies and the doctor allows him to rely on a tradition of loyalty to his interests.

Humanity. This is the vaguest of the four concepts. The notion is that over and above a right to be treated without deceit or violence, a person has a right to have his full human particularity taken into account by those who do enter into relations with him. It may be that a man has no right to any affirmative consideration at all, but once he has been drawn into a significant nexus, his wants, needs, and vulnerabilities may not be ignored even if his right to autonomy is fully respected and he is treated with complete candor. This too is an important element in the concept of personal care.

Roles and Norms

It has been argued that one of the fundamental ethical questions generated by the doctor-patient relationship arises from the unequal position of the person in need having little choice but to rely upon the professional expert for assistance and relief. In essence, this position of dependence implies that the physician has power(s) over patients, and therefore the question of authority in the exercise of that power becomes fundamental. In the subsection on Clinical Authority we present a brief letter from Brody and Miller criticizing a false dichotomy in an all-or-nothing approach to patient involvement in decision making. Next, there are several selections from an interesting study of doctor-patient behavior in British and American pediatric clinics by P. M. Strong. We conclude this subsection on authority with an insightful review by S. Reichman of the expectations and realities of the relationship from both the patient's and physician's perspectives.

The next subsection, Doctor's Roles, focuses upon the physician's role responsibilities with an intensive account of how these responsibilities are developed during professional training and education. A selection from Strong describes the manner in which teaching occurs in clinics, and other selections focus upon encountering the cadaver, learning how to "interview," and the student's "self-consciousness" about his or her developing role as a physician. The subsection concludes with an account of the team approach to medical "service delivery."

The last subsection is designed to provide a discussion of the patient role. It begins with an article by A. Segall which reviews the influences and adequacy of Parson's account of the sick role concept and relates it to current research on patient behavior. A selection from Ducanis and Golin discusses four types of difficult patients from the team perspective. In another selection they discuss five stages through which a person passes as he or she enters and leaves the sick role. For clinical authority see cases 1, 14, 18, *19,* 21, 23, 25, *26, 27,* 28, *29,* 33, 34, *36,* 37, *38,* 41, *45,* 47, 55, 56, 68, 72, 73. For doctor's roles see cases 6, 14, 17, 18, 20, 23, *24, 26, 27,* 28, *29,* 31, 33, 37, *38, 39,* 40, 41, 45, 47, *50,* 52, 56, 61, *65,* 66, 67, 71, *73,* 74. For patient's roles see cases 14, 15, 17, 20, *27,* 33, *39,* 45, 53, 54, 62, 67, 71, 74.

Clinical Authority

19. *Arrogance* Howard Brody Bruce L. Miller

To the Editor: In his thoughtful essay on arrogance, Dr. Ingelfinger confronts the tension between autonomy and expertise that exists in the physician-patient relation. His description of the patient who personally shoulders all the burdens of medical decision making may have been influenced by his own highly atypical predicament—one doubts that a physician with such an eminent gastroenterologist as a patient could respond in the same way that he or she would respond to other patients. In any case, Dr. Ingelfinger's analysis might be taken to imply a false dichotomy: the arrogant, authoritarian physician who tolerates no patient involvement versus the diffident physician who takes no responsibility for the patient's progress or decline.

It is essential in the role of physician to offer authoritative (not authoritarian) counsel, emotional support, and realistic hope in the presence of fear and uncertainty. A non-paternalistic model of the physician's role requires abandonment of none of these qualities. It does demand that the physician's activities be grounded in respect for the patient as a moral equal, and that they be tempered with the awareness that the physician's values and goals may not match those of the patient. To recommend with firmness and authority a course of action that the patient is then free to refuse is simply to avoid paternalism, not to be paternalistic to some degree.

The major difficulty with Ingelfinger's recommendation is that medical paternalism has so shaped expectations that many patients—even assertive and educated ones—are unable to question or disagree with a physician. In this setting, firm confidence can have the same practical outcome as authoritarian arrogance in inhibiting expressions of the patient's autonomy. To overcome these expectations and to allow the patient's true will and values to become evident may require backing farther away from a firm and confident demeanor and admitting more uncertainty than would be desirable on therapeutic grounds alone. But the conflict between respecting and encouraging autonomy and managing one's communications with the patient to secure maximum therapeutic effect is more apparent than real. At a deeper level, any analysis of what is therapeutic for a given patient must take into account that person's own goals and values, and hence his or her moral autonomy. As a practical matter, the skilled clinician should be able to relate to patients in a way that combines decisiveness and support with disclosure of relevant facts and an openness to further discussion.

Source: *The New England Journal of Medicine*, vol. 304, no. 15, April 9, 1981, p. 920.

20. *A Joint Venture*   P. M. Strong

The right to criticize is often given to only one of the participants in a relationship. One needs a social position from which to do character work, and in many positions "it's not your place to criticize." In the charity format only the doctor had that place. But the bureaucratic format, by treating parents as independent, sensible, and moral, defined them as clients and medicine as a service; and in service relationships the client typically has the sole rights to criticism.

Nevertheless, "reasonable" parental criticism was tolerated and even welcomed, for without it how could rational agreement be reached? Indeed, parents who never had any questions and who accepted everything that staff said might be regarded as old-fashioned. Thus doctors at a Scottish hospital distinguished sharply between their urban parents and those from the remoter rural areas. Here, for instance, is a short passage from a consultation for epilepsy, followed by the conversation between doctor and students afterward:

Dr. I: Well, I think we'll keep him on the X (drug) as he has had another attack.
Mother: Oh, aye, oh aye. That's right, doctor. I think that's for the best. Oh, aye, he should be on it for a long time.

Dr. I: Well, that was a classic patient, what traditionally most patients were supposed to be like, although few are these days. That's the sort of patient Dr. Finlay had. We don't see very many nowadays.
Student: (imitating mother) I know the sort—"Oh, aye, doctor, aye, you're right, doctor, you're so right, aye, you're right."

For some doctors this attitude was a distinct fault in their patients. Some criticized working-class parents as far too accepting of what was said to them, even if they did not display their agreement in such elaborate terms as rural parents. Here, for instance, another doctor contrasts the kind of parents found at different local authority clinics:

Dr. D: The more intelligent people tend to ask far more questions and they're less likely to accept one's answers without querying if there could be an alternative answer. And in this respect, I do think that the population who attend the Green Lane Clinic and some of the other ones, I think they have far too much confidence in us as doctors, they don't realize that we are human and we can fail in things.

Not all doctors shared this attitude. Some saw parental questioning of their decision as a waste of time, since the parents were incapable of judging the wisdom of any one line of action. Others expressed both points of view, pleased that parents took a keen interest in their child's welfare but irritated by those who tried to "score points off them." Nevertheless, even the doctors who were most dismissive of parental questioning did not challenge parents' right to question them, merely the efficacy of their so doing.

Such toleration was normally matched by the careful way in which parents phrased their questions, if they had them. Parental questions were commonly information questions, ones which asked for the doctor's viewpoint but treated that viewpoint as authoritative. Even

Source: P. M. Strong, *The Ceremonial Order of the Clinic: Parents, Doctors, and Medical Bureaucracies*, Routledge and Kegan Paul, London, 1979.

the criticisms were normally indirect and carefully based on appeals to lay, not professional, knowledge.

Such procedures offered at least a chance of rational agreement being produced. Staff were sometimes obliged to uncover criticism and certainly required to listen to it, even if they did not accept it, just as they were obliged to answer questions, even if the detail in which they did so varied considerably. Likewise, although parents had rights to question and criticize, they were obliged to use these in a moderate form which did not challenge the entire basis of the interaction.

This rule of reason meant that staff tolerated almost all criticism, so long as their personal authority was not questioned; and even then they made exceptions and tried to preserve some notion of an alliance. Take first the following instance, which involved a child referred to the neurological clinic for general delay, but who was still being seen at an orthopedic clinic. The child was three years old and not walking, a state of affairs which the doctor blamed principally upon the parents, who carried the child everywhere; blame however was apportioned only by the parents not by the doctor:

Father: What about this leg? We come to the hospital but no one says nothing about it?

Dr. J: Well, he's flat-footed but he's capable of walking, the muscle tone is all right. (Examines child's leg for second time.) He will walk. It's just that he's flat-footed. I think what we'll do is refer him to physiotherapy, umm, to see if we can get him walking.

Father: Well, I'm not complaining but I want an answer. We've been coming up here for some time now.

Dr. J: Yes, he's past his third birthday, isn't he? Yes, I think he needs some physiotherapy.

This example is of additional interest in that although both parents were present it was the father who did the criticism. Such a division of labor was typical of many couples. Although mothers attended far more often by themselves, there were many cases in which it was commonplace for criticism or detailed questioning of staff to be done only on those infrequent occasions when fathers also attended. If it was the father who complained about other services, or demanded to know if a child would ever walk, or what the problem really was, then such questioning, however direct, posed only a marginal threat to the central relationship, that of doctor and mother. Their alliance was still secure, for the criticism was done by an outsider, someone with no great knowledge of either the child or the clinic.

21. *Collegial Authority*　　　P. M. Strong

Every Doctor a Good Doctor

The idealization of staff's technical competence within the bureaucratic format had two distinctive features. First, this character was given quite unequivocally; expertise was displayed rather than proved. In the Scottish clinics observed by this author, doctors' status was warranted simply by their being there, dressed in white coats or dark suits, seated behind desks and being spoken to in a deferential manner by other staff. Second, this expertise had

Source: P. M. Strong, *The Ceremonial Order of the Clinic: Parents, Doctors, and Medical Bureaucracies,* Routledge and Kegan Paul, London, 1979.

a "collegial" rather than an individual character. Doctors were expert because they belonged to an expert profession. In this version, hospitals and clinics were staffed by a uniform body of professionals, each one competent and all with equal access to a standard body of medical knowledge.

The principal method by which individual staff came to represent this collective wisdom was that of avoidance. Just as mother's character and competence went uninvestigated and was thus simply assumed to be good, so the staff's actual competence was ignored. Typically no mention was made of their names, mandate, training, or special interests. No patient ever asked a member of staff where they had trained, what were their precise qualifications, where they had worked before, how many publications they had got, or how long their studies had taken them. More particularly, no parent ever asked how much experience the doctor had in cases of this type. The unimportance of the doctors' biography was summed up in the manner in which introductions and greetings were typically done. Although doctors greeted mothers by name as they arrived, they rarely named themselves. Naming the mother was more than polite, for it had an important organizational purpose. In doing this, doctors could check that this was indeed the person they thought it was. Naming themselves had no such bureaucratic relevance.

This impersonality extended beyond name and personal history to cover the clinic's remit, the doctor's own powers within it, and the history of the service. For example, because they had no power to prescribe, Scottish local authority doctors referred some mothers to their general practitioner, but they did not normally mention why they did so. Nor did they inform parents as to the origin or purpose of total population screening, the nature of the various sources of data from which they derived their information on parents—such as the "At Risk" and "Handicapped" registers which they kept—or the way in which their work was supervised by a superior. Again, just as they did not talk about their own work, so staff did not compare it with that of others.

This idealization of the character and competence of the staff who ran these clinics was complemented by a similar treatment of those who saw children in other contexts. The assumption of collegial rather than individual expertise required a general rather than a personal anonymity. What parents thought of their general practitioner, of other hospital specialists, of local authority doctors and social workers was almost never mentioned; and this silence was maintained even under the most trying of circumstances. "Not in front of the patients" was the rule—even where there were major professional demarcation disputes, or where it was staff's job to check on others' work. The only partial exception was the treatment of health visitors. In three instances, Scottish hospital doctors either initiated or concurred in criticism of these relatively low-status staff. By contrast, when hospital staff referred to other kinds of staff, their comments, though uninformative, were often flattering: "You'll have to see Mr. McIntosh (orthopedic surgeon) about this; he's the expert in these matters." "I think you should see Mrs. Armstrong (physiotherapist) about this; she's very good with children like this."

The general avoidance of comment about other professionals is best illustrated by taking one example in detail: the way in which general practitioners were referred to by both staff and parents in hospital clinics. Not all American parents had such a doctor, but Scottish parents certainly did. It was from him that the hospital doctor most commonly received an initial referral, and most parents saw their general practitioner more often and knew him better than they did the hospital or local authority clinic doctor. Moreover, hospital doctors were obliged to write to the general practitioner after each visit, describing what they had done and advising on further treatment if any. General practitioners were therefore involved in almost every case observed in the study, and yet they were almost never a topic of conversation between staff and parents. This was particularly striking given the fact that clinic doctors sometimes disagreed with the diagnosis suggested by the GP, and on some occasions felt the practitioner to be incompetent. Moreover, whereas clinic staff knew, if only by reputation, most of the staff within their own organization, few general practitioners were known to them. They had therefore little to go on besides the referral note itself, and this was sometimes both brief and opaque. Was this, for example, a rebellious or prestigious parent rather than a mysterious complaint? "This is interesting. The GP's written a letter on his own notepaper rather than using the standard referral letter. I don't know why he's done this."

Despite such doubts, doctors normally made no inquiry into parents' transactions with their general practitioner. They asked neither what he nor the parents had said and they certainly did not inquire into parents' feelings about the relationship. There were only four occasions in which this rule was broken, and then only in part. Each of these involved a major discrepancy between the diagnosis given in the referral letter and that made by the doctor in the clinic; and in each the hospital doctor's version was less serious than that proffered by the general practitioner. Although the three hospital doctors involved did, in these instances, make some inquiry into the previous consultation, they did so in an extremely delicate fashion. They did not point out the discrepancy between their own version and that of the GP; far less did they censure his judgment.

One of the most noticeable features of the ward round on the intensive care unit was the number of mistakes, most of them extremely minor, that were confessed as the route proceeded. It seemed quite routine to make mistakes and there was normally no criticism of those who owned up. Errors were expected, and discussion concentrated on procedures to minimize these in the future. But in clinics errors were never mentioned, unless they were grossly obvious. It was not that staff presented themselves or others as infallible but that such matters were almost never mentioned. Avoidance was the fundamental strategy used by staff to transform their particular capacities and acts into the ideal form suitable for consultations within the bureaucratic format.

Expertise in the Private Format

My description of the "private" format, as I shall term it, is, like my earlier description of the charity format, based on only a very limited number of cases. There may well be other ways of doing private medicine, and it seems quite likely that styles of selling will change from time to time. To repeat an earlier caveat, my analysis is not intended to serve as a full description of the phenomenon but aims merely to bring out the contrasting qualities of the bureaucratic format.

In some respects the private format was similar to that of the bureaucratic mode. However, although doctors were idealized in both, the emphasis in the private format was on the competence of the individual doctor and not on that of the profession as a whole. Doctors within the bureaucratic format were anonymous, but here their skills were personalized. This individual emphasis did not extend to all the features that I mentioned earlier. Private patients did not enquire into staff's careers, their mandate, or their area of expertise, nor did staff themselves typically reveal this information. Similarly, the competence of other medical practitioners was not a subject for staff's investigation or criticism. To this extent staff's competence rested on collegial not individual authority. But various other matters were given a more personal treatment.

The individualization of medical competence within the private format had a variety of aspects. Take first the issue of the doctor's name. In contrast with the bureaucratic format, doctors routinely introduced themselves to private patients. That this was a matter of some importance can be seen in the following quotation. Here a child's grandmother, absent for long stretches in the British colonies, or their remains, and used to a private not a bureaucratic format, sought similar treatment in a Scottish hospital clinic. Several battles were fought over this during the consultation. In this instance the grandmother wanted an introduction, but the doctor at first refused to give one:

Dr. I: (to child) Can I just see you walk?
Grandmother: Am I in the way, Doctor? ("Doctor" was drawn out and said with a markedly rising tone.)
D. I: No, no.
Grandmother: Doctor? . . . (pause) . . . Doctor? . . . (pause) . . . What is your name?
Dr. I: Dr Innes.
Grandmother: Dr Innes.

Moreover, although a doctor's career and qualifications might not be discussed in the private format, they might well be on display. Doctors in the Scottish hospitals and clinics worked in completely impersonal rooms bare of any individual reference; and the same rooms were used by many different doctors for their clinics. This was also true of the main ambulatory clinics in the American hospital, and of the various city and state clinics. But doctors who saw private patients in their own room in the American hospital did so surrounded by certificates. They did not point out the parchments, nor were they a topic for discussion, but they formed a significant backdrop for the consultation, in much the same way as the hospital itself was duly warranted by a framed certificate.

This personalization of medical work extended not merely to the doctors themselves but also to their colleagues and contacts. When Scottish doctors cited medical opinion they talked of "we," not of particular doctors; and similarly, when they referred a child to another hospital for more specialist advice, they named the institution and not the consultant and talked simply of "Great Ormond Street" or "Newcastle." But in the private format doctors talked, not just of hospitals or departments, but of specific experts. The medicine that parents received was directly linked to the "best" available opinion. On this model the medical profession was not simply a collection of unknown experts but was staffed by named individuals bound by personal links. Here, for instance, an American doctor discusses a child's small size with his father, a man of considerable wealth:

Father: So it's a little too early to do this now?
Dr. O: Right. We talk about this problem all the time at the moment, and I've had discussions at X and Y hospital with the experts in the field. I've spoken to A, B and C about it. We're all very interested in it but it's early days yet. . . . Remember, it's not just me who's telling you this, I've talked to lots of people who know more about this than I do. (He names them again, plus some others.) And they all agree that it's too risky at the moment.

Not only did doctors refer to others in these individual terms but so too did parents. In the bureaucratic format parents did not normally imply that they knew their GP personally. Indeed the naming of GPs was typically irrelevant, other than as a means to address letters correctly. In the private format, however, naming was a matter of some importance to parents; and with it went a strong hint of both personal knowledge and an ability to assess the competence of the doctor so named. Here, for example, is a quotation from the grandmother in the Scottish clinic:

Usually we see Dr. Charles about him. He's been the family doctor for years ever since dear old Dr. York died. I don't know why Dr. Charles sent me here. I've got no idea at all. I really wanted a surgical boot for him. I just wanted to go to one of the respectable surgical boot-makers but somehow Dr. Charles sent me along here. I don't quite know why. It may just be wasting your time.

Staff themselves did not actually criticize other doctors, but the fact that they passed favorable judgments on some indicated that there were others who were less deserving of praise, a point which parents readily echoed. Although none challenged the competence of the doctor to whom they were then talking, most made disparaging remarks about others:

Mother: The only trouble is that the treatment will cost so much. The most competent physicians aren't found in institutions (i.e., hospitals).
Dr. T: Well, I don't know about that.
Mother: Well, we've had different ones every time we've been here and they've never been any good. They've never helped.

What was most striking about such remarks in comparison with parents' behavior in the bureaucratic format was the typically bland manner in which they were made. To question others' competence was not a threat to the proper conduct of the consultation: indeed, it was even urged by one doctor:

Mother: We liked him (Dr. Levy) particularly because he was critical of schools and said, "Don't believe what they say." That's what got us here.
Dr. Q: True. It's very important work the Learning Disability Group does in building up consumer appreciation. There's gotta be a dialogue, it's the only way.

That such criticisms were made and even openly appreciated is not surprising given the explicitly comparative stance on which these consultations were based. As good consumers and in their child's best interest, parents were openly shopping around; and such a position was honorable not shameful, something to be revealed rather than concealed:

Intern: How did you get here?
Mother: Well, he's been seeing a psychiatrist and he diagnosed minimal brain dysfunction and prescribed X. But we also want to get Dr. Stein's opinion as we felt we ought not just to have a psychiatric opinion.

Just as doctors personalized their own knowledge, so they warranted their decisions far more systematically than was typical in the bureaucratic format. Parts of the following conversation are like a private tutorial for a favored, if somewhat dim, pupil.

Dr. Q: If he's nearly three years behind then he should be in a full-time class with special education, but perhaps we can explain why he was doing OK in the nursery. (Turns to researcher.) Do you know the work of Piaget?

Researcher: Yes.

Dr. Q: (to parents) Piaget is a Swiss psychologist. He's a far brighter man than me! What Piaget really argued was about how children started off with very concrete thoughts and then over time they progressed to abstract thought. What we want to know is, why hasn't he? As I said, if he really is three years behind then he should be in a full-time class of special education, but he isn't. Why isn't he? I want to know why he's not if he really is this.

Parents: Right . . . (pause . . .).

Dr. Q: (leaning forward to mother and speaking in a slow, intimate voice) Now, you know what a learning disability teacher does, don't you?

Mother: (very hesitantly) He teaches children at a level they can understand.

Dr. Q: (emphatically) That's right!

In summary, whereas doctors in the private format were obliged to tolerate or even welcome criticism of their colleages and had to sell the special quality of their services with some vigor, their expertise was simply assumed within the bureaucratic format and was in need of no such display. In the latter mode, each and every staff member was almost automatically granted an anonymous but collective wisdom.

22. *Medical Control*   P. M. Strong

I have noted how parents, though allies, were nevertheless excluded from the medical college and cast as subordinates. What I have not shown is the extent to which that subordination was manifested within the various activities which made up a consultation. Put another way, we must distinguish between those matters which pertain to actors' overall status within a relationship and those rules which govern their actual participation within the action. The two are clearly related but the one does not follow directly from the other. In some encounters the lowly may be granted considerable speaking parts, while in others their baseness may be reflected both in their exclusion from large areas of the action, and in a heavy control upon those parts which they do get to play.

Here parents were both excluded and controlled. They might be partners but they were not equals, and the imbalance of power within the bureaucratic format was one of its most striking features. Although parents had some rights to question and to criticize, they could use these only within an overall context of medical dominance. The technical authority given to doctors was matched by an equivalent authority to control almost every aspect of the consultations' shape, sequence, and timing.

My emphasis on medical control should not be taken to mean that parents had no power to negotiate with staff. As other work has clearly shown, there are various ways in which patients may influence the course of action within consultation. However, although we still need to know more about such influence, its effect should not be exaggerated. Within the bureaucratic format, and indeed within all the formats discussed here, medical control of the consultation was systematic, all-pervasive, and almost unquestioned.

Source: P. M. Strong, *The Ceremonial Order of the Clinic: Parents, Doctors, and Medical Bureaucracies,* Routledge and Kegan Paul, London, 1979.

Objects of Involvement

In clinics, doctors might do many things. They could break off conversation with a mother to read or write a note, or to look at the child, or to ask the nurse a question, or to teach a student. They were also allowed to be "away" for long periods. Some doctors spent considerable time lost in thought, their eyes unfocused or their fingers drumming. They therefore had a wide variety of sources of involvement within the consultation, and parents typically recognized the legitimacy of such engagement by not "interrupting" doctors when they were so involved. By contrast, parents had no such rights to other activities but maintained themselves in a state of permanent alertness during gaps in the conversation. While the doctor read or wrote mothers waited, ready to spring into conversation when requested to do so. They did not read, smoke, or suck sweets; and talk with their children or their husband was strictly subordinate, or a "side involvement." Many mothers abstained from discussion altogether, particularly with older children. Only if a doctor left the room might a conversation of any normal volume or gesture begin.

Given this suppression of other involvements, it could not be said that staff interrupted parents when they took up their conversation once more, for there was nothing of any substance to be interrupted. Parents were at the doctors' disposal, and talk could begin or end at any time of the doctors' choosing and typically without any need for permission or apology.

The way in which parents were allocated and accepted a dependent role within the consultation can also be illustrated by the highly restricted set of bodily actions in which they engaged. Staff could move freely around the room, now standing up, now sitting down, now looking at this, now doing that, but parents sat in the chairs provided for them and did not move from these except to facilitate medical examination. The one mother who, of her own accord, left her chair and walked round to the doctor's side of the desk was greeted with immense surprise. Some parents even seemed unsure as to how far they could make themselves comfortable. Parents who arrived in overcoats often sweltered in the heated rooms rather than remove them, and one mother who arrived in a thunderstorm sat there and dripped until the doctor asked if she wanted to remove her coat.

Three alternative objects of medical involvement need a further consideration. The first of these, the discussion of medical matters with an audience of colleagues and students, has already been noted. Such discussion was overtly subordinated to the consultation between doctor and parents. Nevertheless, staff's ability to talk with an audience was an important assertion of their power, for such rights were not symmetrical. Some parents talked *at* nurses and other staff as well as to the doctor, but no one except the doctor normally responded, and such communication disappeared into a void. By contrast, staff's right to engage in discussion with others could be used to influence directly their relationship with the parents. In the following instance, the doctor used the researcher to help to pacify a recalcitrant mother who had made a series of complaints in a rather aggressive tone:

Dr. F: Apart from her food, are there any problems?
Mother: Well, there's her sleeping.
Dr. F: Well, what, doesn't she sleep?
Mother: (firmly) Well, she does now because she gets something to make her sleep.

Dr. F grins at the baby and dangles his stethoscope in front of it. He then says to the researcher:

Dr. F: Isn't it marvelous having a baby like this? (Researcher smiles. Mother smiles back at researcher.) But it's not always marvelous. What's this about her not sleeping?

This use of an audience was exceptional. Nevertheless, it illustrates a potential resource that was always legitimately available to the doctor but was rather more dubious if parents attempted it. Including the audience in their remarks was one thing, manipulating them another.

The doctors' power in the bureaucratic format was therefore reinforced by their access to an audience which acquiesced in their handling of the occasion and could be manipulated to further their own ends, a resource which was not available in quite the same manner to the parents.

Two further asymmetries also had important consequences for medical control. The first of these involved children. I have already noted that children were treated as mere side involvements for parents. Staff's authority extended, temporarily at least, to the relationship between parent and child and not just to that between parent and doctor. Indeed, the maintenance of their authority depended on a rigid segregation of parent and child. Staff might interact with the children whenever they chose but parents could not do so. Staff might switch openly between the two; parents must attend to whatever they were bid. Staff might address parents through the child, but they themselves were only to be spoken to directly. Where parents' presence was deemed to affect the relationship between staff and child too greatly, parents were removed from the setting. After the initial visit, both occupational and physiotherapy staff in the Scottish hospital did not permit parents to be present during treatment. Staff were also in charge of the allocation of praise and blame for the child's performance. Further, even though parents might normally be considered to have the most extensive knowledge of their child and to be the best interpreter of their words, actions, and feelings, such knowledge was treated as partial and as able to be overriden where staff saw fit.

When doctors did interact with children, it was parents' duty to assist staff in their management. In this they were principally required to ensure that children recognized staff's paramount authority; or, put another way, they were obliged to underwrite the temporary loss of their own control. Alongside this they were expected to bring the child in a suitable condition for examination or therapy and to aid during these as appropriate, to hold children when they struggled, to encourage them when they failed to respond, and to soothe them when they cried.

Despite this partial removal of the child from their keeping, parents had some rights here. They might still interact with their sons and daughters even though such action was clearly subordinate to, and in the end controlled by, medical staff.

The medical records were a very different matter. For all practical purposes these belonged to the doctor and not to the parents. In the American clinics parents had a legal right to inspect their children's records, but none was observed to ask the doctor if they too might consult the file during the interaction. In all settings the notes stayed with the doctors and in no sense were they common property. Moreover, in many ways the presence of the medical record was as essential to medical interaction as the presence of parents or children.

Where the file for a particular case was not present, as when a child was attending another clinic at a similar time, doctors deferred the case until the file had arrived. If they were forced to carry on without it, as where records had to be acquired from another hospital, they made continual mistakes. Such constant correction challenged their normal professional ease. Proper medicine could begin only when the file as well as the patient was present, for it constituted an alternative biography to that available from the parents, and one that had been medically warranted.

Writing that biography was a medical and not a parental task, and was one of the main tasks in the consultation. Everything that parents said in clinics was for the record. For them to speak was to permit their words to be written down at the doctor's discretion. The presence of the form and of an official pen hovering over it defined the nature of the parental task: the production of brief answers that could be filled in as quickly and efficiently as possible.

The record was not as obtrusive on those other occasions when there was no official form to be completed. When asking questions of parents, doctors would often not address them directly but simply speak as they consulted the file or added fresh contents. Only when presenting their conclusions did they routinely look parents continuously in the face as they spoke. For attention was not guaranteed to parents. Although they had the right to ask questions or introduce topics of conversation, they had no definite rights to an answer. Doctors could demand this of parents but parents could not do likewise, for doctors, as we have seen, had other legitimate objects of attention through which they could ignore their remarks.

Not only did doctors control the medical records and use them to enforce their general control of the encounter, but parents rarely made or at least used any records of their own. There were only seven cases in which parents brought along their own notes, and in three of these it was the doctors who had asked the parents to do this. More importantly perhaps, no parent was ever observed to make notes during a clinic. Doctors wrote down what they said but parents did not reciprocate. Minutes of a kind were kept, but only staff made these, stored them, and had ready access to them.

Not only did staff have special rights to involve themselves in a wide variety of activities, but they also largely controlled the overall timing of the consultation and the scheduling of individual pieces of the action. Thus it was staff who decided when a consultation both began and ended: in only one case in the entire study did a mother rather than a doctor end a consultation. Time was the doctors' and not the parents'. Not only did parents have to arrange to see the doctor and not the other way around, they might also have to wait even where they had been given a set time. Doctors usually apologized for major delays, but parents had no right to interrupt and be seen at the time that had been formally set aside for them. Similarly, once in the consultation it was typically the doctors who scheduled events and not the parents. As such it was doctors who normally made comments like "Right," "Fine," and "OK," which signaled changes in the topic or the action.

Controlling Talk

Just as doctors had special rights to engage in a variety of activities besides talk with parents, and could also largely determine the sequence and timing of those activities, so too they exerted a major control over talk itself. In considering that control, three points need particular emphasis. The first of these is the general absence of small talk from consultations. When staff talked to children all kinds of personal matters might be discussed: their school, Christmas presents, holidays, or favorite television programmes. By contrast, conversation with parents was all of a piece. Normally the participants talked of nothing besides medical matters either before, during, or after the consultation; with doctors there was no pre- or postactivity talk.

Not only was talk confined almost exclusively to medical matters; it was also largely question-and-answer talk, and rights within this were unequally distributed. Doctors by and large asked the questions; parents did the answering.

The third major feature of clinic talk, apart from its specificity and its concentration on medical matters, was the "hidden agenda" to which that talk was directed. Doctors asked for information but they did not normally explain why they needed it, nor did they reveal the criteria by which they judged its relevance. Some doctors might give a brief résumé of their thinking when they produced their conclusions, but no one gave this at the beginning of the consultation or during the actual questioning. Doctors had parents' answers at their own disposal and could do with them as they wished. They could accept them and pass on to something else, or they might make demands for greater precision and even on occasion check this out with the child:

Dr. G: And there's no question of his inhaling or swallowing anything that afternoon?
Mother: No, he didn't have anything in his mouth.
Dr. G: (to child) You're quite sure, Arthur, that you didn't have anything in your mouth and you hadn't swallowed anything?
Child: No.

Similarly, where a doctor was not happy with an answer he might continue to ask the same question until he was satisfied. Just as doctors repeated their questions until they got what they wanted, they also ignored things that they took to be irrelevant and might even interrupt a reply to ask about the matters that really concerned them:

Dr. F: Can he drink from a cup?
Mother: Yes. He's still got a bottle but. . . .
Dr. F: Can he hold a cup?
Mother: Yes, he can manage to hold one.

Not only could doctors make whatever they liked of answers to their questions, since their agenda was largely concealed, but they also used that agenda in an extremely rapid and routinized fashion. Such routinization was most obvious when doctors worked from an official form, but it was equally true of other cases. Each doctor had set methods for handling the kinds of case which he saw and used the same questions and the same formulations, in much the same order, in case after case of any particular type.

Controlling Topics

The right to control the consultation was used to restrict the topics of consultation even more narrowly than has hitherto been mentioned. Clinic action was not only exclusively medical, but also the medical remit was overtly defined in a most limited fashion. Staff focused on the individual case and, within this, on the current physical problems which that case involved. Only in exceptional instances was this focus broadened.

Take first the individualizing tendency of medical work. I noted earlier how in any one consultation staff concentrated on that particular child as if it constituted a world in itself and was not just another example of X or Y. In doing so they avoided the twin dangers of treating the child as either mere work or just clinical material. At the same time this focus also prevented parents from gaining general knowledge about medicine and its ways, and those few parents who dared to seek this were actively discouraged. Take, for instance, this example from the maternity hospital ward round:

Mother: Why do they measure the baby's length?
Dr. K: Well, we measure all children as it is related to their adult height. You probably wouldn't be interested.
Mother: (eagerly) Oh, yes, I'm fascinated by all the things you do, but I just wondered why you were doing it. I must have been about four inches long at birth. I'm so small.
Dr. K: How tall is your husband?
Mother: 5 feet 10 inches.
Dr. K: (tells the mother the average length of children at birth and adds) There's not much variation in this. (The mother smiles eagerly again and looks as if she wants to continue the conversation, but the doctor turns to talk to a registrar.)

Besides the omission of general discussion about medical matters, the range of topics covered was highly restricted. Fundamentally, doctors were interested only in problems. If there was no problem, there was nothing to talk about. Indeed, where the doctor was rushed, this might constitute the end of the interaction. Here, for example, are two fairly typical consultations with old patients on the maternity hospital ward round:

Dr. K: Hello, Mrs Jones.
Mother: Hello.
Dr. K: Is baby feeding OK?
Mother: Yes.
Dr. K: Fine. . . . No problems?
Mother: No.
Dr. K: Super.

We move on to the next bed.

Dr. K: Hello. You're an experienced mother, aren't you? No problems here?
Mother: No.
Dr. K: Fine.

We pass on to the next bed.

Not only were doctors interested solely in problems, but their definition of the problematic was severely limited. This had several aspects. Let us start with child development. This was a matter of major concern in all the clinics, and all the doctors and therapists had some training in the matter. However, staff took notice only of those who were retarded. Although local authority clinic doctors graded the children that they assessed, parents were not normally informed of the grade. Indeed, the fact that the child was being assessed was not normally mentioned. Only where a child was delayed were mothers told the result of the assessment.

Similarly, in all clinics mothers of delayed or handicapped children were routinely given advice on how to aid their child, but no such advice was given where babies were judged to be normal. Children, it seemed, needed to be "brought on" only if they were "behind."

Similarly, doctors normally showed little interest in the everyday difficulties posed by children. As children grew, they created all kinds of new problems for their care and management. Outside clinics, among mothers waiting in the corridor, such problems were a standard topic. "Mother craft" was, however, normally excluded from clinic conversation, even where the doctor felt the mother to be relatively incompetent. This was simply not the doctor's business; it did not fall within their remit and therefore it was not dealt with. Only where it was sufficient to cause a "medical" problem, for example, severe nappy rash, was it raised, and even here its handling was often delegated to others such as health visitors or nurses.

Psychiatric matters were another topic that was normally excluded from pediatric consultations within the bureaucratic format. It is worth noting here that almost all emotional issues were sidestepped and not just those which involved possible psychiatric disturbance. Clinics were not bereft of every emotion, some indeed were marked by jollity, but the emotional range was a foreshortened one. It ran simply from joy to neutrality. Where the occasion was a happy one, both parties might express happiness; where it was not, by and large they expressed nothing. Here as elsewhere doctors set the tone. As we have seen, parents who tried to import a language and emotional tone appropriate to other and more cheerful occasions by laughing or displaying great affection for their child often failed.

Serious conditions were examined without any dramatic comment to the parents, and just as doctors refrained from using such language, so too did almost all parents. Clinics, it seemed, were not places for emotional display. Bad news was broken in a matter-of-fact way and received in much the same fashion. Doctors indicated the tragic nature of events only by indirect means. Some, for instance, used a quieter and more intimate tone of voice. Some parents likewise lowered their eyes, looked embarrassed, and said little or nothing, but almost none displayed any open signs of grief. Only three parents in all were observed to cry and then only briefly. This does not mean that others felt no such emotions, but that clinics were inappropriate places to express these:

Dr. J: I think they often express some of their emotions as soon as they get outside the room. If I go out to get something or to test the urine of the next patient I find them in tears in the corridor, when they would seem nowhere near tears in the room. . . . They demonstrate relatively little in clinic. I'm sure the picture they present at home or on the bus on the way back is quite different.

The absence of open grief in clinics seems linked to the absence of any occasion formally provided for its expression. Having revealed the existence of a serious condition, doctors simply moved on to a discussion of further visits and possible treatment.

Such absence of occasions for grief did not mean that staff were annoyed when it was displayed, for they saw tears as "natural" and as "one end of the continuum." However, they acted as if those who were on the brink of tears would rather not cry if this could be avoided. They therefore carried on with their normal routine, or else, when this became impossible, paused to allow parents a chance to master their emotions.

Grief was treated as a private matter by both sides and not as something that was appropriately expressed in clinics. Even when mothers did cry, their tears were their own affair. The action might pause to allow them to recover, but sorrow was not itself a topic. Doctors did not put their arms round parents in such circumstances, nor did they encourage them to express their feelings further. The most that any doctor did was to murmur softly, "I know, I know." These matters were not entirely neglected, for staff did act where they were particularly worried about parents' reactions; but these were not dealt with in the clinic but delegated to other specialists, such as social workers.

23. *The Physician-Patient Relationship: Expectations and Reality*   Stanley Reichman

Patients and professionals each have expectations concerning the contract between them. Reality, however, often does not meet their expectations. The resulting gap may interfere with the patient-physician relationship. Moreover, the expectations of each are often dissimilar, and neither the professional nor the patient considers these differences, which I shall specify later. Despite the fact that some expectations may even be unachievable, discomfort, anger, frustation, and even hostility may arise from discrepancies between anticipations of entitlement and reality.

Recognizing such sociologic factors, it is not surprising that differing cultures and upbringings may also affect the response and expectations of patients. Consider the contrast between an Oriental who is taught that his illness is caused by wind or rain, a Hispanic who believes in the "hot and cold" theory, a devout religious individual who feels that an external force determines his fate, and an individual who seeks a physician with the expectation of a medical cure regardless of the underlying etiology of his illness.

In addition, acceptable standards for professions create specific professional behaviors, not only through basic education and training, but through requirements of licensure and the cultural determinants of professional societies. In a society such as ours, where we believe in rationality and individualism, is it surprising that different people and groups have different expectations?

The relationship of patient and physician can be viewed as a social system. Patients are expected to be motivated to get well. They must seek technical help and need to trust a physician. Their privileges, when ill, exempt them from normal or social tasks and from the responsibility for their own state. The professional, on the other hand, must act for the welfare of the patient, guide his conduct by the rules of professional behavior, apply a high degree of acquired skill and knowledge to the problems of illness, and maintain objectivity and professional self-regulation. The privileges for the professional include access to physical and personal intimacy, autonomy, and dominance over the patient.

Szasz and Hollender[1] subsequently described three models which depend upon the nature and severity of the illness, upon personality, and upon the preferences of doctors and patients. The active-passive, the guidance-cooperation, or the mutual participation relationships have analogy to and are reminiscent of the St. George model, the military model, and the symphony orchestra that Dr. Mauksch[2] has described. Selection of such relationships or behavior is influenced by the culture from which the professional and the patient come

Source: *Bulletin of the New York Academy of Medicine*, vol. 57, no. 1, January-February 1981, p. 5.

and the expectations of future benefits that each has in the relationship with the other. The dynamics that occur are more of a series of "happenings" than a simple contract.

Initially, a patient comes to a physician's office and says, "I don't feel well," which, translated, means, "Will you help me?" The physician in turn questions, "What is it that you feel is wrong?" which means, "I'll try." Thus, an implied contract is established. McGraw[3] has suggested that such contracts actually become a series of different transactions in which the physician plays the role of "gate keeper" for problem solving and treatment decision.

From the patient's standpoint, advances in medicine have resulted in increasing recognition by patients of conflicts that occur in decision making. Ellen Goodman, in a syndicated article in the Miami *Herald*[4] in February of this year, entitled "New Tests for Doctors: Confidence or Confusion," indicated that doctors who depend on statistics in science "can invite total mistrust or the charge that doctors know nothing. Willingly or not," she goes on to say, "we have to become consumers who treatment-shop, who research disease and 'cures' more carefully than we research the purchase of a dishwasher. And the doctor who asks for our trust is not prescribing certainty, but is guiding us through a thicket of difficult scientific information-forcing and is helping us to be his partners."

The American Society of Internal Medicine represents practicing internists in this country. Their publication, *The Internist,* recently printed a hypothetical physician-patient interview in which compliance is discussed.[5] The physician defines compliance as following orders; the patient disapproves of the term, speaking instead of a "social contract" with her health professional and expressing willingness to follow his advice only after weighing its risks and benefits. Growing adamant, the physician warns that noncompliance can lead to dire consequences, but the undaunted patient, while admitting the possibility of "ill-effects," suggests that noncompliance can sometimes be harmless and even beneficial.

While our subject is not compliance, it is essential that we understand that out of the relationship between the doctor and the patient comes a series of interactions that will affect the outcome of an illness, as well as general behavior promoting health and wellness. Where each participant's perception is at the beginning may well affect that outcome. That the American Society of Internal Medicine emphasizes such conflicting statements is a significant recognition of new requirements for satisfying patient-physician relationships.

Guze suggested four kinds of satisfactions that can be derived from medicine: prestige, income, helping to relieve suffering, and intellectual effort.[6] He points out that prestige and money are not enough for the "long haul." Helping people often makes a physician feel like a god, but this is unrealistic because medicine is a long way from such powers. Self-doubts and frustrations in practice soon destroy such illusions of omnipotence. Guze concludes that cultivating the intellectual side of medicine is the true satisfaction to avoid boredom and frustration and to make the practice of medicine fun for a lifetime. Guze's ideas support the studies of Friedson, who maintained that patients value competence as highly as the medical profession does but, in addition, also value personal interest on the part of the physician for their specific needs.[7] However, they often use the specialist for his competence and the general physician for his personal interest in their welfare.

The ability to communicate, i.e., the methods by which a physician obtains information and feeds back his thinking to the patient, is important in the teaching relationship that must be present between physician and patient. Recent studies suggest that many physicians, particularly during training,[8] fail in this process. If communication, a key element in the diagnosis, treatment, and education of the patient, is impaired, can we expect that holistic medicine, consumer advocacy, and the "wellness" movements will be successful without recognizing gaps between expectations and reality?

To use this expectations-reality concept one begins by defining an expectation as what one would like to have if he could write his own ticket. All of us live with reality, and difficulties sometimes develop because we do not examine our own expectations or desires closely enough.

Table 1 presents a series of expectations for patients. No one patient may ask for all of them nor are they listed in any special order; rather, they are general and theoretically designed to provoke and stimulate discussion. Convenient, comprehensive services which include continuity of care at a reasonabe cost are the major desire. Patients like their doctor to be caring, compassionate, and competent. Competency also includes trust, with the hope to be comforted and possibly cured and to be relieved of the anxiety associated with the fear of being ill. But in this process patients like to maintain control.

Compare these to the professional's expectation (Table 2). Here, instead of services, practice is viewed as the prime concern. Physicians expect that practice will be scientific and intellectually challenging. They view themselves as ethical individuals with high standards who are rewarded financially with a high level of income. Physicians expect that patients will be respectful and compliant and that the physician will maintain autonomy in the process.

Actually, however, services are not always accessible and care is frequently episodic and not comprehensive, although some patients seem to prefer episodic care and there are often expenses with unexpected failures in third party coverage. The professional is regarded as callous or even godlike. That he may not be sufficiently trusted is suggested by the movement to obtain second opinions. Finally, patients often complain that they are dependent and afraid to make their wishes known or to ask questions for fear of appearing to be too demanding (see Table 1).

Physicians, on the other hand, are concerned because of burdensome paperwork, pressures, and problems of keeping knowledge up to date because of the increasingly time-consuming demands of practice. New technological procedures raise ethical questions of performance and decision making, and increasing government controls produce new restraints which affect not only autonomy but ethical decisions. Moreover, rising costs and inflation in a changing health care system affect daily practice. And, finally, patients appear distrustful, forcing defensive medicine, displaying episodic and self-destructive behaviors, and often ignoring specific instructions (see Table 2).

It is this gap between expectations and reality that produces fear, distrust, anxiety, and hostility on the part of the patient and worry, discomfort, frustration, and anger on the part of the physician.

NOTES

1. T. S. Szasz and M. H. Hollender, "A Contribution to the Philosophy of Medicine: The Basic Models of the Doctor-Patient Relationship," *Archives of Internal Medicine*, vol. 97, p. 585, 1956.

2. H. Mauksch, "Sociologic Aspects of Patient Behavior," *Journal of the Association for Hospital Medical Education*, vol. 7, p. 15, 1974–1975.

3. R. McGraw, "Expectations and Responsibilities for Better Health Care," *Journal of the Association for Hospital Medical Education*, vol. 7, p. 15, 1974–1975.

4. E. Goodman, New Tests for Doctors: Confidence or Confusion. *Miami Herald*, February 2, 1980.

5. An Act for Two Players. *The Internist*, November 1979, p. 12.

6. S.B. Guze, "Can the Practice of Medicine Be Fun for a Lifetime?" *Journal of the American Medical Association,* vol. 241, p. 2021, 1979.

7. E. Friedson, *Patients' Views of Medical Prac-*

tice, Russell Sage Foundation, New York, 1961.

8. R.W. Platt and J.C. McMath, "Clinical Hypo-competence: The Interview," *Annals of Internal Medicine,* vol. 91, p. 898, 1979.

TABLE 1. PATIENT—PROFESSIONAL RELATIONSHIP

Expectations	*Reality*
Services will be:	*Services are sometimes:*
Convenient	Inaccessible
Comprehensive	Episodic
Reasonable in cost	Expensive with coverage failures
The professional will be:	*The professional may be:*
Caring	Callous or godlike
Competent	Not trusted
I would like:	*I am often:*
Control	Dependent

TABLE 2. PROFESSIONAL—PATIENT RELATIONSHIP

Expectations	*Reality*
Practice will be:	*Practice is:*
Scientific and intellectually challenging	Stressful keeping up to date with increasing paperwork
Ethical	Controlled by technology and government
Financially satisfactory	Pressured by rising costs and inflation
Patients will be:	*Patients have:*
Respectful	Distrust and force defensive medicine
Compliant	Episodic and self-destructive behaviors: do not follow instructions
I shall have:	*I have:*
Autonomy	Third party, institutional, and patient demands

Doctors' Roles

24. The Professional and Patient Relationship
Tom L. Beauchamp   James F. Childress

Conflicts among Contractual and Role Obligations

In many cases, the health care professional has a duty of care because of an explicit or implicit contract with the patient. But in some cases, the therapeutic contract may actually be with a party other than the patient. The beneficiary need not hold one end of the chain of obligations and rights. For example, if someone promises John Doe to look after his children after his death, we would say that the promisor has an obligation to John Doe although the children are the primary beneficiaries.[1] When parents bring a child to a physician for treatment, the physician's primary responsibility is to the child, whose interests are paramount. Courts have rightly refused to allow Jehovah's Witnesses to reject medically necessary blood transfusions for their children, even though the courts have often allowed adult Jehovah's Witnesses to reject blood transfusions for themselves. In some cases, parents may be charged with child neglect when they fail to seek or permit highly desirable medical treatment, even if it falls short of being necessary to save the child's life. Angela Holder has provided a summary of one such case: "A teenage boy suffered from a massive deformity of the face and neck. He was so grotesque he was excused from school attendance and was therefore illiterate. Surgery could correct the condition but could not be performed without blood transfusions. The mother objected on religious grounds to administration of blood and therefore would not consent to surgery. The court held that he was a 'neglected child' and ordered the surgery performed."[2]

In recent years there has been considerable moral debate about decisions regarding defective newborns who need surgery to sustain their lives. In the much discussed Johns Hopkins Hospital case, a mongoloid infant needed surgery for duodenal atresia. The parents refused to grant permission for the surgery, and the infant died of starvation after several days. In some cases, physicians or hospitals have gone to the courts to gain permission to provide the medical treatment refused by the parents. Such interventions are probably more common among physicians and hospitals in cases of refusal of treatment on *religious* grounds, partly because the health care professionals rarely share these belief systems. In cases where parents appeal to the best interests of the child and to familial interests, such as the prevention of disruption and strain on financial resouces, physicians appear to be more willing to support the familial decision to refuse treatment. Of course, there may be major disagreements about what would be in the child's *interest,* or in the family's *interest,* but the point is that many physicians appear to be more comfortable with such judgments about interests than with refusals on religious grounds.[3] Our own view is that physicians have a primary responsibility to the patient, even if a third party establishes the initial contract. The physician ought to act in the patient's

Source: Tom L. Beauchamp and James F. Childress, *Principles of Biomedical Ethics,* Oxford University Press, New York, 1979.

best interests, even when it is necessary to seek a court order to authorize surgery, a blood transfusion, or whatever. Other familial interests such as avoiding the depletion of financial resources should not be considered until a certain threshold is reached, viz., when significant patient interests would not be served by continued treatment or by a particular treatment.

The above examples focus on the conflict between the interests of the patient, the beneficiary, and the wishes of the contractor with the health care professional. In another major type of conflict it may be less clear exactly what the health care professional owes the "patient." Examples include a physician's contract to examine applicants for positions in a company or to determine whether applicants for insurance policies are good risks. In such cases, the health care professional may rightly not think of the person he examines as his patient. He has certain responsibilities of due care, but they may not be as comprehensive or as stringent as the responsibilities that obtain in the ordinary physician-patient relationship. They would include care in the examination so as not to injure the individual—e.g., by exposing him to excessive x-rays. From a legal standpoint, the health care professional in some jurisdictions may not even have a duty to disclose the discovery of a disease to the examinee. For example, in one preemployment physical examination, x-rays indicated that the woman who was subsequently hired had tuberculosis, but the physician and employer did not disclose these findings to her. After three years, the employee became ill with tuberculosis and was hospitalized for a prolonged period. In this case, the court held that the woman's only recourse was Workman's Compensation. The court did not allow her suit against her employer and the physician who examined her, on grounds that there was no established patient-physician relationship, and hence no duty to disclose the information to her.[4] From a moral standpoint both the employer and the physician had a duty to disclose this information in order to prevent harm to her; they did not merely have a duty to benefit her. Furthermore, one could argue that the employer and the physician had no right to withold this information, because the woman had a moral right to it.

What does this moral duty of disclosure require in conflict situations where some institutional interests might be at stake? Suppose a company requires regular physical examinations of all employees by a company physician. The physician's contract requires him to inform the company about employees' health conditions that might bear on their work. If the company uses materials that might be hazardous to the employees, e.g., kepone or benzene, and the physician discovers symptoms of a disease that might be directly related to working conditions, what obligation does he have to report these findings to the employees as well as to the company? Does he have the same obligation if the employer expressly forbids such disclosures to employees? Health care professionals, we suggest, have a moral responsibility to oppose, avoid, and withdraw from contracts that would force them to withhold information of significant medical benefit to examinees.

In another type of situation, a health care professional may be under contract to, or otherwise obligated to, an institution to provide *care* for a group of individuals. In these cases, there can be no doubt that physicians, for example, owe "due care" to these individuals who are their "patients," despite the third-party contract or obligation. Examples include health care professionals in industries, prisons, and the armed services. In these settings, care of the patient may come into conflict with needs of the institution. The patient's needs generally should take precedence, but not always. Difficult cases may emerge, for example, on the battlefield. Triage in the battlefield setting may be different from triage in the peacetime emergency room. In the former setting the needs of the military may dictate that certain patients be given priority even when medical needs establish a different priority. In a celebrated example, when penicillin became available for use in North Africa in World War II, a difficult allocation decision had to be made because the supply was severely limited. Authorities decided to give the available penicillin to soldiers suffering from venereal disease rather than those who had been wounded on the battlefields. The former, they reasoned, could be restored to fighting capacity more easily and effectively than the latter. It is not possible to generalize from the battlefield to ordinary medical practice. Even on the battlefield, however, medical needs should not be wholly subordinated to military needs. For example, conventions regarding the laws of war hold that the fallen enemy soldier with medical needs is to be given equal consideration along with one's own comrades.

Similarly, the two roles of research scientist and clinical practitioner may come into conflict. As an investigator, the physician acts to generate knowledge that can lead to progress in medicine that will ultimately benefit individual patients. As a clinical practitioner, he acts in the present patient's best interests. Both these roles may function to "benefit the sick," but the scientific role aims to benefit statistical lives in the future, while the clinical role seeks to benefit particular patients now. Responsibility to future generations thus may come into conflict with "due care" for particular persons who are subjects as well as patients. The Declaration of Geneva of the World Medical Association affirms that "the health of my patient will be my first consideration." Yet, can this principle be affirmed under all conditions in the context of research involving patients as subjects? If not, should it be sacrificed or at least compromised in order to benefit more people in the future?

Controlled clinical trials are considered important and even necessary in order to make sure that an observed effect, e.g., reduced mortality from a particular disease, is really the result of a particular treatment rather than some other variable that the researcher might have missed, e.g., other conditions in the patient population. Among the controlled trials to determine the effectiveness and safety of treatments and procedures, the randomized clinical trial (RCT) is widely used. Instead of trying to match patients for variables so that some of the matched patients can receive A and some B, the RCT randomly assigns patients to different therapies or placebos. Randomization is used to keep variables other than the treatments under examination from distorting the study. It is often preferred to observational or retrospective studies on the grounds that its results have a higher degree of validity by virtue of its elimination of bias in assignment and reduction of extraneous variables. Thus, it appears to offer a sound inductive technique to validate knowledge.

Many questions can be raised about RCTs: are they as essential as their proponents say? Can they be used without compromising acknowledged responsibilities to patients?[5] The increased probability of their results is only a matter of degree, and there might be reasons for preferring a less conclusive method if it would more fully respect our duties to current patients. Proponents of RCTs often argue, however, that RCTs do not violate moral duties to patients, because there is genuine doubt about the merits of existing therapies or of standard and new therapies. No patient will receive a treatment that is known to be less effective or more dangerous than another available alternative. Because current patients, in effect, are not asked to make any sacrifices, who could object to the use of RCTs? After all, they will in addition benefit future patients. It is, of course, possible that treatments rarely exhibit such perfect balance, especially if all the patient's circumstances are considered. Rarely would a physician be willing to determine by chance which treatment a patient receives except in the context of RCTs.

A vivid recent example indicates some difficulties in the use of RCTs. A controlled, double-blind experiment on a new drug, adenine arabinoside (ara-A), indicated that it is an effective treatment for herpes simplex encephalitis. Of the ten people who were given the placebo, seven died. Of the eighteen who received ara-A, five died, seven recovered to lead reasonably normal lives, and six had serious brain or nerve damage. The ten who received the placebo also were given standard treatment, which mainly consists of palliative efforts. (No treatment prior to ara-A had been found to be effective.) Because ara-A had already been shown to be effective and nontoxic in other localized herpes simplex hominis infections, and because no other treatment prevented mortality and serious brain and nerve damage, moral questions arise about giving anyone the placebo. The experiment was stopped early, but it remains unclear whether it was necessary to have a placebo group instead of historical controls.

Even when there are no scientific or ethical grounds for opposing a particular randomized clinical trial—for example, of two treatments that are roughly equal in safety and efficacy—patients may have strong preferences for one or the other. Suppose that two surgical procedures for treating the same disease appear to have the same survival rate (say, an average of 15 years), and suppose we propose to test their effectiveness by an RCT. The patient might have a preference if treatment A has little risk of death during the operation but a high rate of death after ten years, while treatment B has a high risk of death during the operation or postoperative recovery but a low rate of death after recovery (say, for 30 years). A patient's age, family responsibilities, and other circumstances in life might lead him to prefer one over the other. [6] While a research institution could legitimately accept only patients who were willing to participate in certain research projects related to their own diseases, patients in other types of settings should be able to choose between treatments whenever both treatments are available.

Since patients commonly assume that decisions about their treatment are made in their best interests, and not in the interests of a research design, the physician-researcher should disclose all the alternatives to patient-subjects so that they can make an informed judgment about participation. One relevant item of information is the method of allocation to a particular treatment. Some contend that disclosure of such matters would cause distress that would be harmful to patients or would lead some patients to refuse to participate in the research. They also argue that disclosure of such matters is not necessary, since the patient does not need to know how the allocation is made between two treatments that appear to be equally effective and/or harmless. However, since the physician-researcher is a double agent, holding dual responsibilities, he has a fiduciary duty to inform his patient-subjects of everything that is relevant to their own decisions and, in particular, that might involve the physician-researcher in a conflict of interest. [7] The duty of disclosure persists throughout the period of the research and requires that the patient-subject be informed about developments that might be relevant to a decision to withdraw.

Physician-researchers also face difficult questions about whether to stop an experiment before it has been completed, and even before there is enough information to have preliminary data accepted. If a physician determines that his patient's condition is deteriorating and that the patient's interests dictate withdrawal from the research, he should be free to act on behalf of the patient, assuming, of course, that he does not act in opposition to the express wishes of the patient. Some research designs take advantage of emerging evidence to alter the protocol; some play the winner by utilizing what appear to be the best therapies until they fail. But in an RCT, particularly if it is a double-blind study, it may be difficult to determine whether the experiment as a whole should be stopped merely because some physician-researchers insist that they have enough evidence already. One proposal to handle the ethical conflict involves a differentiation of roles; it recommends an advisory committee to determine whether to continue or stop a trial. Such a committee "must consider the impact of its decision on the treatment of future patients. Although an individual physician may only be responsible for treating his current patients, the advisory committee must act as if the care of future patients rests in their hands, because their recommendations are likely to influence therapy for the many patients to follow."[8]

The proposal of a differentiation of roles by using an advisory committee may be procedurally sound, but it fails to resolve the ethical questions. Instead, it relocates them. Even if occupants of different roles represent different interests, e.g., the physicians represent current patient's interests, while the scientists and the advisory committee represent future patients' interests, it is still necessary to determine when it is legitimate to impose certain risks on current patients in order to benefit future ones. It must be determined whether medical knowledge and scientific progress with their undisputed benefits are optional or mandatory, whether the increased probabilites of the knowledge gained by randomized clinical trials are worth the moral costs, and whether the benefits outweigh the burdens. When the physician charged with the care of particular patients is convinced that their interests are being sacrificed for the benefit of others, he should not surrender his judgment to the advisory committee. He should remain a patient advocate. In other cases, an institutional review board may determine that the research fails to offer patient-subjects adequate protection from harm, and it should demand revisions in the research protocol and possibly should refuse to allow the research.

Some hold that the researcher-physician's commitment to the welfare of his patients offers the best protection, even in a research project authorized by an institutional review board. Others, however, contend that we should differentiate roles so that physicians do not use their own patients in research. Their point is not that a person cannot be both an investigator and a clinician, but that a person should not assume both roles for the same patient-subject.[9] A similar argument supports not allowing the physician who is going to transplant a kidney from a A to B to determine when A is dead. Proposals for procedures will depend in part on conceptions of human nature and convictions about the importance of reducing conflicts of interests. In many cases role-differentiation may obviate some of the moral conflicts. Nevertheless, answers to procedural questions will not be satisfactory unless we also have answers to more substantive questions. What is at stake is not merely who can and should protect patients' interests, but how much weight should be given to the interests of current patients and how much to future patients. Our view is that medical knowledge and scientific progress are important but often are optional. Generally the broader duty of beneficence is less stringent than the duty to "benefit the sick," who already have a special relationship with health care professionals. This conclusion should not be construed to subvert research. Rather, we should promote research methods that will enable us to pursue knowledge while simultaneously protecting the interests of current patients.

NOTES

1. See H. L. A. Hart's discussion in "Are There Any Natural Rights?" *Philosophical Review*, vol. 64, p. 175, 1955.

2. Summary of *In re Sampson*, 317 NYS 2d, NY 1970, by Angela Holder, *Medical Malpractice Law*, p. 17, John Wiley & Sons, New York, 1975.

3. See, for example, Anthony Shaw, "Dilemmas of 'Informed Consent' in Children," *The New England Journal of Medicine*, vol. 289, p. 885, October 25, 1973.

4. Holder, in *Medical Malpratice Law*, p. 19, John Wiley & Sons, New York, 1975.

5. A thorough and helpful study of randomized clinical trials appears in Charles Fried, *Medical Experimentation: Personal Integrity and Social Policy*, American Elsevier, New York, 1974. For other criticisms, see Milton C. Weinstein, "Alloca-

tion of Subjects in Medical Experiments," *The New England Journal of Medicine*, vol. 291, p. 1278, December 12, 1974. For defenses of RCTs, see David P. Byar et al., "Randomized Clinical Trials: Perspectives on Some Recent Ideas," *The New England Journal of Medicine* vol. 295, p. 74, July 8, 1976, and several writings by Thomas Chalmers, including Thomas C. Chalmers et al., "Controlled Studies in Clinical Cancer Research," *The New England Journal of Medicine*, vol. 287, p. 75, July 13, 1972, and L. W. Shaw and T. C. Chalmers, "Ethics in Cooperative Clinical Trials," *Annals of the New York Academy of Science*, vol. 169, p. 487, 1970.

6. See Weinstein, op. cit., p. 1280.

7. See Fried, op. cit., p. 71.

8. Byar et al., op. cit., p. 78.

9. See Fried, op. cit., p. 160.

25. *Responsibility: Medical Students*
David E. Resser   Andrea Klein Schroder

Rich was a freshman when he had this experience:

My wife and I were coming home from a movie. Up ahead we saw that there'd been an accident. A woman had been hit by a car. She was lying on the pavement and a crowd of people was standing around her. I felt my heart leap into my throat.

My first reaction was, this isn't really happening. Then I heard myself saying, "What's the difference, we can just drive on, the ambulance will be there soon anyway.

But then I realized, "You're a doctor! You *have* to stop!"

I tried desperately to remember what I knew. I raced through my mind trying to remember the details of the one lecture we had received on emergency first aid. We had received that lecture more than 6 months ago."

When Rich stopped, his worst fears were not confirmed. The woman had suffered a head injury but was conscious. She was reluctant to go to a hospital, and Rich was able to use his authority as a medical student to insist that she go. "Well," she said, "If you really think it's necessary, Doctor." Thus, he learned that his responsibility turned out to be neither as all-encompassing as he had feared, nor as insignificant as he sometimes imagined.

Nowhere in medicine are the paradoxes more exquisite than in the area of responsibility. At one extreme, students have quite exaggerated notions of their ultimate power. They imagine the practice of medicine as a war constantly being waged on the very cusp of life and death. The training that most students receive in university and charity hospitals, where patients are critically ill, tends to reinforce this harrowing view of responsibility. Usually, students anticipate a time—typically the first day of their internships—when they will have to

Source: David E. Resser and Andrea Klein Schroder, *Patient Interviewing: The Human Dimension*, Williams & Wilkins, Baltimore, 1980.

know everything and be able to do everything, responsible for saving a half a dozen lives a day. Sometimes, faculty reinforce this frightening fantasy.

As the student's sophistication increases, he begins to realize that responsibility is a concept that goes far beyond TV heroism, however. It is an idea filled with excruciating paradoxes. The student comes to understand that he will be responsible not only for handling the occasional fearsome emergency but also (far more often) for knowing when not to do something. When does a doctor decide not to prolong a child's misery with one more anticancer drug? When does one write the order in a patient's chart, "no heroic measures," or a similar code phrase meaning "allow the patient to die"? When does a doctor decide *not* to take responsibility?

> Quinn was a senior student on surgery during an especially hectic admitting night. The hospital was a county hospital, located in a notoriously dangerous section of town. It was Saturday night, the night which the surgery residents cavalierly called "the weekly meeting of the Los Angeles gun and knife club." Two gunshot wounds and a serious stab wound had come up to the floor in rapid succession. In addition, a young woman with a painful breast, presumed to be due to an abscess, had also arrived.
>
> During a hasty 10-minute dinner break, the chief resident had distributed responsibilities. By the time it was decided who would operate on whom, there were no residents left to take care of the young woman with the breast abscess.
>
> "Why don't you do that down in the treatment room, Quinn?" the surgery resident suggested.
>
> Quinn was reluctant. "Well, maybe you'd better help me do my first one."
>
> "Nonsense," the chief resident said. "Here I'll show you!" He then drew a hasty diagram on a napkin with his ballpoint pen showing the presumed location of the abscess and how to make an incision. "Just get to the loculated fluid," he said. "And don't forget to put in a drain."
>
> Two hours later, the resident had to be called out of surgery to come down to the treatment room. Quinn had managed to make a mess of things. The "abscess" had turned out not be an abscess at all, but a cyst. Quinn's incision had led to a futile groping about for the site of loculated fluid. In addition he had nicked a small artery which he couldn't tie off.
>
> In the end, no mortal harm was done, but the patient had been terribly frightened, subjected to unnecessary pain, and probably had been given a needlessly disfiguring scar.
>
> Quinn was very hard on himself. "How stupid of me!" he ranted to himself. "I should have been responsible enough to say no."

There are many things to say about this disturbing vignette. Quinn himself probably hit on the most important point when he recognized that responsibility also involves knowing one's limitations. Certainly, the system that Quinn found himself in did not make this any easier.

Finally, responsibility is not restricted to knowing what to do (and what not to do). Too often, doctors tend to gravitate toward action. Frequently, the real responsibility that a physician should assume has less to do with action than with his willingness to stand by his patients, making a personal, human commitment to them.

Learning a true sense of responsiblity is not easy. Students find that they often vacillate between extremes of excessive detachment and excessive involvement. They struggle with the need to be committed to their patients on the one hand while preserving some sense of serenity in their personal lives on the other. At times they feel terribly vulnerable, stripped of their psychological epidermis. At other times, they feel excessively detached, as though they are clanking around in a suit of psychological armor, effective but unwieldy, and purchased at the price of their humanness.

In my view a major responsibility of ICM courses involves helping students to define responsibility in its most human terms. A further goal should be helping students to integrate growing responsibility in a way that permits the excitement and joy that come from a commitment to patients to flourish. It is unquestionably in this growing ability to be close to patients, and truly responsible for them, that the doctor will discover his greatest meaning. Many current ICM courses represent a heartening step in this direction. More still needs to be done, however, to build on the foundation of the first two years. Students in their junior and senior years, interns and residents are also entitled to help in mastering their responsibility in a way that is enriching rather than traumatic.

26. *The Client and the Team Approach*
Alex J. Ducanis　Anne K. Golin

The models of the client role and the client-professional relationship examined in this chapter focus on the traditional dyadic relationship between the "sick" person and an individual who attempts to help. Although this has been the most common pattern of medical services and has generally served as a model for other professionals in their relationships with clients, there are a variety of service delivery systems available today that reflect different models of the client-professional relationship. This includes, of course, the team approach.

The most pronounced shift in the traditional Western therapeutic dyad is probably a departure from the dyad itself. Increasingly, the patient is involved not in an isolated two-person social system but in a medical team effort in which the physician is first among equals rather than unique healer. A paramount issue of the future may be the redefinition of the doctors' role as a collaborative one and the patterning of team medicine for maximum therapeutic efficacy. The future of medical practice will probably rest on a detailed meshing of medicine, nursing, social work, administration, and perhaps even social science.

What kinds of changes in the relationship between client and professional result from the team approach? We can see a number of possible effects. First, it might be expected that the degree of dependency in the relationship between client and professional cannot be as great when a number of health agents are involved. Thus, although *more* professionals are involved, and consequently clients may have a better chance of finding one with whom they can develop a comfortable relationship, the strength of each of those relationships is likely to be less intense than if only one team member were clearly involved with the client. This dilution of the relationship affects both patient and professional. While the patient whose welfare rests on a number of professional workers may feel less dependent on any one of them, the professional may at the same time experience less personal responsiblity for

Source: Alex J. Ducanis and Anne K. Golin, *The Interdisciplinary Health Care Team*, Aspen Systems Corp., Rockville, Maryland, 1979.

the client and perhaps even feel a diminished sense of accomplishment when treatment is successfully completed.

Second, clients' lessened dependency on any one member of the team and the fact that at times they may receive contradictory information from various team members suggests that the treatment process might become more confusing for some team-treated clients. Illness and hospitalization generally produce heightened anxiety and a sense of helplessness in the client, and the client may feel an increased need for structure and for clear communication. If the patient is unsure which team member can be asked to supply clarification and additional information, the team situation could create more problems for the patient.

Third, members of the team, particularly if it is a strong, cohesive working group, may find that their primary job satisfaction has shifted from working with clients to working with other team members. Since goals for the client have now become team goals, reaching those goals may no longer give the same sense of personal reward, but are now important in terms of the *team's* accomplishment. The team may actually become more important to the professional than the client.

Fourth, clients may be given more responsibility for their own care and be expected to play a more active role than in the past. Clients may more often be included as active participants in team conferences and asked to play a major role in decision making and treatment planning.

Fifth, the family is also more likely to be included in the planning process if a team is involved. Since a number of specialists are concerned with all aspects of the client's functioning, inclusion of appropriate family members seems a natural step.

Finally, the overall quality of care received by the client may well be better with a team approach than with a traditional dyadic relationship. Both the treatment of existing conditions and the prevention of potential problems may be more effective under an interdisciplinary team, thus enhancing the client-professional relationship.

While many clients will welcome such changes, some may find them disturbing. For example, patients identified as *primary* (i.e., those who expect to have primary needs taken care of by the hospital) may not welcome the more active role implied by the team concept. Such patients tend to look upon the doctor as omnipotent and seem to find that reassuring. On the other hand, *instrumental* patients view the "good" patient as one who is relatively autonomous and self-sufficient rather than submissive and compliant.

The view of the client as an active participant in treatment is not a new one. Not all professionals have adopted the hierarchical, asymmetrical dyad as a model of client-professional interaction. Psychotherapists and counselors have traditionally tended to emphasize the need to develop a therapeutic relationship in which the client assumes a major responsibility for treatment and plays an active role. Most striking in the "nondirective" or "client-centered" approach, this view is held to some extent by most proponents of psychotherapy. The increasing popularity of family therapy and group therapy reflects further departures from the asymmetrical dyad.

Clients may serve as comanagers in their rehabilitation. Such a relationship connotes active participation by *both* client and specialist, enchances the client's self-respect, and increases motivation. Furthermore, the counselor often does not have sufficient knowledge to make important decisions affecting the client's future, and some decisions may well fall within the "inalienable rights" of the client to self-determination.

More recently, legislation has specified the participation of clients and family members in treatment and educational planning. For example, Individualized Written Rehabilitation Programs require the signature of the client receiving services from the state-federal rehabilitation programs. Similarly, Public Law 94–142 requires parental approval of a child's Individualized Educational Program (IEP) if the child is receiving special education services, and provides for due process hearings if the parents do not support the decisions reached.

For the team member, the changing role of the client may be a mixed blessing. While many professionals welcome a more active role for their clients, the client's participation in team meetings sometimes calls for adjustments that may be difficult for some members. When clients become members of the team, team interactions may become more inhibited, communication may become more formal, and reports may be considerably abbreviated. In extreme cases the team conference may become a mere formality, with the real decisions made outside the team meeting. Sometimes the addition of clients to the team can be seen as primarily a political move designed to shift the balance of power in the team, "open up" the decision process, or respond to consumer pressure.

Finally, it should be reemphasized that whatever the role of a particular client vis-à-vis the professionals on the team, the client remains the major focus of the team's efforts. The problems presented by the client define what the team is to do and who is to do it. If the client is dependent on the team for treatment and care, the team is equally dependent on the client for its continued functioning. The client *is* the reason for the existence of the team.

27. *For the Sake of the Child*　P. M. Strong

Observation of a Scottish clinic demonstrated that, although staff felt an obligation toward individual patients, many other motives also influenced their work: their career, academic interest, personal schedules, professional advancement, scientific development, departmental rivalry, and general policy matters. All these perspectives could be brought to bear on any one patient and each case was of more or less collegial interest as it combined these various qualities.

Such interests were, however, not relevant within the bureaucratic format and many would have destroyed the world which it contained. Just as staff never questioned the good character of parents, so too their own motivation went unremarked. Parents were never told that their child's complaint was boring or routine, and on only a handful of occasions was any comment made on its fascination. Words like "odd" or "unusual" were only very rarely used, while the work which any case involved or the degree of disruption it caused were largely hidden. The existence of other patients or of other demands upon their time were not topics of conversation with parents. In all this, each case was overtly treated as a world in itself. The present consultation stood alone, detached from other medical pursuits. Staff's interest in the general was subordinated to the particular, to this child, to whom they, like the parents, were now apparently devoting all their skill and attention.

Source: P. M. Strong, *The Ceremonial Order of the Clinic: Parents, Doctors, and Medical Bureaucracies,* Routledge and Kegan Paul, London, 1979.

This general strategy of avoidance fitted well enough with the medical anonymity required to sustain collegial authority. However, just as there were certain occasions when it was difficult to idealize parents' character, staff's character could also be threatened. Here too, not everything could be readily ignored, and special procedures were necessary to smooth over and nullify the more intrusive aspects of medicine.

For example, in most of the settings parents did not see staff in private. There was normally a medical audience present, usually a nurse, often some students, occasionally other doctors; and the simple presence of colleagues or apprentices created the continual possibility of collegial discussion between them. Indeed this was often essential, particularly since teaching was a central activity in both the hospitals. As it was teaching that created the greatest threat to the idealized moral commitment of staff to the individual child patient, I shall treat this in detail, and this case must serve as an example of the challenge that any kind of collegial discussion presented.

Teaching was especially revealing of much that was not normally mentioned. First, from the perspective of medical training, patients and those who accompanied them were best viewed as "living textbooks," as empirical instances of types of phenomenon. Medical problems were of interest, not because this or that patient suffered from them and wished to be cured of them, but because this was the kind of problem students were obliged to learn about. Second, medical teaching in such contexts involved the doctor's own actions quite as much as any patient's condition. It was a highly reflexive act. Not only did doctors describe the medical phenomena under investigation, they also spelled out their own involvement in the proceedings: how they had done this and why they would now do that.

Teaching could therefore be a most elaborate affair. Doctors might sketch in the general background to a clinic and discuss their general mandate, the types of patient seen there, hospital policy for these, and referral patterns to and from the setting. More specifically, doctors could detail the nature of particular problems, their various causes, incidence, and prognoses, and then describe how to recognize them, the various tests to use, their reliability, and the reasoning that lay behind them. Instructions might also be given on how to read a file or a referral letter, how to get a history, and how much trust to place in it. In other words, good teaching necessarily involved making explicit many of those things that were typically concealed from parents. The difficulties that the revelation of these matters might cause were presented in a particularly acute fashion in the settings observed in this study. Teaching on these cases involved hot medicine, rather than the action replay or cold medicine found in some forms of bedside teaching. Here new diagnoses were actually made, fresh problems discovered, and binding decisions taken.

The principal method used to overcome the dangers of collegial discussion was the careful segregation of such talk. This was done in a number of different ways. In all but the American amphitheater clinics, one staff member was clearly in control of the interaction. In the Scottish settings, the audience never spoke to or examined the patient without the doctor's permission, and such permission was a rarity in all but the maternity hospital ward round. Scottish students, with this one exception, had no right to speak to the doctor in front of parents, save when spoken to; and the remarks made to them were normally statements, not items of conversation which required a reply. Medical discourse as opposed to medical pronouncement was therefore a great rarity. The same rule applied in most of the American settings. Interns or residents might talk directly with parents in the presence of their "chief," since they had conducted the workup, but detailed medical discussion about the case was usually avoided.

Such avoidance was possible because in most settings parents and staff were readily segregated. Detailed teaching in the Scottish clinics could be done in the gaps between patients, while in the American ambulatory clinics staff left the cubicles each time they wanted a private discussion: "We'll be back in a minute" was the refrain which punctuated the parents' sojourn. Parents had the right to object to teaching. One mother, who complained afterward to a nurse, was seen in private from then on, the researchers too being barred. Similarly, when an adolescent boy complained about being taught on in the American hospital the doctor and students withdrew.

These procedures minimized the amount of collegial discussion that took place in front of parents, while some doctors rarely taught openly on children. The staff in the Scottish neurological clinic thought their cases were too serious for overt teaching, and one of them eventually banned students altogether. In four settings, however—the special nursery follow-up clinic, the amphitheater clinics, the maternity hospital ward round, and one of the Scottish general medical clinics—large amounts of such discussion were held in front of parents. Despite this, staff in all settings indicated that their clinical discussion was subordinate to their interaction with parents. The clinical format coexisted with the bureaucratic format, but it was a side event. Thus, where doctors talked with students or with other staff they typically did so quietly and at the margin. In the amphitheater clinic, staff discussion was usually confined to those on the stage and was conducted in whispers. In the general medical clinic, junior doctors who wished to discuss their cases with the consultant waited quietly at the side until he had noticed them; they did not themselves interrupt his conversation with patients.

Overt teaching was similarly given a secondary place. Some teaching comments were made in ways that fitted in naturally with the conversation with parents, the doctors' statements serving as remarks to both the mother and the students. Here are examples of how this could be done, one from history taking and the other from an examination.

Dr. F. Is she walking yet?
Mother: She's walking round the furniture.
Dr. F: Children usually walk round the furniture before they walk properly.
Dr. F: (lifts the baby) That's a nice straight back. Right! (He puts the baby back down.) Well, he can sit but he's a little off balance. He's got good head control. He doesn't wobble at all. Hello! Hello! (The baby smiles.) You get nice easy social smiles.

Such smooth welding of the two activities caused no offence, but where staff engaged in any detailed teaching with students something more was needed. Here they commonly indicated that a break in the action was occurring and asked for parents' forgiveness: "Excuse me a minute." Such apologies were particularly elaborate in the Scottish maternity hospital ward round where, given the Nightingale ward system, there was no private place in which teaching could be done in between seeing patients. Here, for example, are a doctor's comments from the beginning, middle, and end of a case in which the doctor demonstrated how to conduct the examination of a newborn baby:

Dr. K: Hello, Mrs. Angus. You don't mind all this congregation, do you?
Mother: No.
Dr. K: (inspects the notes and makes comments to students, then says in aside) I'm sorry this is going to take a wee while.
Dr. K: OK. Thanks very much. I hope we haven't mesmerized you.

Apart from its subordinate place being indicated, many aspects of the clinical format were transformed when it was used in parents' presence. As may be seen from the examples of history taking and examination, staff's comments related almost entirely to the good things that might be said about a child.

Even here the version of medicine that was displayed was heavily bowdlerized. Personal challenge and enthusiasm, rivalry, and career aspirations were all carefully removed, and the resulting discussion had the gravity and moral purpose of some lay versions of "science." Such discussion was therefore highly reassuring. At first sight, it might seem to threaten the overt order of the occasion by revealing what went on behind the scenes. But the "private" action that was thereby disclosed was of the highest moral seriousness. Teaching might take up a large proportion of the time spent with some mothers in the maternity hospital ward round but, since it necessarily involved the spelling out of medical practice and manners, it could be used to display the highest motives and principles. The generalizing interest of the clinical format could therefore be shown to be relevant to a mother's own child.

Dr. K: He's still looking a bit yellow, isn't he?
Mother: Yes.
Dr. K: (to students) You know, don't you, that in newborn babies jaundice, what we call physiological jaundice, reaches a peak at the fifth or sixth day and then goes down. Everyone says that the peak is at five days but we've studied our own figures and found that many peak on the sixth day. So give it the fifth or sixth day. When you've had sufficient experience at handling these babies and you know that it's the third day, if it's a mild case, you can say leave it till tomorrow and test it then, but if you do have any doubts, it's important to test it right away.
Dr. K: (to nurse) It is jaundiced a bit. It's very mild at the moment, but if it gets any yellower, tell Dr. James here. Otherwise we'll look at it tomorrow. Bye, Mrs. Morrison.

In this, Dr. K not only instructed the students to be cautious, watchful, and take nothing on trust, but demonstrated to the mother that this was staff's own attitude. They had not just gone along with what "everyone says" but had conducted their own studies and produced a revised analysis. Their constant thought about such babies had resulted in better care for all. Thus, when the doctor gave the nurse instructions at the end of her lesson, her words bore a special meaning. They were not just an order but the embodiment of caring, concerned, and technically sophisticated medicine. In this manner, teaching, for all its emphasis on the general, might nevertheless serve to display the personal concern for advanced knowledge that was more typical of the private format.

28. Becoming a Doctor
David E. Resser   Andrea Klein Schroder

The Cadaver As Patient

A phenomenon that we sometimes see during the dissection of the cadaver is the development of a distorted perception of what the doctor's "ideal" patient should be like. The cadaver can leave the physician longing for similar attributes in his later living patient. Our first patient is silent. He does not protest. He demands no attention, no reassurance, and he never fights back. With this patient, the doctor is always right. Or if he isn't, his patient never says so. Some doctors do in fact seem to get angry at their difficult living patients because they do not display the passive, uncomplaining qualities of their first dead patient.

Obviously, this model of the doctor-patient relationship is limited. It is a model in which the doctor acts upon his patient, who in turn receives his actions passively. Although it certainly represents one aspect of the doctor-patient relationship—the most obvious example is surgery—there are other modes of interaction that are as important in medicine. One is the model of mutual collaboration, in which the patient is seen as an active participant and collaborator with the doctor in the process of his treatment. The cadaver obviously has a very limited contribution to make here.

The Student's Self-consciousness About His Role

One outspoken but apprehensive student said to her preceptor: "You've brought a patient in here for us to examine. At least to talk to. You've implied that he's going to see a doctor. But the fact is, we're not doctors, and I think this is an exploitation. It's for us—it has nothing to do with the patient. Really," she half joked, "the patient would get about as much value from spending a half-hour with the gas station attendant across the street."

This is false, and her preceptor hastened to tell her as much. But it is how many students feel, at least some of the time. The beginning student, as he approaches his first patients, does not know how to regard himself. Is he an intruder? A learner? A data collector? A sympathetic listener? A detached "scientist" scrutinizing an object of interest? A friend? An impostor? Or is he the victim, along with his patient, of a contrived learning situation into which both student and patient alike have been forced?

The answer is all of these, at least to some extent—all, except a doctor. There is almost universal consensus on this among students: however else they may regard themselves, very few students view themselves early in their training as doctors, albeit beginning ones, with something unique and important to offer their first patients. Almost always, preceptors try to argue them out of this point, emphasizing that students are indeed physicians, though still in training, and will be seen by patients this way. Students in turn invariably react in one of two ways: either they feel the preceptor is trying to toss them a bone to make them feel better, or they suspect that he is encouraging them to be phony and to misrepresent themselves to their patients.

The student in his first interviews is faced with a very difficult task. Limited in his knowledge of pathophysiology, he listens to patients describe signs, symptoms, and technical

Source: David Resser and Andrea Klein Schroder, *Patient Interviewing: The Human Dimension*, Williams & Wilkins, Baltimore, 1980.

procedures, frequently with greater comprehension than he himself possesses. Even if he is only attempting to understand the patient as a person and to empathize in a general sense with how illness has affected his patient's life, the task is not easy. Interviewing a patient is no ordinary conversation, and a great deal is going on. It can be quite difficult to listen on many levels at once—to listen to the emotional tone of what a patient is saying, to the content of his communications, to the process by which his remarks come up, to the mood in the room, and to a host of other subtleties that transpire during the interview. On top of this, the student typically is being watched by his preceptor, by his peers, and in a real sense by himself. It sounds almost glib, in such a situation, to assert that the best way to hear and perceive most in an interview is to be able to listen with a relaxed receptiveness! This is hardly a stance that one can expect a student to attain. During his initial interviews, the student is bound to feel somewhat uptight, which can't help but constrict his receptivity to some degree.

Beyond the complexity of the task to be performed, students also feel self-conscious. Typically, a student feels that he is on trial. The competitive system that got him into medical school and keeps him there obviously does little to allay these concerns. Even with the most encouraging and uncritical preceptor, however, many students turn out to be their own harshest critics—critics who watch vigilantly to see what kind of doctor this student will be, how patients respond to him, how good he looks in front of his peers.

Medical students throughout their training constantly find themselves in the unenviable position of being neither fish nor fowl. They barely get used to the routine of the basic science years when they are thrust into their clinical years. They have barely mastered those before they are "back to go" as interns. In the beginning years, when most introductory interviewing courses are taught, generally students are closer to identifying with patients than they are to thinking of themselves as physicians. Many of us have had the experience of being a patient. At the very least, we can readily imagine what it would be like. When students go up on the wards for their first interviews, they naturally feel helpless and out of place. They are foreigners in a milieu that seems to operate smoothly, incomprehensibly, and very much without them. The strangeness of a modern medical ward and the mysterious new technology that is everywhere conspire to make the student feel like an outsider in a foreign country. This enables most students to feel a very special sensitivity for bewildered and "lost" patients in this same situation. Such empathy can often contribute greatly to the unique relationship a medical student offers his patients, although he does not often value it highly. To begin with, he recognizes that he is not a patient. More important, he is trying to struggle his way out of the role of "complete novice" and to begin to see himself as a physician. Feelings of helplessness and bewilderment are seldom comfortable. In his new role, as awkward and uncomfortable as a new white coat, the student finds himself already estranged from his earlier nonmedical identity yet not integrated into a new one. In this awkward hybrid state, the student must perform the difficult task of trying to reach out and make contact with patients. It is clearly no wonder that students have a terrible time appearing "natural" with their first patients, much less feeling natural.

This inevitable self-consciousness in turn creates a kind of psychological "Heisenberg principle" in which the student's inevitable tendency to observe himself leads to a powerful interruption of his natural abilities to relate to people. Some of the old and comfortable ways of relating to people that he brings to training must in fact be given up and replaced by other skills as he begins to interact with patients as a physician. However, much of the native empathy and compassion for people that the student brings with him is valuable.

When increasing self-consciousness alienates the student from his own empathic abilities, the experience can be unnerving.

Fears and Fantasies About What Constitutes Professional Behavior

What is a doctor? Even in simpler times than these, people's perceptions of doctors were enigmatic, extreme, and often paradoxical. Is the doctor a wise, sympathetic healer who sits patiently at the bedside sometimes holding his dying patient's hand? Or is he the austere, emotionally unapproachable "brain surgeon" who nevertheless performs brilliant and miraculous operations? Images of the wise, humane physician commingle uneasily in our minds with the image of Dr. Frankenstein, the scientist who flirted with life's ultimate mysteries, who had commerce with forces dark and uncontrollable. In our current social climate, the paradoxes are even more abundant. The glowing accolades that accompany medicine's unparallelled technical advances coexist with an increasingly restive and suspicious public image of physicians as greedy, technologically obsessed, compassionless, incompetent, and grandiose. It is no doubt inevitable that anyone linked as closely with the fundamentals of human existence as a doctor would be perceived with such ambivalence. At no time in history have the paradoxes been more abundant and seemingly irreconcilable.

The physician himself is not immune to these fragmented and conflicting views of what a doctor really is. Doctors at all levels of training and experience are currently experiencing a considerable crisis of identity, self-esteem, and purpose. The beginning student is particularly vulnerable. In the midst of this confusion, the student has a strong and understandable psychological need for an image of stability, coherence, and confidence. Just as societies in times of great turmoil turn to strong charismatic leaders, so do students during a period of major internal upheaval and loss of identity search for some strong, charismatic image of the ideal physician.

The images, myths, and fantasies about this figure change over time for each student and vary considerably in their details from student to student. The common thread that links all students, however, is the wish for a model to aspire to and perhaps initially to imitate until its ideal characteristics can be internalized.

Three "caricatures" of the charismatic physician are identified below—there are doubtless more. They are the wise professor, the humane generalist, and Captain Medicine. Not only do these three images often commingle in a student's mind, but, more importantly, each figure is perceived with some ambivalence, as we shall see.

The wise professor. These are older clinicians, usually men, often department heads, almost always full professors. Often they wear long white coats and have at least some distinguished trace of gray. Typically they have achieved national prominence in some specialized area of research, but they also retain stature as senior clinicians.

Viewing them from afar, students see in such mentors symbols of absolute calm, inner equanimity, and unflappable self-assurance. These traits are most appealing at a time in the student's development when they hardly characterize his own experience.

On the other hand, students can perceive these same professors at other times in a very different, and negative way. They are the aloof administrators cut off from real patient care. They are the scientists, more interested in research than in human beings. Finally, like all patriarchal symbols, the wise professor walks perilously close to the "dottering old fool." It is not uncommon for a student's image of one of these heroes to be shattered when he hears younger house staff say that this professor is, in fact, totally out of date and hasn't written "anything worth a damn" in the last 10 years.

The compassionate generalist. Call him Dr. Welby or Dr. Jones. For most medical students, as for much of society, there runs a deep respect and affection for our image of the wise, humane, warm family doctor. The recent resurgence of interest in family medicine among many medical students doubtless reflects this respect and perhaps a longing to get back to "the basics." As the popularity of the TV show made clear, the basis of our longing for this archetypal hero runs deep. Take the lovely, famous poem by Robert Frost, "Stopping by Woods on a Snowy Evening," which we believe was written about a country doctor.

> Whose woods these are I think I know.
> His house is in the village though;
> He will not see me stopping here
> To watch his woods fill up with snow.
>
> My little horse must think it queer
> To stop without a farmhouse near
> Between the woods and frozen lake
> The darkest evening of the year.
>
> He gives his harness bells a shake
> To ask if there is some mistake.
> The only other sound's the sweep
> Of easy wind and downy flake.
>
> The woods are lovely, dark and deep.
> But I have promises to keep,
> And miles to go before I sleep,
> And miles to go before I sleep.

Certainly the poem is about much more than just a country doctor. Very possibly this briefly serene, solitary man symbolizes the artist himself midway in the journey of his own life. But it is also an apt symbol for the dedication, tolerance of fatigue, endless patience, and fundamental loneliness that we associate with the country doctor.

It is often the image of the compassionate generalist that most shapes a student's notion of physicianhood prior to beginning medical training. In most training centers, however, generalists are nowhere to be found. Thus, the image of the generalist's good qualities becomes based more on fantasy than on actual exposure to real models. In contrast, students also hear a great deal that is pejorative.

The compassionate generalist is referred to by many house staff as "the LMD" (local medical doctor)—a dumb jerk who is so out of date with recent journals that he can't order the right tests and sends his disasters to the medical center to be saved when it's all but too late. He is also a money grubber, an excessively affluent businessman of medicine who owns two Cadillacs and a funmobile. Finally, he is an ignorant sentimentalist—a hand holder—because he lacks the skills and technical expertise to cure his patients of rare diseases. Many of these negative stereotypes are reinforced by the third charismatic type.

Captain Medicine. In our experience, it is the interns and residents who ultimately exert the most powerful influence as role models for medical students. This is less apparent in the first 2 years of medical education, when a great deal of time is taken up with basic science lectures. The clinical courses that are offered in these first 2 years—notably, introduction to clinical medicine courses—are typically taught by faculty. Early in the student's education, however, the image of the house officer emerges vividly. He is the exhausted yet somehow dashing figure toting a bellboy and dressed in surgical greens. He is the one who knows just what to do when that disastrous motorcycle accident is brought into the emergency room. He starts the IV, gives the bicarb. He administers the cardiac massage. It is he who seems comfortable with the catastrophic, overwhelming, and unimaginable. It is he who has the latest journal article at his fingertips. Always, the student remembers that it is this figure who the student will become in just a few short years.

During the junior and senior years, resident house staff exert a truly profound influence on medical students. Here is a description by one of the authors of his impression of house officers when he was a junior student.

> I remember those weeks vividly. The sounds and smells . . . I have never felt so help-less or inadequate . . . perhaps I was too impressionable. As I look back on the experi-ence, it's clear I wasn't emulating the medical techniques of house officers, but rather their style of adaptation to stress. It was very strange. Under normal circumstances I would have seen these people for what they were: students a little older than I with strengths and weaknesses of their own. But somehow my sense of inadequacy at that time made it necessary to take them for models.
>
> Basically what I learned from my young mentors was that preparing oneself for an admitting night . . . is like preparing for battle. We don callousness like a suit of armor (DER).

House officers epitomize both the best and worst of medicine. A seasoned third-year sur-gery resident may well be at the pinnacle of his emergency room prowess; his technical skills, his knowledge of the latest procedures, and his ability to implement them can be awe-some. At the same time, he may be callous, brusque, and harsh to the people entrusted to his care. Overwhelmed by the demands placed on him—for omniscience in the face of sleepless-ness, omnipotence in the face of overwhelming suffering—the house officer is not at a stage in his own development that permits him to be receptive to himself, warm, or well rounded.

Perhaps, partly from his own sense of guilt, this house officer is often prone to mock such qualities in other physicians. Generalists are handholders. Older clinicians are "behind the times." Medical students who show too much feeling for their patients are "impressionable" and "green."

It is important to remember that, in a world increasingly populated by technologists and machines, the most precious gift a doctor has to offer a patient is still himself. Rediscovering the therapeutic potential of one's own personality, therefore, is one of the important goals of any introductory interviewing experience.

Formal and Informal Groups

Often it is a doctor who can best understand another doctor. Students should not be excessively hard on themselves, therefore, when they find that most of their friendships form with fellow students. The worry about narrowness aside, a great deal that is supportive and growth-promoting can come out of such friendships.

At the University of Colorado Medical Center, students spend much of their first 2 years in assigned laboratory spaces called "UTLs." Often informal groups spring up among students who are physically clustered together in this manner. Each section of a UTL begins to take on its own life, developing its own rules, jokes, and history. The bonds, though informal and often expressed through humor, can be intense.

These students are not simply engaged in bull sessions. Rather these informal networks help the students support each other through the turmoil of change. Lack of support is one overlooked reason why students so often experience the beginning of their clinical rotations as traumatic. In addition to their greatly increased patient responsibilities, students also feel isolated, torn away from the informal support groups they had developed during the basic science years.

One might ask, therefore, why more effort isn't made to formalize such support groups. Why, for instance, are opportunities for medical students, interns, and residents to share their experiences with each other almost nonexistent? The party line states: No time—too busy! But probably a more fundamental reason is the deeper myth of the physician as lone soldier, the solitary hero who fights his battles alone, the Spartan who may bleed inwardly but never lets it show. This myth, in my view, is destructive, not only to the student's sense of well-being but ultimately to patients. A doctor who believes that sharing feelings and seeking support is a "weakness" is apt to transmit this prejudice to his patients. How can such patients then be expected to open up and trust?

Human Limitations and Vulnerability

Each student must come to terms with his own personal limitations. The fact is, students are not all alike, nor will they be when they become doctors. The sheer vastness of medicine has promoted a trend toward specialization and subspecialization. As one academic physician, an individual with many publications on hepatic biochemistry, put it, "I'm a liver man."

This physician went on to say, quite candidly, that he knew he couldn't master everything, but he could "know everything there is to know about the liver." At one level, this reasoning is logical. It certainly provides patients with experts for almost every conceivable problem (at least if they are fortunate enough to be located close to a university medical center in a major urban area). On the other hand, specialization has tended to fragment medicine and fracture the continuity of patient care. The sad situation of a patient with half a dozen specialists who doesn't know the name of his doctor is lamentably common. The current interest in a more holistic approach to medicine is a response to this.

Despecialization is probably not the answer to medicine's current problems. Specialization seems to be a necessary, inevitable response to the current knowledge explosion.

At the same time, students should anticipate the real allure of closing one's mind to certain types of experiences prematurely, out of anxieties over personal limitations. Some students have great gifts of memory that enable them to do well on basic science tests. Others have exceptional manual dexterity and thus may be spared the awkwardness that many students feel when they begin to do technical procedures. Still others have great natural capacities for empathy and can relate comfortably to patients in a clinical setting from the beginning.

Each type of student may at points be tempted to cope with his overall sense of limitations by channeling his aspirations and interests toward what he naturally does best. Thus, the empathically gifted student with a humanities background may assert, "I don't need to learn all that biochemistry, anyway. I'm going to be a psychiatrist." Similarly, everyone knows the would-be surgeon who, in his freshman year, has already picked out his residency and can't be bothered with patient interviews because "that isn't real medicine anyway."

Students who "specialize" prematurely as a defense are attempting to cope with a reality that medicine thrusts on all of us—we can't be perfect, we can't know everything. This can be an especially painful realization for men and women in their twenties. As Gail Sheehy has pointed out in *Passages,* the twenties are that period of life when people feel they can do anything; all it seemingly requires is hard work, endurance, and a faith in what one (secretly) believes are his own limitless capacities. According to Sheehy, most adults begin to reconcile themselves to their limitations during their thirties and forties, when it begins to dawn on them that the choices they have been making have also been denials of other cherished wishes.

By contrast, this normally gradual maturational insight dawns on medical students more abruptly, long before their thirties and forties. Students quickly realize that there is too much to learn, that the field is too vast and bewildering in its dimensions ever to be mastered. For the many students who have considerable talents in areas quite removed from medicine, medical training can require some hard choices.

Uncertainty About How To Proceed Technically With Patients

The most immediate concerns students have prior to beginning an interview are pragmatic. How do I introduce myself? What if the patient says he doesn't want to be interviewed? What happens if I don't understand his disease? What happens if I say something to upset him and make him feel worse? What happens if he has a cardiac arrest and drops dead in the middle of the interview? The questions seem endless. In fact, the issue of how to begin with patients is as fundamental as how to think of oneself as a physician. How does one approach the patient in a physicianly way? How does one convey his sense of competence? No interview outline, however well considered and inclusive, can accomplish this. There simply is no armamentarium of sure-fire techniques that the student can bring with him. It is impossible to be fully prepared for the fluid, unpredictable process of any physician-patient interaction.

In some ways, the best advice prior to any interview is, "Just go and do it." Yet such advice does not seem to convey empathy when it is offered, and students generally feel frustration when preceptors keep reminding them of how stressful and ambiguous the process is. Students want answers! Surely something can be written down in black and white that is more precise than generalities about one's emerging identity, changing role experiences, and the like. Students may well appreciate that there is no foolproof map to lead them through the thicket of questions and technical considerations that arise. At the same time, the wish for some concrete guidance is reasonable. In this section, therefore, we will address a number of beginning issues that students commonly face.

Introductions. The question of how to introduce oneself to the patient immediately raises a knotty issue—should I say I'm a doctor? Current educational trends suggest that the student be completely honest. But what is being "completely honest?"

> "Good morning, Mrs. Smith, I'm Mark Brown, a medical student—a freshman medical student. This is only my first month of school and this is an introductory course. I really don't know much about medicine but they told me I should come here and interview you to ask you how you feel about your illness and all—ah, that is, if it's all right with you?"

While this seems a bit exaggerated in print, it is, in fact, typical of the way students tend to introduce themselves. Why? Are such lengthy disclaimers really for the patient's benefit? In our view, medical students often have a greater need to disclose their novice status than is necessary for the patient's understanding or comfort. They may do this to protect themselves. It is as though the student is issuing a disclaimer: "I'm not really a doctor so don't expect anything from me." This reduces the student's anxiety, but is it, in fact, truthful? Do patients really perceive medical students as being little different "from the gas station attendant across the street"?

The answer is, no. For most patients, the exact nature of the medical hierarchy, and different people's status in it, is never entirely clear. This may not be ideal, but it tends to be a fact. With the exception of certain chronic patients who have had complex ongoing care in teaching hospitals, most patients have little grasp of the difference between an intern and a junior student much less between a junior student and a freshman. As uncomfortable as this may feel, most patients regard medical students as doctors. They confer on the student both the prestige and responsibility that the title Doctor demands.

We recommend, therefore, that introductions be brief: it is sufficient to identify oneself as a medical student and then to give a brief statement of the purpose of the interview. If the purpose is to talk about the patient's response to his illness in general terms, then say so. If the intended scope of the interview is broader, including the obtaining of a medical history, it is sufficient to say, "Good morning Mr. Smith. I'm Mark Brown, a medical student, and I'd like to spend some time talking with you about the troubles you've been having." Such an introduction is sufficiently general to permit the patient to begin where he wishes—either with the specifics of the medical history or with different concerns. The doctor later has plenty of time to focus in on more specific concerns.

Many students feel a need to include some statement that the interview is taking place as part of a course. This is often defended in the name of honesty, yet it is open to question. Sometimes students do, in fact, obtain important information about the patient that becomes a part of his record and may influence his management. Furthermore, telling the patient that the interview is for a course may be one more way the student has of minimizing the prestige and responsibility that he is endowed with. Still, if students wish, it is perfectly acceptable to say that the interview is part of a course.

The question of introductions raises another controversial issue. It is the current trend for students to introduce themselves as Mr., Ms., or Mrs. Interestingly, 10 years ago the trend was quite different and students were encouraged from the beginning to call themselves doctors. Has this change come about to protect the patient from deception? Is it a reflection of our greater enlightenment and humility? Perhaps. But we would at least like to raise the question of whether calling oneself Mr. or Ms. isn't potentially as misleading to a patient as calling oneself "Doctor." In legal terms, a medical student presumably becomes a doctor on a given day in June when he graduates. Or does he? Is it rather when he receives his state license? After internship? After completion of house staff training? Even legally, the issue is not clear-cut. Ethically, it is even more cloudy. Most physicians train for a minimum of 8 years. At what point along the continuum are they doctors? Obviously, the answer is—at all points. The limits a student places on his interventions and responsibilities should depend more on his own grasp of his limitations and capabilities than on an official title. A junior student alone on a ward will conduct a cardiac arrest until more help arrives, if he must. Is he not a doctor? On the other hand, a second-year medical resident may wisely defer to a more experienced house officer in performing a tricky liver biopsy. Is he any less a doctor? If, then, patients tend to regard students as doctors; if, in fact, the student assumes a responsibility the minute he introduces himself to the patient—to listen, to attempt to understand, perhaps to contribute to the information on the patient's chart—which then is really more misleading, to call oneself Mr. or doctor? We raise the issue not to encourage deception. We know full well that most students prefer to begin calling themselves doctors after receiving their M.D. degree, usually at the beginning of an internship. This is reasonable enough. We have dissected the question at some length because this seemingly simple content issue—like so many others in medicine—is far more complicated when one takes a deeper look.

The white coat. We recommend that students wear white coats during their patient interviews. We recognize that this is not the prevailing trend at many medical centers, where "appropriate dress" is the rule of thumb but not specified. Nevertheless, we consider the white coat a reassuring symbol of physicianhood for the patient. As in the matter of calling oneself "Doctor," some students argue that wearing a white coat is deceptive. To the contrary, we feel that *not* wearing one is an act of denial and is inconsiderate to the patient.

Consider the patient's vulnerability. He may be told that he is going to be interviewed by a medical student, "a young doctor," or "a student physician." However it is defined, 9 times out of 10, the patient anticipates an interview with "a young doctor." He expects to disclose feelings and intimate details about himself that are private and personal and may leave him feeling vulnerable. Yet, patients are generally willing to do this because they are speaking to a doctor. In this sense, we feel that donning a white coat is a symbolic act of commitment—an expression of the student's willingness to be responsible to the trust the patient places in him.

Despite this logic, some students may still choose not to wear a white coat. Sensible standards of dress should then be a minimal requirement. For men, this means a clean, pressed pair of slacks, shirt, and tie; for women, a dress, a skirt and blouse, or a comfortable yet not excessively casual pair of slacks and blouse or sweater. Again, however, we recommend the white coat; though it has fallen out of popularity, it remains a potent symbol of physicianhood to most patients. The use of a name tag is also strongly recommended.

Confidentiality. In a busy medical center, it is common to overhear clusters of doctors inappropriately discussing their patients in public places. Often the details they discuss are intimate, specifically identifying, and quite frightening to the visitors and nonmedical personnel who crowd into the elevators and cafeteria lines with them. How this loss of consideration has become so widespread raises some disturbing questions about the way most medical centers are run. It goes without saying that patient confidentiality is an absolute expectation for anyone treating patients but most especially for physicians—including student physicians.

In many ways, the importance of a commitment to confidentiality is internal. In reality, a casual reference to some patient, spoken too loudly in the elevator, is apt to be forgotten by whoever overhears. But the student's commitment to honor his patients' communications as a sacred trust—this attitude is directly related to an emerging sense of oneself as a doctor.

Students sometimes have questions about where to draw the line. Talking among peers is appropriate in one setting, yet not in another. Furthermore, should the student go home in the evening and discuss the matter with his or her spouse? One could answer this rigidly with a resounding, no! Never! But the truth is, almost every student (and, for that matter, every physician) at some point discusses a case with his or her spouse. It is doubtless wrong to do so. Yet we physicians sometimes strap ourselves with Draconian standards of perfection that are hard to fulfill. A student may well go home at night feeling exhausted yet quite overstimulated. The spouse may be the only person to turn to and share with. Similarly, it is often very difficult for the nonmedical half of a relationship to be left in the dark about the exciting and intense activities that comprise the medical student's days. Therefore, there are no absolutes. However, a good rule of thumb is: no patient should ever be identified by name, and any discussion of patient contacts with close friends or spouses should be general and focus more on the student's side of the experience than on anything specific about the patient.

Finally, it is well known that doctors frequently group together and joke about patients. In the safety of a back room, they laugh about someone, call him names, make wisecracks. It is easy to condemn such behavior; yet one must understand the plight of the physician. Overwhelmed and overloaded, he can sometimes find relief in camaraderie through humor, even sarcastic humor. It can provide a useful release that then enables the physician to return to work and behave in a humane and professional way with a difficult patient. Yet students should also be aware that jokes, casual or cruel jargon, and slang can quickly lead to a mind set in which physicians begin to think of patients as "crocks," "turkeys," and "gomers." If doctors think of patients this way, they are bound to treat patients that way, and if they do treat them that way, they are bound to get a response in kind; and thus the vicious cycle is completed.

Confidentiality and the highest level of respect for the patient's dignity are therefore worthy aspirations. Although we all fall short of this goal at one point or another, we should try to discover the underlying frustration that motivates such humor. Perhaps in finding an answer to this question we may find a way more effective than mockery to cope with a difficult patient.

Closeness. Many students wonder about the appropriate distance to set with a patient. Usually patients tend to set the distance themselves, though some patients tend toward one or the other extreme. Some, for example, stand excessively aloof. Others become excessively regressed, demanding, and clinging. Students likewise have different degrees of tolerance for closeness. A bit of "chemistry" goes into this. Some students, for instance, can tolerate angry, hostile patients better than seductive ones, while others find their undoing in excessively dependent, clinging patients, and so forth.

Generally, the experienced clinician develops a capacity for empathy that permits fluid shifts between closeness and detachment. At different times during an interview, an experienced interviewer can be almost at one with the patient emotionally, identifying with his pain and inner suffering, then shifting quickly into detachment and objectivity—sliding back and forth along an axis of closeness-distance as the situation warrants. This is far more difficult for the beginner. Typically, early in clinical exposures, students find themselves vacillating between overidentification with patients and excessive aloofness and detachment. One student referred to this as "not knowing how to regulate my empath-o-stat." In fact, the problem of establishing a balance may be another important motivation for the laughter and gallows humor that we hear among physicians. It is possible that caustic, barbed humor is a way physicians have of mitigating the excessively tender feelings that patients may arouse.

The concrete questions that students raise about closeness are many: Should I sit on the patient's bed? Should I hold his hand if he cries? What if the patient asks me to hug her? As much as he would like specific guidelines, the student will probably appreciate that there really can be none. In general, professional contact should be conducted primarily through words. A great deal of empathy and concern can be communicated to most patients through language alone. Occasionally, holding a patient's hand or a reassuring touch are both necessary and appropriate. The student should be cautious, however, because body contact is a potent intervention that often has significant, though sometimes unconscious, meaning to a patient. This is an area that takes time to master and one in which the understanding of an experienced preceptor can be especially helpful.

Another specific question that many students have centers around self-disclosure. Patients can, and frequently do, ask students questions about themselves. These can range from the quite chatty to the very intimate. How and when does a student respond to these questions, if ever? Again, there are no absolute rules. Some students seem to try to caricature the physician as a psuedo-Freudian statue who stonewalls every personal question. Obviously, this is rude and unempathic. At the other extreme, some students seem ready to answer every question that a patient asks, from the state of their marriage to the age and health of their parents, without ever asking why the patient seems to want to know all these things. A general principle (alas, not a rule) is that less self-disclosure is preferable to excessive self-disclosure. The doctor-patient relationship is one in which the doctor must be essentially unselfish and focus primarily on the patient. Sometimes this must be said to a patient so he will understand.

Similarly, students may find themselves having strong feelings about patients. Some patients evoke great feelings of tenderness, admiration, protectiveness. Others may evoke frank feelings of contempt and revulsion. Sometimes students wonder whether to share these feelings with patients. Generally, however, it is unwise to tell patients directly how one feels about them. There are usually more tactful, therapeutic ways of transmitting the same information. Take, for instance, the highly demanding, interrogative patient who keeps asking detail after detail regarding the medical student's exact level of expertise and training. The student may feel, "I'm getting increasingly annoyed with this man's attack on my credentials, on my right to be here interviewing him." To say so directly might well be honest, but it would not be especially helpful to the patient. Recognizing the feeling, however, the student could well say, "You seem to be concerned, Mr. Jones, about whether or not I will be able at my level of training and expertise to understand you. In fact, it sounds to me like you're worried about whether the entire staff is up to the task of helping you as much as you need and deserve." In both interventions, an awareness of an intense feeling leads to a response to the patient. But in the second response, the intervention is shaped in a way that does not specifically disclose the student's angry feelings toward the patient or needlessly put the patient on the defensive.

29. *The Sick Role Concept: Understanding Illness Behavior* Alexander Segall

How well (if at all) does the Parsonian sick role model apply to the study of mental illness? Blackwell[1] explored adult expectations about entering the sick role for physical and psychiatric dysfunctions and reported that the rights and obligations of the sick role (as described by Parsons[2]) apply directly to physical conditions, but not to psychophysical and psychosocial conditions. A major finding of this study was that the extent of societal agreement about admission to the sick role decreases as the social and psychological aspects of the condition increase. Consistent with this finding, Denzin and Spitzer[3] also argued that the medical sick role, particularly the classic Parsonian formulation, is not adequate for predicting psychiatric patient role behavior.

Recognizing that there is a difference between the medical sick role (i.e., Parsons' model) and the psychiatric sick role is only the first step. The next is to articulate clearly the dimensions of the psychiatric sick role. Sobel and Ingalls[4] attempted to measure the sick role as seen by a variety of participants in the doctor-patient relationship (i.e., psychiatrists, psychiatric patients, physicians and surgeons, and medical and surgical patients) and suggest a number of areas in which the medical and psychiatric sick roles differ.

In the case of a physical condition, the situation is relatively clear. Something is wrong with the individual's physical functioning (for which he is not responsible), and he would consult a physician as soon as possible. However, when the condition also has psychological connotations, the question of personal responsibility arises. To what extent is the individual responsible for both causing and coping with mental illness? In this situation, the social norms related to adopting the sick role become uncertain. On the one hand, the individual is still expected to try to get well (i.e., seek professional help) but, on the other hand, he must be prepared to face the potential stigma and rejection often associated with being formally labeled mentally ill.[5]

According to the Parsonian model, the occupant of the medical sick role is exempt from performing "normal" social roles. He is expected to seek technically competent help and to "cooperate" in the process of getting well. The medical patient is expected to cooperate by being passive, submissive, and generally dependent upon the doctor. In contrast, it has been argued that it is important that the mentally ill individual not be exempted from all his social responsibilities while he tries to get well.[1] Furthermore, the characteristics of the medical patient, just described, tend to be viewed as undesirable features for the psychiatric patient. Research findings "indicate that on the parameters of helplessness, passivity, submission, and dependency, the psychiatric role tends to be in opposition to the medical role."[4] The psychiatric patient is generally expected to be active, independent, and self-

Source: *Journal of Health and Social Behavior*, vol. 17, p. 163, June 1976.

directed in interacting with his doctor. The medical and psychiatric sick role models, then, entail rather different types of reciprocal relationships between doctor and patient.

Variations in the Medical Sick Role

As previously stated, the sick role concept has been utilized in the study of many different types of physical conditions. How well does the Parsonian conceptualization (which is best typified by the temporary, acute physical illness episode) apply to chronic illness or permanent physical disability? Kassebaum and Baumann,[6] using the concept of the sick role as a point of departure, attempted to investigate the dimensions of this role model as it applies to chronically ill patients. Their findings indicate that sick role expectations vary among patients with different types of illness. Indeed, the chronically ill patient differed from the "ideal-type model" (based on the acutely ill patient) in a number of important respects. For example, Kassebaum and Baumann point out that chronic illness by definition is not temporary. Consequently, the role expectations that one should try to get well, overcome the condition, and resume functioning in a "normal preillness" capacity are inappropriate. In the case of chronic illness, the individual is faced with the necessity of adjusting to a permanent condition, rather than striving to overcome a temporary one. Furthermore, since many chronic patients (e.g., diabetics) are ambulatory, exemption from performing usual social roles is more often partial than total.

Callahan et al.[7] also examined the sick role in chronic illness and came to similar conclusions. For example, they argue that it is a mistake to cast the chronically ill in the traditional sick role (for many of the same reasons outlined by Kassebaum and Baumann). Furthermore, there is still no clearly developed social definition of the role of the permanently disabled or chronically ill and this will remain unchanged until efforts are made to achieve "a deeper understanding of the dynamics involved in the sick role as played by the chronically ill."[7]

The general tendency has been to treat physical disability (like chronic illness) as an extension of the sick role, i.e., a subtype. For example, some authors argued that to understand the problems of physical disability, role theory must be employed. However, a respecification of the basic Parsonian model is required if the sick role concept is to become relevant for the study both of the chronically ill and of the physically disabled. Clearly, the underlying assumptions based on the temporary nature of illness must be modified and the Parsonian view of the sick role extended.

This rather versatile conceptual model has also been applied in a number of other contexts: (1) Aging and the sick role—Lipman and Sterne[8] point to the need to modify the Parsonian paradigm to include cases in which the sick role is not a temporary state, e.g., the aged, as well as the mentally retarded and the physically handicapped. In their opinion, "the Parsonian scheme is deficient in that it omits the terminal case." They propose instead a "terminal sick role" model, which they feel is more appropriate for the study of the aged. (2) The sick role during pregnancy—Rosengren[9] used the Parsonian model to guide his investigation of the sick role expectations held by pregnant women. (3) Alcoholics and the sick role—Roman and Trice[10] contend that placing the deviant drinker or alcoholic in the sick role may serve to legitimize the "abnormal" use of alcohol by removing the individual's responsibility for engaging in this behavior. However, Chalfant and Kurtz[11] used the Parsonian conceptualization in their study of whether alcoholics are viewed by social workers as legitimate incumbents of the sick role and found that very few of the social workers accept the alcoholic as legitimately ill, because of their feeling that the alcoholic is responsible for his condition. This finding seems to reflect the underlying societal ambivalence toward the alcoholic and alcoholism.

Sociocultural Differences in Behavioral Expectations

Although limited and unclear, the existing research evidence offers little support for Parsons's sick role formulation. For example, Twaddle[13] reported that many of the respondents he interviewed did not perceive the rights and obligations of the sick role in a manner consistent with Parsons' conceptualization. In fact, he concluded that "while Parsons may have successfully described the nature of the role, as defined by many Americans, when the elements he posited are treated discretely the total configuration seemingly applies to only a minority."

Segall[12] explored the sick role expectations held by hospitalized female patients and found only one clear-cut area of agreement between the respondents' perception of how a person should behave when sick and the Parsonian model. The vast majority of the patients agreed that to be ill is "inherently undesirable," and that the occupant of the sick role should strive to achieve a state of "good health." It is important to note that while few of the patients disagreed completely with Parsons' conception of the sick role, their responses did not support strongly all the dimensions of this role, as originally outlined. Clearly further research is required to determine: (1) how closely general public perception of the rights and duties of the sick role correspond to the Parsonian conceptual model, and (2) the extent to which shared expectations in regard to the sick role are affected by sociocultural factors.

Adopting the Sick Role

In past research, willingness to adopt the sick role has generally been operationalized as willingness to consult a doctor. For example, Mechanic and Volkart[14] measured "tendency" to adopt the sick role among male college freshmen by asking them if they would report to the University Health Services in three hypothetical situations (e.g., if feeling poorly, temperature of 100°). Similarly, Phillips[15] investigated the "inclination" of married females to adopt the sick role by asking them what they would do in four hypothetical situations (e.g., trouble sleeping at night, no appetite). Those respondents who indicated that they would seek medical help were considered to have a willingness to adopt the sick role. A major weakness of this type of study is that only one dimension of the individual's willingness to adopt the sick role has been investigated, i.e., "tendency" or "inclination" to consult a doctor.

In Parsonian terms, the occupant of the sick role must be prepared to: stop performing many daily activities, become dependent upon others for his well-being, and utilize professional medical care facilities. Clearly, it is possible to accept some but not necessarily all the dimensions of the sick role. Consequently, attempts to measure willingness to adopt the sick role must: (1) specify which dimensions are being considered, and (2) attempt to develop more comprehensive measures that would include all facets of the sick role. In addition to exploring willingness to visit a doctor, it is equally important to know if the person is actually ready to relieve himself of normal role obligations (e.g., be absent from work), and at the same time become dependent on others.

Another limitation of research in this field is that attempts are often made to measure willingness to adopt the sick role, without first carefully specifying the nature of the role expectations held by the respondents. Just what type of behavioral pattern is the individual willing (or unwilling) to adopt when sick? The respondents' expectations in regard to the kind of behavior perceived as appropriate for a sick person (and those with whom he/she interacts) must first be understood if expressions of willingness to adopt the sick role are to be meaningfully interpreted.

NOTES

1. B. L. Blackwell, "Upper Middle Class Adult Expectations about Entering the Sick Role for Physical and Psychiatric Dysfunctions," *Journal of Health and Social Behavior,* vol. 8, p. 83, 1967.

2. Talcott Parsons, *The Social System,* Free Press, New York, 1951.

3. N. K. Denzin and S. S. Spitzer, "Paths to the Mental Hospital and Staff Predictions of Patient Role Behavior," *Journal of Health and Human Behavior,* vol. 7, p. 265, 1966.

4. R. Sobel and A. Ingalls, "Resistance to Treatment: Explorations of the Patient's Sick Role," *American Journal of Psychotherapy,* vol. 18, p. 562, 1964.

5. K. T. Erikson, "Patient Role and Social Uncertainty—A Dilemma of the Mentally Ill," *Psychiatry,* vol. 20, p. 262, 1957.

6. G. G. Kassebaum and B. O. Baumann, "Dimensions of the Sick Role in Chronic Illness," *Journal of Health and Human Behavior,* vol. 6, p. 16, 1965.

7. E. M. Callahan, S. Carroll, P. Revier, E. Gilhooly, and D. Dunn, "The Sick Role in Chronic Illness: Some Reactions," *Journal of Chronic Diseases,* vol. 19, p. 883, 1966.

8. A. Lipman and R. S. Sterne, "Aging in the United States: Ascription of a Terminal Sick Role," *Sociology and Social Research,* vol. 53, p. 194, 1969.

9. W. R. Rosengren, "The Sick Role during Pregnancy: A Note on Research in Progress," *Journal of Health and Human Behavior,* vol. 3, p. 213, 1960. Social Instability and Attitudes toward Pregnancy as a Social Role," *Social Problems,* vol. 9, p. 371, 1962.

10. P. M. Roman and H. M. Trice, "The Sick Role, Labelling Theory, and the Deviant Drinker," *International Journal of Social Psychology,* vol. 14, p. 245, 1968.

11. H. P. Chalfant and R. A. Kurtz, "Alcoholics and the Sick Role: Assessments by Social Workers," *Journal of Health and Social Behavior,* vol. 16, p. 66, 1971.

12. Alexander Segall, "Sociocultural Variation in Illness Behaviour, unpublished Ph.D. dissertation, Department of Sociology, University of Toronto.

13. A. C. Twaddle, "Health Decisions and Sick Role Variations: An Exploration," *Journal of Health and Social Behavior,* vol. 10, p. 105, 1969.

14. D. Mechanic and E. H. Volkart, "Stress, Illness Behavior and the Sick Role," *American Sociological Review,* vol. 26, p. 51, 1961.

15. D. L. Phillips, "Self-reliance and the Inclination to Adopt the Sick Role," *Social Forces,* vol. 43, p. 555, 1965.

30. *The Client*   Alex J. Ducanis   Anne K. Golin

The health team is essentially client-centered; that is, the client is the primary focus of the team's attention. This does not rule out the possibility that at times the client may actually raise barriers that interfere with the effective functioning of the team. In fact it is *because* clients play such a central role in the team system that they can create such major difficulties.

Source: Alex J. Ducanis and Anne K. Golin, *The Interdisciplinary Health Care Team,* Aspen Systems Corp., Rockville, Maryland, 1979.

Client-related Barriers

Professionals hold certain expectations for "good" patients. Some hospital staff see "problem patients" as those who demand a great deal of attention. When patients are seriously ill they are not held responsible for their demands, but patients who demand attention solely through complaints and uncooperative behavior may actually receive less adequate services because of the staff's attitudes.

Not only the "problem patient," but other stereotyped patient types, may also hinder the team's efforts, directly or indirectly. Let us look briefly at some of the ways these patient-helper interactions may reduce the team effectiveness. Four patterns can be identified, along with some techniques for coping with them.

The problem patient. That a patient is considered a problem by the team is often recognizable by the members' reaction when the client's name is brought up in the team meeting. Certainly, some team discussion of the problems raised by such patients may serve to diffuse some of the negative feelings staff members develop in working with them. Sometimes information contributed by other team members can in part explain some of the client's deviant behavior and may help change the team's attitudes toward the client. It is particularly important that the team leader keep discussion of the problem patient within reasonable bounds so that the team's resentment and frustration are not exacerbated by the team meeting rather than alleviated through the discussion. The team leader can help the group maintain some degree of objectivity toward the client, and most important, *avoid decisions about the patient that are essentially punitive rather than treatment-focused.*

The manipulative client. The client who is accused of being manipulative is one who is adept at playing off one team member against another, in the same way that children sometimes learn to pit mother against father. "Dr. Smith said I could leave the hospital this afternoon" may be a straightforward statement of a fact, or it may be a subtly distorted version of what Dr. Smith actually said (or didn't say). Like the problem patient, the manipulative client may evoke a host of negative emotions from various members of the team. However, the team approach intrinsically offers certain advantages in working with patients who seek to play on the inconsistencies of the system. If the team has agreed on a course of action and team members jointly support the plan, there should be fewer contradictions and inconsistencies for such a client to seize on. More important, the team meetings can help staff members better understand the needs of certain clients to maintain a sense of control when placed in what may be helpless and dependent positions. The team may be able to identify other legitimate ways the patient can exert power in the system without resorting to game playing.

Sometimes staffers' perceptions of the patient are so different that misunderstanding can easily develop. Some team members may be overly protective of the client, while other members feel that such behavior is "naive and unprofessional." These issues may need to be addressed directly by the team leader before the dissatisfaction can spread. In any case, the client should not become a divisive factor that disrupts the cohesiveness of the team.

The yea-sayer. The "yea-saying" client is one who is unusually compliant in responding to the team's efforts. While this may sound like the behavior of a "good" client, in fact the client's excessively compliant and passive behavior may at times cause problems for the team. Just as a shy and withdrawn child may be overlooked in a classroom of aggressive fifth graders, so the client who always accepts whatever the professionals say may not be receiving adequate attention from the team. Team meetings may focus on clients who are management problems of one sort or another, and the yea-sayer simply does not come up. A schedule for reviewing clients can ensure that every client receives some attention at the team conference.

Another problem with yea-saying clients is that it may be difficult to determine just what the clients themselves want. Their tendency to agree with every suggestion made by the staff can lead to considerable confusion and even conflict around goal setting and long-term planning. As with the manipulative client, it is particularly important that the team agree on a consistent course of action. Otherwise, it might be discovered that the client has agreed to two or more different, perhaps even inconsistent, plans.

The unmotivated client. In truth there is no such thing as an unmotivated client, since any client who is alive—eating, breathing, sleeping—is obviously motivated. The label generally refers to a client who is not motivated to the degree expected or in the direction expected by the team. Such clients tend to be the source of considerable frustration and may even elicit widespread hostility among team members. The ultimate punishment for the unmotivated client is discharge from the program or agency. "We want to make room for another client who will get more out of being here," is the comment frequently heard. In many circumstances this is a reasonable alternative for the team to consider.

Sometimes, however, spending some time on the problem in a team conference will lead to a better understanding of the client's dynamics and resulting behavior. Perhaps the client is acting out of anxiety and fear of failure, and by not really trying the failure is averted. In other cases, lack of incentives rather than lack of motivation may be the crucial factor. Working together, the team may be able to reduce the client's anxiety, provide appropriate rewards, or modify the environment in some way so that the client can cope more effectively with the demands of the agency and the expectations of the team.

When teams use labels such as "manipulative" or "unmotivated" in referring to clients, team members sometimes get the impression that the client's behavior has somehow been "explained." It is important to recognize that such labels add nothing to an understanding of the client's problems; the labels should not become an excuse for inaction. "Since she isn't motivated, we really can't do anything for her," is a common statement. The team can serve to explain to its members the danger of using vague generalizations as a basis for decision making and can provide a broader information base on which decisions can be made.

31. *The Sick Role*   Alex J. Ducanis   Anne K. Golin

Freidson discusses the difficulties inherent in understanding the doctor-patient relationship and suggests that Parsons' analysis is based on ideal expectations rather than actual behavior. He suggests also that Parsons' definition of the sick role is drawn from the physician's perspective rather than from the perspective of the patient, the nurse, or any of the other involved parties. The doctor-patient relationship is seen by Freidson as a compromise of "conflicting needs, demands and forces." As Wilson and Bloom summarize it, "in place

Source: Alex J. Ducanis and Anne K. Golin, *The Interdisciplinary Health Care Team,* Aspen Systems Corp., Rockville, Maryland, 1979.

of the mutuality and reciprocity dynamics of the Parsonian analysis, Freidson substitutes hostility, ambivalence, and conflict." To understand such relationships, according to Freidson, we must look at the expectations of all the involved parties and the "social structure in which those perspectives are located," as well as the situations in which the doctor and patient find themselves. Thus, "the model of the structure of the doctor-patient relationship must encompass two distinct social systems—a professional system containing the doctor and a lay system containing the patient." Using the referral mechanism as the point of departure Freidson discusses in some detail how the patient moves through the lay-referral and professional-referral systems in the course of diagnosis and treatment.

Another approach to the patient role in the treatment process has been developed by Suchman, who identified five stages in the sequence of medical events as the patient moves through the medical care system. Beginning with a definition of "illness behavior" first proposed by Mechanic and Volkart as "the way in which symptoms are perceived, evaluated and acted upon by a person who recognizes some pain, discomfort, or other sign of organic malfunction," Suchman looked at illness behavior in terms of patterns in the "seeking, finding and carrying out of medical care." Suchman's five stages and the decisions involved in each are:

1. Symptom experience stage. A middle-aged man wakes up with a scratchy throat, a ten-year-old boy comes home from school flushed and feverish, or a housewife notices pain and stiffness in her back: these are examples of the symptom experience stage. This is the period in which the potential patient first becomes aware of symptoms of illness and decides that something is wrong. The physical experience of pain or discomfort, the individual's interpretation of that experience, and the emotional reaction to it are the major elements of this beginning stage. Once the person is aware of symptoms, some evaluation of these symptoms takes place as the individual (or individual's family) decides on the next step. The person may react by denying the symptoms or delaying further action or may accept the symptoms and move on to the next stage.

2. Assumption of the sick role. At this stage the individual seeks temporary "provisional validation" as a sick person. Family and friends may be asked to diagnose or evaluate the individual's condition and attest to the illness. Self-medication may be tried if the symptoms are not too severe. The man with a sore throat decides to stay in bed, the young boy is given aspirin and orange juice by his mother, and the housewife lies down with a heating pad while her husband cooks dinner. In the latter two cases, if the mother and the husband do not accept the validity of the claim to the sick role, the boy and the housewife will not be relieved of their normal responsibilities. At this stage the individual must decide if he or she is sick and needs professional care.

3. Medical care contact. If the symptoms persist or become more severe, the individual is likely to formally enter the professional medical care system. Only the professional can offer authoritative validation of the sick role. Thus the patient or patient's family calls the doctor or goes to the clinic for further diagnostic evaluation. The decision to seek medical care is an important one, but "once the decision to seek care is made, the initial medical contact is fairly well routinized and offers little difficulty to the patient."

4. Dependent patient role. By deciding to seek treatment and entering the medical care system, the individual becomes a patient. At this point the patient must decide whether to give control to the doctor and follow treatment procedures. The extent to which this dependency creates problems for the individual will vary from patient to patient. For some patients the "secondary gain" involved in the dependency of the patient role may actually interfere with recovery; for others the dependency may be more unbearable than the illness itself. Many people in our society seem to find this stage particularly difficult to accept.

5. Recovery and rehabilitation. The course of the patient's illness may be long or short, mild or severe. However, in most cases the patient will eventually relinquish the "sick" role and return to normal activities and responsibilities. The middle-aged man goes back to work, the young boy returns to school, and the housewife resumes her normal routine. The decision to give up the patient role normally marks this stage. But in the case of long-term rehabilitation, a "process of resocialization may be necessary through which the incapacitated individual must learn to establish new relationships with those around him." In the case of chronic illness, this stage may present serious medical problems. However, most individuals welcome this stage and return rather easily to former roles.

Segall reviews 20 years of research on Parsons' concept of the sick role and concludes that "the extent to which this theoretical model contributes to a greater understanding of the way in which the sick person actually thinks, feels and behaves still awaits empirical verification." The Parsonian concept, according to Segall, is best illustrated by "temporary, acute physical illness," and evidence suggests that the sick role is affected by social, cultural, and personal factors as well as by the nature of the illness.

The importance of such factors is illustrated by the work of Zola, who interviewed patients of different ethnic groups about their symptoms. Comparisons of Irish and Italian patients showed a pattern of differences in the complaints presented (even when the disorder was the same), with the Irish patients "limiting and understating their difficulties and the Italians spreading and generalizing theirs." Zola attempts to account for these differences in terms of the cultural differences between the two groups. As Zola points out:

> While there has long been recognition of the subjectivity and variability of a patient's reporting of his symptoms, there has been little attention to the fact that this reporting may be influenced by systematic social factors like ethnicity. Awareness of the influence of this and similar factors can be of considerable aid in the practical problems of diagnosis and treatment of many diseases, particularly where the diagnosis is dependent to a large extent on what the patient is able and willing, or thinks important enough, to tell the doctor"

Gordon demonstrated the importance of socioeconomic status in validating an individual as "sick." There were no differences between socioeconomic groups in terms of behavioral expectancies of the sick person once the definition was made, but differences were found by Gordon in the "conceptions of who is and who is not sick." Gordon's findings support the idea of a "sick role" that is used when the prognosis is serious and uncertain. In cases where the prognosis is known and not serious, the set of behavioral expectations are referred to as the "impaired role," and persons seen as occupying this role are under social pressure by others to maintain normal activities.

In a more recent restatement of his concept of the sick role, Parsons points out that he had never intended to restrict the concept of the sick role to "deviant behavior" or to acute illness. Nor did he mean to imply that the role of the patient is completely passive. Indeed with less acute illness, the active participation of the client may be substantial. However, Parsons contends, the patient-physician relationship is basically an asymmetrical one, since "there must be a built-in institutionalized superiority of the professional roles, grounded in responsibility, competence, and occupational concern." He views the relationship between the full-time career professional and the lay person (client) as inherently asymmetrical and hierarchical with respect to issues concerning health and illness, in the same way that there is a built-in asymmetry between professor and student or lawyer and client.

Professional–Patient Communication

Although the knowledge and techniques required for the successful practice of medicine are highly scientific and technologically based, the fact remains that these services and procedures are performed upon people in the most intimate and personal circumstances. As can be inferred from the prior sections, the basis for this relationship relies very heavily upon *communication*. Medical success may be definable in most situations in terms of biomedical parameters, but "success" in terms of patient satisfaction, physician gratification, etc., relies most upon the success of the "relationship." Also, many aspects of treatment itself rely upon the cooperation of the patient in conscientiously following prescribed therapy, such as taking drugs as prescribed or returning for follow-up visits, matters which require trust in the physician and satisfaction with the relationship.

Too often texts reduce the "issue" in communication to the decision whether to tell the truth about a particular diagnosis or procedural outcome. Although this is a focal moral problem, it cannot be separated from the general mode of communication with patients throughout the whole range of information sharing. Thus, we have provided selections which focus upon the actual character of communication in clinical situations. The student must not forget that it is never a matter of simply telling the truth about a fact and leaving a patient with it. Information is communicated over time, in segments, after events that are constantly changing the "truth"; it is communicated as part of an emotional interaction that must also be understood for its messages and for the way in which it supports the therapeutic process itself.

The section begins with an abstract discussion of fidelity by Beauchamp and Childress, which is then related to several cases and clinical situations. This is followed by several studies of doctor-patient communication by Korsch, Gozzi, and Francis and by Strong, all of which are based upon studies that include communication with parents as part of pediatric medicine. There is then a selection by Novack et al. on the physician's expressed attitudes toward telling cancer patients their diagnosis which reports a reversal of earlier studies in which physicians were inclined not to tell the actual diagnosis. Also included are a number of letters on the topic. (See cases *3*, 4, 17, 18, 23, 24, *25*, 27, *28*, 29, 32, *35*, *37*, 47, *50*, 52, 56, 61, 64, 71, 72.)

32.

The Professional and Patient Relationship
Tom L. Beauchamp   James F. Childress

According to Paul Ramsey, the fundamental ethical question in biomedicine is: "What is the meaning of the faithfulness of one human being to another?" While Ramsey interprets faithfulness along such theological lines as covenant-fidelity, it is commonly expressed in nontheological language in terms of duties of fidelity.

Because duties of fidelity arise from *voluntary* actions, such as making contracts, they cannot be used to explicate all the moral requirements in biomedicine, e.g., the duty of nonmaleficence. Nevertheless, they play a central role in biomedical ethics.

Several moral conflicts emerge within relationships between health professsionals and patients. For example, the principle of veracity may require nondeception, yet the health care professional may determine that the use of a placebo would actually be in the patient's best interests. Other problems stem from a conflict of claims between patients and other individuals, or perhaps society itself. For example, it may be difficult, if not impossible, in some cases to respect the rule of confidentiality while also protecting other individuals and the society and in other cases to meet the needs of a particular patient while also satisfying the demands of a research protocol.

It is commonly agreed that we have a duty of veracity, i.e., a duty to tell the truth and not to lie or to deceive others. But as Henry Sidgwick observed many years ago, "it does not seem clearly agreed whether Veracity is an absolute and independent duty, or a special application of some higher principle." Sidgwick's observation still holds. One contemporary philosopher, G. J. Warnock, has included the principle of veracity as an independent principle ranking with beneficence, nonmaleficence,

and justice. Others have held that the principle of veracity is derived from other principles, such as respect for persons or fidelity or utility. Whether the duty of veracity is independent or derived, it does express several other principles and values.

Three arguments for the duty of veracity are particularly applicable to the relationship between health care professionals and patients. The first argument holds that the duty of veracity is part of the respect we owe to persons. As Alan Donagan writes:

> Relations between human beings are largely carried on by means of language; and much of what is communicated in language consists of expressions of opinion about what is the case. Unless it is required by a specific moral precept, nobody has a right to know another's opinion. The respect owed to other human beings includes respect for their liberty to withhold their thoughts when it is not their duty to divulge them; but, if anybody chooses to divulge his thoughts, the respect he owes to his audience requires that the thoughts he communicates must really be his.

Within biomedical contexts, respect for persons is commonly expressed through the principle of autonomy. Not to solicit *consent* for treatment from patients or for participation in research from subjects is to violate their autonomy and to fail to respect them as persons. But consent cannot express autonomy unless it is informed, and it therefore depends on communication and ultimately on truth-telling. Thus, a duty of veracity can be derived from a principle of respect for persons or autonomy.

Second, some philosophers, including W. D. Ross, argue that the duty of veracity

Source: Tom L. Beauchamp and James F. Childress, *Principles of Biomedical Ethics*, Oxford University Press, New York, 1979.

is an expression of the duty of fidelity or promise-keeping. When we use language to communicate with others, we implicitly promise that we will speak truthfully, that we will not lie by misrepresenting our opinions, and that we will not deceive our listeners. Our participation in society and our shared language engender a duty of veracity because of an implicit contract that is created. This contract generates the expectation that we will speak truthfully. Within biomedical contexts, it is sometimes possible also to point to a more specific though still implicit contract or promise. By entering into a relationship in the context of therapy or research, the patient or subject not only retains a general right to the truth but gains a special right to the truth regarding diagnosis, prognosis, procedures, etc.

Third, relationships of trust between human beings are necessary for fruitful interaction and cooperation. At the core of such relationships is confidence in and reliance upon others to respect the principle of veracity. This form of argument, commonly used by rule utilitarians, holds that lying can undermine relationships of trust and produce undesirable consequences. For example, relationships between health care professionals and their patients and between researchers and their subjects ultimately depend on trust. Lying thus fails to show respect for persons and their autonomy, violates implicit contracts, and also threatens relationships based on trust.

Despite these arguments for the duty of veracity, the various codes of medical ethics tend to omit this duty. The Hippocratic oath does not impose it, nor does the Declaration of Geneva by the World Medical Association in 1948. According to the Principles of Medical Ethics of the AMA, the physician has discretion about what to tell his or her patients. There is no clear duty of veracity in these codes. In sharp contrast, one recent Patient's Bill of Rights holds that a patient has a right "to informed participation in all decisions involving his health care program," a right "to know what research and ex-

perimental protocols are being used" in the facility and what alternatives are available in the community, a right "to a clear, concise explanation of all proposed procedures in layman's terms, including the possibilities of any risk of mortality or serious side effects, problems related to recuperation, and probability of success," and a right "to know the identity and professional status of all those providing service."

These differences between codes of medical ethics and the Patient's Bill of Rights in part reflect differences between physicians' and patients' perspectives—both of which are probably too limited. Physicians often think in terms of patients' needs and interests. This can lead them to a paternalistic stance rather than to an emphasis on patient autonomy. Patients, on the other hand, frequently think in terms of rights more than in terms of needs and interests. These different perspectives are reflected in surveys of medical and lay views about telling the truth to cancer patients. According to one study, the majority (88 percent) of physicians tend not to disclose a diagnosis of cancer to their patients. According to another study, the majority of lay people (82 to 98 percent) indicate that they want to be told the truth if they have cancer.

What does the principle of veracity entail and how much weight does it have? Like other duties, veracity is prima facie, not absolute. Nondisclosure, deception, and even lying can sometimes be justified when veracity conflicts with other duties. In many areas, but especially in disputes about veracity, moral debates involve the definition or description of the act as well as its justification. Let us consider "lying." We define "lying" as telling another person what one believes to be false in order to deceive him. So defined, "lying" would only be prima facie wrong and thus could be justified in some circumstances. If, however, "lying" is defined as intentionally withholding the truth from a person who has a right to it, then "lying" could be construed as absolutely wrong. The latter definition incorporates moral elements since it holds that the truth is due some persons but not others. It "resolves" moral dilemmas by redefining them, for some statements that would be described as lies according to our definition would not be lies according to this definition.

Although lying has attracted more attention and discussion than other ways of departing from the principle of veracity, it is in fact only one species of deception. It is distinguished from other species because it involves statements and because it is intentional—one cannot accidentally tell a lie. Deception is broader and encompasses many acts other than lying. For example, when a physician gives his patient a placebo, he may or may not lie to the patient. The duty of veracity requires nondeception, as well as truth-telling, but nonlying deception probably does not threaten the relationship of trust as much as lying, because lying means that an agent asserts what he believes to be false in order to deceive another.

The duty not to lie to or otherwise deceive others is stronger than the duty to disclose information to others. The duty to disclose depends more on special relationships than does the duty not to lie or deceive others. In a therapeutic relationship, for example, the patient entrusts his care to the therapist and has a right to information that the therapist would not be obligated to provide to total strangers. It is difficult to conceive of a positive duty to promote the truth by providing information apart from special relationships.

Both lies, as we have defined them, and other forms of deception are prima facie wrong and stand in need of justification; but they can sometimes be justified. We shall now consider some arguments for limited nondisclosure and deception in *therapeutic* settings.

The first argument for nondisclosure of some diagnoses and prognoses in the therapeutic setting represents what Sidgwick called "benevolent deception." It holds that disclosure of a diagnosis of cancer, for example, would violate the duties of benficence and nonmaleficence by causing the patient anxiety ("what you don't know can't hurt you"), by causing the patient to commit suicide, etc. One objection to this argument is based on the uncertainty of predicting consequences. Samuel Johnson made this point:

> I deny the lawfulness of telling a lie to a sick man for fear of alarming him. You have no business with consequences; you are to tell the truth. Besides, you are not sure what effects your telling him that he is in danger may have. It may bring his distemper to a crisis, and that may cure him. Of all lying, I have the greatest abhorrence of this, because I believe it has been frequently practised on myself.

Such an objection is especially applicable to act-utilitarian approaches to truth-telling. The more telling objections to "benevolent deception" stress violations of the principles of respect for persons and fidelity as well as the long-term threat to the relationship of trust between physicians and patients.

In one case a radiologist did not warn his patients of the possibility of a fatal reaction to urography on the grounds that it would not benefit them to know and might be dangerous. He contended that if he had told the woman who died of the possible fatal reaction, she would have become upset. He would then have convinced her that the probability of benefit outweighed the slight chance of a fatal reaction. Thus, he argued, telling her would only have upset her and would not have changed the outcome. Even if such cases do not seriously threaten the relationship of trust, they involve violations of the principles of fidelity and autonomy. In particular, the radiologist denied the patient information necessary for informed consent and violated her right to make her own assessment of the risks and benefits. (Of course, not all possible information is necessary.)

A second case represents another instance of "benevolent deception." A retired army officer was having chronic pain after several abdominal operations. He had lost weight and was depressed, unkempt, and socially withdrawn. He was admitted to a psychiatric ward which had the clear expectation of reducing his reliance on Talwin to relieve his pain by substituting pain control. Nevertheless, the patient insisted that he needed his medication to control his pain. After group consultation, the therapists decided to withdraw the Talwin by gradually substituting saline, but without informing the patient. The substitution was effective, and although the patient was angry when he was told three weeks later, he asked that the saline be discontinued. He was able to control his pain and to resume relatively normal functions. The therapists justified this deceptive use of a placebo because of its "high probability of success." While it is tempting to justify the means by the ends, especially when they are successfully realized, alternative nondeceptive means might have worked. The prima facie duty of veracity dictates a search for available alternatives even if they sometimes require more time, energy, and money. Furthermore, on utilitarian grounds this deceptive use of a placebo may have long-term negative effects on the patient's self-image and may damage his trust in health care professionals.

A second argument for nondisclosure and deception is that health care professionals cannot know or cannot communicate the "whole truth," and if they could, many patients and subjects would not be able to comprehend and understand the "whole truth." Such an argument does not, however, undermine the duty of veracity, understood as the duty to be truthful, for this duty requires that health care professionals disclose as completely as possible what a reasonable patient would want to know and what particular patients want to know.

A third argument for nondisclosure and deception is that some patients, particularly the very sick and the dying, do not really want to know the truth about their condition, despite what opinion surveys seem to reveal. According to this line of argument, neither the duty of fidelity nor the duty of respect

for persons requires truth-telling, because patients indicate by various signals—if not by actual words—that they do not want to hear the truth. To the rejoinder that many and perhaps most patients appear to want disclosure of relevant information, proponents of this third argument for nondisclosure hold that the patients they have in mind *really* do not want to know even when they say they do. Claims about what patients really want are suspicious, and there is no moral alternative in such cases to respecting the autonomy of competent patients by acting on their expressed wishes and wants. Also, this third argument sets dangerous precedents for paternalistic actions, even if it is a correct view of patient wishes and wants in some cases.

In some instances, of course, patients genuinely do not want to know. For example, some patients with a high risk of developing Huntington's chorea, an incurable genetic disease, indicate that they would not be interested in a simple, safe, and accurate predictive test if one were developed. In one sample, 23 percent of the high-risk respondents indicated that they might not take such a test. In other cases, patients who suspect that they have cancer explicitly ask not to be informed of the diagnosis and prognosis. What should health care professionals do when patients ask not to be given certain information? Some writers go so far as to argue that a patient has a *duty* to seek and appropriate the truth—not merely a *right* to the truth. But to force unwanted information on a patient is generally to act paternalistically and to violate that patient's autonomy. To force a person to confront the truth seems to be an act of disrespect, though it might on occasion be justified—e.g., in cases of weak paternalism where a person acts from false beliefs. However, respect entails allowing persons to exercise the right not to know whenever they are adequately informed and are acting autonomously.

If the disclosure of information in part depends on a duty of fidelity, what responsibility does a health care professional have when a test undertaken for a specific purpose reveals information not specifically requested by the testee who might, however, be very interested in the information? In a case discussed by Robert Veatch, a forty-one-year-old woman had unexpectedly become pregnant and was referred by her physician to the Human Genetics Unit in order to determine whether her fetus might have Down's syndrome (or mongolism). Because of her age she was considered to be at high risk of having a mongoloid child. The woman underwent amniocentesis, in which a sample of amniotic fluid surrounding the fetus was withdrawn by a needle for purposes of a biochemical or chromosomal analysis. The test showed that the fetus did not have Down's syndome. There was no *extra* 21st chromosome. But the sex chromosomes were abnormal. They were XYY, rather than the normal patterns of XX for female or XY for male. There is considerable debate about the significance of the extra Y chromosome. Although some studies show that XYY males tend to commit more violent crimes, other studies reject those findings. What should the genetic counselor do? Would he fulfill his duty of fidelity and disclosure if he only reported that the fetus did not suffer from Down's syndrome? Or is he also morally required to report the other findings? Does the woman have a right to obtain this information even though she did not specifically request it? Does the fact that the correlation between the XYY chromosomes and antisocial behavior is not established make his disclosure even more risky since it (1) could lead to an abortion or (2) could be a self-fulfilling prophecy if the woman did not abort? Should the patient have the right to make her own decision about the significance of this information? If the duty of veracity is based on respect for persons and their autonomy, a strong case can be made for disclosure. However, there are cases in which nondisclosure might be preferable, and there are, of course, many ways of disclosing the truth with compassion and sensitivity.

33.

Teaching Students How to Talk and Act with Patients
Howard Brody   Elliot S. Dacher

Howard Brody

To the Editor: The recent article on teaching interactional skills by my professors, Drs. Werner and Schneider,[1] makes an important point: medical students can be taught interviewing skills in a structured manner because recent research has clarified what these skills consist of. The course described, emphasizing interactional analysis, in conjunction with later courses emphasizing interviewing content, combines to teach the student how to get information out of a patient. An equally important problem in medical practice is how to get information into the patient, after a diagnosis is reached and a management plan selected. To my knowledge, no course in the skills required here now exists in a medical school.

An increasing amount of research has dealt with patient education by the physician on a one-to-one basis. Many researchers studying "patient compliance" have committed the error of concentrating on the patient's behavior and neglecting the physician's contributions. Of the studies that analyze the doctor-patient interaction as a whole, those by the Korsch group are perhaps the most impressive. It is of interest that many of the techniques applied by Werner

Source: *New England Journal of Medicine*, vol. 291, no. 7, August 15, 1974.

and Schneider in teaching students were also used by the Korsch group in their research.

Given this growing data base, medical educators ought to be designing training programs for medical students in the skills required for patient education. The present trend seems to assume that the possession of a medical degree automatically renders a person competent to inform and educate patients about their health problems. This is as unwarranted as the assumption that a doctor of philosophy is automatically qualified to teach college students.

Elliot S. Dacher

To the Editor: I read with much pleasure the article by Werner and Schneider. Although I applaud their achievement, I am less than assured about the ultimate success of their endeavor. They clearly recognize that a successful doctor-patient relation underlies all attempts at delivery of good medical care. We all recognize, however, that the next 5 to 10 years of students' training will in all aspects be such as to negate the possibility that they learn to understand the dynamics of the doctor-patient relation and apply it in their daily practice.

They will be taught to become "organ oriented" rather than "patient oriented," and "cure" oriented rather than "care" oriented. They will learn the skills of "roundsmanship" rather than those of "patient interaction," and how to call a psychiatric consultant rather than "waste" an hour. They will never be taught how to deal with aging, sexual problems, patient compliance, death and dying. They will be taught by academicians whose education has been similarly aborted.

In short, the doctor-patient relation is the foundation for the delivery of ongoing comprehensive medical care and its elements must be taught and emphasized throughout training. In the final analysis, it must be as prestigious and rewarding to establish an effective and meaningful relation with a patient as it is to come forth with a quick, bright answer on rounds.

NOTE

1. A. Werner and J.M. Schneider, "Teaching Medical Students Interactional Skills," *New England Journal of Medicine*, vol. 290, p. 1232, 1974.

34.
Gaps in Doctor-Patient Communication
Barbara M. Korsch   Ethel K. Gozzi   Vida Francis

Eight hundred patient visits to the walk-in clinic of the Childrens Hospital of Los Angeles were studied by means of tape recording the doctor-patient interaction and by follow-up interview. Seventy-six percent of the patient visits resulted in satisfaction on the part of the patient's mother; in 24 percent there was dissatisfaction. A number of communication barriers between pediatrician and patient's mother were found to contribute significantly to patient dissatisfaction: notably lack of warmth and friendliness on

Source: *Pediatrics,* vol. 42, p. 855, 1968. Copyright 1968 by the American Academy of Pediatrics. The authors wish to express their gratitude to Milton Davis, Ph.D., for his most helpful consultations; to Dr. R. Mickey at University of California, Los Angeles, Health Sciences Computing Facility for statistical counsel; to members of the pediatric and nursing staff of the Childrens Hospital of Los Angeles for their patience and cooperation; to the research team, Barbara Freemon, Marie Morris, and Elaine Aley, for their

the part of the doctor, failure to take into account the patient's concern and expectations from the medical visit, lack of clear-cut explanation concerning diagnosis and causation of illness, and use of medical jargon.

The Patient's Expectations

Patients' expectations from the visit and the strong influence of mutual expectations on doctor-patient relationships have been investigated at length. Patients' expectations may relate to the doctors' "expressive" role, i.e., they may look for kindness, understanding, emotional support. Some patients emphasize that they expect explanations about the disease and its seriousness. Other patients simply state that they expect competence in their doctors or symptom relief for themselves.

Patient Satisfaction

It seems appropriate to point out first that, although many communication breakdowns were documented in the study, satisfactory and effective communication was the rule and not the exception. After all, 76 percent of the patients were satisfied with their visits. The wisdom of using patient satisfaction as a yardstick to measure the effectiveness of doctor-patient communication may be questioned, especially since insufficient data are available at this time to demonstrate how and when patient satisfaction correlates with follow-through on medical advice.

At present the findings concerning patient satisfaction are being correlated with those on compliance. Even now it can be stated that there is no simple, direct correlation between satisfaction and compliance with medical advice, and the dependent variables will have to be looked at separately as well as together.

Patient Expectations

From a practical point of view, one of the most relevant results from this investigation is the documented need for attention to the patient's own ideas about the illness and the family's expectations from the medical visit. It has been shown that important and highly relevant information concerning patient fears and expectations is readily obtainable with the simplest interview questions which could easily be incorporated into regular medical visits. It has also been demonstrated that currently these concerns are given insufficient attention during doctor-patient consultations. Some of the recorded patient visits suggest that, rather than adding to the physician's burden, attention and recognition given to these topics makes for shorter patient visits. Once the mother's urgent needs are met she seems more attentive and amenable to the physician's ideas and plans. Balint[1] has stressed the patients' need to have a name for their illness before they can proceed. The present findings bear this out in that a failure to receive a clear diagnostic statement was definitely associated with patient dissatisfaction. Yudkin[2] suggested that often there is a "second diagnosis" in addition to the ostensive chief complaint which needs attention. Some of the "main worries" mentioned in this report would seem to represent such initially non-expressed urgent needs of the patient which it behooves the physician to elicit. These might fit into Yudkin's category of the "second diagnosis."

Diagnosis and Cause

Previous explorations[3] on patient expectation had suggested that, whereas adult patients more often seek symptom relief for themselves, pediatric patients' parents have a need to learn the cause, "what brought it

continued invaluable assistance; and to Anne Hinton, Myrene Smith, Irene Dalzell, Muriel Schuerman, and Leah Martin for past help in the project. Appreciation is expressed to Miss Coralee Yale for her competence and enthusiasm in the preparation of computer programs.

on?" and so forth in order to feel satisfied
and reassured. It can be speculated that this
relates not only to the wish to prevent
similar problems in the future but also to a
need to be relieved from feelings of self-
blame. Whatever the basis, the investigation
reported here illustrates amply that the
parents of pediatric patients are concerned
with causation and often need a clear statement from their physician in order to be
satisfied and reassured. A question might be
raised as to the harm of allowing persistent
uncertainty concerning cause and unabated
feelings of self-blame on the part of the
mother. There is clinical evidence that, in
addition to the anxiety and distress of the
parents, these feelings lead to overprotection
and inappropriate behavior on the part of
the parents in handling the child's illness
which may be harmful and should be avoided
if possible. The present investigation suggests that clear discussion of causation of
illness and relief of feelings of self-blame
on the part of the parents may aid in preventing undue parental anxiety and over-
protective behavior.

Expressive Versus Instrumental Functions of the Physician

Some of the findings presented can be
regarded profitably in the light of Parsons'[4]
separation of instrumental and expressive
functions of the physician. Only 54 of the
800 respondents in the study group seriously questioned the technical competence
(i.e., the instrumental functions) of the
pediatrician whom they had seen, and only
six mothers felt that the pediatrician's
handling of the child left something to be
desired. However, there were a considerable proportion of mothers who wished for
more warmth, greater show of concern,
and more friendliness for themselves from
the physician. A different sample of pediatric patients who have a long-standing relationship with a particular doctor might
experience a higher degree of friendliness,
warmth, and sympathy. Still, to judge by

the public protest over the inhumanity
and impersonality of present-day medicine,
the problem does exist when one looks at
medical and pediatric care on a broader scale.
A recent study by Charney et al.[5] illustrates
that long-standing relation with a pediatrician
correlates with follow-through on medical
advice. Long-term compliance cannot be
estimated on the basis of the present study.
Patient satisfaction, on the other hand,
is related to the expressive role of the doctor without a question of a doubt.

Patient Attributes

The only specific attribute of patients
with higher education demonstrated in
this study is that they are more prone to
express their fears and hopes to the doctor and that they have a better chance
of having them responded to or dealt with.
However, the study does not support the
view that patients' health behavior in the
threat of an acute illness can most frequently be explained on the basis of their
socioeconomic, ethnic, religious, or educational background. These findings, like
the results of Davis,[6] are encouraging to
contemplate at a time when health care is
being offered increasingly to groups in
the lower educational and economic strata.
These findings should also be heeded by
all those physicians who will readily admit
that they spend more time and give more
explanations to patients who seem more intelligent and more educated. As pointed
out by Samora et al.[7] and Seligmann et al.,[8]
physicians tend to underestimate the patients' understanding and medical information, and this leads them in turn to give
less information to these patients, which
clearly leads to a kind of vicious circle
in which those most in need of education
from their physician are apt to receive
the least. Taking all this into consideration,
it seems important for physicians and
other health workers to give the patient the
benefit of the doubt and to give their
medical explanations with as much enthusi-

asm, albeit in a somewhat different manner, even with those who seem less responsive and less well informed.

Physician Attributes

The physicians in the study were generally homogeneous in training and background; hence, no significant inferences were made concerning specific physician attributes in relation to patient responses and satisfaction. As has been presented, every physician in the study had both satisfied and dissatisfied patients, and, incidentally, there was also variation in compliance. It is clear from all aspects of the study that patients' individual needs vary greatly and that no one pediatrician can meet them all. Some patient expectations are so unrealistic and their problems are of such a nature that no pediatrician can fulfill them in a short encounter. It has often been suggested that the known presence of a tape recorder in an examining room would make the pediatrician "do better." This assumes that unobserved pediatricians are not trying to do their best but do know how to do better. This was not an assumption to which the research team subscribed, and hence it came as no surprise that there was no increase in patient satisfaction or in compliance in the group of patients whose visits were tape-recorded.

Utilization of Doctor's Time

Evidence that a doctor-patient communication can be satisfactory and effective in as little as 5 minutes is of practical interest. Inferences must be drawn from this with reservations, however. It is possible that an already effective consultation between doctor and patient might be even more satisfactory if more time were available even though more time, as such, is not enough. One thing is clear, however, that much time is lost in ineffective verbalization, especially on the part of the doctor, and that the time the patient and doctor spend in the same room is of lesser import than how they spend this period of time. It would

seem also that a few minutes spent in getting acquainted with the patient's ideas and expectations would save the physician time later on and make for a more satisfactory doctor-patient relationship.

One observation that is hard to describe without lengthy examples from the case records is that many physicians lose time by letting themselves be trapped into what can only be described as arguments and quarrels with the patients. These take time and are ridiculous. For instance, a mother will describe what she calls "vomiting" by her baby. The physician corrects her and informs her that "regurgitation" is the proper term for what she has described. She counters that she thought it was vomiting. He argues back, and many, many precious minutes pass while he lectures and she attempts to describe things in her original language. Most likely the mother will leave the doctor and tell the sympathetic listener in the waiting room that the doctor never did understand what brought her to the doctor or that her child was vomiting. Another time-consuming and unnecessary activity during physician's consultation with pediatric parents is repetition. Especially when they feel that a mother does not comprehend them, physicians repeat their own words sometimes three or four times, apparently hoping that the mother will accept and understand them the next time even though she did not do so before. On the contrary, it may be assumed that, if certain formulations are unacceptable to the mother the first and second time, another approach must be needed. Repetitions from the mother are also a sign that communication is not taking place. If she asks the same question two or three times, although the doctor believes he has already answered it, something has gone wrong either in his interpretation of the question or in his approach to the answer. Perhaps she is one of the mothers who has a "second diagnosis" or a "hidden agenda." Whichever of these alternatives applies, repetition alone will not meet the previously unmet needs.

NOTES

1. M. Balint, *The Doctor and His Patient and the Illness,* International University Press, New York, 1957.

2. S. Yudkin, "Six Children with Coughs—The Second Diagnosis," *Lancet,* vol. 2, p. 561, 1961.

3. Unpublished data.

4. T. Parsons, "Illness and the Role of the Physician," *Journal of Orthopsychiatry,* vol. 21, p. 452, 1951.

5. E. Charney, R. Bynum, D. Eldredge, D. Frank, J. B. MacWhinney, N. McNabb, A. Schneider, E. A. Sumpter, and H. Iker, "How Well Do Patients Take Oral Penicillin? A Collaborative Study in Private Practice," *Pediatrics,* vol. 40, p. 188, 1967.

6. M. S. Davis, "Deviant Interaction in an Institutionalized Relationship: Variations in Patients' Compliance with Doctors' Orders," International Sociological Association, Evian, France, September 1966.

7. J. Samora, L. Saunders, and R. Larson, "Knowledge about Specific Diseases in Four Selected Samples," *Journal of Health and Human Behavior,* vol. 3, p. 176, 1962.

8. A. W. Seligmann, Neva E. McGrath, and L. Pratt, "Level of Medical Information among Clinic Patients," *Journal of Chronic Diseases,* vol. 6, p. 497, 1957.

35.

The Social Context of the Clinical Interview
Allen J. Enelow   Scott N. Swisher

The private physician conducts most extensive medical interviews in his office, his most congenial environment. It is here that he feels most at home and where, consequently, his most spontaneous behavior is likely to occur. Both the doctor's and the patient's behavior will be influenced by the way the office is used. Both can communicate more freely if the setting of the interview is a quiet consulting room with reasonably comfortable furniture and if there are few or no interruptions. While it is perhaps easiest to secure the conditions for a successful interview in the physician's office, it does not necessarily follow that these conditions will exist. Many physicians permit the telephone and office personnel to interrupt their interviews, do not allow sufficient time for the interview, or narrowly limit the topics discussed. Some physicians make a practice of conducting interviews in their examining rooms, where the patient is partially clothed or under a drape sheet on the examining table. The patient rarely feels at ease under such circumstances. He is likely to feel both powerless and self-

estranged without the clothing which announces his identity to others and confirms it for himself. The social distance between the doctor and the patient is likely to be increased. Docility, obedience, embarrassment, and efforts to please the physician will reduce the amount of information from the patient and sometimes bias it.

The least suitable setting for the outpatient interview is probably the clinic of a large public hospital. The physical setting is likely to be uncomfortable and unattractive and is likely to afford little privacy. The physician is usually on a tight time schedule. Both the physician and the patient are likely to be caught in a maze of bureaucratic procedures, and frequently both are aware that the patient will see a different physician on his next clinic visit. Usually the interview brings together a doctor and patient of quite different sociocultural backgrounds with the many attending difficulties. All these create problems that require a great effort on the part of the physician and the other health workers, if they are to be overcome. While it will probably require a

Source: Allen J. Enelow and Scott N. Swisher, *Interviewing and Patient Care,* Oxford University Press, 1972.

major organizational overhaul to provide comprehensive, coordinated patient care in municipal health care systems, an effective interview on the part of a clinic physician can go a long way toward providing the basis for such care to the patients he sees.

Alienative Features of Health Care

Alienation refers to feelings of disconnectedness from, and disenchantment with, one's society and its organizations, values, and norms (or standards). Sociologists identify four facets of alienation: feelings of powerlessness, normlessness, meaninglessness, and self-estrangement. One of the reasons for the alienating quality of health care is lack of continuity and coordination in the highly specialized health services received by patients. They are frequently made to feel not only that they are overlooked as a person or viewed only as a human body but that they are regarded as a set of organ systems, each in the hands of a different medical specialty. The interface between the patient and the health care system is the interview, and it is almost decisive in determining whether these problems will be overcome in the patients' treatment.

Seeman and Evans[1] state that medical care "represents a microcosm of the alienative features" of mass society in that it is a situation with "low control over one's fate, heavy reliance upon specialized experts, bureaucratic authority, and the loss of community ties."

The patient may feel alienated in the hands of private physicians in those situations, far too common, where he must suffer long periods of waiting in reception areas and examining rooms, where he may be under treatment simultaneously by four or five medical specialists whose communication is faulty if not altogether absent, where he may understand little of what is done to him and where he must wait days, weeks, or even months for an appointment with an overworked physician. However, the hospital and its associated clinics are usually even more likely to create feelings of alienation. The patient is usually admitted to the new and strange hospital environment when illness has already rendered him relatively helpless and attacked his self-concept. In this setting, the patient feels normless, which means he has no set of standards to which to relate his behavior. Many of his usual standards of personal conduct—including bodily modesty, personal self-care, pursuit of useful activities, and self-direction in his personal affairs—no longer apply. He realizes this but has difficulty responding as he is now expected to. He is not permitted to help himself, but how much help is he permitted to ask of hospital personnel? Are there still rules of modesty he is expected to obey? If so, which and how? He is expected to report his symptoms, but how freely may he do so without being accused of complaining? He is cut off from those to whom he usually expresses his fear and despair but how freely may he speak about these to hospital personnel? These and many other questions perplex and stress the patient as he attempts to meet the expectations of hospital personnel in his new role of hospital patient.

Powerlessness is another aspect of alienation commonly engendered by the hospital setting. He has little or no control over what happens to him. Every detail of his life is regulated by doctor's orders or hospital regulations. He is admitted and discharged at the will of the authorities and must conform to hospital regulations and arrangements about meals, medications, diet, and visitors.

A sense of meaninglessness often numbs hospital patients. The reasons for the regulations and procedures in a bureaucratically organized hospital, and much of his medical treatment as well, may remain obscure to the patient. He is incapable of engaging in many of the activities and social relationships which lent meaning to his life or is prevented from doing so by the restrictions imposed by the hospital. Alone in a sterile atmosphere isolated from friends and family, subjected to strange and often painful procedures, life itself may become meaningless to the patient.

Self-estrangement is also sometimes part of the hospital experience. A sense of unreality may pervade the self when one is deprived of one's own clothing and other possessions and of the support of customary relationships. Hospital personnel do not treat an individual as he is accustomed to being treated, and in the role of patient, he is not in a position to exhibit many of the personal qualities and capacities which ordinarily elicit responses that support his sense of self.

The interviewer in the hospital situation has his own set of problems. The private physician making hospital rounds usually feels less at home than in his own office. Given the changing roles of physicians in hospitals he may be engaged in role conflicts with the hospital administration or the burgeoning staff of new health personnel. He must adjust his practice to the hospital's bureaucratic procedures, and his practice is more open to the scrutiny of his colleagues than it is when he is in his office. The staff physician, the nurses, and other personnel may feel more comfortable in the hospital, but they also have many problems which make effective interviewing difficult. Hospitals are usually understaffed, which means that health professionals are tightly scheduled and overworked. Large teaching hospitals are likely to foster segmented care and divided professional responsibility through their highly specialized services, making it difficult for any single professional to have the rapport with a patient that develops with successive interviews.

The immediate situation provided in a hospital is likely to be unfavorable for an effective interview. The patient is more frequently than not in a ward or shared room, and hospital personnel or visitors may interrupt the interview. The patient is usually in bed while the interviewer is clothed and mobile. In this situation, some interviewers stand at the foot of the bed, some at the

side of the bed, and some sit on or near the bed while talking to the patient. In each case, the effect on the interview varies. The physical distance from the patient has an effect on the emotional distance; they vary directly with each other. The standing physician speaking with a patient who is lying down creates a status difference that reduces communication. The physician who is sitting and close enough to touch the patient will be helping to create an atmosphere that is supportive and that encourages communication.

Each health care delivery system defines the task of the health professional with respect to the patient's care somewhat differently. This definition affects the information to be obtained in the interview and the quality of the relationship formed with the patient. In general, the larger and more complex the health care system and the more specialized the service provided by the individual health worker, the more difficult it is to provide continuity and coordination of health services and the more alienative is the process of health care. The scope of the interview will ordinarily be defined by the nature of the service to be performed. The laboratory technician about to draw blood will probably conduct a brief interview obtaining information immediately relevant to the procedure, putting the patient at ease, and, if required, relieving his anxiety about the procedure. The more comprehensive the professional's responsibility for the patient, the more comprehensive the interview required. Health care systems in which the patient is seen many times by different individuals in circumscribed interviews contribute to feelings of alienation.

NOTE

1. M. Seeman and J. W. Evans, "Alienation and Learning in a Hospital Setting," *American Sociological Review*, vol. 27, p. 772, 1962.

36

Reaching Agreement   P. M. Strong

This selection discusses those features of communication between doctors and parents of patients in which adjustments are made to sensitive information. When parental doubts were to be amplified rather than dismissed doctors proceeded more slowly and indirectly. Dr. G did not repeatedly probe the parents about their doubts or worries; he merely asked them a question which might lead to such talk, as might his own statements and the various demonstrations he provided, such as the book and the walking. Doubts and their discussion were allowed to develop gently over time. Thus, although agreement was certainly a high priority for staff, search is perhaps too active a word to describe their method in such cases. Agreement here was stalked rather than sought after; doctors lay in wait and watched, and the end was no sudden spring but a gradual luring toward acceptance.

For what was at issue was the parents' whole conception of the child: its present, its future, and their own future as well. And, whereas normalizing a child might be done in a session, as might the revelation of minor illness, stigmatizing a child could take many months or even years. Although it is conventional to refer to the telling of bad news as something that occurs at one point in time—"When they told me"—such a description does not capture the complex nature of the process by which such news was broken here. To some extent this depended on clinical uncertainty. As doctors saw a child over time, so they gained a more accurate version of the child's condition and capacities. Just as crucially, however, the stages depended on the doctors' belief that bad news should be broken slowly, that parents had to prepare themselves for the worst, that they could not take everything in at once, and that the news staff had to tell should match parents' expectations:

Dr. J: She's a very nice mother. I think what we're trying to do is to introduce her very gradually to the fact that the child is very small, though we know she will look like a circus dwarf. You know the sort of child I mean? Well, we haven't really told the mother that. We've just said that she's going to be very small. Anyway, she seems to be a candidate for delayed development and there's also this increased intracranial pressure, that's going to be a problem. Now at six months I saw her, that was at the special nursery follow-up clinic and she had a head-lag there, but of course then it wasn't necessarily developmental delay. So we saw her again at eight months, and by then she had got some head control but she hadn't her setting balance. She had some hand movements and was vocalizing all right. So that seemed to be on the credit side. But at ten months we found that she wasn't sitting. The mother feels that otherwise she's doing all right there. She's not a very bright thing but I think in this case she's a pretty good judge of what the situation is. Then she was referred here. There has been this query about brain damage but we've not mentioned any of this to the mother. In fact the child had this very bashed-about head, she looked really awful when she was born.

The breaking of bad news was therefore an extremely delicate operation, in which staff probed to see how much parents suspected; produced some information and

Source: P. M. Strong, *The Ceremonial Order of the Clinic: Parents, Doctors and Medical Bureaucracies,* Routledge and Kegan Paul, London, 1979.

saw how they reacted; elaborated if they were challenged; withdrew slightly if the parents looked angry, and so on. Staff played a waiting game, not enforcing their own definition of a child but always leaving a part to be negotiated in each consultation, trying to build on last time's definition, but first waiting to see how parents commented on what had happened in the intervening weeks or months. As far as the two can be separated, the movement was from diagnosis to prognosis, first indicating what the child was and then saying what it would be. The movement from one to the other varied with the parents' receptiveness. No parent was told everything immediately, but some achieved detailed and dispassionate discussion far more quickly than others. The following example indicates both the difficulties that might be faced and the way these were surmounted by making little agreements at each stage. The excerpts are from three consecutive consultations.

This was the child's first visit to the neurological clinic. He was four months old at this point and had already been seen three times at the special nursery follow-up clinic. The mother had several other children, was highly competent, and had made detailed comments on some of her child's problems. She had not, however, noticed the more serious ones, the child's spasticity and microcephaly. In his summary, the doctor started out by appealing to the shared agreement on the child's delay and then moved on to his own diagnosis. But this was phrased tentatively and the entire discussion of the child was in the present not the future tense:

Dr. I: He is very behind in what he's doing *of course* (my emphasis) and although you yourself are not very impressed with it, I think that his muscles are rather stiff. He does have some spasticity, this is what it's called.

Four months later, at the next visit, the mother indicated at the very beginning of the consultation that she was skeptical if her boy had made any progress and the doctor's own history-taking revealed very few signs of this. This time he looked toward the future in his summary:

Dr. I: Well, I don't find anything new. From what you say he has made a very, very slight progress, not very much, not very much, but a little. . . . I hope that there will be further progress, and don't be too upset if it is slow. It looks as if Alan is going to be handicapped to some extent.

On the third visit, eleven months later, the mother talked freely of the child's severe handicap: "He's absolutely ruined." The doctor's summary was in turn far more specific about the future than on the previous visit.

Dr. J: He's a long way off walking now. I don't know if he ever will. He's got to get sitting balance first, if . . . (pause) . . . When he gets near weight-bearing age we might ask the orthopedic surgeons if there is anything that can be done to improve the mechanical performance of his feet. He seems well, he's avoiding any deformities, but he's certainly got quite a way to go before he's got complete head control. His head is lagging back a bit. The next stage after that is sitting balance, he's nearly got head balance. (The child is in sitting position.) How long can he stay like this? Just for a few seconds?

Mother: Yes, for a few seconds and then he keels over.

Dr. J: So we want to work on sitting balance and then the next stage is weight-bearing, but he's a long way off that at the moment. OK, that's fine. At present you are quite happy coping with him at home?

Mother: Oh, yes (cheerfully).

Even at this stage some matters went undiscussed. The doctor did not press the mother on her ability to cope, though privately he felt her to be unrealistic. Further, the full extent of the child's handicap had not yet been revealed. The microcephaly had not been mentioned nor, as can be seen, was any detailed statement made about the child's mental abilities. Although the mother defined the child as "ruined" at one stage in the conversation, she was eager to try to bring him on. Such eagerness was treated as laudable but unrealistic, and an indicator that she had still not grasped the true nature of her son's injuries. More detailed discussion was thus postponed until the mother herself clearly accepted such facts, that is, until a "reasonable" discussion of the child was possible and reasoned agreement could be reached. Parents and staff preserved their alliance and its rational form by seeking agreement only when this could readily be made.

37.

Changes in Physicians' Attitudes toward Telling the Cancer Patient

Dennis H. Novack   Robin Plumer   Raymond L. Smith
Herbert Ochitill   Gary R. Morrow   John M. Bennett

A number of surveys since 1953 have investigated the physician's approach to the cancer patient regarding the issue of disclosing the diagnosis.

Of 442 physicians surveyed through the mail in 1953, 31 percent said they always or usually tell the patient, while 69 percent said they usually do not or never tell the patient. Of those who generally did not make the diagnosis known, exception occurred when the patient refused treatment or needed to plan. Of those inclined to share the diagnosis, reluctance arose when they were discouraged by the family or afraid of the patient's response.[1] In 1960, of 5,000 physicians, 16 percent said that they always told the patient, and 22 percent responded that they never told the patient. The rest sometimes told the patient. Their decisions were influenced by such factors as the stability of the patient, the insistence by the patient or family, the necessity for the patient to put affairs in order, and the unavailability of anyone else who could be told.[2]

In Oken's[3] survey of 219 physicians at Michael Reese Hospital, based on questionnaires and personal interviews, 90 percent generally did not inform the patient. Although more than three-fourths of the group cited clinical experience as the major determinant of their policies, the data bore no relationship to length of experience or age. Many showed inconsistences in attitudes, personal bias, and resistance to change and to further research, suggesting that emotion-laden a priori personal judgments were the real determinants of policy. Underlying were feelings of pessimism and futility about cancer.

By 1970 a questionnaire survey responded to by 178 physicians showed that 66 percent sometimes inform the patient, 25 percent always tell the patient, and only 9 percent never tell the patient.[4] This suggests

Source: *Journal of the American Medical Association*, vol. 241, no. 9, March 2, 1979.

This study was supported in part by grants R18-CA-19681 and CA11198 from the U.S. Department of Health, Education, and Welfare, and the Rochester Plan at the University of Rochester, Rochester, N.Y.

Donald Oken, M.D., and George Engle, M.D., provided valuable suggestions during preparation of the manuscript.

Copies of the questionnaire used can be obtained from Dennis H. Novack, M.D., P.O. Box 432, University of Virginia Medical Center, Charlottesville, Va. 22908.

a modification of previous practice. To assess whether this represents a genuine change, the present survey was undertaken.

Results

Two hundred seventy-eight, or 40 percent usable responses, were returned from a single mailing. In comparing the 1977 and 1961 populations, the present sample had a mean age of 37 years and was 91 percent men, while the 1961 sample had a mean age of 50 years and was 97 percent men. Oken reported that the great bulk of physicians in the sample were in active private practice in addition to taking a regular part in the teaching program. Two-thirds of the respondents were older than 31 years and were involved in the practice of their specialties. Many took an active role in the hospital's teaching program.

Of those who responded, 98 percent reported that their general policy is to tell the patient. Two-thirds of this group say that they never or very rarely make exceptions to this rule. This stands in sharp contrast with Oken's 1961 data, which showed that 88 percent generally did not tell the patient, with 56 percent saying that they never or very rarely made exceptions to this rule.

No differences between specialties were found, with the exception that the pediatricians, while reporting that their usual policy is to tell the patient, make exceptions to this rule more frequently than other physicians. With minor exceptions this lack of specialty difference was a consistent finding for all questionnaire items.

The results seem to indicate that the many factors that went into the decision to tell the patient influenced not only whether a physician would tell the patient but also the manner in which he made the diagnosis known, perhaps influencing the timing or wording of the communication.

The four most frequent factors considered in the decision to tell the patient were age (56 percent), intelligence (44 percent), relative's wish about telling the patient (51 percent), and emotional stability (47 percent).

Four factors most frequently believed to be of special importance were the patient's expressed wish to be told (52 percent), emotional stability (21 percent), age (11 percent), and intelligence (10 percent).

As before, clinical experience was given the major credit in both studies, with more than 90 percent citing it as a source and more than 70 percent citing it as a major source. As in Oken's data, analysis of the age of respondents citing clinical experience as a major policy determinant showed that younger physicians were just as likely to cite clinical experience as their seniors. Seventy-four percent of our group (and 86 percent of Oken's group) said that their policy had not changed in the past.

Thus, as in 1961, it appears that personal and emotional factors are of major importance in shaping policy, perhaps even more so in the present study. Subsequent to the general inquiry, "How did you acquire your policy?" it was specifically asked if personal issues were determinants. Seventy-one percent of the 1961 survey and 92 percent of the current survey reported that personal elements were involved.

Responses to the last two survey questions are perhaps indicative of the conviction with which the present policies are held. One hundred percent (vs. 60 percent of the 1961 sample) indicated a preference for being told if they themselves had cancer. One hundred percent thought that the patient has the right to know.

Comment

There appears to have been a major change in physicians' attitudes concerning telling patients their diagnosis of cancer. Even if only those physicians who believed strongly about telling the patient responded to our survey, there has still been a significant change since Oken's study. Indeed, there is some evidence that our results may be representative of more widely held views.

Therapy for many forms of cancer has notably improved in recent years. Oken's data suggested that the great majority of physicians believed that cancer connoted certain death. As many patients shared this pessimism, this common belief was often an effective deterrent to free communication. Today advances in therapy have brought longer survival, improved quality of life, and, in many cases, permanent cure. Physicians believe they can offer their cancer patients more hope.

There has been an increase in public awareness of cancer at many levels. The media are constantly presenting evidence of the ubiquity of carcinogens. Public figures such as Betty Ford and Happy Rockefeller spoke openly about their malignant neoplasms. The American Cancer Society publicizes the "Seven Danger Signals of Cancer." Perhaps all this has led to a lesser stigmatization of cancer, a greater ease in talking about its reality, and a greater awareness of its signs and symptoms.

Oken suggested that most physicians thought that the diagnosis of cancer, with its expectation of death, deprived the patient of hope, and hence they were reluctant to tell cancer patients the diagnosis. Our data suggest that this attitude has also changed. Even when death is expected from the disease, physicians are nevertheless telling their patients the diagnosis. Perhaps improved therapy allows physicians to be overly optimistic with their patients.

Perhaps more patients are being told because more need to know. Many university hospitals are major clinical research centers, and patients who agree to participate in research protocols must be told their diagnosis to satisfy the legal requirements of informed consent. At the University of Rochester, in 1975, 15 percent of patients with all newly diagnosed cancer participated in national protocols.

It is impossible to know to what extent the literature on telling the cancer patient has shaped attitudes. If it has had any effect, however, it would be in the direction of encouraging frankness. This has been more recently reaffirmed by Cassem and Stewart,[5] who, in suggesting a general policy of frankness, cite two sets of empirical studies. The first set includes those studies in which patients were asked whether or not they should be told. These indicate overwhelming positive favor for telling. The second set looks at the effects of telling on patients and their families. These studies dispelled the myth of the harm that telling the patient might engender.

The comments of some of our respondents indicate that the present reversal in attitude is due, in part, to more sweeping social changes. The rise in the consumerism movement and increasing public scrutiny of the medical profession have altered the physician-patient relationship. In this era of "patients' rights," an attitude of frankness feels right and, indeed, given the current disputatious atmosphere of medical practice, may be the safest one to adopt.

Many questions remain. Do physicians tell patients they have "cancer," or are euphemisms such as "tumor" or "growth" still widely used, and if so what does that mean for the communication process? Are changing attitudes on telling the patient accompanied by the emotional support that a patient's knowledge of his diagnosis may demand of a physician? Saunders[6] wrote, "The real question is not 'What do you tell your patients?' but rather, 'What do you let your patients tell you?'" Now that we tell our patients more, are we also listening more? Unfortunately one survey cannot answer these questions.

Is the present policy of telling the patient the best policy? The majority of our respondents cite clinical experience as shaping their present policy, even though most of them have never had experience with another policy. The majority of Oken's respondents also cited clinical experience in shaping the exact opposite policy. While not discounting the value of clinical experience, its use as a determinant of policy must be called into question.

Our data suggest that, as in Oken's study, the present policy is supported by strong belief and emotional investment in its being right. One hundred percent of our respondents stated that patients have a right to know. Yet in asserting this in a blanket manner, are physicians sometimes abdicating a responsibility to make subtle judgments in individual cases? Do patients also have a right not to know?

Is it possible to determine who should be told what, when, and how? What are the criteria by which we judge if telling is right? Patient evaluation in future studies on telling might include assessments of compliance with the medical regimen, quality of communication with physician and family members, ratings of adjustment to illness, or psychological tests of depression and anxiety.

Our respondents' written comments seem to indicate that the current policy of telling the patient is accompanied by increased sensitivity to patients' emotional needs. There is some evidence that telling is the best policy.[7] Yet how rational is the process of deciding what to tell the patient with cancer? Even though the policies have reversed, many physicians are still basing their communication with cancer patients on emotion-laden personal convictions. They are relying on honesty, sensitivity, and patients' rights rather than focusing on the following relevant scientific psychological question: Does telling the diagnosis of cancer help or harm (which) patients and how?

NOTES

1. W.T. Fitts Jr., and I.S. Ravdin, "What Philadelphia Physicians Tell Patients with Cancer," *Journal of the American Medical Association*, vol. 153, p. 901, 1953.

2. D. Rennick (ed.), "What Should Physicians Tell Cancer Patients?" *Nuclear Medicine Materials*, vol. 2, p. 51, 1960.

3. D. Oken, "What to Tell Cancer Patients: A Study of Medical Attitudes," *Journal of the American Medical Association*, vol. 175, p. 1120, 1961.

4. H.S. Friedman, "Physician Management of Dying Patients: An Exploration," *Psychiatry in Medicine*, vol. 1, p. 295, 1970.

5. N.H. Cassem and R.S. Stewart, "Management and Care of the Dying Patient," *International Journal of Psychiatry and Medicine*, vol. 6, p. 293, 1975.

6. C. Saunders, "The Moment of Truth: Care of the Dying Person," in L. Pearson (ed): *Death and Dying*, p. 49, Case Western Reserve University Press, Cleveland, 1969.

7. B. Gerle, G. Landen, and P. Sandblom, "The Patient with Inoperable Cancer from the Psychiatric and Social Standpoint," *Cancer*, vol. 13, p. 1206, 1960.

38.

Do Patients Feign Ignorance?   Jonas Brachfeld

To the Editor: I was interested to learn that across the ocean[1] the same patient posture ("my doctor ain't telling me nothing") prevails as in the United States. In this country, various health professionals, but particularly the nursing profession, have managed to turn this intriguing problem into the latest growth industry—patient education and teaching.

It is a common experience to find patients who claim complete ignorance about why they have been admitted to a cardiac-care unit when one knows that the reason has been explained to them time and time again. The concept of denial is often considered a satisfactory explanation for this phenomenon. I am not so sure. I suspect that frequently the claim of ignorance is an acceptable way for patients to try to relate to personnel. Patients cannot expect the busy doctor or nurse to take time off simply to chat about the latest football scores or the situation in Iran, but they can always get attention if they request information about their diseases. I have frequently demonstrated to nurses that the patient is not as confused and ignorant as is believed: when asked what the monitor, the wires, and the oxygen are all about,

Source: *New England Journal of Medicine*, vol. 302, no. 14, April 3, 1980, p. 817.

he admits quite readily that all this obviously is needed for the treatment of his heart attack.

I submit that we can delegate to others the responsibility of patient monitoring, defibrillation, emergency drug therapy, and many other procedures, but that the ultimate role of the physician in giving reassurance and comfort must be confronted. To divert a patient toward the health educator or the "patient-teaching" nurse may pro-

vide a lot of factual data but will make the patient who longs for the nurturing figure of the authoritative physician even more frustrated.

NOTE

1. J. Lister, Compliance in Clinical Care—Congress in Vienna—Health Services Quangos, *New England Journal of Medicine*, vol. 301, p. 1226, 1979.

39.

Talking to Patients   Margaret Izzo   Cheryl Tabatabai

Margaret Izzo

To the Editor: I write concerning Dr. Brachfeld's letter in the April 3 issue. Dr. Brachfeld makes the statement that patients who ask questions are not seeking information but are instead seeking reassurance. He also points out that this reassurance is better given by the physician than by the nurses, whom the good doctor apparently sees as persons of some technical competence but of dubious value in other aspects of health care.

The idea that independent nursing intervention can lead to improved patient care is being investigated with increasing frequency and with positive results.[1,2] This concept, along with the growing philosophy of health self-care, makes Dr. Brachfeld's assertion that it is the ultimate role of the physician to give comfort appear outmoded and inappropriate.

Work with patients faced with illness has demonstrated that they deal with the resulting threats to their well-being by means of a series of coping mechanisms.[3,4] This series often begins with denial or repression and proceeds through identification of self as a "sick person" to information

seeking and planning for changes necessitated by disease or treatment. This method enables the patient to adjust gradually to disease in a way that is relevant to his experience. It dictates that those attempting to help the patient accommodate to his illness approach him in different ways during its progression. Most (if not all) schools of nursing train nurses in using such approaches.

I agree that there may be times, especially in the acute phases of illness, when a patient may seek reassurance that he will, in time, be "all right." He may even seek communication with a nurturing and authoritative figure.[5] Whether this figure needs to be the physician, however, remains open to debate.

NOTES

1. I.V. Miller and J. Goldstein, "More Efficient Care of Diabetic Patients in a County-Hospital Setting," *New England Journal of Medicine*, vol. 286, p. 1388, 1972.

2. E.C. Perrin and H.C. Goodman, "Telephone Management of Acute Pediatric Illnesses," *New England Journal of Medicine*, vol. 298, p. 130, 1978.

3. D. Hamburg, B. Hamburg, and A. de Goza,

Source: *New England Journal of Medicine*, vol. 303, no. 4, July 24, 1980, p. 227.

"Adaptive Problems and Mechanisms in Severely Burned Patients," *Psychiatry,* vol. 16, p. 1, 1953.

4. E. Kubler-Ross, *On Death and Dying,* Macmillan, New York, 1969.

5. V. Carson and K. Huss, "Prayer—An Effective and Therapeutic Teaching Tool," *Journal of Psychiatric Nursing and Mental Health Services,* vol. 17, p. 34, 1979.

Cheryl Tabatabai

To the Editor: I believe that Dr. Brachfeld is missing the point when he contends that patients often feign ignorance of their conditions and treatments to gain more attention from their physicians. When patients repeatedly ask the same questions, it is frequently because their requests for information have been met by the kind of response that Dr. Brachfeld provides: "the monitor, the wires, and the oxygen" are needed "for the treatment of [the patient's] heart attack." For an educated patient, this hardly constitutes a complete explanation; it is, in fact, a response more appropriate to the questions of a small child, and it smacks of paternalism when proffered as an answer to the queries of an adult. This is not to say that an extensive clinical rationale need be provided to the patient, but it would seem that the health educator and the "patient-teaching" nurse are more on target than Dr. Brachfeld when they respond to patients' questions with comprehensive, factual data in a form comprehensible to the layman. Few people, least of all physicians, like to feel ignorant about things that affect their lives profoundly. When physicians can put aside their arrogance and realize that most patients seek thoughtful, straightforward, and reasonably detailed information about their conditions, and not just comfort from the "nurturing figure of the authoritative physician," they may find that their communication problems, as well as patients' claims of "complete ignorance," even though explanations have been offered "time and time again," will disappear.

Institutional Responsibility

Increasingly health care is being delivered in institutional contexts. Although the private practice office of the physician is still the major source of health care for middle- and upper-income individuals, the major source of primary and acute care for the large numbers of indigent patients occurs in hospitals, outpatient clinics, and emergency rooms. Regardless of economic class most individuals now die in hospitals, fighting the last stages of one of the major chronic diseases: cancer, heart disease, stroke, kidney failure, etc. Even office-based practices are changing into group plans with their own clinic facilities or competing with large prepaid health "maintenance" organizations. For a profession whose basic moral codes have been developed against the model of an interpersonal face-to-face relationship, many questions are raised by the employment of the physician in these large structures. Szasz addressed this in "The Moral Physician," and the writers included in this section discuss the issue directly. Pellegrino argues that the individuals running these large organizations have a direct moral responsibility for *all* aspects of the medical care delivered within their walls by all of the staff, both professional and nonprofessional. He takes issue with Fried, who argues that the physician should limit his responsibility to the face-to-face relationship of "personal care," and delegate concern for the broader policy matters to administrators. Conversely, he continues, these administrators are not responsible for care decisions on the level of particular patients; rather their responsibility is to populations. Rosenberg discusses the possible conflicts that can be generated by the divided loyalties of physicians practicing in prepaid group plans. Drucker and Dubler discuss special features of health care in the context of prisons. (There are a number of other institutional contexts which the student may be interested in studying, for example, the armed forces, long-term-care nursing facilities, religious institutions, and corporations.) (See cases 14, *16*, *18*, *24*, 25, 26, 29, 30, 40, *52*, 63, 70.)

40.
Hospitals as Moral Agents Edmund D. Pellegrino

Because of the urgent and intensely human milieu within which it operates, the hospital must be among the first to attend to its institutional moral obligations. It can, in fact, be the paradigm for others.

In discussing these obligations, I shall reflect on three questions: First, what is the actual nature of the human relationship between a patient and a hospital in today's system of health care? Second, what obligations are derived from the nature of that relationship? And, third, what are some of the practical implications of these obligations?

*Institutional Ethics: What It Is;
What It Is Not*

I hold the traditional view of ethics as the systematic search for generalizable and rationally justifiable principles on how we ought to live and act in various relationships with our fellow men. Ethics is, therefore, a branch of practical philosophy. It includes the analysis of ethical statements but is not limited to that analysis. Ethics deals with what "ought" to be rather than with what "is." Institutional ethics, from this view, consists of the general normative principles which define the way institutions "ought" to act with respect to their obligations. It is a branch of social ethics in that it pertains to men when they act as members of a group rather than as individuals. The problems of institutional morality, those which emerge from the actions of organized groups, are more complex than those of individual ethics. What an institution must decide is whether it sanctions absolute or limited pluralism, and whether, on this or that issue, it will take some specific stance to which it feels morally obligated above others. Institutions, as we shall examine further, will be called upon increasingly to make their moral choices more explicit than has been customary.

Nor is institutional ethics to be equated with meeting only the legal requirements for accountability. Many obligations which derive from the nature of the hospital's mission in society are now being transferred to the realm of law. This is a forceful commentary on the tardiness of hospitals in sensing what should be ethical obligations. I refer to the sharpening of the definitions of legal and fiscal accountability of board and administrators for quality of care, protection of the rights of consent, managerial efficiency, equity in provision of services, and assuring rights of due process. Most of these obligations would have, and should have, been derived from a conscious reflection on the moral obligations implicit in what hospitals are all about. Their translation into legislation and patient pleas for a variety of bills of rights are signs of the ethical lassitude of our institutions.

But, if these rights and obligations are now being expressed in law, is this not sufficient? A brief look at the distinction between law and ethics will make the answer clearer. Law and ethics may often coincide, but they are not necessarily and always the same. In fact, as recent history shows, they may often be antipathetic.

Law is in many ways the *coarse* adjustment of society to assure that certain obligations are fulfilled. Law, for example, can guarantee the validity of consent or minimum standards of quality by requiring hospitals to follow and record certain procedures

Source: Edmund D. Pellegrino, *Humanism and the Physician,* University of Tennessee Press, Knoxville, 1979. Based on a speech entitled "Hospitals as Moral Agents: Some Notes on Institutional Ethics," *Proceedings* of the Third Annual Board of Trustees/Medical Staff Executive Committee Conference sponsored by Saint Joseph's Hospital in Saint Paul, Minnesota, on March 26, 1977, pp. 10–27.

and by imposing penalties for violations. But law, by its nature, seeks standardized and bureaucratized, often impersonalized solutions. What is transferred to law is by definition taken out of the realm of the voluntary recognition of moral responsibility. Something subtle and exquisite is lost.

Ethics, on the other hand, is the *fine* adjustment of men for the voluntary assumption of obligations because they are demanded by the very nature of certain relationships between humans. Ethics sets a higher ideal than law simply because it is not securable. An ethically sensitive institution takes the full dimension of the medical encounter into account—all those things which flow from the existential condition of humanity in the state of illness.

Law and ethics can reinforce each other, as do the coarse and fine adjustments of the microscope. Law assures that patients' rights will be protected from those who do not act from ethical motives; ethics guarantees that the institutional conscience will transcend law and attend to obligations whether covered by law or not. It also guarantees that law is applied humanely, always in the spirit of serving individual needs rather than justifying itself.

Neither should ethics be confused with etiquette, the niceties of conduct between institutions and professionals which protect their mutual self-interests. Even in the so-called ethical treatises of the Hippocratic Corpus, these domains are confused. Intermingled with a few true ethical principles are many more precepts as to the physician's mien, conduct, and comportment with patients and families, and courtesies he should afford his fellow physicians. In our times, the proscription against advertising or unseemly publicity and the rules for enlightened self-interest which govern the inevitable but subtle competition between institutions or professionals are in the "etiquette" category. There may be fragments of moral issues here, but they are not mandatory obligations whose violation undermines professional authenticity.

Finally, institutional ethics does not imply that a single rigid set of principles be uniformly practiced by all hospitals. This is manifestly impossible in a society with such a wide range of values as ours. Indeed, our moral pluralism may itself require some declaration by the institution of its values, if the patient's own values are to be fully protected.

We must look first at the genesis of the hospital's moral obligations as an institution to the patient. I find it useful to begin at what I call the hospital's "profession." By this, I mean that a hospital, by the very fact of its existence, makes a declaration—that is, it professes to concentrate and make available those resources which a person can call upon when he is ill. Implicit in that profession is the promise to assist the person in the condition of illness to regain what he has lost—his health—at least to the maximum degree possible.

If it is a community, voluntary, non-profit hospital, the hospital makes a second declaration, namely, that it is available to all, that it will not profit from the patient's need, and that its self-interests are subservient to the community.

The hospital usually makes its resources available through the medium of the physician. But he too makes a public declaration that he possesses skills he will put at the services of those who are ill. In doing so, he incurs all the moral obligations traditionally delineated in professional codes of ethics: he must be competent, act in the patient's interest, never do deliberate harm, protect confidentiality, and treat the patient honestly, considerately, and personally. These obligations bind the physician within the hospital as they do in his office.

In using the hospital, however, the physician takes advantage of a community resource which he has not personally provided. The community places this resource in the trust of a board of directors, who act as surrogates for the community. The physician's moral obligations to the patient are no longer solely his concern. They now occur within an institutional framework, which modulates the relationship with his patient two ways. First, the physician's decisions directly or indirectly affect others. And, second, he shares his responsibilities with the institution through its board, which must carry out the obligations it incurs by virtue of its own declaration.

As a matter of fact, today an increasing number of patients now enter the same relationship with a hospital which formerly was obtained solely with physicians. The patient with no personal physician, or whose physician is unavailable, or who has an emergency expects the hospital to assume the same obligations for his care a physician would. When the hospital assigns a physician, technician, or nurse, it carries out its moral obligations through them, but it is not absolved of responsibility for how these obligations are fulfilled. When physicians are full-time employees of the hospital, the corporate obligation of the hospital is even more direct.

It is clear from the foregoing that hospitals as well as physicians incur serious moral obligations by the special nature of the fact of illness and the profession they voluntarily make to heal and assist. The central moral obligation is to make that profession fully authentic by fulfilling the expectations implicit in a relationship of such great inequality as exists between the helper and the one to be helped. A little closer look at the nature of the obligations themselves is now in order.

The Nature of Institutional Obligations

We have space to illustrate only a few of the specific obligations which flow from the special relationship between patients and those who profess to heal. Some have been touched upon already.

First, it seems clear that the institutionalization of so many aspects of medicine increasingly demands a moral relationship between the patient and the hospital which can be very similar to the patient/physician relationship. This means a great deal more than simply providing the setting in which medicine can be practiced safely and competently, as well as assuring its managerial efficiency and fiscal integrity, although the

latter too are obligations. What is called for is a sharing of the same range of ethical responsibilities which have traditionally been implicit in the relationships between physician and patient. The board of trustees must feel moral as well as legal responsibility for the actions of the professional and nonprofessional workers within the hospital walls. This responsibility, even in presumably professional matters, cannot be delegated. Institutional morality, by necessity, must concern itself with every facet of the corporate life of that institution.

The result should be an overlapping and sharing of moral obligations in which the professional and the institution check and balance each other more intimately than is now customary. On this view, I take some exception to Professor Charles Fried's recent analysis of the partitioning of responsibilities between physicians and hospital authorities. He assigns the hospital directors the bureaucratic decisions—those affecting efficiency, equity, and allocation of resources—and excuses them from responsibility for the personal dimensions of care given. The latter he assigns wholly to the physician, excusing him from concern with allocational decisions and suggesting that he must work within the framework of efficiency/equity decisions made by administrators or government.

Fried's division of responsibilities is reasonable so far as primary operational emphases are concerned. But these domains must not be compartmentalized; they must always be in dynamic equilibrium with each other. On the theses I am suggesting here, physicians and hospital directors are morally bound to see that their areas of primary responsibility do, in fact, interact. Each must fulfill the ethical obligations for the whole of what patients have a right to expect. The patient must be provided the knowledge necessary to participate rationally in the decisions which affect him. He must know what is wrong, what can be done, what the chances are for success, the dangers of treatment, the alternative procedures. The physician and the hospital share this obligation to enable the patient to make as free and rational a choice as possible. The obligation goes well beyond the mere legal requirement for valid consent. It demands consent of the highest quality and fullest sense of self-determination by the patient. The right to refuse specific treatment must be protected as well. The physician, the patient, and the hospital share obligations to each other, but because of the patient's vulnerability his needs are foremost.

This particular obligation assumes exquisite significance when a decision involves a moral question—a situation increasingly more pertinent as the capabilities of medicine expand the ways human life can be altered, shortened, or extended by technologic means. The questions in this realm are already matters of widespread public debate: abortion, continuing or discontinuing life-support measures, treatment or nontreatment of terminal or seemingly hopeless patients, participation in experimentation, and the like. The choices involve an intersection of the patient's values and those of the physician and the institution. Respect for the patient and humane treatment demand that these values be respected and that the patient be given the opportunity to act as his own moral agent if he wishes.

There are clear indications that more and more patients will wish to be their own moral agents and not delegate this agency to physicians as in the past. We live in a democratic society in which there is no uniformity of opinion on most medico-moral issues and no recognized authority to settle differences in ethical beliefs. There is also a growing tendency to distrust experts and institutions. The traditional moral authority of the physician has already been substantially eroded. Under these circumstances, the moral responsibility of hospitals, like that of the physician, must be to make its values clear so

the patient can make his own choice among institutions. We can foresee a time, not too far distant, when hospitals will have to declare their positions on the major medico-moral questions for the patient's guidance. Catholic hospitals have customarily done so on certain specific procedures.

There is room for considerable variation in ethical practices among hospitals. A democratic society should offer each patient the possibility of care in institutions that declare the same moral values he holds. This right can be actualized only if boards of trustees are willing to state clearly, in more specific terms than is now the case, the ethical principles to which they subscribe.

Unanswered Questions with Practical Implications

Many practical questions remain. How does the hospital balance its moral obligations to individuals who work for and with it and its obligations to those it serves, including the community as a whole? How are obligations defined and deployed among professionals, nonprofessionals, and administrators? What mechanisms can be designed to implement the hospital's moral agency? What is the best way to allocate moral responsibility in team care? The team is, after all, a transitory, mini-social system operating within the hospital. It illustrates in microcosm the difficulties of the ethics of group actions. How are conflicts of values and principles among individuals in the institution resolved? To what extent and to what degree of specificity should the institution declare the values it subscribes to? How are the legal and ethical values of everyday decisions reconciled with each other? Law may lag behind ethics in some instances. Can an institution take a stance which society has not yet sanctioned in law?

41.

Medical Care in General: The Hospital and the Obligation of Bureaucrats
Charles Fried

The Hospital

Those giving service in a hospital are generally under the control and direction of chiefs of service, chief medical officers, or boards of trustees whose responsibility is explicitly a corporate responsibility. These doctors do not have patients in the sense that they administer care in a personal, face-to-face, one-by-one fashion. Their responsibility is to a defined group of patients, and the nurses, interns, residents, and others act under the specific direction of what one might call these group doctors. Now the position of the intern or resident who is charged with giving the front-line care in a hospital is consequently rather ambiguous. In terms of medical ethics and law he does assume a personal professional obligation to the particular patient when he treats him. If his standing orders were to give what would be found to be improper attention, I would assume that like any other subordinate he would be personally liable for any actions which he knew or ought to have known were negligent or improper, even though his actions might also make those on whose orders he acted similarly liable.

The problem before us, however, rarely if ever involves doing something actively improper (we will come back to this when we deal with experimentation specifically) or even anything falling below a standard which in a court of law or in the proceedings of a professional society would be found to be unprofessional. Rather we are concerned with adjusting the level of care and attention the intern, resident, or nurse can give when his time and attention represent scarce resources in the hospital. At the very least, a subordinate who consistently gave more care and attention to fewer patients than the overall staffing needs of the hospital required would find himself looking for another position. And where the question is one of ordering tests, surgical procedures, and the like, the directives of group supervisors could hardly be systematically circumvented.

These interrelations are illustrated when we consider the norms for average length of hospital stay in various classes of conditions. For instance, should hospitalization last for two, three, or four weeks after an acute coronary episode? For the patient of a private physician it is up to that private physician to determine the length of stay. For a ward patient or a patient who is in some sense the patient of the organization hospital norms are likely to be determinative. Indeed such norms will exert influence on the private physician, as well, since as a physician with admitting privileges in the hospital he is under considerable pressure not to stray too far out of line with the standards set by his colleagues, particularly where there are waiting lists for entry into the hospital and a failure to abide by these guidelines would prejudice the chances of other doctors' patients' finding hospital beds. Also various financial intermediaries have referred to such norms in determining what level of hospital charges they would stand ready to assume.

Since those on the front line of patient care in hospitals are under the control of hospital administrators (even though many doctors will in fact occupy both roles at different times of the day), we should turn to those administrators' principles of choice. Most hospital administrators are severely

Source: Charles Fried, *Medical Experimentation: Personal Integrity and Social Policy,* American Elsevier Publishing Co., New York, 1974.

constrained at least in their choice of goals: The kind of hospital, its geographical area, its mode of financing are usually beyond their control. That is why so much even of the recent literature on hospital administration is concerned with ways of cutting costs, given the system and level of benefits the hospital is bound to offer. There is very little systematic explicit consideration of ways to choose between possible benefits, except perhaps in respect to quite marginal issues. Where such decisions are made it is often in terms of pricing policy: What services and what categories of patients will in effect subsidize what others, how much free care will be offered and to whom, and the like. This does not necessarily suggest simply an unwillingness to face hard choices. Rather it may reflect a partial adherence by hospital administrators to the model of personal care. Like private physicians they continue to hold themselves out as offering their traditional services and the only allocational devices resorted to are queuing (waiting lists) and financial barriers. The effect of these is that when someone does not receive help no one in the hospital is in the position of saying that he cannot help because he does not want to; it is only because he cannot. And as financial barriers are dropped through the intervention of government aid and private insurance there are shifts in what constitutes the best possible hospital care. The fact that "good care" has required progressively shorter periods of hospitalization after normal delivery or after acute heart attacks may surely be attributable at least in part to the pressure of rising costs.

At the other extreme, when capital improvement decisions or expansion decisions are called for, something approaching the optimization model is far more explictly in play. The decision not to undertake a particular kind of service, say heart surgery, is recognized to entail the loss of a certain number of statistical lives, but the justification is that the scarce resources available to the hospital can be better used in other ways. Yet here too the adherence to the model is less than complete, for hospital administrators generally think of themselves as serving a particular, traditionally defined community irrespective of whether other communities receive anything like adequate care. Indeed one might analogize the hospital's attitude toward "its" community to a doctor's obligation to "his" patients. The obligation, once undertaken, is binding, but the assumption of the obligation is itself a far more discretionary, arbitrary matter.

The Obligations of Bureaucrats

If the fulfillment of their obligations by primary care providers results in disparities between the care received by the rich and the poor or maybe just between the lucky and the unlucky, if queuing is the determinative distributional device, it is the responsibility of those at the secondary and tertiary levels to remove the disparities. For it is their responsibility to provide for the welfare of populations as a whole. As we have seen, the objects of their humanity can only appear to them as groups and abstractions, and indeed any concern for particularity on their part is nothing other than corruption and arbitrariness.

This is not to say that for bureaucrats there are not moral constraints on the pursuit of the greatest good of the greatest number. Their systems must be adequate and efficient, but above all they must be just. The systematic, general character of the constraint of distributive justice makes it the ethical consideration specifically directed to those who design and operate systems, while its application grows unclear and anomalous when it is proposed for those who confront only particular individuals in discrete cases. Other virtues, other claims predominate at that particular level.

Thus, the issue of fairness, of justice, is of particular concern to the health care bureaucrat. It is his regulations, resource allocation decisions, his incentive structures which will determine the circumstances, the quantity of resources, and the length of the queues when doctors encounter patients and assume obligations to them. It is the task of bureaucrats to define the level of training and the allocation between generalists and specialists. Therefore, it is up to these bureaucrats to arrange things so that the benefits of primary care are distributed in a fair and equitable way. While I have argued that it is not the responsibility, indeed it is inimical to the responsibility, of the physician to seek to implement some overall notions of fairness in the ways in which he provides care to individuals, it does not at all follow that stringent obligations of this sort do not rest on the higher-level bureaucrat. If minimal health care might be regarded as a good which cannot be subdivided past a certain point, so that the attempt to make it smaller and go around to more people would destroy it entirely, this does not at all imply that the overall system should not provide the appropriate amount of this good or distribute it as fairly as possible among the population.

Finally, it is worth making quite explicit

a moral assumption of the foregoing argument. I readily concede that everything need not work out for the best in the far from perfect world we have been considering. It is possible that government officials will stupidly or corruptly fail to perform the functions on which the fairness of the outcome of the total system depends. The result will be suffering and privation. Does that show my argument is wrong, that primary care providers should abandon in such cases the obligations of their roles? Why? Who says that it is a test of a sound set of moral principles that pain is reduced in it to a lower point than in all competitors? That is not my view. We must reduce the suffering of men, but not so much because suffering is bad as because it is human beings who are suffering. Consequently it is more important that we retain respect for our own and each other's humanity as we relieve suffering than that suffering be relieved. After all, suffering like death will always be with us.

42.

Prison Health Care
Ernest Drucker   Nancy N. Dubler

Surprising as it may seem, the inmate of a correctional institution has *more of a right to health care* than most other citizens in this country. Take the case of Sylvester Jones, Number 76A-4725, an inmate at State of New York—Ossining Correctional Facility—Sing Sing. Mr. Jones has a crippling neurological problem which, during his time at Ossining, was cared for by the health staff of that institution. Recently Mr. Jones became eligible for consideration for parole. But, in the absence of family and friends on the outside who can care for him, his medical condition is delaying the Parole Board's consideration. No outside health care institution is *obligated* to care for him and there is no

one on the outside from whom he can *demand* health care. As of this writing he is still in prison because, with few exceptions, U.S. citizens have no guaranteed right to health care. Prison inmates are one of these exceptions.

We choose Sylvester Jones' story to begin this discussion of health rights of inmates because it demonstrates that access to health care is not a universally accepted right in this society. But exactly because there is no such right on the outside which could be used as a basis of comparison, inmates must understand their special health right well enough to enforce and defend it.

Inmates in prisons, jails, and detention

Source: *Fortune News,* The Fortune Society, New York, September 1978, p. 1.

centers have a right to health care under the 8th Amendment of the Constitution of the United States, which prohibits "cruel and unusual" punishment. The cases which have established this constitutional right argue that putting someone in a prison where he can't secure his own medical care obligates the prison to provide care. Failing to do so *is an excessive and disproportionate punishment* which was not included in the sentence of the court. Furthermore, over the years, the courts have reasoned that to provide *grossly inadequate medical care* offends the sense of "fairness," "decency," and "dignity" which are the standards against which punishments are judged for acceptability. Grossly inadequate medical care is therefore also a "cruel and unusual" punishment and is prohibited by law.

This distinctive right, a prisoner's legal right to health care, has a relatively brief history. Indeed, the first Supreme Court case squarely on health rights of prisoners was in 1976—the case of *Estelle v. Gamble* (95 S.Ct.285 (1976)). This means that the definition of the extent and nature of the right to health care in prisons is still an open issue being actively considered by modern courts. Let's look at what the courts generally agree upon as the right of prisoners to health care, keeping in mind that every case is an opportunity for determining just what the right will mean in practical terms.

The Supreme Court's ruling in *Estelle v. Gamble* states that the prison must "provide medical care for those whom it is punishing by incarceration," and that the "deliberate indifference to the serious medical needs of prisoners" constitutes the "unnecessary and wanton infliction of pain . . . proscribed by the Eighth Amendment." Technically that is the baseline of the constitutional right of inmates to health care. But cases which have been brought by inmates and by prisoners-rights groups in various federal courts have already begun to provide a more detailed description of these rights and are continuing to do so. These cases, unlike the Supreme Court, do comment on specific rights: the right to *a regular health care pro-*

gram within the institutions (i.e., a clinic, infirmary, or regular physician); the right of the inmate to have *a routine relationship with health-care personnel* (i.e., regular access, regular intake physicals, and responses to complaints, not just to emergencies and injuries); the *right to have diagnostic testing done* when necessary based on the complaints of inmates (i.e., laboratory tests, x-rays, etc.); and the right to have *medical care which goes beyond what the prison itself can provide* (i.e., the use of outside specialists, hospitals, or emergency rooms where needed). This list of health rights will grow.

Inmates should also be aware that there are several professional organizations which have studied the problems of prison health-care and have produced reports and studies to serve as guidelines for defining basic standards of medical care in American prisons. These organizations include the American Medical Association, the American Bar Association, the American Public Health Association, and the Law Enforcement Assistance Administration. Their findings and reports should be familiar to inmates, their councils, and health workers concerned with protecting the health rights of inmates because, like the court cases, they form the basis of legal and professional discussion about what "minimal standards" and procedures in prison health should be.

However, despite the law and despite minimal standards, *in real life* the inmate's right to health care is not easily defended. Past court rulings can be broadly or narrowly interpreted and applied or ignored in similar cases. Likewise professional standards can look good on paper but bear little relation to the daily reality of prison life. Consider the following actual cases:

Case 1. A prisoner at a state correctional institute in New York hurt his ankle while playing basketball. He thought it was a strain and that it would go away on its own, but after a day the ankle began to swell and become painful. He went to see the prison doctor, who examined it and said that in all likelihood it was not broken but merely a twisted ankle and would respond to aspirin, the use of an Ace bandage, and ice pack treatments. The inmate thought he should have an x-ray of the ankle but the doctor was quite certain that it was not broken and did not require an x-ray. No x-ray was done.

Case 2. An inmate at a city jail had a chronic back problem which required a hard sleeping platform and lighter work. The beds and springs in this jail were old and saggy and he'd been working at a heavy work detail with heavy lifting. No bedboards were available, work details were controlled by the C.O.'s, and the nurse said there was nothing she could do about it.

Case 3. A lifer at a federal penitentiary had a history of epilepsy and without medication had been known to have dangerous seizures. He went twice daily for his anti-convulsive medication but one day had a bitter quarrel with the C.O. on his block—the C.O. "never showed up" to take him for his afternoon dose. He got desperate, started a fight with another C.O., wound up in solitary, and suffered a convulsion.

Case 4. A prisoner's outer ear was cut off in a fight. The prisoner and his ear were brought to the prison hospital, where the ear was thrown in a garbage can before the inmate's eyes, the doctor, sewing up the stump, said, "You won't be needing this anymore."

Are these inmates protected under the 8th Amendment right to health care? The answer is *probably no* for cases 1 and 2 and *probably yes* for cases 3 and 4.

In the first two, the inmate does not have a claim that his constitutional right to medical care has been violated. Even though he disagrees with the competency of the physician, the diagnosis or the treatment, that disagreement in and of itself does not give rise to a constitutional claim. The courts have been very careful in defining the right to health care in such a way that it would not require them to review every dispute of this sort between patient and doctor. But when does the quality of medical work become so inadequate that it constitutes denial of the right to health care? Cases 3 and 4 have been heard in federal court

and decided in favor of the inmates. These two cases *were* found to be deprivations of constitutional rights because they involved *"denial"* of medical care or because the care was so "callous and indifferent" as to constitute denial. But, in cases 1 and 2, the inmates would, as things stand now, have no legal recourse in the federal courts.

Now, most inmates, like other citizens, do have a right to sue their doctor—even a prison doctor—for malpractice. But the issue of malpractice in prison medicine is not a *simple* one because for all intents and purposes inmates have no real recourse to the usual legal process as a means of demanding good health care or being compensated for bad medical care. While most inmates *technically* have the right to sue for malpractice the likelihood that it would produce results is almost nil. Private lawyers are generally not willing to take such cases from prison inmates and Legal Aid is specifically prohibited from doing so.

Since the federal courts have ruled that issues of the quality of treatment are not in their jurisdiction and since the right to sue for malpractice is not really open to prison inmates, some other strategy must be taken to ensure the right to health care. Finally, inmates must realize that only through opening up discussion of this issue and working collectively can any progress be made in defining the right of prisoners to health care in a way that will matter.

Inmates' complaints about the health care in prisons often focus on access to services; long waiting periods; staff whose cultural origins or language make it impossible to understand an inmate's complaints; staff whose attitude indicates a disregard or disrespect for the inmates; inappropriate treatment; insufficient use of diagnostic tests and outside consultants; lack of feedback to inmates about test results; etc. These grievances are familiar to anyone who knows prison health services, and many of them are also true of medicine on the outside.

These concerns, which clearly relate to good and decent medical care, are not necessarily covered by the constitutional right of an inmate to such care. The individual problems are not usually serious enough to be considered violations of the 8th Amendment's prohibition on cruel and unusual punishment, nor do they result in the kind of clear physical damage to a particular patient which might be grounds for a malpractice suit. These issues are issues having to do with the *quality* of health care for the general inmate population. However, there has recently been an important case involving both constitutional and quality or care issues—the case of *Todaro v. Ward,* (431 F.Supp 1129, (SDNY.1976), and 565 F2d 48, (2nd Cir.1977). *Todaro* is important and positive because it focuses on issues which are generally considered *quality of care* and places them within the constitutional right of the inmates. It is also discouraging because such a case requires extraordinary legal planning, strategy, and perseverence to accomplish its goals.

The Todaro case. In 1974 a lawyer from the Prisoners' Rights Project of New York's Legal Aid Society became aware that there were some serious problems with the health care at Bedford Hills, a medium-security women's prison in Westchester County. Using letters, interviews with inmates, and telephone conversations, that lawyer, Eric Neisser, now a professor of law, began to compile a substantial file on health care at the prison. These grievances and the pattern of poor quality of care that they seemed to show so disturbed Neisser that he went to the rest of the staff of the project with his file; the staff agreed that they should launch an investigation of the claims and test if the systematic pattern of violation of *good* health care was also a violation of the *right* to health care for the 400 women at Bedford Hills.

After 1½ years of careful work Neisser and Ellen Winner, another lawyer from the staff of the project, went to court with 26 plaintiffs from Bedford Hills "on behalf of themselves and all other persons similarly situated." This case is known as *Todaro v. Ward* because Todaro was the first of the plaintiffs on the list and Benjamin

Ward, then the Commissioner of Corrections for New York State, was the first of the defendants. The *Todaro* case demonstrates the need for inmates and their advocates to go beyond the case-by-case, incident-by-incident grievance machinery. *Todaro* was a class action suit and its intent was to bring about improvements in the health care for *all* inmates at Bedford Hills. Neisser and Winner were able to satisfy the Federal District Court of New York that "certain aspects of the medical care at Bedford Hills are constitutionally inadequate, cause needless suffering and violate the rights of the plaintiff's *class* under the 9th and 14th Amendments of the United States Constitution." In other words they extended the "right to health care" to issues of health delivery service and to issues of quality of care.

Very specific claims were made based on the accumulated experience of hundreds of Bedford Hills inmates and supported by the testimony of expert witnesses in medicine and corrections. Some of the these claims dealt with the inadequacy of:

1. The x-rays and x-ray machine
2. The quality of care in the sick wing (infirmary)
3. The sick call procedure
4. The diagnostic testing and follow-up

The evidence offered to support these claims described women with acute symptoms left untreated for weeks or months; nurses' examinations conducted through locked doors and wire-mesh screens with no privacy; medications dispensed without obtaining prior records and with no systems for ongoing record keeping; patients in the sick wing locked behind doors in acute illness or even during convulsions with no help possible or available. Because these complaints were so specific and so well documented, the court did more than simply find the defendants guilty. It finally ordered the defendants, officials of the Department of Corrections of the State of New York and of Bedford Hills, to change the way medicine is organized and practiced at Bedford

Hills. Accordingly the court's orders are very important, and we reproduce them in some detail here:

Ordered that defendants, their successors in office and all officials, employees, agents and others acting in concert with them who have notice of this judgment are enjoined to comply fully and promptly with each and every part of the following order:

Ordered that. . . .

I. X-ray equipment

A. No member of the plaintiff class (hereinafter inmate) shall be exposed to any Bedford Hills x-ray machine which does not meet state standards and has not been inspected and certified by the appropriate certifying state agency.

B. All x-ray machines . . . shall be inspected . . . for safety and adequacy within 30 days of the entry of this judgment.

C. Defendants shall provide counsel for the plaintiffs with copies of all inspection reports concerning x-ray machines.

II. Sick Wing

A. 1) Sick wing shall not be used for boarding any types of persons other than medically sick patients, except psychiatric patients may be temporarily boarded in the event the mental hygiene satellite clinic is full. The provisions of this judgment do not govern psychiatric care and treatment.

2) No inmate shall be placed in an individual locked room unless she has been admitted to sick wing from segregation. . . .

B. The solid door at the end of the sick wing corridor shall be permanently removed and only grated doors permitting visual observation of the entire corridor may be employed at the end of the corridor. . . .

C. A nurse's station shall be established within or immediately adjacent to sick wing and shall include all necessary emergency equipment, medication, and supplies. . . .

D. Defendants shall maintain at all times a functioning mechanical buzzer or bell call system which can be operated by each inmate in sick wing directly from her bed and the terminal of which will be within the nurse's station and within the direct hearing of a medical staff member. . . .

E. In addition to the nurses' and corrections officers' regular daytime rounds which the Court found were being conducted at the time of the trial, doctors rounds of sick wing shall be conducted daily. . . .

F. . . . A record shall be maintained of all rounds of sick wing conducted by either medical or correctional personnel. . . .

III. Sick Call—Physician Referral Procedures

A. . . . all inmates who request to be seen by a physician must be seen by a licensed physician by the next day. . . .

B. . . . inmate requests for a physician examination must be medically evaluated and screened and appointments scheduled according to urgency of need in accordance with the following procedures:

1) Medical evaluation and screening (hereinafter screening) shall be performed at a time and place separate from the administration of medication;

2) Screening shall be conducted by licensed medical personnel . . .

3) Specific written protocols, defining the evaluation procedures to be followed at screening . . .

4) Screening shall be readily available to all members of the plaintiff class . . .

5) . . . screening shall be conducted in a facility permitting both confi-

dential communication between
the inmate and the screening medical staff member and physical
examination in privacy, relevant
to the physical complaints presented by the inmate.
6) The screening staff member
shall have immediately available
(medical equipment) a thermometer, a sphygmomanometer,
tongue depressors, . . .
7) The medical record of the inmate being screened shall be available at the time of the screening
. . .
8) The staff member doing the
screening shall determine by when
the inmate will be seen by a
physician . . .
9) The screening staff member or
the staff member preparing the
physician appointment list shall
prepare a list each day of all inmates who have been screened,
and the nature of the problems
presented.
IV. Diagnostic Test Orders and Doctor
Appointment Follow-Up
A. Unless a diagnostic test is to be
performed the same day it is
ordered, the inmate shall receive,
at the time the test is ordered, a
written notice of the date, time,
and place of the appointment for
the diagnostic test ordered by a
medical staff member, along with
written instructions regarding any
dieting or other preparations required for the test . . .
B. The results of all diagnostic tests
shall be reviewed by a medical
staff member on the date they are
available to or received by the
faculty . . .
C. Inmates shall receive written notice
of all normal test results within
ten days of the faculty's receipt of
such results;
D. Unless an immediate physician appointment is needed, inmates shall

be seen by the doctor ordering the
test within ten weekdays of the
facility's receipt of abnormal test
results for a personal explanation
of any abnormal results and the
doctor's determination of appropriate follow-up, if any, on those
results;
E. At the time of the order for re-
appointment with a physician, inmates shall receive a written notice
of the date and time of the re-
appointment, signed by a medical
staff member, and all such reap-
pointments shall be entered in the
chronological doctor's appointment book required by paragraph
III(B) (9) above;
F. Defendants shall maintain a laboratory order book. . . .
V. Audits and Record-Keeping Procedures
A. Defendants shall maintain such
records as are necessary to effective and meaningful auditing of
the performance of the medical
care delivery system at Bedford
Hills. . . .
B. Every three months for the first
year after entry of this judgment,
every six months for the second
year after entry of this judgment,
and once during the third year
after entry of this judgment, qualified personnel shall conduct, at
defendants' expense, an audit of
the medical care delivery system
at Bedford Hills. . . . including, but
not limited to, review of all
records mandated by this judgment, review of 20 randomly
selected inmate medical charts,
inspection of all medical facilities and equipment, and such
personal observation of medical
procedures and interviews with
medical staff and inmates as the
auditors shall deem appropriate.
A written report concerning the
completeness of medical records

and the adequacy of such records and procedures to implement the requirements of this judgment and containing recommendations for changes to achieve those requirements more efficiently and speedily shall be made to counsel for both sides, within 45 days of each audit.

(The above is taken from the Judgment of the United States District Court for the Southern District of New York, Judge Robert J. Ward presiding.)

Thus the *Todaro* case adjudged the entire system for delivering health care at Bedford Hills to be constitutionally inadequate and ordered specific institutional changes to improve the quality of care for all women at that prison. The problem with the *Todaro* case is that it required years of lawyers' time, masses of expert testimony and tens of thousands of dollars to accomplish this goal and such resources are rarely available. Even at Bedford Hills, however, eighteen months after the judgment and three years after the trial, the implementation of these orders is still not complete. It finally took a contempt hearing and an implicit threat to hold prison officials in contempt to force them to hire two additional nurses and to make much needed physical improvements in the sick wing. Almost 4 years after the initial complaint and 1½ years after winning the case, the lawyers at the Prisoners' Rights Project are still fighting to get Bedford Hills to provide decent health care to its inmates. However, the *Todaro* case does give a good idea of the kinds of changes that can be won in regard to quality of care in serious situations through legal action, and does provide a measure of hope for the future. Inmates must know that quality of care issues are coming under constitutional protection.

Quality of care issues in prisons. But, for the inmate, the question still remains: How does one maximize the quality of health care in a prison? If you are a patient on the outside you can do several things if you're not satisfied with the quality of care you are getting from your doctor. You can find a new physician, you can complain to the local medical organization, you can refuse to pay the bill and, if you feel that damages have resulted from physician's actions, you can sue for malpractice. You may not be successful through any of these routes but at the very least you will not be forced to continue getting medical care from someone you dislike, distrust, or believe to be incompetent. The inmate does not have these options and must therefore see that health care in prison is as good as it can possibly be—not just for himself but for everyone. In this way prison is like other communities dependent on public institutions for health care. Most ghetto communities rely on overcrowded emergency rooms, public clinics, and hospitals for their medical care. Long lines and longer waiting periods are common, there is generally no choice of physician, the care is often impersonal, and finally, little can be done about individual dissatisfactions with the quality of that care. In such communities today, there is a growing awareness that consumer involvement is one way to get better-quality health care for everyone. Consumer involvement on the outside means membership on hospital committees and boards or on local health planning agencies; it means active lobbying for needed new programs and for maintenance of existing services in the community. But what does consumer involvement mean in a prison?

We think it means that prison inmates must organize around health. Inmates must take a more active, more positive, and more collective interest in the health care system of their prisons. They must become more sophisticated and selective consumers of the limited health services available to them, must learn about health and disease, about their own bodies, and must understand what modern medicine *can* and *cannot* do. Most important of all: both inmates and professionals working in prison health must insist that prison health services function to serve inmates' health needs, not as an arm of corrections and not to extend the punishment of prison to the care of patients.

Conflict between Plan Advocate and Patient Advocate
Conrad Rosenberg

In general the conflicts we will be reviewing originate in three areas, the classical patient-physician relationship, be it fee-for-service or prepaid, those unique to the patient who perceives himself locked into a delivery system that is strange to him, and those of the physician who is part of and accountable to an organization and the patient.

The first group are those that are the rather traditional ones that exist in most physician-patient relationships and in fact are generic to most situations in which one person is a recipient and the other the provider of a service. They usually originate in differences in expectations. The studies periodically emanating from medical economics identify long waits in making appointments, long waits in the office waiting for the physician, not enough time, not enough caring, not enough explanation as the complaints of fee-for-service which have their counterpart in prepaid practice. To our advantage in prepaid group practice we do not have to contend with the rage felt by patients resulting from the frustrations that are part of completing claim forms and their subsequent rejection or very partial reimbursement.

But there are situations specific to HMOs that express themselves in the form of patient testing. The new member may be suspicious about the system. He is certainly entitled to be questioning about this new method of securing care. He may just put his toe in to see what the water is like or jump in and come up either smiling or sputtering. He is presenting himself to a system, an organization that in its very name, health maintenance organization, suggests delusions of grandeur. In solo practice the referral is to an individual physician recommended by family, neighbor, or the local shopkeeper.

That absence of positive feeling at start-up in the group model is rapidly dissipated once the two parties have met. By and large, after the second and third visit the relationship in prepaid practice is much the same as that in fee-for-service and is less a function of the system than the personality of the two parties involved.

There is a further problem. Not only has the member joined an organization new to him, but because of enrollment procedure he is locked into this system until the next enrollment period. Compounding the problem may be the fact that he may have brought along a reluctant spouse, reluctant to give up a previous patient-physician relationship. Understanding these doubts that may arise in some patients, recognizing they are expressions of concern directed toward a new concept and its implications helps in their resolution. The provider is not the source of the patient's anxiety but is the recipient of the members acting out this uncertainty. Recognizing its dynamics permits resolution of the issue by being a caring, informative provider and not picking up gauntlets thrown in your general direction but not really at your feet. There are days when it is difficult to remember that the vast majority of people prefer amicable relationships.

There is still another locus of conflict. It is internal to the physician and is the result of the physician's having two loyalties. His most important, his primary one, is that of patient advocate. Nothing really supersedes that role. Secondarily, but still important, is his loyalty to the HMO, of which he is a key member, ably supported by other staff, the prime provider and the irreplaceable part of the system. He will be called upon much more than his fee-for-service colleague, to say no to the patient,

Source: HMO Primary Care Conference, Philadelphia, May 1980.

to deny the patient testing and consultation which the patient may feel he needs, deserves, or even wants merely because he believes it is paid for. The physician in fee-for-service solo practice has less difficulty with this problem. He too sees himself as the patient advocate but usually disassociates his activities as having an impact on the rest of the community, for that is a rather large, poorly defined population of people "out there."

It is his inability to identify with this large community that permits his extravagant use of diagnostic procedures, treatment modalities, and hospital days. As a result, controls come from outside in the form of utilization review committees and PSROs. The fee-for-service physician senses minimal or no conflict and as a consequence experiences increasing regulation on the part of government and third-party payers. The physician in prepaid practice, however, has quite a different experience. He must distinguish the relevant from the irrelevant for he is more sensitized to the existence of options and their consequences. His community is smaller than all of society and because he can identify with his microcosm, the choices become more apparent. Having made his value judgment, he must act as the advocate of the patient. His training, his ability to live at peace with his decisions, all relate to his willingness to be governed by the primacy of the patient's need. But he then must go on to a second level of advocacy, a role not assumed by the solo practitioner. He is required to understand, accept, and participate in an accountability to the HMO, to all the other subscribers of the group. It is their money, their health dollars, that he will be spending wisely or poorly. It requires an individual who is not only competent to make appropriate decisions but has the stamina to stick with those decisions and not capitulate for peace at any price. We have been charged by all members of our HMO to invest their health dollars to their best interest, and when they are squandered, whether it be inappropriate and excessive utilization of services or poor management,

which is part and parcel of the same issue, we are doing our patients a disservice. In the November 3, 1979, issue of the *Canadian Medical Association Journal,* there is an editorial referring to the study of the Canadian Task Force of experts that was assembled, and after three years of study, proposed what they felt to be appropriate standards for health assessments. From that editorial: "Clinical diagnosis is a curious mixture of thoughtful search and decerebrate routine . . ." Decerebrate routine—what a wonderful term! It should be listed on laboratory requisition slips in place of the SMA-12. The conflict is not you versus the patient but rather your having to choose between obsessive behavior sometimes euphemistically referred to as thoroughness, together with patient pressure on the one hand, and your considered assessment of appropriate care on the other. It should be illegal, at least unethical, to request an alkaline phosphatase as part of a periodic health assessment without specific indications. The domino effect existed in medical practice long before it became part of the jargon of geopolitics. The slightly elevated alkaline phosphatase is repeated and again slightly elevated, demonstrating the wonderful capacity of the well-run automated laboratory to reproduce error. What next? Let's skip separating liver or bone as the cause of the so-called elevation. On to the liver scan with its report of nonspecific, nondiagnostic changes. By now the patient's anxiety has been raised to a level where we must continue. A brief hospitalization for liver biopsy. The patient awakens in the middle of the night to void, forgets the hospital bed is higher than his own at home, falls, is found on the floor stunned, confused, kicking off his pajama pants which are now wet with urine, and is labeled as a seizure disorder. You may continue with your own scenario.

We are all familiar with the delightfully erudite essays of Dr. Lewis Thomas which have appeared from time to time in the *New England Journal of Medicine* and collected in his two volumes, *The Lives of a Cell* and *The Medusa and the Snail.* At a recent meeting honoring the memory of Dr. Caldwell Esselstyn, one of the founding fathers of prepaid practice, when Dr. Thomas was asked to comment on HMOs he did not discuss cost containment or the quality or the comprehensive nature of prepaid care. His comment was merely that "the problem is not access, but egress from the health care system." Another commentator, supporter but not an uncritical one of the British National Health Service, described an employee of a crematorium happily looking out at the blue sky. The author questioned the worker as to what it was that appeared to please him so. The response was "I have never seen so much go in and so little come out."

Conflict may originate with our dependence upon each other. With that mutual accountability comes stress. The loner, sitting in his own office, practicing in his individual fashion, keeping scrupulously complete records or writing them on 3 x 5 cards, manages to remain essentially free of all forms of peer review. The physician, the nurses, the physician assistant practicing in a group or in association does not have that luxury. But accountability is old hat to us whether it be to patients, to peers, to family, to chairmen of departments or deans of schools, or to police cars with radar equipment. Many of us feel that accountability is not so terribly onerous and that it is acceptable by the mature individual as long as it is not unreasonable. We expect others to be accountable for their behavior as it impinges on our good and welfare and are prepared to return that same courtesy. For some, however, this is a difficult situation. Group practice, or

practice in an association, is not for all providers, just as membership is not for all patients. There are ground rules for all activities, and our ability to identify them, adjust to the reasonable ones, and modify the unreasonable ones, is part of a mature society rather than an adolescent state. The collegial relationship, the opportunities for ongoing education that come by virtue of shared experiences, the quality of life which has as its goal the maximum fulfillment of one's self as a provider of care, the elimination of the role as a vendor of care are ample rewards for what has been described as conflicts.

While it is appropriate to accept the concept of constraints, they should be understandable and reasonable. If not, one should do what one can to modify them. One has the right to expect there will be no obstacles to our practicing our professions, each to the best of his ability, without concern regarding the patient's ability to afford necessary services. We are entitled to a milieu that makes practice attractive, enjoyable, dignified. There is nothing inappropriate in insisting that there be ego gratification and not blind adherence to some formulation we poorly understand. It is our responsibility to be participants, not mere providers, actively sharing in the responsibility of seeing the HMO achieve its objectives and experiencing the pleasure of making available to a vast community of people health care that is concerned and responsive to their needs.

A final quote:

If I am not for myself, who is for me?
If I care only for myself, what am I?
If not now, when?

Professional Accountability

The prior sections have presented a variety of ideals, models, and accounts of actual behavior and beliefs defining the responsibilities and duties of the physician and patients. In this section we provide selections which address how the practicing physician is held accountable to these rules, norms, and laws.

Perhaps the major mechanism by which order is maintained in a profession as well as society at large is by the voluntary conformance of individuals to their laws and ideals. We begin this section with two selections that discuss various features of the notion that the physician's voluntary concern for the patient's best interests may be compromised either by the structure of the hospital environment itself or by the threatening aspects of the legal "malpractice" climate used to enforce medical law. Annas and Healey argue in favor of patient rights advocates because they believe that in fact most patients do not receive full recognition of their rights in large institutions. By contrast, Tancredi and Barondess discuss the claim that physicians are forced to provide too many tests and are too cautious as a result of the way in which litigation is used to punish the few negligent physicians. They find that reliable data are scarce and that the topic is complicated by the possible benefits for individuals of what might be seen as "defensive" only with respect to broad categories of patients.

There are many laws specifying standards for physicians in various situations and with respect to varying levels of expertise and certification. Many of these are discussed by Holder as she reviews the notion of due care based upon the rules that have emerged from case litigation.

Two selections concern professional enforcement of discipline. Derbyshire discusses the role of the designated agencies in enforcing regulations and standards and discusses serious deficiencies in their performance. A position paper by the Council on Mental Health follows; it discusses the "sick physician" and presents possible model statutes for medical practice to be recommended by state and county medical societies. (See cases 7, 18, 37, 38, 41, 45, 52.)

44.

The Patient Rights Advocate: Redefining the Doctor-Patient Relationship in the Hospital Context
George J. Annas   Joseph M. Healey, Jr.

We begin with two fundamental propositions: (1) the American medical consumer possesses certain interests, many of which may properly be described as "rights," that he does not automatically forfeit by entering into a relationship with a doctor or a health care facility; and (2) most doctors and health care facilities fail to recognize the existence of these interests and rights, fail to provide for their protection or assertion, and frequently limit their exercise without recourse for the patient.

Because a sick person's first concern is to regain his health, he is willing to give up rights that otherwise would be vigorously asserted. Moreover, the doctor-patient relationship as it exists in the hospital—where the most critical decisions are made and where most people receive their primary care—effectively removes the patient from any participation in the medical decision-making process. This article argues that one does not relinquish basic human rights upon entering a health care institution, that these rights can be protected without fear of decreasing the efficacy of medical treatment, and that protecting these rights requires a return of medical decision-making power to the patient and a legal redefinition of the doctor-patient relationship. The foundation for protecting the patient's interests within the health care facility is a clear, comprehensive statement of the rights of the patient. A statement alone, however, is neither self-enforcing nor does it guarantee protection of the patient's interests. To ensure such protection, this article suggests the patient rights advocate as an enforcement mechanism.

Legal Redefinition: The Legacy of the American Legal System

It is necessary at the outset to dispel the common objection that the legal system has no legitimate interest in "interfering" with the doctor-patient relationship. Even a cursory glance at the legal history of the past century demonstrates the weakness of this argument. In myriad situations, the judiciary, the legislature, and the chief executive have exercised novel and widespread control over previously protected relationships. For example, the enactment in 1935 of the National Labor Relations Act substantially redefined the employer-employee relationship, and subsequent amendments and judicial decisions continually refined and adjusted the balance of power between labor and management. Similarly, the federal securities acts have made far-reaching changes in at least two fundamental corporate contexts—the relationship between a corporation and its shareholders and the relationship between a purchaser and a seller of securities. In both cases, the courts and the Securities and Exchange Commission have been quick to redefine further the relationship in order to implement more effectively the purposes of the federal legislation. In the field of consumer law, courts and legislatures have reshaped the right-duty relationships between buyer and seller and between debtor and creditor.

The foregoing are but a few examples of the many individual relationships that have been redefined by governmental bodies. Hopefully these examples make it clear that the prior establishment by law or custom of

Source: *Vanderbilt Law Review*, vol. 27, 1974.

a relationship is not in itself sufficient justification for its unchanged continuation. Moreover, when basic constitutional rights or fundamental human fairness provide sufficient justification, the legislature, the judiciary, and the executive can and will act to redefine the relationship. These observations suggest that a legal redefinition of the doctor-patient relationship is neither a radical nor an unprecedented suggestion.

Rights and Duties

Attempts to redefine the balance of power between doctor and patient and between hospital and patient focus on the limits of personal interaction delineated by such concepts as rights, duties, privileges, and liabilities. The right-duty concept affects at least three specific areas of decisions concerning the health care of the individual: the right to the whole truth, including information that is part of medical records both during and after treatment; the right to privacy and personal dignity; and the right to retain self-determination. The manner and extent to which these rights exist and are in need of protection can be seen by considering the interaction between the health care facility and the patient in chronological form. In the following list, the word "right" is used to denote those rights that would be recognized at law as well as those that should be recognized either at law or as a matter of internal hospital policy.

Selection of the health care facility:

Does the potential patient have a right to know the available medical resources within the community?

Does the potential patient have a right to know what research and experimental protocols are being used by the doctor and by the health care facility, and to know what alternatives exist for treatment?

Does the potential patient have a right to know in advance what rights are afforded him as a patient at a medical facility?

Does the potential patient have a right to the highest-quality medical treatment available?

Does the potential patient have a right to the highest degree of care without regard to the source of payment for that care?

Does the potential patient have a right to complete secrecy concerning the source of payment for treatment and care?

Entering the health care facility:

Does the patient have a right to prompt attention in an emergency situation?

Does the patient have a right to know the identity and level of professional training of all those providing treatment?

Does the patient have a right to have each and every form that must be signed carefully explained and the significance of each consent clarified?

Does the patient have a right to a review of his preliminary diagnosis to protect against premature labeling of his condition?

Does the patient who does not speak English have a right to an interpreter?

While in the health care facility:

Does the patient have a right to a clear, complete, and accurate evaluation of his condition?

Does the family of the patient have a right to a clear, complete, and accurate evaluation of his condition?

Does the patient have a right to all the information contained in his medical record?

Does the patient have a right to discuss his condition with a consultant-specialist at his own request and expense?

Does the patient have a right to a detailed explanation, in layman's terms, of every diagnostic test, treatment, procedure, or operation, including alternative procedures, costs, risks, and the identity and qualifications of the person actually performing the procedure?

Does the patient incapable of informed consent have a right to the appointment of a guardian who is not a member of his family?

Does the patient have a right to know whether a particular test or procedure is for his benefit or for educational purposes?

Does the patient have a right to refuse any particular drug, test, or treatment?

Does the patient have a right to both personal and informational privacy with respect to the hospital staff, other doctors, residents, interns, and medical students, any type of researcher, nurses, and other patients?

Does the patient have a right of access to the "outside world" by means of visitors and a telephone, or to limit such access as he sees fit?

Does the patient have a right to refuse to leave the health care facility if he feels it would seriously endanger his health?

Does the patient have a right to leave the health care facility regardless of physical condition or financial status?

After termination of the hospital-patient relationship:

Does the patient have a right to a complete copy of the information contained in his medical record?

Does the patient have a right to continuity of care by means of access to the doctors who provided treatment while he was in the health care facility?

The Traditional Doctor-Patient Relationship and Attempts to Resolve Health Care Conflicts

The traditional doctor-patient relationship model takes a "doctor knows best" position for granted. The individual doctor evaluates the needs of the patient, determines what the patient can be told, and provides only that information. The health care facility carries out the wishes of the doctor. All major medical decisions are made by the doctor, who derives his authority and responsibility from the traditional concept of the doctor-patient relationship. This formulation, however, has failed to keep pace either with the parallel historical developments in areas such as employer-employee relationships discussed above or with developments in the field of medicine itself.

As technology has increased the doctor's ability to deal effectively with more health-threatening situations, it has also widened the gulf between doctor and patient. More problems can be diagnosed and treated,

the doctor's time is more in demand, and he has less time to spend with his patient to develop a working relationship of trust and mutual respect. As medical advances become more subtle and complex, explaining diagnoses, procedures, treatments, and alternatives to the patient becomes more difficult. Concurrently, widespread publicity—especially through television and newspaper coverage of medical breakthroughs and portrayal of medical crisis resolutions in fiction—generates greater public expectations. Though some way must be found to restore the expectations of the medical consumer to reality, there is a sense in which such expectations represent the inadequacies of the present doctor-patient and hospital-patient relationships. The doctor's position has been strengthened and the patient's weakened by technological advances; it is no longer beneficial to the patient to maintain the doctor-patient relationship of 140 or even 40 years ago. Too much has changed.

Nevertheless, physicians continue to argue that the "traditional doctor-patient relationship" must be maintained at all costs. Although the tremendous changes in the content and context of that relationship over the past century seem to undermine this argument, the advantages from the doctor's perspective of maintaining such a "traditional" relationship are many. Accountability for actions is likely to be restricted to peer review. Public scrutiny of medical decision making is likely to be minimal. Autonomy of action is likely to be maximal. Patient-consumer influence on services rendered is not likely to be significant.

The maintenance of the traditional doctor-patient relationship in a modern hospital context has generated many problems that characterize present-day medical decision making. First, both the decision maker—the party with the actual power to make a treatment decision—and the person or entity whose interests command the decision maker's loyalty are ambiguously identified. The existence of research in which the decision maker is involved and the decision maker's own biases, factors that may bear directly on the treatment decision, may not be apparent. A pediatrician may be responding to the interests of the parents rather than the child, for example. The recent kidney and bone marrow transplantation cases questioning the appropriateness of a guardian's consenting on behalf of an incompetent or minor donor illustrate the conflicts inherent in the existing structure. Second, the attending physician controls pertinent medical information, thereby limiting the ability of the patient or other interested persons to enter into the decision-making process. Third, the present system lacks systematic reporting or review of the ultimate treatment decision, and peer review mechanisms are unsatisfactory. Often, the only way a person can determine relevant facts about a past decision is to institute a malpractice action and gain the desired information through discovery procedures. Finally, the current decision-making process permits the doctor to justify his decision on grounds of "quality of life," resource allocation, societal goals, and other public policy issues, all of which determinations are usually best left to judicial and legislative bodies.

Public relations persons, nurses, or unit managers who lack both autonomy and authority, however, are unable to respond to the problems raised by the traditional medical decision-making process. Moreover, they usually cannot discover who has the power to make a treatment decision, where the decision maker's loyalties lie, who controls the pertinent information, whether there is any reporting or review of the treatment decision, or on what basis the treatment decision is justified. These persons owe primary loyalty to the health care facility, not to the patient. In the event of a conflict, their first responsibility must be to their employer. Without the ability to devote all possible energy and influence to protecting the patient, the third party becomes a barrier rather than a shield. The Patient Service Coordinator for the New York Hospital

has described this intermediary as "someone who will greet the patient with a smile, listen to him, get to know him as a person, and be his voice." While such a person may be needed, the role described is extremely limited and does nothing to resolve the problem characteristics of the traditional doctor-patient relationship. When an individual is sick, dying, or both, he needs more than a "placebo-practitioner" to hold his hand. He needs to know that he can count on the loyalty and judgment of a competent person who, at his direction, has access to his medical records and to staff consultants, and who can and will give him straight, unbiased answers to his questions. Anything less means that both his health and his human rights are potentially in danger.

The twelve-point "Patient's Bill of Rights," promulgated by the American Hospital Association on January 8, 1973, follows the pattern of the Joint Commission and Beth Israel statements. It is vague and does not provide an enforcement mechanism. Furthermore, the premise of the document is that the provider decides what rights the patient-consumer should have. In the field of landlord-tenant law, it would seem clearly anomalous to permit the landlord alone to determine tenant rights. In the health care field, however, such provider dominance over the consumer is so commonplace that it is seldom even commented on. Johnny Carson's January 9, 1973, parody of the document emphasized this irony when his own list of "patient rights" concluded that "the patient has a right to assume that if he is in a coma he will not be used as a door jamb."

The collections of minimal "rights" currently being promulgated by health care facilities remind one of the free enterprise, human-rights-be-damned philosophy of Ayn Rand, restated for the medical profession by Dr. Robert M. Sade in his "Medical Care as a Right: A Refutation." Unable to distinguish between the sale of bread and medical services, Dr. Sade fails completely to consider the human rights of patients while they are under medical care. We do not need more lists drawn up by health care providers. We need a clear, carefully articulated catalogue of hospital patients' rights, presented from the patient-consumers' perspective. To ensure that these rights are protected, a properly functioning mechanism within the health care facility is needed.

The Patient Rights Advocate

This section and the next present a mechanism within the health care facility capable of assisting the patient in decisions affecting health care and a model bill of patient rights that provides the legal foundation for the patient advocate system (*see appendix, ed.*). The introduction of these proposals into the hospital context is designed to benefit doctor and patient alike.

The goals of a patient rights advocate system are:

To protect patients, especially those at a disadvantage within the health care context —the young, the illiterate, the uncommunicative, those without relatives, those unable to speak English—by making available an advocate and a series of decision-making procedures.

To make available to those who seek it the opportunity to participate actively with their doctor as a partner in a personal health care program.

To restore medical technologies and pharmaceutical advances to proper perspective by deflating the exaggerated expectations of the modern American medical consumer.

To reflect in the doctor-patient relationship the reality of the health-sickness continuum, and to assert the humanness of death as a natural and inevitable reality.

To this end, we propose a "patient rights advocate," an individual whose primary responsibility is to assist the patient in learning about, protecting, and asserting his or her rights within the health care context. The advocate exercises, at the direction of the patient, powers that belong to the patient. To a large extent, these powers are rooted in the rights that the patient possesses and include:

Complete access to medical records and the authority to call in, at the direction of the patient, a consultant to aid or advise the patient.

Active participation on those hospital committees responsible for monitoring quality health care, especially utilization review and patient care.

Access to support services for all patients who request them.

Participation at the patient's request and direction in discussion of the patient's case, especially before decisions must be made and alternatives chosen.

The word "advocate" is used deliberately. In its classical sense, "advocare" means "to summon to one's assistance, to defend, to call to one's aid." Connotations of "adversariness," of contentiousness, and of deliberate antagonism are unfortunate, for they involve not the concept of advocacy per se, but the manner in which the advocate pursues his duties. Yet most of the criticism directed against the patient rights advocate has concerned the alleged introduction of conflict into the hospital setting. The advocate as adversary could confront the hospital with a number of problems. The relegation of all serious decision making to adversary proceedings, for example, would raise many questions: How can an independent decision be reached? Should the doctor retain final authority to do what he judges to be in the best interests of the patient? Who would define what is "serious?" How could such a program be supervised? Would a state of paralysis engulf the health care facility?

Such criticism, however, seems less a reaction to the concept of the patient rights advocate itself than to one manner in which the advocate could discharge his responsibilities. The advocate could, for example, function instead as an ombudsman. In this role he would seek out broad problem areas, research facts, publicize grievances to appropriate audiences, and make suggestions about resolving those problems. He would not participate, however, in the actual resolution. This conduct would provide active representation without direct personal influence on the outcome of the decision. While this approach would eliminate the problems created by an adversary system, the danger is that such a person would have no influence upon important decisions.

A third suggestion would combine aspects of both the adversary and ombudsman approaches. While acting as an ombudsman available to all patients who desired his services, the advocate could compile lists of recurring situations in which the rights of patients are affected and classify them according to seriousness. In a special category, for example, would be matters like transplantation and the refusal of life-sustaining medication or procedures. In each case fitting this category, the patient's interests would be represented by an advocate in an adversary hearing. An appropriate tribunal might be a decision-making committee like the kidney or heart transplant committees that select donors and recipients, or a policy-setting committee like the executive house staff. For less serious situations, other appropriate safeguards would be established. In both instances, an open process in which the patients' interests are represented would replace current covert policies for dealing with "difficult" cases.

It is essential to have as many advocates as necessary to ensure a functional patient-advocate ratio. The advocate would interview the patient at the time of arrival at the hospital, present a packet of materials including an explanation of the patient's rights, and remain available at all times via telephone. He would perform additional services for all those who request them and also provide objective information to members of the community who want to know before entering the health care facility how a particular problem is treated and whether alternatives are available. The advocate would also make daily rounds.

Case 1: The Emergency Room

Paul, a ten-year-old boy, had a seizure at his home and passed out. His father

picked him up and rushed him to a police station. The nearest hospital was a private institution. Paul had been receiving treatment at the County Hospital, which was some distance away. The police said they could not take him there because it was out of their district. When they arrived at the private hospital. Paul's father was subjected to an interview about his finances and insurance. No one would look at Paul until his father had answered such questions as: "Do you own your own home?" "Who is your employer?" "How long have you worked there?" The interviewer also refused to call the County Hospital. In frustration, Paul's father left the emergency room at the hospital and drove the long distance to the County Hospital. In the course of his trip, he passed several hospitals but was afraid to stop because of the possibility that they would treat him as the first hospital had. He arrived at the County Hospital, where his son died within an hour.

This case illustrates the tragic results that occur when a hospital places housekeeping chores above medical duty in an emergency situation. An advocate could have asserted the right of the patient to receive emergency care promptly without reference to ability to pay. Failure to provide an opportunity to assert that right was a significant factor in the loss of a life. An advocate could have played a key role in saving it.

Case 2: Diagnostic Tests

Patient 2, a professor, was admitted to the hospital for a series of tests to determine the identity of the condition from which he was suffering. A neurologist and three medical students ran him through a neurological examination. In his words: "I got a reinforcement of the sense of not only am I a patient who is supposed to behave in a certain way, but I'm almost an object to demonstrate to people that I'm not really people any more. I'm something else. I'm a body that has some very interesting characteristics about it. . . . I began to feel not only the fear of this unknown, dread thing that I have, that nobody knows anything about —and if they know, they're not going to tell me—but an anger and a resentment of 'Goddamn it, I'm a human being and I want to be treated like one!' And feeling that if I expressed anger, I could be retaliated against, because I'm in a very vulnerable position."

Some of the frustrations of Patient 2 could find an outlet in a patient rights advocate. The advocate would be a person to whom the patient could talk without fear of retaliation; a person who could pull his medical records and tell him whether or not a diagnosis had been made; a person who, on behalf of a busy medical staff, could take the time to explain the reason for the tests, why medical students were present, that he could have them excluded if he wished, and that notwithstanding his attitudes toward the medical staff or his expressions of fear and resentment, no retaliatory action would be taken against him. Tension and conflict would be reduced and the quality of medical care improved.

Case 3: Childbirth

Mr. and Mrs. 3 have attended classes on natural childbirth. They have discussed the matter with the doctor in the outpatient clinic of the hospital where the child will be delivered. The hospital has a policy of allowing the husband in the delivery room "at the doctor's discretion." They enter the hospital and spend three hours together in the labor room. As she is being transferred to the delivery room the doctor (a resident) says to the husband, "Sorry, you can't come in, you make me nervous."

In the delivery room Mrs. 3, who has previously given birth by the natural method in England, demands that the stirrups be removed. The attendants laugh at her and hold her down as her wrists are strapped to the table by leather thongs.

The current system offers Mr. and Mrs. 3 little, if any, recourse. Under a patient advocate system, an advocate assigned to the maternity ward would be in charge of advising the medical personnel about the couple's desires concerning natural childbirth, would make whatever preparations were deemed necessary, and would be present at the parents' request to ensure during birth that the father was not denied access to the delivery room and that the mother was not subjected to coercion or ridicule—a function probably unnecessary if the husband were allowed to be present in the delivery room as a matter of course. The advocate would function similarly in the emergency room to eliminate delays when possible or to provide an interpreter when needed. Again, the advocate would improve the resulting doctor-patient relationships.

Case 4: Breast Cancer

Ms. 4 enters the hosptial to have a breast biopsy. She is extremely nervous and upset. She is asked to sign a consent form that she doesn't understand. She is assured it is "routine" and signs it. When she sees her doctor she asks him about the alternative methods of treatment available if her tumor turns out to be malignant. He tells her that he does only radical mastectomies, but that she shouldn't worry before they know whether her tumor is malignant or not. The doctor then leaves the hospital for the day. Patient 4 continues to think about her condition and asks the nurse what will happen if her tumor is malignant. Specifically she wants to know if the doctor will immediately proceed with the mastectomy while she is still unconscious. The nurse says that this should be discussed with the doctor.

Currently, the patient's only recourse is either to try to get her doctor on the phone or to wait until the next day when she hopefully will see him again before the biopsy. Moreover, no one is presently available to explain the consent form to her. A patient rights advocate, on the other hand, would be present to explain consent forms and their implications to all patients required by the hospital to sign them. Additionally, the advocate would have provided the patient with a list of questions to ask anyone requesting that she sign such a form:

What treatment does the doctor want to use and why?

What alternative treatments are available and why is the method chosen superior to others?

What are the risks of having the procedure and of not having the procedure?

Is the procedure experimental?

What is the name and status—doctor, intern, resident, or medical student—of the person who will perform the procedure?

What are the side effects and how long will they last?

How much will it cost?

What will be the duration of hospitalization?

What will be the permanent effects?

What are the possibilities of a complete cure?

Had Patient 4 asked her doctor these questions initially, and had the doctor responded to them, the difficulties she is now experiencing would not have occurred, and conflict and tension between her and her doctor would have been significantly reduced.

In all these examples and in myriad others, a patient rights advocate with the powers outlined above could have effectively improved doctor-patient communication and improved the quality of medical care delivered. The recent series of informed consent cases has demonstrated that the old adage "good medicine is good law" is no longer universally true. Courts likely will more and more frequently allow juries to decide, without the aid of any expert testimony from the medical profession, what patients should be told about their conditions. As this trend continues, attempts to characterize the perpetuation of low standards of doctor-patient communication and the exclusion of the patient from important medical decision making

concerning his treatment as "standard medical procedure" will no longer provide any protection against legal liability. Therefore, hospitals considering the adoption of a patient rights advocate system should recognize not only the public relations value of such a move, but also, from the perspective of resolving doctor-patient grievances at the hospital rather than in the courts, the legal wisdom as well.

Our proposed system requires a person whose primary responsibility and loyalty are commanded by the patient alone and who can be fired only upon patient complaint. Beyond that, however, there is no single set of qualifications for the advocate. The advocate will deal with people of varying degrees of education and ability to communicate and of different ethnic, religious, and social backgrounds. Some knowledge of law, medicine, and psychology would appear essential, but the extent to which formal education would prepare a person for this job seems minimal. Some commentators have suggested a highly clinical, interdisciplinary program centered about our teaching hospitals. Experience here would seem the best teacher.

Financing and supervising the advocate program and deciding who should pay the advocate for his work also present enormous problems. The preferred situation would provide support and supervision from such outside organizations as the Department of Health, Education, and Welfare, the state department of public health, a consumer affairs office, Blue Cross, a statewide medical foundation, or a health consumers group. If there is no alternative to making the advocate a member of the hospital administrative staff, it is imperative that he or she be accountable only to the patients served.

Different approaches may be needed for different types of institutions. Proposals for legal advocates in mental health institutions, for example, have made substantial progress and contributed significantly to the civil rights of mental patients. The problems of people in such long-term facilities are, of course, different from those in general hospitals where the average stay lasts eight days, and variations of the system may also be necessary in the nursing home context, in the health maintenance organization context, and in the neighborhood clinic con-text. No matter which method is chosen to implement the patient advocate system, however, the key to its success will be the patient-centered bill of rights it seeks to enforce.

45.
The Duty of Care   Angela R. Holder

General Definition of the Term "Due Care"

Once a physician-patient relationship has been established, the physician is obligated to diagnose and treat the patient's illness or injury with "due care." Failure to do so constitutes "negligence" for which the patient may recover monetary damages.

All negligence actions are a species of tort law, which is defined as "a violation of duty imposed by general law or otherwise upon all persons occupying the relation to each other which is involved in a given transaction." Negligence in particular is defined as "the omission to do something which a reasonable man guided by those ordinary considerations which ordinarily regulate human affairs, would do, or the doing of something which a reasonable and prudent man would not do." All negligence actions are therefore predicated on the allegation that the party who claims damage was owed some duty by the other and that the duty was breached, causing injury. In any automobile accident litigation, for example, the plaintiff claims that the defendant owed all others on the road a duty to drive safely and that he breached that duty, thus causing the accident.

The standard used by courts in determining whether or not there has been a breach of duty in any negligence action is the "reasonable man" rule. If the reasonable, prudent man would have avoided the difficulty, the defendant will be held to have been neg-ligent. On the other hand, if the reasonable man would have acted the same way the defendant acted, no negligence can exist as a matter of law even though the plaintiff's injury may be quite genuine.

These basic principles of negligence law are applied in cases in which a patient alleges that a physician has in some manner been negligent in diagnosing or treating the patient's complaint, but in any type of professional negligence action against a professional person, including physicians, lawyers, architects, and others, the concept of "the reasonable man" becomes the "duly careful member of the profession." Two old and very famous decisions in cases which alleged that physicians had been negligent established the definition of medical malpractice which is now accepted by the courts of all states:

As early as 1898 the highest court in New York established the basic definition of medical negligence in *Pike v. Honsinger*. The patient had been kicked in the knee by a horse and claimed that the defendant had set it in a negligent manner, resulting in a failure of the bones to unite. The court said:

The law relating to malpractice is simple and well settled, although not always easy of application. A physician and surgeon, by taking charge of a case, impliedly represents that he possesses, and the law places upon him the duty of possessing, that reasonable degree of learning and

Source: Angela R. Holder, *Medical Malpractice Law*, John Wiley and Sons, Inc., New York, 1978.

skill that is ordinarily possessed by physicians and surgeons in the locality in which he practices, and which is ordinarily regarded by those conversant with the employment as is necessary to qualify him to engage in the business of practicing medicine and surgery. Upon consenting to treat a patient, it becomes his duty to use reasonable care and diligence in the exercise of his skill and the application of his learning to accomplish the purpose for which he was employed. He is under the further obligation to use his best judgment in exercising his skill and applying his knowledge. The law holds him liable for an injury to his patient resulting from want of the requisite skill and knowledge or the omission to exercise reasonable care or the failure to use his best judgment. The rule in relation to learning and skill does not require the surgeon to possess that extraordinary learning and skill which belong only to a few men of rare endowments, but such as is possessed by the average member of the medical profession in good standing. . . . The rule of reasonable care and diligence does not require the use of the highest possible degree of care and to render a physician and surgeon liable, it is not enough that there has been a less degree of care than some other medical man might have shown or less than even he himself might have bestowed, but there must be a want of ordinary and reasonable care, leading to a bad result.

The Supreme Court of Indiana expanded on this definition in 1938. *Adkins v. Ropp* involved a patient who had lost the sight of one eye. He claimed that the defendant had been negligent in removing a foreign body from it and the eye had then become infected as the result of the negligence. The defendant argued that the infection was an unavoidable result of the original injury. The court said:

When a physician and surgeon assumes to treat and care for a patient, in the absence of a special agreement, he is held in

law to have impliedly contracted that he possesses the reasonable and ordinary qualifications of his profession and that he will exercise at least reasonable skill, care and diligence in his treatment of him. This implied contract on the part of the physician does not include a promise to effect a cure and negligence cannot be imputed because a cure is not effected, but he does impliedly promise that he will use due diligence and ordinary skill in his treatment of the patient so that a cure may follow such care and skill, and this degree of care and skill is required of him, not only in performing an operation or administering first treatments, but he is held to the like degree of care and skill in the necessary subsequent treatments unless he is excused from further service by the patient himself, or the physician or surgeon upon due notice refuses to further treat the case. In determining whether the physician or surgeon has exercised the degree of skill and care which the law requires, regard must be had to the advanced state of the profession at the time of treatment and in the locality in which the physician or surgeon practices.

In law, negligence is not by any means limited to situations involving carelessness. For example, a physician who does not have the training to perform a given procedure or who does not ask for the necessary information on which to make a diagnosis may be extremely careful as he deals with the patient and in fact his care may meet the highest possible standards, but he may still be negligent if he does not refer the patient to a specialist.

Thus, simply put, the physician must have adequate knowledge and skill and use it with adequate care in his dealings with a patient. "The reasonably prudent physician or surgeon, acting under the same circumstances" is the standard by which his conduct will be judged.

An electrocardiogram made when a patient complained of chest pains indicated possibly serious cardiac abnormalities. The physician did not tell the patient anything about the results, nor did he prescribe rest or any treatment. A week later when the chest pains recurred and were worse, the patient called him and the physician told him to go to the hospital. He did not, however, tell him to go in an ambulance, so the patient walked down several flights of stairs and rode to the hospital in his car. Examination revealed that he had had a heart attack several days before. Open heart surgery was required to repair the damage. He sued and recovered damages from the physician. The court held that a duly careful, reasonably prudent physician would have told his patient about the electrocardiogram results and would have hospitalized him immediately.

A draftee during the time of the Viet Nam war arrived at his preinduction physical examination with a letter from an orthopedist saying that he had a knee injury. A chest x-ray at the examination indicated a serious abnormality, but the man was not told about it. When he received a letter stating that he had failed his physical, he assumed that his knee was the cause. Six months later he was ordered to report for reexamination, and while holding his folder, read the radiologist's report of the abnormality. He went immediately to his family physician, who found a malignancy. He died and his widow sued the government for malpractice. The court held that even in the absence of a physician-patient relationship, due care required the Army physicians to inform the man of his condition since it was admitted that treatment at the time of the x-ray would have saved his life.

Application of the Principles of Due Care

Certain factual situations are quite common in medical malpractice suits. Thus in many areas there are general guidelines from many judicial decisions as to what acts constitute due care as a matter of law.

The obvious first step in determining due care is consideration of the amount of skill possessed and used in treating the patient. A physician may be liable either for failure to know what he is doing, if a reasonably prudent physician would have known, or he may be liable if he knows what to do, but for some reason does not do it carefully or omits doing it at all. "Skill and knowledge" as discussed in the definitions of due care usually includes the former, "diligence" the latter. A physician may, for example, be liable in negligence if he is remiss in his obligation to realize that he is not capable of treating the patient and should therefore send him to a specialist. A physician whose native language is not English would probably be found liable if his difficulties with the language prevent him from reaching any understanding of the patient's complaints and as a result he administers the wrong treatment no matter how skillfully he applies it. Both those problems would involve lack of skill. Failure to visit a hospitalized patient sufficiently frequently to keep aware of his problems, on the other hand, would constitute lack of diligence.

Nonphysicians who attempt to treat diseases, once they come within the boundaries of the practice of medicine, are held to the same standard of skill and knowledge as a physician. A chiropractor, for example, is judged by the knowledge of other chiropractors as long as what he is doing does not involve the practice of medicine. If he ventures into diagnosis or treatment of a medical problem, the law requires him to be as knowledgeable and able to treat the patient as a physician would be. If he cannot comply with this standard, he cannot later defend himself on the ground that he did not know what he was doing because of his lack of education.

A college undergraduate doing an independent project for a biology course got permission from his teacher, a Ph.D. biologist, to take blood samples from other students. The samples were to be drawn by the student in the teacher's office. The student had worked as a lab assistant at a hospital and had drawn blood, but did not know first aid or how to take a pulse. The teacher gave him no instructions and was not present when the samples were taken. One of the students whose blood was drawn fainted and knocked out six front teeth. She sued the university and the professor. In upholding the jury's verdict in her favor, the court held that withdrawal of blood is a "medical function" and that it was the duty of the professor to see that the same standard of care, including having a place to lie down available and knowledge of what to do if someone fainted, would be used as would be used if a physician had drawn the blood.

Nonphysician health professionals are held to the standard of skill, care, and knowledge possessed and used by the "reasonably prudent member" of their professional group as long as the activity undertaken is one commonly performed by members of the group. A nurse performing a function usually performed by other nurses, such as giving injections, is held to the standard of care of "the reasonably prudent nurse." On the other hand, if she undertakes to diagnose a condition and prescribe medication, she would be held to the standard of the reasonably prudent physician, since those activities are usually considered "practicing medicine," not "practicing nursing."

Women who worked at a women's health center but who were not licensed physicians or nurse-midwives delivered babies at their "patients'" homes. They were convicted of practicing medicine without licenses, although they argued that childbirth is a normal function, thus they were not "treating disease." In upholding their convictions, the appellate court pointed out that they were obliged to know signs of complications and deal with them, and thus the women they delivered might be damaged by their lack of skill, care, and knowledge. The statute was thus upheld as constitutional.

Since there is frequently less than unanimous opinion in the medical profession on the best method of treating a given problem, a physician is generally free to adopt the one of several alternative treatments he thinks best as long as the patient understands the risks and benefits of each, and gives a genuinely informed consent. As long as the course of treatment chosen is one which is accepted by a "respectable minority" of the medical profession, the courts regard it as an approved one.

A physician did not administer a relaxant drug to a patient prior to an electroshock treatment. A fracture resulted. At the time of the incident there was honest disagreement among recognized psychiatric experts as to the side effects risk of the medication. The court held that failure to give the medicine was not negligent.

A patient's sciatic nerve was damaged during hip replacement surgery. He sued the surgeon, and presented an expert witness who testified that there were two methods of performing the procedure and that he used the other because there was less danger of nerve damage. The court noted that evidence of a difference of professional opinion is not evidence of malpractice and said "Differences of opinion are consistent with the exercise of due care or even the highest degree of care." The action was dismissed.

Defining a "respectable minority," however, is one of the more complex questions confronting a court in a case of this type.

A physician whose method is either unknown to or disapproved by his peers may well find himself presumed to be negligent if the patient suffers damage, particularly if he did not follow the usual methods of treatment prior to the use of his own innovations. Use of an unproved method of treatment which damages the patient without a truly informed consent by the patient, given with a clear understanding that the method of treatment is unproved, is usually considered negligent even if it is carried out with the highest possible degree of care.

Of course the degree of innovation which is legally acceptable is largely determined by the patient's condition. If the ailment is not serious, presumably negligence would be found if innovation in treatment causes damage of any sort. On the other hand, where the patient is critically ill or not responding to the standard treatments for the condition from which he suffers, use of unproved methods might well be justified as long as the patient or his family understands that the treatment is unproved and the consequences thereof are not predictable.

A teenage boy died as the result of an unorthodox orthopedic procedure. His parents had consented to the surgery but were not told that it was experimental. The surgeon was found liable for his failure to disclose that fact to the parents.

A patient broke his ankle. A year of treatment by standard methods did not result in any improvement. Several physicians advised him to have it amputated. Another surgeon performed an unorthodox operation. Eighteen months later the ankle was amputated. The court held that under the circumstances the new and unorthodox procedure was justified as last resort and all that had resulted from its failure was what would have happened sooner without it.

Due care may require the prudent and careful physician to consult with other medical practitioners in many situations. He may, for example, be required by principles of good medical practice to contact for information or instructions a physician who has previously treated the patient.

A patient had had a piece of bone removed from his nose and his optic nerve was unprotected. He consulted another physician a considerable time after surgery for treatment of asthma. He told the second physician about the nasal surgery and the name of the surgeon who had performed it. The second physician did not call the surgeon to inquire about the operation or any of its effects. During his treatment of the asthmatic condition,

the optic nerve was damaged and the patient lost the sight of that eye. The court held that the physician's failure to consult with the prior surgeon before beginning treatment constituted negligence.

In some cases, the physician may be obliged by the principles of due care to consult with another physician on his diagnosis or plan of treatment even though the second physician is not asked to take over responsibility for the case. Many decisions discuss the necessity of consultation when a diagnosis is uncertain.

Consultation on treatment may also be required if the physician knows or should know that his methods of dealing with the case are proving ineffectual.

After an operation in 1952, a surgeon knew that the patient's wound drained constantly but did nothing about it. In 1961, the patient's children took her to a specialist, who removed a sponge from the incision. The court held that the surgeon was negligent in failing to consult with someone in the face of abundant evidence that something was wrong.

In some situations the physician has the duty to refer the patient to a specialist for diagnosis or treatment and to allow the specialist to take over the case. If a physician who is not a specialist in the field of the patient's illness knows or should know that treatment by a specialist is reasonably available and would benefit the patient, he is negligent if he does not advise the patient of that fact.

A woman had a hysterectomy. The surgeon was a general surgeon, and the operation took place in a hospital with limited facilities. The following day she vomited frequently and the surgeon realized she had peritonitis. Six days later he arranged for her transfer to a specialist in a larger hospital. The specialist operated and removed a gangrenous bowel, but she died of a kidney problem caused by the infection. The court held, in her husband's suit against the surgeon who had performed the hysterectomy, that the failure to send her to a specialist as soon as her condition demanded it was negligent.

However, before a nonspecialist can be found liable for failure to refer a patient, the circumstances must be such that the duly careful generalist should have known that a problem existed which he was not equipped to solve.

Symptoms of a simple and widespread eye ailment are virtually identical to glaucoma. The general practitioner who treated the patient for the common complaint did not realize that glaucoma was present until severe and permanent damage to eyesight had occurred. The court held that he was not liable for his failure to refer the patient since his original diagnosis was reasonable.

A great many cases in which it was alleged that the nonspecialist was liable for failure to refer involved fractures. In general, if an orthopedist is readily available, a general practitioner would be well advised to make referrals in all cases of suspected broken bones.

A physician who knows what is wrong with a patient and exactly what treatment is necessary may have an obligation to refer the patient to a hospital which has better facilities or equipment than are locally available.

A general practitioner attempted to remove a foreign object from a patient's eye. Symptoms presented evidence of a detached retina, but he did not have the instruments necessary to make a conclusive diagnosis. By the time the patient consulted a specialist her vision was permanently damaged. The court held that the general practitioner was negligent in failing to send her to someone who had the specialized instruments required.

In an emergency, of course, a different situation is presented. A physician in a small hospital unit might in fact be considered

negligent if he sent a patient to a larger hospital if the patient's condition would be jeopardized by the move. In that situation, good and careful medical practice would require only that the physician do the best he could with whatever equipment he had at his disposal.

In most cases, if a physician refers a patient to a duly qualified specialist of whom there is no reason to suspect negligence and the first physician's involvement with the case terminates at that time, any negligence by the specialist is not imputed to him and he is not liable for it. When the referring physician continues to participate actively in the care of the patient, however, he may be jointly liable with the specialist.

If his assistance is entirely directed by the specialist, as in a situation in which he assists in surgery planned and carried out by the specialist, or if the specialist assumes all decision-making responsibility, however, the referring physician probably would not be liable even if he continued to visit the patient in the hospital or involved himself in other cooperative ventures to that extent. The controlling factor, therefore, in any question of joint liability in a referral situation is the extent of participation by the referring physician in diagnosis and treatment.

One of the most important duties a physician owes his patient under the general concept of due care is his obligation to keep abreast of new developments in medicine.

A hospital was liable for the negligence of one of its staff physicians who set a fractured leg in an emergency. The physician admitted at the trial that he had not read a book on orthopedics in 10 years, but he had not asked for consultation when obvious postoperative signs of difficulties developed.

Medication permanently affected a patient's eyesight. Medical literature had contained numerous articles indicating the possibility of such a side effect but the physician who prescribed it had not read any of the articles. The court found that he was negligent in failing to keep up with and be aware of developments in the field.

What may be accepted as the most advanced practice of medicine or surgery at one time in a physician's career may be swiftly outdated by new discoveries and advances, and it is his obligation to render treatment to his patients based on adequate understanding of those new developments.

A common defense to an allegation by a patient that the physician has been negligent is a showing that customary and approved practice in the community was followed. Where a physician can show that he has followed the practices and treatment methods commonly employed by his local peers, he is usually not considered negligent. However, in recent years courts have begun to realize that the local custom itself may be negligent and if it is, the fact that the negligence is widespread is no defense.

A patient went into shock following surgery. The surgeon did not visit him for 12 hours. Although he showed that the local custom was to deal with this problem by telephone, he was still found liable for the patient's death.

A patient fell during x-rays. The radiologist was not aware that part of her complaint was "dizzy spells." Even though local custom did not make history taking the radiologist's responsibility, the court held that he had been negligent in failing to question her.

Therefore, while adherence to the usual practice by which the local medical community deals with a problem is ordinarily a good defense to a charge of negligence, "everybody does it" is no excuse if "it" is in fact a sloppy or careless practice.

Two ophthalmologists saw a young woman at frequent intervals from 1959 to 1968. They fitted her with contact lenses and gave her routine eye examinations. At her last visit, the ophthalmologist, for the first time, did a glaucoma pressure test. The test showed that the patient, then 32, had glaucoma. She sued them for damages and alleged that an earlier diagnosis would have improved her chances for successful treatment. Medical evidence was not disputed that the standard practice of the duly careful ophthalmologist not only in the community but nationwide was to do testing only of patients age 40 and older. In finding the ophthalmologists liable, the Supreme Court of Washington imposed strict liability, rather than negligence, since "negligence" implies moral blame. The court conceded that the ophthalmologists acted reasonably and in conformity to standards of the specialty, but pointed out that they, and not the patient, should bear the loss resulting from omission of a simple test.

As might be expected, this decision engendered considerable comment in both law and medical journals. It has not, however, been followed in any other case arising in any other jurisdiction. The general rule remains that in the absence of medical evidence that standard practice is actually negligent, conformity thereto is a good defense.

Due care obligates a physician to follow up on his patient's progress. He must be sure, for example, that his patient understands his instructions pertaining to medication, restrictions on activities, return visits, and the like. If the patient is a child or young adolescent, of course, the physician must communicate instructions to the parent as well as to the child. If the patient is senile or otherwise incompetent, instruction must be given to a family member or other responsible adult. If the patient has difficulty with English, the physician must present the instructions until he is sure that they have been understood. If there is any question of illiteracy, oral instructions corresponding to any written ones, such as those on medication labels, must be given.

If people who are caring for a patient are not trained health professionals, the physician must make quite sure that they understand how to respond to any problem and what they are to do for the patient. On the other hand, a physician does have the right to assume that a nurse or other trained person will use ordinary standards of professional knowledge if caring for a patient at home.

If any medication is prescribed which might affect a patient's ability to drive a car or to participate in similar activities in which the physician knows or should know that he is likely to be engaged, the physician is absolutely obligated to explain this to him. If a patient becomes drowsy as a side effect of the medication while driving, falls asleep at the wheel, and has a wreck, not only will he have a malpractice suit against the physician, but any other persons who are injured would have an action against the physician as well.

If the patient's condition is such that driving could endanger him or others, the physician is also negligent if he does not instruct the patient to stop driving until he is well.

If instructions are given and the patient disobeys them, of course, he and not the physician is at fault when his condition does not improve. It should be remembered, however, that a sick or frightened person may not be capable of the same kind of common sense, judgment, or intelligence he exhibits when he is well. For that reason, in order to prevent any misunderstanding in the patient's mind about what he has been told to do or to refrain from doing, a physician should make a habit of having patients repeat instructions back to him to be sure they understand. A physician may, however, tell a mentally competent patient to "call me if you need me" and assume that the patient will do so. The physician need not call or visit the patient to ask how recovery is progressing if he has no reason to believe that there is any problem.

A physician is also obligated to pay attention to patients' complaints. Failure to listen to what a patient is trying to tell him about any symptoms or changes in condition could result in the physician's remaining unaware

of early indications of serious problems. While obvious schedule disruptions would occur if a physician tried to talk to all patients who call him at his office, telephoning a drugstore to prescribe medication on the basis of what an office assistant tells him the patient says his symptoms are is potentially dangerous for that reason. A better practice is for the physician himself to return the call when he has time to talk to the patient.

Another type of failure to communicate with and listen to the patient which may result in serious consequences is a failure to take an adequate medical history or to make reasonable inquiries about the circumstances of the illness.

A diagnosis was made on admission to the hospital that a patient suffered from delirium tremens. In fact the patient was almost a teetotaler. After death an autopsy revealed a massive subdural hematoma. Since the physician who made the diagnosis could have made immediate inquiries about the patient's drinking habits from members of the family who were at the hospital, failure to do so was held to be negligent.

A man who was in a wreck in the middle of the night was brought into the emergency room and was treated and admitted by an orthopedist. His leg and wrist were both broken. The orthopedist casted the leg, but decided to wait to see if the wrist required surgery. A day later he decided that it did, but the operation was not considered an emergency procedure. Hospital rules required all surgical patients to have preoperative histories and physicals, and the orthopedist wrote orders for a resident to do it. The resident did, and specifically indicated that the patient was vomiting frequently. The report was not, however, attached to the chart, and the orthopedist did not look for it or talk to the resident. The patient aspirated, and died following surgery. The widow sued the surgeon, and the court held that he had been negligent in failing to know the preoperative condition of his patient.

Of course all patients do not recover from their problems. Physicians are neither magicians nor insurers of their patients' good health. Some conditions refuse to respond to all known methods of treatment and some patients exhibit idiosyncratic reactions to established and accepted methods of cure. The legal definitions of due care and negligence are such that no inference of negligence is raised from the fact that a patient's condition did not improve. A poor result is never sufficient in and of itself to establish negligence by a physician or surgeon. As long as the treatment was proper, there is no malpractice regardless of the outcome of the patient's illness.

A very old decision from the Minnesota Supreme Court gave an excellent summation of the legal principles to be applied in case of bad result:

Physicians and surgeons deal with progressive inductive science. On two historic occasions, the greatest surgeons in our country met in conference to decide whether or not they should operate upon the person of the President of the United States. Their conclusion was the final human judgment. They were not responsible in law, either human or divine, for the ultimate decree of nature. The same tragedy is enacted in a less conspicuous way every day in every part of this country.

A physician is also not liable for an honest error of judgment. The law does not demand infallibility of any physician. If he complies with recognized standards, a simple error will not subject him to liability. In retrospect he may realize that his judgment was wrong, but as long as it was reasonable, he is not liable.

A patient was burned during x-ray treatments. In finding that there was no negligence, the court said:

Physicians and surgeons must be allowed a wide range in the exercise of their judgment and discretion. In many instances there can be no fixed rule to determine the duty of a physician but he must often use his own best judgment and act accordingly. By reason of that fact, the law will not hold a physician guilty of negligence even though his judgment may prove erroneous in a given case, unless it be shown that the course pursued was clearly against the course recognized as correct by the profession generally.

The Locality Rule

Until quite recently, as a matter of law comparison was made of the due care exercised by the particular physician in reference to that of other physicians in his geographical area. The standard test was "that degree of care which other physicians exercise in the same or similar communities." The skill and knowledge of a physician were compared only to other physicians in the same geographical area on the theory that physicians practicing in isolated rural areas, for example, should not be expected to be as well trained and up to date as a physician in an urban environment. This rule does remain strictly adhered to in a few states, but it has been completely abrogated in others and, in general, even where it is still theoretically accepted it has been modified. In most jurisdictions today, the local standard of practice is considered only one factor presented for the jury's determination and is not in and of itself determinative of the presence or absence of negligence.

Most states now make the comparison on the basis of the "professional area," those centers to which a patient can be easily transferred for treatment, as opposed to the strict geographical area. There is no longer any reason why a small-town physician cannot practice at the level of competence of his urban counterpart. As early as 1940, the Supreme Court of North Dakota pointed out that with the advent of rapid transportation and communication, horizons of physicians have been widened and even the physician in the smallest village now has access to all medical journals, opportunities for continuing education, and larger medical centers to which he may refer patients. The intellectual borders of the physician's community have been extended far beyond those remotely conceivable a century ago when the locality rule was devised and when it was both fair and reasonable.

Some courts in fact have adopted the position that the old interpretation of the locality rule gives rural physicians an undue and unfair advantage over urban physicians. In one decision, the Supreme Court of Washington pointed out that the small-town physician should not enjoy a legal advantage not given to other small-town tort defendants and should not be able to rely on being "a little more careless" there. The decision pointed out that small-town residents who drive cars and cause automobile accidents are not allowed greater latitude for either carelessness or incompetence than urban drivers enjoy when sued for damages.

The standard to which a specialist must adhere is quite a bit broader than that which courts consider reasonable to expect from a nonspecialist. The result of the differing standards of course means that in a given situation a specialist may be found negligent, whereas a general practitioner who did the same thing would not.

Even a specialist is not presumed to guarantee that his patient will get well. As long as he observes the required standard of care, neither a specialist nor a general practitioner is liable for an error of judgment.

Courts in most states have now completely abandoned the locality rule in regard to the standard of care required from a specialist. The specialist is increasingly assumed to adhere to national standards in his field, and numerous decisions have pointed out that the usual reason a patient consults a specialist in the first place is to have his problem treated by someone who is abreast of all advances.

A pediatrician failed to make a standard PKU test on a newborn. The baby had the disease, and the delay in diagnosis caused permanent impairment. Evidence that such tests were not made in the community's hospitals was not disputed, although the parents showed that they were in general use throughout the country. The court held the pediatrician to the national standard and found him negligent for failing to make the test.

Since eminent specialists often disagree on the merits of a particular treatment, of course failure to follow majority opinion as to a given method does not presume a specialist to be negligent. The respectable minority rule within the members of the specialty will control.

Hospitals, too, are held to a standard of care in safeguarding the welfare of their patients. Although small community hospitals are not expected to provide the facilities, equipment, or expertise of major teaching institutions, and thus are judged by the standards of the "community of similar institutions," there appears to be an increasing tendency by courts to expand that definition. In particular there is an increasing willingness to hold hospitals accredited by the Joint Commission on Accreditation of Hospitals to a national standard of care in those matters in which JCAH standards are relevant.

Proximate Cause

Even if a patient can prove that a physician or surgeon did not meet the required standard of care, he cannot recover damages unless he can also prove that the negligence caused him injuries which would not have occurred in its absence. Even if there is clear-cut proof of misdiagnosis, for example, the patient must prove that his condition was worsened by the error before a jury can, as a matter of law, award him pecuniary compensation. This requirement of proof between cause and effect is known as the legal concept of "proximate cause." No matter how negligent the physician may have been, harm must be shown to have resulted before damages may be awarded.

Where a patient is so ill or so severely

injured that death may be imminent, if negligence occurs in the course of treatment and the patient dies, damages will not be awarded unless the survivors who bring the action can prove that the deceased probably would have survived in the absence of the malpractice. In many cases, particularly those in which patients have been critically injured in automobile accidents, this may in fact be quite difficult to prove.

A 16-year old boy was hit by a car while riding his bicycle. His mother took him to the emergency room, where the physician on call gave him a cursory examination and sent him home. The boy died a few hours later. Autopsy revealed that he had had a massive skull fracture. The mother sued the physician, and expert testimony proved her allegations that failure to examine the boy more carefully was clear negligence. Her case was dismissed, however, because none of the experts could testify that he would more probably than not have survived such a severe head injury even if he had had proper care.

If the initial injury or illness is not considered life-threatening, however, the causal connection between severe damage or death and negligence is correspondingly easier to demonstrate.

A patient died after a tonsillectomy. Evidence indicated that the cause of death was probably the manner in which the anesthetic had been administered. Since there is rarely a substantial likelihood of death after having one's tonsils out, the court assumed that there was a causal connection between the negligence and the death, even in the absence of exact and specific proof of what had gone wrong.

Delay in diagnosis may also be negligent and yet not be established as the proximate cause of damage to the patient. In innumerable fracture cases, in particular, a great many of which involved fractured hips, the problem was not discovered until long after the original evaluation of the injury. In numbers of these cases, the physicians have submitted evidence that a high percentage of such fractures never heal properly even with an immediate diagnosis. Courts have therefore been reluctant to conclude that the delay caused the outcome.

Since the sick or injured patient has something wrong at the time he consults the physician, numerous decisions involve attempts to determine if the poor result of treatment was caused by the physician's negligence or the preexisting condition of the patient. Before any patient can recover damages, he must eliminate his condition as the probable cause of the failure to recuperate fully.

An automobile accident victim had a broken leg. By mistake, the cast was put on the wrong leg and the error was not discovered for 10 days. Since the residual stiffness of the leg was as likely to have been caused by the accident itself as it was by the error, no proximate cause of damage was shown against the orthopedist.

After a hysterectomy damage was discovered involving the patient's left ureter. The patient alleged that it was sewed or crushed during surgery. Evidence for the surgeon indicated that the condition was as likely to be a natural swelling following surgical interference. The court held that no proximate cause was shown.

In most situations, expert medical testimony must be presented in order to prove that a negligent act and not the preexisting illness was the proximate cause of the patient's condition.

Where there may be two or more causes for a bad result of treatment, the jury is charged with the responsibility of choosing between them. Although proof beyond a reasonable doubt is not required in order to allow the patient to recover damages, he does bear the burden of proving all the facts which he alleges indicate negligence. The defendant, in most cases, does not have to prove that he was not negligent. The evidence presented by the plaintiff must be "substantial" and causation must be shown to be at least a "reasonable probability" before damages can be awarded.

Proof of Negligence

Since the standard of care in suits against medical practitioners is the reasonably careful physician or surgeon, specialist or not, in most cases the plaintiff is required to prove both that standard and the defendant's deviation from it by the use of expert testimony. Expert testimony is given by another physician. If the case involves a specialist, the expert witness is usually, but not always, from the same specialty. The expert witness must be familiar with the procedure involved in the case, but in most jurisdictions he does not necessarily have to perform it himself as a regular part of his practice. Thus a specialist in one area of medicine is allowed to testify against a specialist in another as long as the subject matter of the suit is common to both.

If the court requires application of the locality rule in a malpractice case, the expert, no matter how well qualified, must testify that he or she is in fact familiar with the standard of care in that community or at least in similar communities. This not infrequently results in dismissal of a plaintiff's case because the expert is on the faculty of a medical school and in some cases is acknowledged to be the ranking national expert on the subject, but has never practiced in a small community similar to the one in which the patient was treated.

The expert witness explains to the court and the jury what the standard of care should be in the situation at hand and gives his opinion on how well the defendant met the standard. If a physician wishes to defend on the grounds that he was not negligent, he usually presents expert medical witnesses of his own to rebut the testimony of the plaintiff's experts. If he wishes to present an affirmative defense, that is, if he wishes not only to deny that he was negligent but to show that the plaintiff caused the problem

himself or to make some other affirmative response to the charge, he is required to bear the burden of proving such a defense and almost always would use expert witnesses to do it. Since a jury of laymen is not considered competent to know the standard of care in a complex matter of medical diagnosis or treatment or whether the defendant complied with it, as a matter of law the jury usually cannot render a verdict against a physician without expert testimony on behalf of the plaintiff indicating that the expert believes the defendant to have been negligent.

A physician's own statements contemporaneous with the event or in court on cross-examination indicating that he was negligent can in some cases be substituted for the requirement of an expert witness for the plaintiff. In some states the defendant may be asked on cross-examination what the standard of care in the situation should have been.

Some areas of negligence are so obvious that courts have held that laymen can understand them without expert help and therefore no expert witness is required. This is the doctrine of *res ipsa loquitur*—the thing speaks for itself.

Where the accident is one which does not usually occur in the absence of negligence, the apparent cause was within the exclusive control of the physician, and the patient could not have contributed to the difficulties, the doctrine may be applied. This rules out most cases of misdiagnosis, since such may occur without any lack of due care.

The usual example of the use of *res ipsa loquitur* in a malpractice case is one in which a sponge or other foreign object is left in a patient's body during surgery. The jury is considered qualified, without the necessity of expert explanation, to conclude that something is wrong when a sponge is left. Furthermore, in these cases the surgeon is in control of the instrumentalities and it can hardly be the patient's fault. Paralysis after spinal anesthesia is another common situation in which expert testimony is not usually necessary to prove negligence. The risks of more complicated medical procedures, such as laminectomies which may result in paralysis, are usually not considered sufficiently obvious, however, to allow a jury to infer negligence from the event itself.

In most states, in a case in which *res ipsa loquitur* is utilized, the jury may, but is not required to, infer negligence from the

mere existence of the situation. In a few jurisdictions, however, presentation of a *res ipsa loquitur* situation raises a presumption of negligence, meaning that the jury is obliged to find in favor of the plaintiff unless the physician presents a satisfactory explanation other than negligence of how the event occurred.

46.

Medical Ethics and Discipline — Robert C. Derbyshire

The hospitals, organized medicine, and the state licensing boards are the main agencies responsible for enforcement of discipline in the medical profession, thus guarding the public against unethical and incompetent physicians. These agencies have been critically examined in an effort to determine whether or not they are properly performing their functions. Serious deficiencies have been found in all, and the reasons for them analyzed. Suggestions are made for improving the all-important self-policing procedures of the medical profession.

In the United States today the most important agencies concerned with medical ethics and discipline are the hospitals, organized medicine, and the state boards of medical examiners. How well are they doing their jobs? Are they doing everything possible to uphold the ethical standards of the medical profession? If they are not doing their jobs, why aren't they? Finally, what can they do to improve their procedures?

Although the "Principles of Medical Ethics" of the American Medical Association serves as a guide to acceptable behavior for physicians, the medical practice laws go beyond this. Most of them define some variety of unprofessional, immoral, or dishonorable conduct as a cause for disciplin-

ary action. Only ten laws, however, refer specifically to unethical conduct.

Effectiveness of Disciplinary Agencies

How effectively are the various disciplinary agencies upholding standards? First the hospitals. During the past few years they have definitely improved their disciplinary procedures. This can be attributed both to the Joint Commission on Accreditation of Hospitals and to the courts. The establishment of tissue, audit, and professional review committees has at least made the hospitals aware that ethical problems do exist, but enforcement of professional standards is no better than the effectiveness of the committees, and this varies widely. The hospital administrators, however, are assuming more responsibility for the performance of their staff members since they were jolted by the landmark decision of *Darling vs. Charleston Memorial Community Hospital.*[1] This stated essentially that the hospital administration can be held responsible for the competence of staff members.

Regardless, many hospitals are lax in regard to the physical and psychological standards of staff members. If professional incompetence is classed as a cause for action,

Source: New Mexico Board of Medical Examiners, Santa Fe. Read in part before the Fourth National Congress on Medical Ethics, Washington, D.C., April 26, 1973. *Journal of the American Medical Association*, vol. 228, no. 1, April 1, 1974.

certainly a person who is physically or mentally handicapped is guilty of unethical conduct if he undertakes procedures beyond his capacities. A large number of hospitals do not demand certificates of competence from the physician who wishes to resume practice after suffering a severe illness. Regan's suggestion[2] that hospital bylaws should provide that staff members be required to submit reports of physical examinations at specified ages is indeed sound.

Although many accredited hospitals may be adequately handling problems of medical ethics, there are still the so-called fringe hospitals that are not approved by any recognized professional evaluating body. Granted that they are inspected by licensing agencies, their evaluation is primarily concerned with the adequacy of fire escapes and the width of doors rather than with professional standards. Consequently, these institutions are havens for unethical and incompetent doctors.

The accredited hospitals often fall down in their duty to discipline the unethical physician by protecting him. While they may attempt to control certain aspects of misconduct of their staff members, such as alcoholism or drug addiction, it is common practice for the hospitals to permit the errant staff member to resign voluntarily. While this serves the immediate purpose of removing him from the staff, the authorities have placed nothing official in the record. Therefore, if the member moves to another locality and a second hospital or licensing board inquires about him, the answer is that he voluntarily resigned from the staff and there is no derogatory information on his record. The usual reason given privately for this is that the authorities did not want to interfere with his means of livelihood. Should this be permitted? Isn't protection of the reputation of the physician, when it is a reputation for incompetence, flagrant disregard of an obligation to protect the welfare of the public?

There are varying degrees of incompetence or unprofessional conduct, many of which do not require the approach of the prosecu-

tor. If the potential danger is not great or the offender is just beginning to show signs of difficulty, members of the staff can informally take preventive or corrective measures. For instance, a friendly talk over lunch may be sufficient.

Disciplinary Functions of Organized Medicine

How well is organized medicine performing its disciplinary functions? For several years, the medical societies were asked to report their disciplinary actions to the American Medical Association, but in 1969, the Department of Medical Ethics abandoned this project as a waste of time. A large number of societies reported no actions at all, while others submitted incomplete reports. The latest figures available were for 1968, when 33 state medical societies reported no procedures whatsoever.[3]

When grievance committees were first inaugurated, they were hailed as representing a great step forward. They have not lived up to their potentials, however. Notable is their lack of initiative and action so that their main function is the adjudication of disputes over fees and squabbles between physicians.

In 1960, the AMA became so concerned about the problems of medical discipline that it appointed a special investigative committee. The committee report[4] reflected broad dissatisfaction with its findings. Of particular concern was the refusal of local medical societies to act. On the recommendation of the committee, the bylaws of the AMA were amended to provide for "original jurisdiction" by the Judicial Council when necessary. To date, the Council has used this power only once.

Medical societies complain because they have little or no authority to discipline unethical members. Moreover, they point to the fact that their most severe penalty, expulsion, does not stop an individual from practicing, but they fail to realize that they have important investigative functions that they are not using effectively.

An Example of Laxity in Disciplinary Functions

An example of the failure of organized medicine to act was disclosed recently by the *New York Times*. A New York physician was alleged, over a period of many years, to have been treating patients with large doses of amphetamines, in some cases with disastrous consequences. The *Times* editorially questioned the fact that medical organizations had not looked into his activities long ago.

Over the byline of Lawrence K. Altman, in the *Times* of Feb. 25, 1973, there is a summary of the case. The reasons for lack of action on the part of the New York County Medical Society were as follows: (1) Investigations are hampered because of lack of manpower. (2) Most physicians are reluctant to initiate complaints and testify against fellow physicians. (3) The final regulatory power lies not with the medical society but with the state government.

The *Times* article further states that although several physicians knew about the physician's practice, as they had treated some of his patients for toxic psychotic reactions resulting from amphetamines, not one complained to the medical society, the reason being, "Some said discussion of another doctor's cases would be a breach of medical ethics." To which Walter H. Judd, MD, Chairman of the AMA Judicial Council replied, "Any physician who gave 'medical ethics' as his reason for not naming to proper authorities any doctor who he knew dispensed amphetamines liberally was not following the profession's established medical ethics but was failing to follow them" Now, at last, the Board of Medical Examiners is investigating.

By no means is the New York County Medical Society the only one that is lax in disciplining its members. This account is merely a case illustrative of certain unsolved problems that have been brought to light by the *Times,* but some good has come of the investigation. The newspaper later quoted the chairman of the censors of the medical society as saying, "We should be grateful because the case opened the eyes of many doctors to the functions of the medical society."

At the 1972 clinical session of the AMA, the Council on Mental Health submitted a report based on several studies of drug dependence and alcoholism among physicians. It stated in part,

> Peer referral for help usually reveals an entrenched "conspiracy of silence." Physicians strongly resist recognition of the fact that any of their members can become ill. This unwillingness to speak out should be abandoned by members of hospital staffs and other colleagues of the ill practitioner, substituting, perhaps, a "conspiracy of constructive compassion."

Does organized medicine adequately discipline unethical physicians? The answer is no.

The Boards of Medical Examiners

The final disciplinary bodies, arms of the state governments, are the boards of medical examiners. Rightfully, the boards seldom concern themselves with minor breaches of ethics. They are mainly interested in violations of the law. It is here that the legal definition of ethics, assuming acceptance of the concept expressed earlier, is synonymous with unprofessional, immoral, or dishonorable conduct. The boards should be the final guardians of the public, but are they?

In considering the boards, conclusions are easier to reach than in the case of the other agencies in that firm data are available. In 1969,[5] a study of disciplinary actions of boards of medical examiners during the preceding five years disclosed that the boards had taken a total of 938 formal actions varying in severity from revocation of licenses to simple reprimands.

During the recent hearings held by the Department of Health, Education, and Welfare Secretary's Commission of Medical Malpractice, several witnesses bitterly attacked the boards of medical examiners. The most vehement criticism came from an attorney who stated that the licensing board of his state (with a physician population of

2,600) had failed to discipline a single physician in the past 15 years, despite the submission of many complaints.

Problems with State Medical Licensing Boards

One fault of the system was found to be incomplete reporting, causing unjust accusations against some boards. Moreover, the situation appears worse if only a single year is examined; a balance may be established over a five-year period. Questionnaires were sent to the secretaries of all the state boards including that of the District of Columbia. Thirty-six replies were received. Combining these results with those previously reported to the Federation of State Medical Boards of the United States, it was possible to add 11 more states, bringing the total to 47.

The number and types of disciplinary actions of state boards from 1968 through 1972 totaled 1,033. Probation heads the list with 400, while 297 licenses were listed under revocation, and 110 were suspensions. Reprimands, often unimportant, numbered 198. These were included, as they did constitute official acts of the boards. Twenty-eight physicians were classed under voluntary surrender of licenses. Therefore, adding these actions to those found in a former study, the boards took 1,971 formal actions against physicians during the past ten years. Considering the fact that there are more than 300,000 physicians in the United States, 0.66 percent of them had difficulty with licensing boards throughout the ten-year period.

During the past five years, seven states with a physician population of more than 23,000 have reported no disciplinary actions whatever. California, with a physician population of approximately 33,000, reported a total of 194. Some of the other large states reported an amazingly small number. For example, one state with a physician population of 17,000 took only six actions, all reprimands. At the opposite extreme, a state with a total of 1,200 physicians reported 25 actions. Excluding California, the five

largest states with a total physician population of 104,000 reported only 140 actions. In other words, 0.58 percent of the California physicians were disciplined, while in the next five states, the percentage was 0.11 percent. Obviously, there is wide variation in the diligence of the state boards in investigating and punishing unethical physicians.

Obstacles to Disciplinary Action

The reasons for the actions were difficult to obtain. In the 442 cases reported, there were 19 different causes of action. Violation of the narcotics laws constituted 48 percent of the total. Although this is a high proportion, it belies a favorite criticism leveled at the boards—they never take action for anything but drug addiction. Granted that narcotics addiction is an occupational hazard for physicians, the fact that 52 percent of the legal procedures is for other causes refutes this accusation.

Boards of medical examiners encounter many obstacles in the investigation and prosecution of unethical physicians. Difficulties arise from politicians, hospital staffs and administrators, the courts, and even from members of the medical profession. Occasionally, the boards are defeated in their aims by the medical practice laws.

The politicians cause trouble mainly in the initial licensing of physicians. Anyone with experience in medical licensure will attest to the fact that politicians from the local through the national level frequently exert tremendous pressure on the boards to license unethical or incompetent doctors. Influence is brought to bear under the guise of helping minority groups or of furnishing medical care to needy communities. Unfortunately, boards sometimes succumb to such pressure and license physicians of questionable ethics and competence. Almost invariably the board members live to regret such leniency.

The problems caused by hospital staffs and administrators have been mentioned previously. A common reason given for shielding the unethical physician is the fear of lawsuits, which often borders on paranoia, but if the hospital authorities have taken proper official action adhering to their bylaws, their chances of being sued are remote. Legal authorities confirm that the fear of suits is indeed a myth. They could find only one case of a successful suit against a public official, a judge, who was found to have acted through malice.

The legal paranoia also extends to private physicians. Many times boards receive calls from them both about applicants for licensure and physicians already licensed. They make outrageous statements about their moral character. Will they put their allegations in writing? Indeed not! Moreover, few will consent to testify at a hearing. Ignorance regarding due process is widespread among the profession. Many members mistakenly believe that the mere voicing of a complaint is sufficient to revoke a license.

Laws and the Courts

While all medical practice laws mention some kind of unethical conduct as grounds for disciplinary proceedings, there is wide variation in the laws, regulations, and policies. Too frequently, the holder of multiple licenses can have his certificate in one state revoked and then move to another state and begin his unethical practices all over again. For instance, in one state drug addiction is grounds for revocation, while in another it calls for reprimand and surrender of the narcotics stamp only. In fact, dilapidated addicts with revoked licenses have been allowed to practice in other states with full knowledge of the authorities. One extreme case involved a physician who practiced in a town near a state line. When his license was revoked in his state of residence, he merely moved his office across the state line and continued to prey on his unsuspecting patients.

The lack of enumeration of professional incompetence in the laws has long been a weapon of defense attorneys who have used it to acquit their clients. An important exception to this was a ruling of the Kansas Supreme Court.[6] The Court overruled the trial court in reversing a decision of the board of medical examiners that had revoked a physician's license for extreme incompetence, supported by the testimony of expert witnesses. The Supreme Court stated that the law could not practically list every act or course of conduct that might disqualify a physician from practice. "No conduct of practice could be more devastating to the health and welfare of a patient or the public than incompetency. Integral to the whole policy the legislature had in mind must be the power of the board to protect against it."

The courts often interfere with the prosecution of the unethical physicians. Serious difficulties arise when the order of the board is stayed pending formal appeal. Judges sometimes grant stay orders ex parte, that is, without hearing the board's arguments. Furthermore, if the district courts should overrule the board's decision, the stay order will remain in effect until the case is settled by the Supreme Court. Therefore, it is often possible for a doctor whose license has been revoked to practice for many months before the matter is finally settled. For example, one physician obtained an ex parte stay order that remained in force for almost two years before the Supreme Court finally upheld the board. During this time, he killed at least two patients and severely injured several more, two of whom sued him for malpractice. The remedy for this obviously lies with the legislatures. They have the authority to outlaw the granting of stay orders ex parte, and they should do so.

An interesting sidelight of the study of medical discipline was the number of instances in which the accused physician had appealed to the courts and with what degree of success. In the past five years there have been 38 appeals. In ten instances, or approximately one quarter of the total, the courts overruled the boards. This is a respectable record, and one might conclude that the boards have expert legal advice, that they move only when the evidence is sound, or both.

Comment

To the question, "Are the boards of medical examiners adequately disciplining unethical physicians?" the answer must be, on the whole, no. Granted that in ten years they took 1,978 actions, the startling figure of only 140 actions in states with 104,000 physicians makes one wonder how many unethical physicians go undetected and unpunished.

One of the most glaring faults of the whole system, involving all the concerned agencies, is the inadequate reporting of disciplinary procedures. The biographical section of the AMA is a well-established repository for actions that have been taken against unethical physicians, but its effectiveness is limited by the reluctance of disciplinary bodies to submit reports.

The medical profession has long insisted that it can best police its own ranks, and it should. Yet, unless all the agencies involved in medical discipline work together to im-prove their methods, outsiders conceivably could take over the control of medical discipline. This must not happen.

NOTES

1. *Darling vs. Charleston Memorial Community Hospital,* 211 NE 2d 253, 1965.
2. J.F. Regan, "Physical Disability and Professional Incompetence," *Federation Bulletin,* vol. 53, p. 318, 1966.
3. 1968 disciplinary report, Department of Medical Ethics. *Journal of the American Medical Association,* vol. 210, p. 1092, 1969.
4. R.W. McKeown, "Present Status of Medical Discipline," *Federation Bulletin,* vol. 48, p. 132, 1961.
5. R.C. Derbyshire, *Medical Licensure and Discipline in the United States,* p. 79, Johns Hopkins Press, Baltimore, 1969.
6. *Kansas State Board of Healing Arts vs. Foote,* 436 P2d 828, 1968.

47.

The Sick Physician
Report of the AMA Council on Mental Health

Accountability to the public, through assurance of competent care to patients by physicians and other health professionals, is a paramount responsibility of organized medicine.

Occasionally such accountability is jeopardized by physicians whose functioning has been impaired by psychiatric disorders, including alcoholism and drug dependence. An equally important issue is the effective treatment and rehabilitation of the physician-patient so that he can be restored to a useful life.

A sampling of boards of medical examiners and other sources reveals a significant problem in this area. Also indicative of the problem, and the difficulty organized medicine has in coping with it, are the numerous requests for guidance received by the American Medical Association.

The Council on Mental Health makes the following observations and recommendations:

1. It is a physician's ethical responsibility to take cognizance of a colleague's inability to practice medicine adequately by reason of physical or mental illness, including alcoholism or drug dependence. Ideally, the affected physician himself

Source: A report of the AMA Council on Mental Health, approved by the Board of Trustees and by the House of Delegates, November 1972.

should seek help when difficulties arise. Often, however, he is unable or unwilling to recognize that a problem exists. When exhortations by family and friends are ineffective and when the physician is unable to make a rational assessment of his ability to function professionally, it becomes essentially the responsibility of his colleagues to make that assessment for him, and to advise him whether he should obtain treatment and curtail or suspend his practice.

In carrying out this task, advising physicians should begin with informal talks and proceed to more formalized approaches only as necessary and according to the following sequence:

(a) Discussion of the problem with other physicians who are in close working relationship with the affected physician, to the end that they will exert their influence in a positive and beneficial manner.

(b) Referral of the problem to the medical staff of the hospital on which the affected physician serves.

(c) Referral of the problem to a specific committee of the state or county medical society if the physician is not a member of a hospital staff, or if the staff is unable or unwilling to act. It should be one created exclusively for the purpose, not an existing one, such as an ethics or a grievance committee. Its function should be to determine whether the physician is suffering from a disorder to a degree that interferes with his ability to practice medicine. The committee should comprise examining physicians including, but not limited to, psychiatrists and neurologists. In carrying out its function, the committee should be guided by procedures that are appropriate to the local situation as worked out by the state or county society.

(d) Referral of the problem to the appropriate licensing body in the state if the physician is not a medical society member, or if the medical society is unable or unwilling to act. The licensing body should have a committee comparable to the one established by the medical society.

2. Spouses can be helpful in bringing physicians into treatment. The spouses should become as fully informed as the society's members about the overall problem and the medical society's approach to its solution. The Woman's Auxiliary should be asked to take an active part in this educational program.

3. AMA's Office of the General Counsel should be requested to draw up a model law to deal with physicians who have such problems, and to disseminate that model to state and county medical societies for legislative action in their jurisdictions.

4. Educational programs should be developed for the medical student and the physician in training, emphasizing their high vulnerability to psychiatric disorders, alcoholism, and drug dependence.

Scope of the Problem among Physicians

The literature since at least the mid-1950s presents numerous reports on studies of drug problems among physicians; several of the reports will be cited here. The number of physicians reported in each study is small, but the findings are consistent.

In 1964, Modlin and Montes[1] noted that estimates of the incidence of narcotic addiction in physicians varied from 30 to 100 times that found in the general population, and they classified such addiction as an occupational hazard. They found that narcotic addiction ordinarily depends on three conditions: (1) a predisposing personality, (2) the availability of narcotics, and (3) a set of circumstances that brings 1 and 2 together. They further noted that the majority of the 30 physicians studied consistently denied serious addictive difficulties and shared the illusion that they could stop using drugs at any time they wished. Reports from England, Germany, Holland, and France indicate that, of the known drug addicts, about 15 percent are physicians and that an additional 15 percent are members of the nursing and pharmacy professions.

In 1969, Vaillant et al.[2] reported a pro-

Disciplinary Action Against Physicians

State	Period of Study (Years)	Average Annual Active Registration	Condition		
			Alcoholism	Drug Dependence	Other Mental Disorders
Arizona	11	1,627	53 (3.2%)	28 (1.7%)	22 (1.3%)
Connecticut	6+	4,682	NA	42 (0.9%)	NA
Oregon	10	2,388	55 (2.3%)	48 (2.0%)	21 (0.9%)

spective study carried out over a 20-year period that showed that a group of 45 physicians took more tranquilizers, sedatives, and stimulants than 90 matched controls. As college sophomores both groups had been selected for the study because of better-than-average physical and psychological health. The physicians drank alcoholic beverages and smoked cigarettes to the same extent as the controls.

Reporting later on a similar controlled study, Vaillant et al.[3] noted that physicians, especially those who treat patients, were more likely than nonphysicians to be involved in heavy drug and alcohol use and to have relatively unsuccessful marriages. The presence of these occupational hazards, however, appear strongly associated with life adjustments before medical school, and those physicians who had the least stable childhoods and adolescent adjustments seemed to be especially vulnerable to these hazards.

Figures obtained from three state boards of medical examiners, shown in the table, give the percentage of the total of actively practicing physicians in each state subject to disciplinary action for alcoholism, drug dependence, and mental disorders for the period of study noted. In 11 years, nearly 2 percent of Arizona's physicians came before the board for disciplinary actions because of drug dependence; in 10 years a similar proportion of Oregon physicians; and in about 6 years, almost 1 percent of Connecticut's physicians.

Thus, in just a decade, 118 drug-depen-

dent physicians have been brought before their disciplinary bodies in three of the smaller states, with an equal number of physicians appearing for alcoholism, and a smaller but significant number for other mental illness.

In 1958, the California State Board of Medical Examiners estimated that at some point in their careers 1 to 2 percent of the physicians in that state abused narcotics. Currently that board handles 125 disciplinary cases a year, well over half of them involving narcotics.

Apart from the cases of alcohol and drug dependence that come before disciplinary bodies with relatively high frequency, there are, as in the general population, other less visible diagnostic entities of mental disorders occurring with perhaps greater frequency among physicians. Specific studies of the epidemiology of mental disorder in physicians are few, but Duffy,[4, 5] in a survey of physicians treated at the Mayo Clinic, found the following diagnoses (in order of prevalence): affective psychosis, psychoneurosis, schizophrenia, personality disorder, and organic brain syndrome.

The psychotic reactions, without question, impair the ill physician's judgment and ability to practice, and a psychoneurosis or a personality disorder of sufficient degree can constitute a similar risk to the safety of the patient.

Suicide is generally accepted to be one of the major behavioral consequences of mental illness. Demographic data were compiled on

249 physicians listed in the *Journal of the American Medical Association* obituary columns from May 1965 to November 1967 as having died by suicide.[6] Suicides exceeded the combined deaths from automobile accidents, plane crashes, drowning, and homicide. In addition, 56 deaths were reported as possible suicides. The total of all these violent deaths is 534, or over 5 percent of all the physicians' deaths during that period, according to Blachly et al.[6]

The mean suicidal age was 49, at or near the usual productive peak for a physician. Abuse of alcohol or drugs was an important factor in two-fifths of the cases, and depressive illness was very common. Medical specialty was an important variable: Suicide ranged from a low of 0.01 percent among pediatricians to a high of 0.6 percent among psychiatrists.

About 100 physicians commit suicide annually, equivalent to the size of the average medical school graduating class. The comments of two widows of physicians who died by suicide[6] were: "I sought a colleague but for reasons of his own, he would not try. Could there be a board or group of doctors to whom a wife can turn?" and "If it were possible to have a telephone number available to persons in remote areas as this, and trained personnel who would help, suicides such as his could be prevented. *This was such a waste!*"

No information could be found on the incidence of organic brain syndromes among physicians; but no county medical society can disclaim knowledge of this slowly developing and chronic disorder in one or a few of its members, usually associated with advanced age or gradual impairment of cerebral blood supply. Watchful colleagues can usually protect the patients concerned, but eventually a crisis develops because of a major omission or commission, an improper prescription or dosage, or a frank error in practice judgment. Acute organic disorders, as with psychotic illness, may cause a rapid change in physician behavior that is less amenable to controlling intervention by colleagues.

Programs by State Medical Societies

Threat of suspension or revocation of the license to prescribe narcotics or the license to practice medicine may, in some cases, be an incentive toward rehabilitation or a deterrent to drug abuse. In many other cases, however, it may work against the physician admitting to himself or to others that he has a problem.

A letter to the Council, quoted here in part, is illustrative:

I am a member of your association and I should greatly appreciate any information relating to the all-too-common problem of physicians becoming addicted to narcotics.

As can be surmised I had such a problem myself for one year and have been free of drug abuse for six months. The wrath incurred shall be many years in subsiding, however. I found much help from a few MD's who (themselves) had overcome such a problem—really more help than from psychiatrists, who tend to categorize the physician with the street-dwelling heroin pushers. I spent a month at the Federal Narcotics Hospital at Fort Worth, Texas, and I found I barely spoke the same language.

One of the many things to be warned against is the insidiousness of onset and the inevitable denial which follows—especially with the most commonly used drug, meperidine.

Another physician, a drug-dependent pediatrician, writing in a medical news journal,[7] stated:

I am that common but rarely mentioned problem, the drug-addict doctor. Depending on whom you talk to, I am an amoral bum, an ill-used and tragic figure, an embarrassing statistic, a blameless sick man, or a disgrace to the profession.

Actually I am none of these things or perhaps a little bit of all of them, but eight years of fighting the problem have made one thing discouragingly clear:

the most enlightened medical profession that civilization has ever known, in the wealthiest country in history, doesn't know how to treat me, and really doesn't want to know. The profession that has for generations battled to keep the government from intervening between the doctor and his patient is content to let a federal tax agency tell it what to prescribe for me.

The Council sent a letter to all state medical society executives noting its interest in drug-dependent, alcoholic, and psychiatrically disordered physicians and inquiring whether any state or county medical society has established an outstanding and effective program for handling the difficult and serious problem of such physicians. Of 54 societies canvassed (including Puerto Rico, the Virgin Islands, the Canal Zone, and the District of Columbia), 37 responded. Seven of the respondents indicated that there is an active committee at the state level charged with the problem, and that the state either has, or has pending, a "sick doctor statute." Another seven reported having no active program but indicated that either some related action was pending or they had been stimulated into initiating action on the basis of the letter of inquiry. The remaining respondents (23) stated there was no county or state society program directed at such a problem, and three went so far as to deny vehemently that any such problems even existed in their states. It could be surmised that among the nonrespondents—almost one-third of the total number of state associations—there is an indifference about these problems, or a denial of their existence.

The San Francisco Medical Society has activated an advisory committee for physicians. Its purpose is "to serve physicians who have emotional problems. Other physicians may contact the committee when they feel that a colleague is in need of its help. The physician in question will then be contacted, confidentially, in an effort to help him understand his problem."

A similar group in Oregon (Friends of Medicine), having both physicians and lay members and somewhat broader goals, has evolved outside the structure of organized medicine in the belief that the group is more effective and more acceptable to the sick doctor if it is not under the aegis of a medical association or a board of medical examiners.

The "Sick Doctor Statute"

The pioneering effort in the development of a "sick doctor statute" came in the 1969 Florida legislature, which revised grounds for professional discipline under the medical practice act of that state to protect the public further against the incompetent or unqualified practice of medicine.[8]

A similar "sick doctor statute" became law in Texas in 1971. Prior to the passage of the legislation in these two states, as in most states today, disciplining a practitioner of the healing arts was predicated on his commission of misconduct on one or more of a variety of specified grounds, provided that fault could be proved against the practitioner. In most states, even though a physician's fitness or ability to practice may be substandard, no violation of the applicable medical practice act occurs unless his alleged misconduct violates a specified standard of behavior. Such a law leaves a board of medical examiners impotent in its desire to protect the public against a physician's incompetence or inability to practice medicine, unless the physician has also committed an act predicated on fault. Many state laws have a provision automatically suspending a physician's license if he is adjudged mentally incompetent or is committed for psychiatric care, but as is well known, such a last-resort legal action rarely occurs in the case of a physician-patient.

The "sick doctor statute" defines the inability of a physician to practice medicine with reasonable skill and safety to his patients, because of one or more enumerated illnesses. It eliminates the need to allege or prove that a physician's clinical judgment was actually impaired or that he actually injured a patient. The defined inability can be the result of organic illness, mental or emotional disorders, deterioration through the aging process, or loss of motor skill. Further, the inability can arise from excessive use or abuse of narcotics, drugs and chemicals, alcohol, or similar types of material.

The act provides that, prior to board action against a physician, there must be probable cause of his inability to practice medicine with reasonable skill and safety to his patients. The intent of this provision is to protect physicians from harassment by capricious accusations.

If probable cause is shown, the physician is required to submit to diagnostic mental or physical examinations. He has given implied consent for such examination, under this statute, by using his license to practice or by registering his license annually. The doctrine of implied consent is further used in the law to remove privileged communications that ordinarily exist between physician and patient. A physician so ordered to examination waives this legal privilege, thus making available to the administrative trial records of the examiners' consultation and diagnostic tests, and testimony.

The accused physician has the right to receive copies of the examining physicians' reports and diagnosis, and there is provision for his taking the deposition of his examiners. Further, his own medical expert may present testimony.

Following the hearing, if the board determines that the physician is indeed unable to practice, it may suspend his license and, in addition, place him on probation. The board may compel a physician to seek therapy from a physician designated by the board, or it may restrict his areas of practice to those in which he is still believed to be competent. Suspension of licensure privileges is specified to be only for the duration of impairment, and the sick doctor is guaranteed the opportunity to demonstrate to the board that his license should be reinstated when he is competent to practice again.

A further provision, again protecting the ill physician, is the guarantee that neither the record of the proceedings nor any unfavorable order entered against him can be used against him in any other legal proceeding, such as malpractice action, a divorce proceeding, or a suit to challenge his testamentary capacity.

During the first year after its enactment in Florida, the statute was most frequently used for physicians manifesting incompetency due to excessive use of drugs or alcohol. These are the most common disciplinary problems coming before medical boards.

A departure from the usual centralized medical examining board approach is found in the Medical Practice Act of Delaware. About 12 years ago, a medical censor committee was created in each Delaware county, consisting of three members of the county medical society, appointed by the medical council or board from a list submitted by the medical society. The powers delegated to these committees include those of subpoena and discipline of the allegedly incompetent physician, subject only to the approval of the medical council. It seems doubtful that this decentralization, though closer to a peer-review mechanism, would be entirely desirable, since it places considerable power in the hands of persons who might be inexperienced in such matters, however well they might know the ill physician.

A desirable feature for inclusion in the medical practice act of all states is found in the existing codes of Arizona and Virginia. In both jurisdictions it is mandatory that any licensed physician report to the board of medical examiners any information he may acquire that tends to show that any physician may be unable to practice medicine safely. It also provides for civil immunity under the law for any physician so reporting in good faith.

In cases of drug-dependent physicians, all state boards of medical examiners would be wise to follow a supervised rehabilitation program of sufficient duration to give the physician every opportunity to remain drug-free. Representative of a number of state boards pursuing such a course is California. A former member of the board, Dr. William F. Quinn, states:

We've found that rehabilitation is facilitated by allowing the doctor to practice medicine. So, with first offenders, the board takes away the doctor's narcotics stamp and revokes his license, but places a stay of execution of the revocation. The sword of revocation hanging over him is very effective, much more so than the seemingly more charitable approach of issuing warnings and reprimands for first offenders. The temptation to return to drugs is just too strong for a doctor to resist testing the board.

After a second offense, Dr. Quinn noted, 85 percent of the violators have their licenses immediately suspended or revoked. A recent study by the California board showed rehabilitation to be successful in 85 of 100 physicians on probation for abuse of narcotics. Of the remainder, ten returned to use of drugs and five committed suicide.[9]

The Undergraduate Problem

Of particular concern for the future are the incidence of use of, and the attitude toward, psychotropic substances among medical students and physicians-in-training. These young men and women progress into the area of total, unsupervised responsibility for patient care, where impeccable judgment and unclouded thinking are the primary bulwarks protecting them from malpractice.

A statement by the AMA Committee on Alcoholism and Drug Dependence reads, in part

> Because physicians are accessible to most types of dangerous drugs and because they often work under sustained pressure, which may enhance the seeking of drugs for relief, physicians appear to be a high-risk population in terms of exposure to drug abuse. This potential should be clearly recognized by medical students and there should be opportunities in the curriculum for them to explore their personal posture with respect to drug use and, if desirable, its impact on their role as therapists.

Medical students also should have opportunities to discuss these matters *in confidence* with appropriate experienced physicians.

Conclusion

In dealing with a "sick doctor," the preparation of guidelines to assist organized medicine to deal with the problem first necessitates delineation of boundaries of responsibility.

First, the primary responsibility for ensuring safe, competent care to the patient population affected must be reemphasized. Parallel to that concern is the welfare of the ill physician, his family, and his colleagues.

The physician-patient is first in the hierarchy of responsibility. As with the lay patient, the drug-dependent or alcoholic physician must recognize that he has a mental disorder and communicate with a competent source of assistance; he must voice his chief complaint and seek help.

Experience in such situations is often disappointing as the physician-patient denies he is ill, lacks insight into his problem, avoids medical assistance, and minimizes his problem outright. Therefore, an element of coercion is often necessary. The family is more often than not ineffectual in exerting pressure, which must then come from some other source.

Peer referral for help usually reveals an entrenched "conspiracy of silence." Physicians strongly resist recognition of the fact that any of their number can become ill. Members of hospital staffs and other colleagues of the ill practitioner should be willing to speak out, substituting, perhaps, a "conspiracy of constructive compassion."

The Council on Mental Health has therefore recommended the following referral pattern: If the individual physician cannot be persuaded informally to seek help, the problem should be taken up by the medical staff of the hospital; if that avenue is not feasible, a specially designated committee of the state or county medical society should be consulted; and if the medical society is unable or unwilling to act, the matter should be referred to the appropriate licensing body in the state.

Notes

1. H.C. Modlin and A. Montes, "Narcotic Addiction in Physicians," *American Journal of Psychiatry*, vol. 121, p. 358, 1964.

2. G.E. Vaillant, J.R. Brighton, and C. McArthur, "Physicians' Use of Mood-Altering Drugs," *New England Journal of Medicine*, vol. 282, p. 365, 1970.

3. G.E. Vaillant, N.C. Sobowale, and C. McArthur, "Some Psychological Vulnerabilities of Physicians," *New England Journal of Medicine*, vol. 287, p. 372, 1972.

4. J.C. Duffy, "Emotional Illness in Physicians," *Medical Tribune*, March 26, 1967, p. 15.

5. J.C. Duffy and E.M. Litin, "Psychiatric Morbidity of Physicians," *Journal of the American Medical Association*, vol. 189, p. 989, 1964.

6. P.H. Blachly, W. Disher, and G. Roduner, "Suicide by Physicians," *Bulletin of Suicidology, National Institute of Mental Health*, December 1968, p. 1.

7. Anonymous, "What It's Like to Be a Doctor-Addict," *Medical World News*, vol. 7, p. 57, July 1, 1966.

8. J. Nesbitt, "The Sick Doctor Statute: A New Approach to an Old Problem," *Federal Bulletin*, vol. 57, p. 266, 1970.

9. J. Middleton, "Drug Abuse—Growing Occupational Hazard for Doctors," *Hospital Physician*, vol. 6, p. 60, October 1970.

48.

The Problem of Defensive Medicine

Laurence R. Tancredi   Jeremiah A. Barondess

Recent years have witnessed a progressive increase in the number of malpractice claims brought against physicians;[1] some estimates have placed the rate of increase as high as 10 percent annually. In addition there have been a number of well-publicized high awards, some in the million dollar range. Recoveries of this order of magnitude are thought by many to encourage yet more malpractice suits. One derivative of these trends has been a marked increase in malpractice insurance premiums,[2] which have risen from a total of about $60 million per year in the early 1960s to an estimated current total well in excess of $1 billion anually.[3] Some specialists, such as orthopedic and plastic surgeons, pay as much as $40,000 per year for malpractice coverage in some parts of the country.[4] These costs are, to a large measure, passed on to the patient, and inevitably affect the overall cost of medical care.

In addition to the significant impact that medical malpractice suits are having directly on the cost of medical care, many believe they are having an even more profound indirect effect on these costs by inducing physicians to resort to defensive medical practices. These practices are said to occur when specific diagnostic and treatment measures are employed explicitly for the purposes either of averting a possible lawsuit or of providing appropriate documentation that a wide range of tests and treatments has been used in the patient's care. Defensive medicine, according to the Secretary's Commission on Medical Malpractice, can be characterized as either positive or negative.[5,6] Positive defensive medicine is the use of diagnostic or therapeutic measures to protect the physician or health care provider from being found liable. Many of these measures are felt to be unnecessary for the proper care of the patient. Negative defensive medicine, in contrast, refers to the withholding of diagnostic or therapeutic techniques that might be medically justified in light of the patient's

Source: *Science*, vol. 200, no. 4344, May 26, 1978.

physical condition but are accompanied by more than the usual risk of an adverse outcome and could thus serve as the basis for a malpractice suit. Positive defensive medicine may not only result in an inflation of health care costs through the overuse of laboratory and treatment facilites but may also expose patients to the risks of adverse outcomes from the procedures themselves. Negative defensive medicine has minimal, if any, effects on health care costs but may result in suboptimal medical care for the patient by denying a potentially beneficial diagnostic or treatment procedure.[6]

The medical and health care literature is replete with references to the impact of defensive medicine on the cost and quality of patient care. Some have concluded that defensive medicine is so pervasive in the medical community as to suggest that the actions of as many as 70 percent of the physicians in this country are influenced by the fear of litigation.[5] The effect of these practices on the cost of medical care has been estimated to be considerable. The Health Insurance Association of America has indicated that defensive medicine induced by fear of malpractice suits may itself create annual costs of $3 to $6 billion.[3] In 1975, the former Secretary of Health, Education, and Welfare, Caspar Weinberger, indicated his belief that as much as $7 billion a year may be spent on defensive medicine that provides no benefit to the patient.[7] Others have disagreed, pointing out the lack of good studies documenting the extent of defensive medicine, and suggesting that its effects are probably small relative to both the cost and the quality of patient care.[6, 8] Somers has suggested that defensive medicine and medical malpractice are being used as convenient scapegoats for the ever-expanding costs of medical care and has suggested that a more significant factor in these escalating costs may be the fact that hospitals derive financial benefit from introducing new technologies into their practice settings,[1] thus creating incentives for increasing the range as well as the utilization of laboratory tests in hospitals.

A Review of the Data

The studies conducted to assess the extent and nature of defensive medicine have created more controversy than resolution of the issue. One of the more frequently quoted addressed only indirectly the issue of defensive medicine. This study involved examination of the effectiveness of x-rays in the evaluation of head injuries.[9] A prospective study was conducted, requiring the cooperation of physicians working in the emergency rooms of two academically associated hospitals. These physicians were asked to complete a form describing the severity of patients' injuries, the likelihood of a skull fracture, and the reasons for ultimately requesting that an x-ray examination be performed. In 1 year 1500 x-rays were ordered and evaluated by radiologists. Ninety-three fractures were discovered; diagnosis of 28 of these fractures (30 percent) resulted in an alteration of the course of treatment. The researchers identified 21 specific clinical findings—for example, the presence of neurologic abnormalities and vomiting—that were associated with a high yield of skull fracture on x-ray examination. Had these criteria been applied to the study group, about 100 x-rays would have been ordered, and would have documented 92 fractures. Those patients who presented with, at most, one or two of the index clinical findings would have fallen into the low-yield group, and could have been effectively treated without a skull x-ray; of the 435 patients who would have fallen into this group, only one presented a fracture. The researchers argued that x-rays of this low-yield group could have been omitted or possibly deferred without creating any adverse effects on the patients. Because the researchers found no clear reason for ordering these x-rays, they concluded that medical-legal reasons must have been operating, and that the excessive use of x-rays in the emergency room situation reflects the defensive practice of medicine. A separate study of skull x-rays in children suffering from head trauma arrived at the same conclusion. In this study, 570 children consecutively admitted to an emergency room after head trauma had skull x-rays performed. Only one of these x-rays actually resulted in affecting the treatment that the child received.[10]

Studies such as these reflect the difficulty in determining when use of diagnostic procedures is motivated by concern about lawsuits. The physician confronted with the individual patient must make a diagnostic judgment on which to base a therapeutic action. Ancillary examinations such as skull x-rays are seen by many as reducing the degree of uncertainty in such a situation. It seems at least as likely that forces such as these are operative; the ready assumption that legal considerations are paramount seems at best simplistic. A recent study of the efficacy of diagnostic radiological procedures resulted in different findings and conclusions.[11] In an evaluation of x-ray practices in emergency rooms seven common procedures were examined—x-rays of the skull, cervical spine, lumbar spine, chest, abdomen, extremities, and kidneys (by intravenous pyelogram)—which constitute approximately 90 percent of the radiologic studies ordered in the emergency room. A total of 8658 cases were studied, of which 1039 involved skull x-rays. It was concluded that at most only a small fraction, perhaps 5 percent, of those x-ray examinations had had little or no input into the choice of diagnoses by the primary physician. At the time the clinicians requested the x-rays they were substantially uncertain about the accuracy of their diagnoses. Medical-legal reasons were infrequently suggested as the basis for request of an x-ray examination. However, when medical-legal reasons were cited by the clinicians, the influence of x-rays on diagnostic reasoning was still present, although, perhaps, to a somewhat smaller degree.

Attempts to Determine Extent of Defensive Medicine

In addition to the studies on the utilization and efficacy of x-ray diagnosis there have been several attempts to address directly the extent to which defensive medicine

operates. The first of these was conducted in 1970 by the *Duke Law Journal*.[6] Ten medical specialties were selected for study because they include procedures which, when used, might reasonably be considered to be motivated by the threat of medical malpractice. Hypothetical situations were constructed around these specialty disciplines, and questions were asked pertaining to the use of specific procedures. The questionnaires relevant to each of these ten specialties were sent to 100 practitioners in each of two states—California, where malpractice insurance rates as well as number of malpractice claims are high, and North Carolina, which ranks relatively low in both.

Of more than 1500 questionnaires that were distributed, approximately 54 percent were returned. The results indicated that the malpractice threat does influence practitioner decision making, but particularly in the direction of practicing positive defensive medicine, which might lead to enhancement of the quality of care. Even so, this influence is not as great as previously estimated by others. In fact, the overall assessment suggested that procedures thought to result from fear of malpractice suits are not frequently performed by the practitioners of the various specialties selected. Paradoxically, physicians in North Carolina, where the malpractice threat is significantly lower than California, actually followed the practices outlined in the questionnaire more often than did those in California.

This survey of physicians, although it represents a very small sample in each specialty, supports the position that the practice of defensive medicine is by no means extensive, and is probably not a contributing factor to the escalation of medical care costs in this country. Other factors, such as the lack of meaningful cost constraints on physicians, the demands of patients for what they perceive to be optimum care, and the growing sophistication and cost of new technologies were felt by the journal staff to be more compelling reasons for overutilization of medical resources. Even when physicians acknowledged that they overutilized x-rays, they did not relate this to the threat of medical malpractice suits. As an illustration of this, orthopedists, who are often sued for medical malpractice, were asked whether they would order x-rays under a variety of circumstances. Among the hypothetical situations was one involving a young, healthy, male adult who might have injured his ribs in an accident. A variety of reasons were given by those physicians who indicated they would order an x-ray in these circumstances. Some simply claimed that this was the usual practice that they followed, even though they questioned the cost and efficacy of the x-ray.[6]

Opinion Surveys

Besides these two studies several recent opinion surveys have also tried to assess the extent of defensive medicine. In 1974, more than 4000 randomly selected physicians were questioned regarding 15 specific actions that might be taken to lessen the chance of a malpractice suit.[12] Of approximately 1400 who responded to the questionnaire, 80 percent indicated that they had taken at least one of the 15 measures presented (such as referring more cases, using consultations, being more selective in accepting new patients, and ordering diagnostic tests), because they were sensitive to the possibilities of a legal suit. Many of the physicans, however, indicate that some of the actions that they took for the purpose of avoiding a malpractice suit also turned out to be highly beneficial for the patient. In a 1976 study of the response of physicians to the increase of insurance premiums in California, investigators surveyed third-year resident physicians, as well as medical and specialty societies in that state, and found that the threat of medical malpractice had not had a significant impact on medical practice.[13]

Last year, the American Medical Association Center for Health Services, Research, and Development participated in a survey of 500 physicians regarding the practice of defensive medicine. Of 111 who responded, 76 percent indicated that they are now practicing defensive medicine; 92 percent indicated that they are more aware of the possibility of a suit than they had been in the past.[14] Nearly 76 percent indicated that they believed that defensive medicine is responsible, in some measure, for the increase in the cost of medical care. Some indicated that it might be responsible for as much as a 50 percent increase.

The Unresolved Issues

The available studies of defensive medicine, as noted, are limited by statistical and definitional difficulties. None is sufficient to characterize the problem of the influence of malpractice suits on medical care. Thus, in both the Duke[6] and Pittsburgh[8] studies, the sample sizes were too small to permit a reliable conclusion. In some of the surveys conducted the small percentage of responses to a wide range of questions precludes placing any reliance on the results.

One of the most difficult issues to be addressed if we are to understand the nature and extent of defensive medicine is that of defining appropriate standards of care for various medical conditions. Standards in most specialties of medicine have not been clearly described, so that what might appear to be defensive medical practice to one clinician may, to another, be quality medical care. The study on the use of skull x-rays in head trauma takes the position that discovering one fracture in 435 x-rays does not justify the extensive use of this diagnostic procedure. However, from the perspective of the physician making a decision about the appropriate treatment of an individual patient,[11] it may be high-quality care to obtain the x-ray in order to reach a greater degree of certainty in the evaluation of the patient's condition. Defensive medicine as a concept is not easily understood in a way that would avert the conceptual difficulties in distinguishing between those acts which are clearly the result of fear of malpractice suits and those which may be perceived as acceptable medical practice.

As pointed out by David Mechanic,[15] much of the argument around the defensive practice of medicine is closely associated with the wide range of disagreement regarding standards of medical practice.[16] To whatever extent they exist, standards of medical care have been focused primarily on the processes of practice rather than the outcomes of medical intervention. Hence, the standards by which physicians are evaluated in terms of malpractice are based on how their diagnostic and therapeutic measures compare with those of other physicians in their locality or specialty. The focus of an individual evaluation tends to center on the process of a physician's judgment and assessment of the patient, rather than on the outcomes of practice. On a broader scale, our traditional approaches to the evaluation of medical practices have sometimes resulted in institutionalizing modalities of care that have later turned out to be of questionable merit in terms of patient outcomes. In other words, the validation of clinical processes is developing slowly, and has proved especially difficult after procedures have been diffused into the care system. One instance of this may be the study by Mather et al. of death rates in acute myocardial infarction, which suggested no advantage in coronary unit care as compared with care at home.[17] Even more striking are the recent studies indicating that coronary bypass surgery may not be as effective as has been thought in the treatment of patients with coronary occlusive disease.[18]

Need for Outcome Assessment

The point is that one cannot handle accurately the issues involved in defensive medicine without having first established epidemiologically the soundness of medical procedures as they relate to specific outcomes in patients. The wide range of disagreement concerning many procedures and practices suggests the need for outcome assessment.

An illustration of this phenomenon can be seen in the increased use of cesarean deliveries in this country. At the 1977 meeting of The American College of Obstetricians and Gynecologists, it was reported that the rate of cesarean sections over the past 10 years has doubled.[19] Some believe that cesarean sections have become more prevalent because of the increasing rate of litigation around birth trauma, and that minimal attention has been paid to the risks, which are not unlike those attending any surgical procedure where anesthesia must be administered. However, there is evidence of a decrease in perinatal mortality coincident with the increase in cesarean births.[20]

The application of fetal monitoring devices during labor has also increased greatly.[20] Although the overall benefits of electronic fetal monitoring have not been clearly established, some argue that the prevention of a percentage of fetal deaths in high-risk groups warrants its widespread use, even though three-fourths of all pregnancies probably fall into low-risk groups that might just as effectively be monitored by highly skilled general nursing care.[20] The physician who uses such precautions may not be doing it out of concern for the defensive medical aspects. The increases in cesarean sections and electronic fetal monitoring illustrate the conceptual difficulties in trying to assess the impact of defensive medicine on medical practice. From one perspective, they can be seen as a direct response to the growing number of suits around fetal injuries. On the other hand, these procedures do enchance perinatal health.

The second major conceptual issue is also related to questions of standards of medical care, and concerns the degree of risk that is acceptable in the physician-patient relationship. Many so-called defensive procedures arguably seem extreme from a statistical standpoint, in light of the benefits they produce. On the other hand, as has been pointed out above, when physicians order such tests, they cannot be aware of which individual may have an altered course of treatment. Furthermore, societal expectations of medical practice demand a high degree of certainty. These factors undoubtedly contribute to the pressures on physicians to employ various tests and procedures that may result in low diagnostic yields.

Conclusion

The definition of defensive medicine is loose and ambiguous; the incentives operating on the physician to conduct a wide variety of laboratory and other diagnostic tests are broader than the threat of medical malpractice suits alone. The studies we have discussed are not definitive, but they do not support the notion of widespead defensive medical practices, nor do they indicate a major impact on the increasing cost of care. At the same time, it is virtually impossible to assess directly the overall impact of defensive medicine, since much of what enters into the decision-making processes of physicians has been determined through the acculturating processes in medical education. The nature of that education is inevitably influenced not only by the scientific knowledge of the day, but also by the range of societal responses to the care being delivered. Hence, individual physicians may be unable to respond accurately to inquiries regarding the extent to which they are being influenced by the increase in medical malpractice suits. Many physicians feel strongly that defensive medicine is an operating factor in medical practice and, although these perceptions may be inflated, they cannot be ignored, as there has been a heightened sensitivity and awareness by all providers of health care of the possibilities of malpractice suits. Even more problematic is the question of whether defensive practices are beneficial for patients or instead result in nonproductive medical activities that are both costly and potentially harmful. The distinction between these two cannot be resolved until standards of care are established for each specialty and for specific medical diagnoses and treatments.

Until we establish the basis for assessing standards of medical care, particularly as they relate to the outcomes of practice, a new study on the role of defensive medicine would probably provide little additional information. One possible exception would be a study that would clarify the nature of medical injuries that occur in various care settings, with particular attention directed to those injuries that result from diagnostic procedures that may be considered to be "defensive" in a variety of circumstances. Clearly defined standards of care may be established in time by professional standards review organizations or groupings within the profession, and may provide a meaningful basis for evaluating overutilization of laboratory procedures and treatment facilities, thereby providing some method for measuring the impact of malpractice suits on medical practice. Perhaps even more important than focusing on the design of studies for assessing defensive medicine would be an examination of the incentive of a medical injury compensation system that would effectively promote positive rather than negative defensive practices. Some of the alterations of the existing malpractice system that have been proposed over the past few years, such as arbitration and automatic systems of compensation, have been geared specifically to that objective.[21] In addition to the incentives of the system, attention must also be directed at developing effective information disclosure methods, so that patients can participate more fully in decisions affecting their medical care. A thorough attempt to educate patients about the benefits and risks of various procedures should not only result in a decrease in the use of negative defensive practices, but may also decrease the number of suits and alleviate concerns about medical liability. Attention should be directed at structuring a fair and equitable system for compensation and patient redress; the problems surrounding defensive medicine would likely be resolved in the process of accomplishing these objectives.

Finally, it should be emphasized that the defensive medicine issue is not the basic problem, but a symptom of it. The underlying difficulty is the parlous state of our compensation system for medical injury; when this has been addressed comprehensively the problems of defensive medicine will fade.

NOTES

1. H. Somers, *Milbank Memorial Fund Quarterly*, vol. 55, p. 193, spring 1977.

2. R. H. Brook, R. L. Brutoco, and K. N. Williams, *Duke Law Journal*, 1975, p. 1197.

3. In *A Review of the Medical Malpractice Problem in the United States* (Health Insurance Associations of America, Washington, D.C., 1975) it is reported that hospitals and physicians together were expected to pay approximately $1.5 billion for malpractice insurance. This was probably a high estimate.

4. Data for California Physicians as of January 1, 1976.

5. *Report of the Secretary's Commission on Medical Malpractice*, DHEW Publication OS-73-89, Department of Health, Education, and Welfare, Washington, D.C., 1973.

6. *Duke Law Journal*, 1971, p. 939.

7. C. Weinberger, *Arizona Medicine*, vol. 32, p. 117, 1975.

8. N. Hershey, *Milbank Memorial Fund Quarterly*, vol. 50, p. 96, 1972.

9. R. S. Bell and J. W. Loop, *New England Journal of Medicine*, vol. 284, p. 236, 1971.

10. *Medical Tribune*, October 26, 1970, p. 1.

11. L. B. Lusted, chairman, Committee on Efficacy Studies, American College of Radiology, "A study of the efficacy of diagnostic radiologic procedures," report submitted to director, National Center for Health Services Research, Department of Health, Education, and Welfare, May 31, 1977.

12. H. T. Paxton et al., *Medical Economics*, September 30, 1974, p. 69.

13. A. Lipson, *Medical Malpractice: The Response of Physicians to Premium Increases in California*, Rand Corporation, Santa Monica, Calif., 1976.

14. *American Medical News*, March 28, 1977, p. 1.

15. D. Mechanic, *Duke Law Journal*, 1975, p. 1179.

16. L. N. Koran, *New England Journal of Medicine*, vol. 293, p. 642, 1975; Institute of Medicine, *The Efficacy of Medical Care: A Review of Current Evidence on Major Procedures*, National Academy of Sciences, Washington, D.C., 1975.

17. H. G. Mather et al., *British Medical Journal*, vol. 3, p. 334, 1971.

18. L. S. Cohen, *Connecticut Medicine*, vol. 40, p. 509, 1976; G. B. Kolata, *Science*, vol. 194, p. 1263, 1976.

19. A. L. Cochrane, *Effectiveness and Efficiency: Random Reflections of Clinical Practice*, Burgess, London, 1972.

20. C. L. Cetrulo and R. Freeman, in *Risks in the Practice of Modern Obstetrics*, S. Aladjen, ed. (Mosby, St. Louis, 1975); see also E. H. Hon and R. N. Petrie, *Clinical Obstetrics and Gynecology*, vol. 18, p. 1, 1975.

21. Congressional Research Service, Library of Congress, "Medical malpractice: A survey of associated problems and proposed remedies," H. E. Schmidt, ed. January 15, 1975), p. 11; C. Havighurst and L. Tancredi, *Milbank Memorial Fund Quarterly*, vol. 51, p. 125, spring 1973.

III. ISSUES IN CLINICAL ETHICS

This section provides extensive discussion of the procedures and features of medical practice which generate ethical controversy. The readings have been organized into five sections, each with a short introduction. In accord with the policy of the text we have selected pieces which provide descriptions of the medical situations at issue and discussion of some alternative courses of action open to the health professional. Certain items advocate specific positions, some merely comment on a recurrent situation, and others analyze the legal and ethical problems in detail. Given the rich diversity of medical practice it is not possible to cover all situations in depth. We trust that there is sufficient material for supporting extensive thoughtful class discussion.

The division into sections follows the major general concerns of practicing physicians and health care providers. First there is the issue of informed consent within the clinical situation. In this section we are concerned to present the diverse ways in which the abstract concept of a person's voluntary participation being expressed in an informed consent is realized in troubling medical situations. Several of the selections focus upon specific cases which by necessity involve a particular type of patient or treatment. However, the issues raised pertain to all kinds of medical care.

The generality of the issue is also characteristic of the next section concerned with the aggressiveness of patient care. This is another notion that derives from the working reality of medicine and far transcends the usual abstract discussion of euthanasia which focuses upon simple dichotomies, e.g., to let die or not. In reality, the physician is confronted by a wide range of treatment choices that provide varying degrees of support to their patients. Further, there are varying degrees of acuteness, irreversibility, chronicity, etc., that raise complex moral problems.

In the third section we provide seven units, dealing with some ethical issues in specific clinical contexts. Noteworthy is the inclusion of a section on placebos which discusses their relevance to medical practice and the question of deception in their administration. There are also selections which discuss the latest technology involved in transplantation, gender identity, and reproduction, as well as the more standard issues of abortion and involuntary psychiatric hospitalization.

The fourth section discusses a subject which is often copresent in many medical care situations, namely, the conduct of biomedical experimentation. There are selections which examine some of the general issues concerned with the justification of experimentation and its regulation, as well as a variety of pieces discussing specific sorts of experimentation, e.g., with the elderly, children, fetuses, prisoners, and with specific disease, such as Huntington's disease.

Finally we conclude with an all too brief section on the delivery of care. Although issues related to this topic were presented under the Right to Health Care in the section on Conceptual Foundations, the items included in this section are intended to focus upon the discussions generated by the development and allocation of important technologies and services, e.g., kidney dialysis, kidney transplant, and heart transplant. There are related selections in the subsection on Transplantation in the section on Clinical Treatments and Procedures above. We would have liked to include a section on the economic aspects of health care. There is a developing literature on the nature of the market mechanism as a basis for regulating the purchase of health care services and products, the incentives and values present in our large insurance mechanisms, the role of the government and "safety-net" policies, and the role of regulation in both the delivery of care and the production of medical products such as drugs and diagnostic equipment. But space limitations prohibit a further extension of the text.

Informed Consent and Refusal of Treatment

In the above section (II.C) on Doctor-Patient Communication we discussed the centrality of communication as a process in the clinical relationship. In this section we focus upon the need for the patient's consent in order to perform most clinical procedures. The receiving of consent is usually understood as a specific *act* of communication, something that occurs at one particular time, either verbally or in written form. The increasing need to document the record of health care for both legal and financial reasons has led to the development of standard forms for consent as well as a large literature on the subject. But as with other aspects of communication, consent is itself a process which occurs over time even when it can be finalized or ritualized in documents and performances. The items on interviewing in the above sections are relevant to these issues.

The selections in this section begin with an account of informed consent by George Annas which briefly reviews the legal doctrine. We then present an extended discussion of the case of David G., a critically burned patient, and a critique of the underlying presuppositions of consent as a procedure by Robert Burt. It is his contention that our medical and legal framework of mandating that consent must be given by a patient or a physician as the act of an autonomous individual judged to be either fully competent to consent, or else judged not competent and placed in the hands of a guardian, is a fiction that does great damage to people placed in life and death threatening situations. He suggests that the presupposition of informed consent, viz., personal identity and autonomy, is not applicable in these critical situations. He recommends that a protracted dialogue, subject to review and to later judgments of a court, be mandated. His position is criticized by Bernard Diamond, who concludes that in such situations the power of the judge should be increased and reinforced by the development of guidelines for appropriate declaratory judgments and guardian proceedings.

Perhaps the major reason cited for compromising the right of the patient to provide consent and to refuse medical treatment is that the patient is not competent to give consent. The notion of "competence" is a psychological one relating to the mental presuppositions for the successful performance of giving an informed consent. The reigning presumption is that all patients are competent to understand the relevant clinical decisions affecting their life and interests, and that it is the physician's obligation to communicate the material facts of the situation in such a manner as to permit them to exercise their competence in making a decision. Physicians often feel that many specific patients are not competent either to "fully understand" the situation or, more radically, to make any decisions concerning their lives. The debated question is whether patients short of the latter case can still be judged not competent enough to provide consent for medical procedures. The selection by Roth et al. discusses various tests of competency. The case discussion by Siegler examines the physician's obligations when a patient's preferences are stated only after the patient is in an extremely debilitated state. There are also some brief items, including a letter, an editorial which expresses opinions on these issues, and an empirical review by Cassileth et al. concerning whether criteria of understanding and recall can be used to indicate success in realizing the goals of informed consent.

We conclude the section with a discussion of a case in which a therapeutic option was chosen by a physician against the advice of a specialist and without informing the patient. The discussion reveals some of the paternalistic assumptions inherent in such a course of action. Each of the remaining selections discusses consent in the context of a specific clinical situation, e.g., emergency treatment, parental consent for infants and minors in pediatric care, and psychosurgery. (See cases *14, 17, 21, 33, 44, 51, 55, 59, 64, 68,* also cases in I.A., above.)

49.

Informed Consent   George J. Annas

The Doctrine

The doctrine itself is relatively simple, requiring physicians to make certain disclosures in lay language to their patients before subjecting them to risky procedures. These are:

1. A description of the proposed treatment

2. Alternatives to the proposed treatment

3. Inherent risks of death or serious bodily injury in the proposed treatment

4. Problems of recuperation that are anticipated

5. Any additional information other phycians would disclose in similar circumstances.

As with any legal rule, there are exceptions. Thus the physician need not generally disclose the above listed information:

1. In an emergency

2. If the patient does not want to be informed

3. If the procedure is simple, and the danger remote and commonly appreciated as remote

4. If in the physician's judgment it is not in the patient's best interest to know, e.g., when the information would so seriously upset the patient that he could not rationally make a decision.

It seems correct to conclude that there are two primary functions of the doctrine of informed consent: to promote individual autonomy, and to encourage rational decision making.

The purpose of autonomy (the "right to be left alone," or the "right to privacy") is to protect the individual's personal integrity by denying anyone the right to invade his body without his consent. Encouraging rational decision making is clearly viewed by courts as a secondary function of the informed consent doctrine. But, in fact, it is an extremely important function since, without rational decision making, the entire doctrine is called into serious question.

Source: *Annual Review of Medicine,* vol. 29, p. 9, 1978.

Hopefully, this self-scrutiny will prevent some procedures from being performed. For example, after a candid review of risks, some patients, based on their personal assessment, might refuse treatment. Informed consent in this instance helps ensure that those who bear the bodily and psychological risks of a treatment will have the final decision as to whether or not it is performed.

The traditional arguments against the patient having a major role in the decision-making process are that (1) the patient will never be able to comprehend the information related; and (2) the information will unduly frighten the patient, and he will therefore not consent to a procedure that actually entails only a minimal risk.

It is the physician's duty to sufficiently inform and educate the patient to enable him to make up his own mind. If the physician argues this is not possible, he may in fact be saying one of two things: he cannot properly explain the risks and alternatives because he does not understand them himself, or he believes if he does properly explain them, the patient will not consent. In either case rational decision making will be promoted by the development of an adequate disclosure statement, and by the requirement that the patient be given final authority.

State Laws on Informed Consent

Prior to 1975 there were almost no state laws dealing specifically with this subject. In 1975 and 1976, however, 18 states, in reaction to the malpractice insurance crisis,[1,2] enacted statutes that either defined or restricted the application of the doctrine of informed consent. Most of the statutes attempt to make it more difficult for a patient to successfully sue a physician who failed to obtain informed consent.

Statutes in nine states, for example, provide that a patient's signature on a consent form shall be conclusive evidence that the information was provided to the patient and that the consent was valid.[3]

In Iowa and Ohio, statutes also contain lists of the types of risks that require disclosure by physicians. The lists are identical; both statutes require disclosure of the following risks: "death, brain damage, quadriplegia, paraplegia, the loss of function of any organ or limb, or disfiguring scars . . . with the probability of each such risk if reasonably determinable."[6,7] Statutes in eight other states are similar to New York's, in which the physician is required to disclose only those "risks and benefits involved as a reasonable medical practitioner under similar circumstances would have disclosed...."[8] Five other states—Colorado, Utah, Nevada, Alaska, and Idaho—(in addition to Ohio and Iowa) adopt their own definitions of informed consent while Pennsylvania and Washington base disclosure on the "risks and alternatives to treatment or diagnosis that a reasonable patient would consider material to the decision whether or not to undergo treatment or diagnosis."[1]

It would be a tragedy if the promotion of a uniform consent form led to making the process itself just one step that both physician and patient come to regard as unnecessary red tape, and, as a consequence, they fail to engage in the dialogue envisioned by the doctrine. Each procedure has its own unique risks, and each patient is in some manner unique. Only by going through the difficult task of tailoring information to fit the procedure and the patient is it likely that either individual autonomy or rational decision making will be promoted. If neither of these functions is furthered, the process becomes meaningless.

Conclusions

While few conclusions can be drawn from this group of statutes, one can see a trend toward treating the written consent form as a complete defense in an informed consent case (barring fraud or misrepresentation). Most legislatures that have acted on this question to date are concerned with *disclosure* on the part of the physician, rather than *understanding* on the part of the patient. In this approach they are consistent with the appellate courts. Some legislatures are less consistent in permitting the physician to limit disclosures based on "standard medical practice" rather than on the patient's need to know. In this regard, many of the statutes must be seen as anti-self-determination measures.

NOTES

1. G. J. Annas, L. H. Glantz, and B. K. Katz, *Informed Consent to Human Experimentation: The Subject's Dilemma*, p. 33, Ballinger, Cambridge, Ma., 1977.

2. Alaska, Colorado, Delaware, Florida, Idaho, Iowa, Kentucky, Nebraska, Nevada, New York, North Carolina, Ohio, Pennsylvania, Rhode Island, Tennessee, Utah, Vermont, and Washington.

3. Colorado, Florida, Iowa, Idaho, Nevada, North Carolina, Ohio, Utah, and Washington.

4. Fla. Stats. Ann., sec. 768. 132(4)(a).

5. Idaho Code 439–4305.

6. Iowa Code Ann. ch. 147 (added by H. B. 803, sec. 16, 1975).

7. Ohio Rev. Code Ann. sec. 2317.54.

8. Delaware, Florida, Nebraska, New York, North Carolina, Kentucky, Vermont, and Tennessee.

50.
David G. and Self-Rule   Robert A. Burt

David G's life exploded in flames when he was twenty-seven years old. He had come home in May 1973 from three years' service as a jet pilot in the air force to join his father's real estate firm. In July the two men went together to inspect some property. When their car failed to start, Mr. G's father lifted the hood to manipulate the carburetor and directed his son to start the ignition. Mr. G did so, and the car suddenly was enveloped by fire. Unknowingly, they had parked the car over a leaking gas main.

Mr. G's father died on the way to the hospital. Mr. G had received severe burns over two-thirds of his body. He was not expected to survive, but he did, though blinded and terribly maimed. From the beginning of his hospitalization he suffered greatly. Doctors believed there was constant danger that fatal infections would enter his extensive open sores. Each day, to guard against this, he was immersed in a chemical-filled tank for excruciatingly painful treatment. Surgeons also performed several operations for skin grafts, for unsuccessful efforts to save his sight, and for restoring some move-

ment to his limbs. Throughout this time, Mr. G had repeatedly expressed doubts about whether he wanted to live. In May 1974—nine months after his accident—he adamantly refused further medical treatment. In explaining this refusal, he described his initial days of treatment in this way:

First of all I didn't want to go to . . . [any] hospital but I was picked up and put in the ambulance anyway, and so was my father and we were taken to the hospital. . . . I told them again that I was burned bad enough that I didn't want them to try to do anything for me and only to keep me out of pain. But they did go ahead and treat me. And although they did not think I was going to make it at the time, they pulled me through. But since then, there is no way I could begin to explain the nightmares and the excruciating pain involved in the first events at [the hospital] that I can barely remember it myself. It was sort of like a dream, and a real bad dream, and I might add that I had a lot of nightmares at the time and I

Source: Robert A. Burt, *Taking Care of Strangers: The Rule of Law in Doctor-Patient Relations*, The Free Press, New York, 1979.

couldn't tell what was really happening and what I was dreaming.

I was dreaming that one of the interns there was using me as a guinea pig for his experiments and him and one of the nurses would get together and at night would cut on me and do other things that were quite painful and I thought this was really happening. Only now that I can look back on it with a clear mind can I say that I know it didn't happen. . . .

I swore up and down that all the nurses were drinking on duty and whooping it up. I was right near the nurses' station and I'm sure they were laughing and talking a lot and I thought they were partying it up with booze.

Mr. G offered this description in a conversation with a psychiatrist, Dr. Robert White. A videotape was made of this conversation and of Mr. G's painful immersion treatment. In this conversation, Mr. G described not only his initial reluctance to accept medical treatment but went further to clearly and eloquently explain why he now wanted all treatment discontinued and wanted to die.

Dr. White was initially brought to interview Mr. G by physicians who asked whether Mr. G might be diagnosed as mentally ill so that the state civil commitment laws could be invoked to force treatment on him regardless of his consent. Dr. White concluded that Mr. G could not be considered mentally ill in the terms of these statutes. Mr. G's lucidity, evident in the conversation transcript, powerfully supports Dr. White's conclusion.

On the face of his statements, Mr. G's intentions might seem quite clear to most observers. He described, as noted, the horrible nightmares of his early hospitalization and the continued pain of treatment. In his conversation, he stated that the initial surgery on one arm had actually decreased his use of it. Although he thought this surgical mishap may have been "just a freak accident," nonetheless he now doubted his physicians' curative capabilities: "I had

lots more faith in what a surgeon could do before this accident than since I have been in the hospital." Mr. G also identified another source for his despair:

[All] my life I have been active in sports. I have played golf, surfed and rodeo and these are things and all that I am doing now. I've played football, basketball in school, ran track and I've been very oriented to athletics in general. And now, I think, at best, I could just be rehabilitated to the extent where I could make it alone rather than be able to do things I really enjoy.

Mr. G's skepticism regarding his physicians' capacities and the worth to him of the maximum curative potential that they promise powerfully supports his choice to end his treatment and his life. At the end of this conversation, Mr. G invoked principles that add great weight to the force of his argument:

What really . . . astounds me . . . is that in a country like this where freedom has been stressed so much and civil liberties, especially during the last few years, how a person can be made to stay under a doctor's care and be subjected to the painful treatment, such as the tankings which are *very* painful, against this person's wishes, especially if he has demonstrated the ability to reason. . . . The way I see it, who is a doctor to decide whether a person lives or dies?

In identifying conflict between a person's wish to die and the doctor's imposition, Mr. G appears to assume that these two are separate people, each of whom can adequately distinguish one's wishes from the other's. This assumption clearly rests beneath the libertarian principle that Mr. G invokes; the idea that one person might be coercing another would be incoherent unless each might conceivably make some choice independent of the other's wishes. In applying the libertarian principle, therefore, it is relevant to ask whether Mr. G conceived himself as choosing death for himself or as choosing death in order to implement others' wishes that he should die. There was contradiction evident in his conversation on this score.

The starkest contradiction I heard in Mr. G's words came in the following exchange:

> Dr. White: Now it's, I think, beyond much question that if you were to leave the hospital and simply go home that within a short time you would die from the infections that would spring up from open burn areas that still remain. Is that what you intend and want, to go home and die?
> Mr. G: Actually, I just want a brief visit to home and I don't intend to die from the infection. I'd use some other means.
> Dr. White: That is, you would intend to do away with your life.
> Mr. G: Yes.

The fact was, however, that Mr. G was so disabled at the time of this conversation that he could take no affirmative action to end his life. The only means available to him were passive—to wait for infection to overtake him—unless someone would act to kill him sooner. Mr. G could not grasp anything with his hands, he could not lift himself from his bed or even move to fall from the bed. He was wholly helpless, wholly dependent on others' ministrations even in the manner that he appeared to choose for his own death—to die, that is, by some means other than infection.

Dr. White pointed to this fact after he asked whether Mr. G would be willing to "wait and see" the results of further surgery on his hands. Dr. White then stated:

> [Y]ou would be able to be up and around sufficiently, to handle things with your hands sufficiently, [so] that if at that point you simply did not want to go on with your life, *you* would be in a position to terminate it if you wish, because as it is now you would be bedfast and would be hard put to do away with yourself even if you were strongly inclined to do so.

Mr. G responded:

> To me, I feel that the chances are so small that the pain and—I mean, that the end result isn't worth the pain involved to be able to get to the point where I could try it out. Ideally, this would be the best thing to do if I could go ahead and see just what things are going to be like after I did get out, and if I didn't like them, as you said, terminate my life then. But I don't wish to go through the pain of having my hands and fingers in traction and learning to walk again, which I never thought of as being a painful thing to do—but especially with my legs it has turned out to be quite painful.

Dr. White then asked a further question, which I think cut more deeply into Mr. G's despair:

> Of course, you are so completely helpless, that is unable to get out of the bed even, by yourself, that you're pretty much at the mercy of all the people around you now as to whether you stay or leave. How do you feel about that?

Mr. G's response to this question revealed the emotional context in which he asserted his principled claim for self-determination, a claim that a moment ago I abstracted from this context:

> It's a really sinking feeling. I have always been real independent and I like to do things for myself. I've had my own ways of doing things and pretty much done as I wished—up to this point. And now I have to rely on someone else to feed me, all my private functions I need help with. And it—what really, I guess, astounds me, I guess I'd say, is that in a country like this where freedom has been stressed so much and civil liberties, especially during the last few years, how a person can be made to stay under a doctor's care. . . .

The force of this libertarian principle is not diminished by insisting that the principle be viewed in the specific way in which Mr. G raised it. Because this principle mandates respect for each person's individual self-determination, careful attention must be given to the individual who claims its application. If we ignored the emotional context in which Mr. G invoked this principle, we would find ourselves purporting to obey the wishes of a caricature, a cardboard cutout, rather than a fully fleshed and recognizable human being.

I do not claim that Mr. G did not want to die or that this wish is an unreasonable or morally wrongful response to the tragedy that fell on him. I do believe that his statements generally—and particularly his specific rejection of death from infection—reveal both his desire to break loose from the helpless passivity imposed by his accident and his belief that he is inextricably dependent on others, in part shown by his rejection of the only means of death available to him without the active ministration of others. His conversation with Dr. White suggests that Mr. G is confused, not so much about whether he wants to die, but about whether others want him to die. At the same time, he appears unwilling to admit this confusion even to himself.

Mr. G could not now see himself. But he could feel his deformed hands against his body, he could imagine how he appeared, he could undoubtedly sense the revulsion (however involuntary) that his appearance inspired in those who saw him. No one stroked his head while he cried in pain. No one held his stumped hand as he was lowered into the tank. No one spoke soothingly to him. The medical technicians around him limited their direct contact with him to quick and painfully administered dabs of ointment. All these facts could press Mr. G to feel shunned by, without sympathy from, others. The blaring rock music from the radio that accompanied his descent into the tank—strapped like an inanimate object onto the stretcher—evoked for me, at least, his nightmare of the nurses "drinking on duty and whooping it up" while he suffered alone. Inevitably, Mr. G must feel a pervasive sense of isolation from others. His blindness alone would bring this. His observation that he was being treated "regardless of [his] feelings" recurs throughout his conversation and is the predominant way that he articulates this notion of emotional isolation from others. A question seems briefly to cross his mind as he speaks: does my "next of kin" want me "here and want me treated," or would I "be held even regardless of this?" I am only suggesting that he feels some nagging doubt about whether they truly wished him well, just as he felt doubt about his surgeon's intentions toward him.

One further remark of his in this conversation amplifies my meaning. Dr. White asked, "What steps are you taking to try and get out of the hospital?" Mr. G replied:

> Well, right now I'm trying to exhaust every legal means that I can find. And I'm working through attorneys and so far I haven't had much luck. It's something that I found out attorneys, at least ethical ones, don't want to touch—probably for fear of getting bad publicity.

I do not think it demeans Mr. G or his family and physicians to suggest that his conscience was troubling him; that he was struggling with the question of whether he deserved to live; that he felt (or feared that he felt) deeply isolated, unloved, and condemned by those around him; and that he sought reassurance against those feelings while attempting to deny that he needed that reassurance. If this is true, his expressed wish to die would have a very different meaning from its first appearance as a self-determining act. From this perspective, that wish would appear more a question to others about their wishes toward him. Particularly because the means of death Mr. G envisioned would require the active collaboration of some other person, that collaborative act would appear conclusively to answer this question.

None of my speculation about Mr. G's motives could support a conclusion that beneath his protestations he "truly" wants to live. It seems to me that he has said quite clearly that he wishes he were dead. The critical ambiguity that I see in his conversation with Dr. White goes rather to Mr.

G's conception of himself as choice maker; that is, it is not clear whether he sees himself as separate from others in exercising choice regarding his future or whether he chooses death because he believes others want that result for him and he feels incapable of extricating himself from their choice making for him. Was he, in other words, implementing his own choice because he saw himself as free to do so, or was he implementing the choice of others because he saw himself as inextricably bound to their choice for him?

Close consideration of Mr. G's claim suggests a general proposition that I will develop throughout: that these distinctions are inherently problematic for any individual to draw in characterizing his own motives and that no individual can rigidly demarcate these distinctions regarding another without pressing both himself and that other into falsely stereotyped roles.

Mr. G is, I believe, palpably confused about whether he is able to conceive of himself as an individual—as a being who is separate from others. In ordinary daily events and interpersonal relations, the distinction between "self" and "other-than-self" seems readily apparent to most people. But Mr. G's circumstances are far from ordinary for him. His sudden and unaccustomed total dependence on others insistently calls into question the psychological basis for his commonsense perception that he has an identity separate from other people and from the external world.

Mr. G's accident did not destroy his belief in his independence. But the accident did break loose his independent self-conception from its customary moorings to his capacities for sight, mobility, and self-care. Dr. White's implicit advice that Mr. G should reach his decision only after he had regained use of his hands and was "able to be up and around sufficiently" had an underlying prescription: that Mr. G should recapitulate the developmental progression that had led from his infancy to his separate self-conception before he or the doctor would be satisfied that his decision was "his own."

My depiction of Mr. G's confusions thus far might appear to point toward a simple solution for legal response to his request to die—the response, that is, already embraced by civil commitment statutes. The considerations that I have set out regarding Mr. G's capacity to conceive himself as a separate and choice-making individual regarding others lie at the heart of clinical psychiatric diagnoses of mental illness. That label has a substantial social pejorative, and it may seem that some new label should be devised to categorize Mr. G's confusion—perhaps "temporary incapacity"—that would not tar him with the mental illness brush. Once this new label is applied to Mr. G, following the kind of analysis of his statements and his general situation that I have set out, a court might rule that the ordinary self-determination norm did not apply to him because he was not sufficiently clear about his own "self-identity" and that others were therefore authorized to decide his treatment for him until his confusion had dispelled.

But this proposed solution contains a critical fallacy. This solution, in common with civil commitment statutes for mental illness generally, rests on the premise that it is possible for two people conclusively to resolve the question between themselves that one is "confused" and the other is not regarding the capacity of both to define themselves as separate and choice-making individuals. I believe this attempt is ultimately fallacious no matter who the two people may be— whether psychiatrist and patient, judge and litigant, parent and child, or indeed, a conscious person and a comatose person.

My assertion—even without this last example—may seem excessively paradoxical. For it is clear that in ordinary social interactions, this kind of differential characterization readily occurs between people— parent/child and conscious person/comatose person may seem to be two obviously justifiable applications of such differentation. But in claiming that these judgments are fallacious, I have a very particular meaning: that no one (whether psychiatrist, parent, or judge) can conclusively characterize himself as a separate and choice-making individual regarding another person when he is perceiving that person as lacking those very attributes; that is, the very act of judgment inevitably evokes the same confusions in the judge.

This proposition may be developed by first of all imagining how lawyers and judges might have responded to Mr. G's claim in litigation. The legal proceedings would most likely have gone forward in this way. Dr. White would indicate his view that Mr. G was not mentally ill. Mr. G would testify, perhaps from his hospital bed with the judge and formal trappings of the law in attendance; he would speak lucidly and even eloquently, as the transcript of his conversation with Dr. White reveals. Mr. G would state his intention to die. He would specifically direct that he no longer be subjected to the daily chemical immersions. He might reiterate his intention to die from some means other than the infection but suggest further, as he indicated in his conversation with Dr. White, that this was a question for future resolution; on the immediate question regarding termination of treatment to prevent infection, at least, he would speak quite clearly.

Could anyone be adequately assured that, in indicating his choice, Mr. G was in fact conceiving himself as making a choice rather than as implementing the choices of others regarding him? Could anyone be assured that all those around him—now including not only his family and doctors but also the lawyers and judge—were not horrified and even repelled by his plight and by him, did not wish that somehow he would go away? Could anyone be assured that the very effort of those around him even to suppress such feelings from their conscious awareness might not betray those feelings to him?

There could be no clear-cut assurances on any of these questions in the formal legal proceedings, because these feelings will inevitably afflict anyone who has dealings with Mr. G. In saying this, I do not mean to impugn anyone's moral stature—and particularly the integrity of his family and physicians who, in fact, dealt with him. I have no special sources of information about any of these individuals to support my speculation. But there are many reasons to believe that anyone dealing with Mr. G would have deeply ambivalent feelings about his prospects for survival.

The videotape tells us what his words alone only hint; that he is a painful, insistent reminder to others of their frailty—an acknowledgment that in the routine of everyday life, is ordinarily suppressed. Others cannot avoid wishing that he and his unwanted lesson would go away. He cannot avoid knowing this of others and wishing it for himself.

If, however, the legal proceeding led to a proclamation that Mr. G were "mentally competent," the law would thereby add its sanction to his explicit claim that he and he alone was choosing death for himself. The law would thus help him and others ignore the extent to which this might not be true. The law would help him and others adopt a rigidly stereotyped view of him as a "self-determining individualist," rather than one who acts only to conform to others' expectations and valuations of him, as the master of his fate rather than fate's victim. His and others' beliefs in the worth and applicability for him of this stereotype would speed him toward his death. In order to see himself as merely the implementer, the instrument, of Mr. G's choice, the judge must conclude that *his* independent personality had no influence in leading Mr. G to this decision.

This choiceless self-conception is a normatively prized role depiction in the legal system. In Mr. G's case, both judge and lawyer could invoke professional norms that would commit them to this self-conception. The lawyer could see himself as "simply an advocate" for his client's wishes. The judge could see himself through a more complex professional role norm but with the same ultimate goal—that he was obligated to set aside his "personal" views of what Mr. G should do and instead to apply standards drawn from "impersonal" legislative and judicial enactments.

This choiceless self-conception underlies the system's claim to constitute governance "by laws not men." A generation ago, the so-called "legal realists" attacked this notion as a hypocritical pretension that permitted judges to mask their personal and political predilections in the supposed impersonal majesty of the law. But why should the legal system rush to answer this unanswerable question simply because Mr. G is attempting to force such an answer from it, as he is attempting with his family and doctors? Why should the legal system accept anyone's invitation to resolve an inherently irresolvable question?

The law's willingness to identify the choice maker exclusively on either side of the doctor-patient transaction is the underlying force that has led to brutal abuse of patients under civil commitment laws. Mr. G's claim that the law should identify him as the choice maker is the mirror image of the commitment laws' assertions and will lead to the same abusive results.

This is the flaw in current proposals that rely exclusively on consent of the blatantly idiosyncratic and apparently threatening individual to govern the occasions for social defensive action. The consensuality norm can easily be used to isolate the idiosyncratic individual from social support in a way that leads to his destruction in compliance with others' wishes in the same way that commitment laws have achieved. This norm lends itself to this purpose because it rests on the conventional premise that self and other can be readily distinguished in social interaction. But that premise is necessarily only partially persuasive to anyone because of the juxtaposition in everyone's mind of thought processes organized around diametrically opposed premises. An attempt by any individual to insist that the self/other distinction can be rigidly maintained among people, an unending attempt to repress all doubts on this score, inevitably leads that individual either to destroy the physical existence of those others whose distinct separateness is so passionately desired or to destroy

himself. That is the future that the proponents of consensuality as the exclusive legitimizing norm for social relations offer to Mr. G., ostensibly for the protection of his freedom to be a self-determining individual.

The notion that physicians are normatively obliged to honor their patients' "self-determination" can reliably forestall this result only if it serves as a continual counterpoint to the contradictory proposition that patients are obliged to obey their physicians' directives. The proposition that patient self-determination should univalently rule the interaction contains the same inherent psychological instability that afflicts the mirror-image notion that physicians should alone dictate the course of treatment. This attempt to impose a polarized stasis, to suppress any conscious awareness of the inevitable intrapsychic experience of alternating power between them mutually to dictate the boundaries of their "selves," unleashes the destructive impulses we have seen.

This is the reason for my conclusion earlier that the central problem in civil commitment laws came from their rigid allocation of choice-making role to one party and choiceless role to the other in a mutual interaction and that the abolition of those laws would reiterate this problem by simply reassigning the same rigid role allocations. From our discussion throughout this book, we can now generalize this proposition as follows. Whenever anyone seeks to conceive himself as either a wholly choice-making or wholly choiceless individual regarding another person, that aspiration reflects the individual's uncertainty regarding the boundaries between his "self" and the other's and an unwillingness consciously to acknowledge his uncertainty.

Courts have now properly emphasized the psychological importance of the countervailing conception; the threat of adverse legal consequences in effect creates psychic stress for physicians that counterposes the stress pushing them toward rigid authoritarianism. But, for the moment at least, many physicians simply feel buffeted by contrapuntal stress rather than soothed by equal stress from all sides. Because physicians (in common with most people) do not enjoy stress, many find attractions in adopting a posture of impotence, which is the mirror-image self-conception of their customary authoritarianism. At the same time, many judges are eager to conceive themselves in this authoritarian mode and to relieve the apparent distress of physicians and patients who appear before them. These judges miscomprehend the underlying psychological forces that have mooted physicians' claims for the univalent choice-making role. They fail to see themselves as participants in a dialogue between physicians and patients, as instruments to unsettle the rigidity of role allocation that the stress of illness provokes in both patient and physician. They see themselves as authoritative dispute resolvers rather than as *agents provocateurs* of disputes between physician and patient on the question whether either one is univalently in command of the other. The contemporary problem in this relationship derives from insufficient dispute on this question; the proper role for courts here is to ensure dispute rather than to join the parties' delusive belief that dispute between them can be conclusively ended. Insofar as judges attempt to describe a static depiction of role allocation for these parties (or to impose it on them), judges will exacerbate the psychological tensions they mean to resolve; they will provoke the destructive impetus of the rigid choice-making/choiceless allocation rather than reliably interrupt it.

The destructive consequences of this misconception are effectively muted when courts are asked to adjudicate disputes between physicians and patients in malpractice litigation long after the resolution of the interaction between the immediate parties. This misconception finds its most destructive expression when courts inject themselves in the middle of a raging controversy between doctor and patient, as between Mr. G and his physicians. The question at issue in that dispute appears to be this: "Is Mr. G or the physicians properly in command of Mr. G?" That question appears capable of some definitive answer at the moment it is posed between them. But the real questions between them are these: "Who is Mr. G? How is his 'self' different from the physicians' 'selves'? Are 'his choices' his or theirs?" These questions are unanswerable at the moment they flare into dispute because this dispute itself is provoked by the stress of his illness, and this stress brings him and his physicians into mutual self-confusions that can be satisfactorily resolved only through continued interaction over time. The dispute can never be conclusively ended. It can only be muted, attenuated, soothed— because the question of separate or fused self-boundaries is never conclusively answered in any interpersonal relation.

The proper role of a court, or of any third party attempting to move the disputants toward satisfactory resolution, is to help them against prematurely abandoning the fluid confusions of identity and power between them that appear to be the very source of their distress, to help them see that ultimately they cannot (and should not attempt to) conclusively answer these questions that seem so urgent at the moment between them.

51.
Assuring Conversation between Doctor and Patient
Robert A. Burt

The following selection utilizes the discussion of Mr. G's case in the preceding article. The touchstone for court interventions in these disputes is to foster and even to provoke prolonged conversation between the immediate parties—not to offer an apparently definitive resolution to the dispute which effectively shuts it off. The rules which courts have recently begun to evolve in malpractice litigation to mandate physicians' respect for patients' "informed consent" can be admirably well suited for this purpose. Increasing conversation between doctor and patient should be the essential effect of these rules. Many physicians (and their legal advisors) unfortunately misconceive or mistrust this purpose and seek to reduce these conversations to stylized monologues in which they recite a litany of the statistics on risks and benefits of the proposed medical intervention and then offer the prospective patient a document for his signature "on the dotted line."

This static conception of the interaction readily becomes a parody; and, indeed, some physicians have viewed the recent court opinions as nothing more than parody by taking them to require that they warn prospective patients even of the statistically identifiable risks of slipping in a hospital shower and thus suffering "medically induced injury." Most patients contemplating hospitalization would not place the prospect of bathroom injury at the top of their list of fears. Some might do so, however; and for those patients, it would be appropriate and important for their physicians to know these fears and to address them.

Some courts and commentators have tangled on the implicit question raised by this example—whether the legal test is "objective" or "subjective" for the adequacy of the physician's disclosure or warning to his patient; whether, that is, the physician is entitled to assume that every patient wants and needs to hear what the "objectively identifiable reasonable man" might require; or whether the physician should be held liable if he failed to disclose what his particular unreasonable patient wanted to hear. This dispute is falsely dichotomous. The physician cannot be obliged to list every possible hazard that any other person might imagine; in that sense, the physician should be able to act on the assumption that all prospective patients are not madmen. But the physician should nonetheless be required to act reasonably in determining whether or not the particular patient before him is mad.

If a patient sues his physician for failure to give advance warning of the possibility that Martians would invade the patient at the point of surgical intervention, the physician might properly rely on the objective reality of the nonexistence of Martians to justify his failure to give this warning. But the physician cannot rely on objectivity for his failure to discern that this particular patient might have had special vulnerabilities on this score unless the physician had acted with reasoned objectivity to learn what particular fears and confusions this unfamiliar patient was bringing to an interpersonal relationship with a stranger.

The underlying impetus of the informed consent requirement should be to press physicians to talk and to listen to the particular patient, not to some statistical abstraction of "patients in general." This very requirement cuts against the psychology of scientific medicine that the practitioner make the therapeutic choices on the basis of statistical abstractions and accordingly conceive

Source: Robert A. Burt, *Taking Care of Strangers: The Rule of Law in Doctor-Patient Relations,* The Free Press, New York, 1979.

himself as interchangeable among "physicians in general." This impersonal conception of the therapeutic enterprise powerfully influences both physicians' and patients' views of the meaning of consensuality in their dealings and can easily lead them to reiterate the static stereotypic depiction of choiceless/choice-making role allocations while reciting the litany of mutual consent and signing a flurry of legalistic documents.

Courts must hold to the conception of informed consent as mandating an ongoing dialogue between a doctor and patient in which the stress of the patient's illness inevitably disturbs any fixed, separate self-conception of either party. It becomes clear that the physician's recitation of risks and benefits and presentation of a written contract form is only one-half of a conversation and the less significant half. The more critical inquiry for the law is: if this recitation is made, what did the patient say in response? This in turn should lead courts to a series of questions pursuing the details of the physician's and patient's conversation.

In many cases—where the patient obviously appears confused or where the physician knows from the gravity of the proposed intervention that the patient must be suffering great stress and confusion—the process of mutual interaction will be greatly time-consuming.

This consumption of time and paper, of emotional energy, may seem burdensome, even wasteful. But this is the only way reliably to countermand the destructive stereotypes implicit in the very therapeutic triumphs of scientific medicine, to ensure that brutal forces that found expression in the Milgram experiments are not increasingly unleashed from the initially hopeful encounters between physicians and patients.*

This same touchstone—to foster and even to provoke prolonged conversation between the parties—yields an organizing principle for the appropriate application of civil commitment laws to persons who refuse to accept treatment prescribed by physicians.

Mr. G's situation can illustrate my vision for reformation of the law. If the civil commitment law provided that a finding of mental illness justified overriding Mr. G's protests only for a limited time period (say, thirty days) and only with treatment modalities that were clearly intended and necessarily limited to fostering conversation between him and his physicians, that would mean Mr. G could be forced to continue the chemical immersions for thirty days and to meet with the psychiatrist and other physicians, but that no law would force him to acquiesce in the operation on his hands. The immersions would not be authorized because they were necessary to keep him alive and thus available for conversation, but rather because the immersions themselves were not central to and did not end the dispute between him and his physicians. A time-limited continuation of the immersions could be seen by both parties as temporizing and thus as an inducement toward, rather than the end of, conversation.

Because of its limited reach, the civil commitment statute would not offer the only or the most important legal framework within which Mr. G and his physicians would measure their respective power to coerce one another. Even if the physicians could obtain a ruling that Mr. G were mentally ill, that ruling would authorize limited treatment only for a limited time. The legal remedies available at the end of this time would be the same as if Mr. G had never been declared mentally ill—a fact which, in itself, might lead Mr. G's physicians to avoid any invocation of the commitment laws even if they believed he might be labeled "mentally ill" under them.

The current rule that physicians have no

---

*In the Milgram experiments subjects were told to administer increasing amounts of electric shocks to volunteers in a learning experiment. Although the subjects could not see the volunteers and were told that the shocks would not cause "permanent damage," nonetheless they continued to follow instructions and increase voltage despite hearing shouts and pleas from the "learners."

authority to detain Mr. G without a judicial commitment order is not peculiar to relations between physicians and patients. This rule is one application of the principle that proclaims individuals' freedom from unjustified imprisonment. The grand tradition of Anglo-American jurisprudence, enshrined in the Constitution, dictates that Mr. G must have access to a judge prepared to issue a writ of habeas corpus to direct the physicians to bring Mr. G into court (literally, to "bring his body") and to justify their detention of him. This remedy sees an independent judiciary as the fundamental protection of the citizen against the state. It is the highest symbolic expression in our jurisprudence of the premise of the impermeable self-boundaries of individualism.

How, then, can some basis be found to accommodate these diametrically opposed and yet equally true premises that men in society conceive themselves at once both willfully separate and inextricably united? The path I have already outlined for the reformation of civil commitment statutes points the way. That reformation applies the premise of organic relatedness, of dissolved self-boundaries, by vesting choice in others regarding a person who is judged to lack conventional indicia of psychological integrity, of individualism. But that reformation sharply limits the consequences of this choice-making/choiceless allocation in order to keep visible for the participants the diametrically opposed allocation and its competing premise of individual separateness. I would apply this same conception to relations between doctor and patient when mental illness is not alleged and commitment statutes are not invoked.

Thus, Mr. G would be entitled to a judicial proclamation ordering his release from the physicians' custody. But this would not be a definitive, timelessly conceived proclamation that would end the possibility of further disputatious conversation between Mr. G and the physicians. The judicial writ would instead be viewed, in effect, as a time-limited expression which will be confirmed, modified, or abandoned in further

negotiations between the parties themselves that only subsequently will be judicially reviewed.

This position finds traditional lawyerly form in two procedural distinctions invoked in many litigative settings: the distinction between rights and remedies and between ordinary and declaratory judgments. The application of these distinctions can be made clear by further consideration of Mr. G's situation.

Assume that Mr. G sought release and the physicians did not attempt to invoke even the limited forced treatment available under reformed commitment laws. In that case, there would be no basis or need for a judicial inquiry into Mr. G's rights: any detention of him would be clearly wrongful and the doctors' continued detention should be identified as such if Mr. G simply requests a habeas writ from a judge. But what consequence should follow if the physicians disregard this judicial proclamation of Mr. G's individual rights? Should the physicians pay monetary damages to Mr. G for the specific injury to him? Should they pay a fine to the state for violating a principle of the social order? Should they be imprisoned?

Any one or all of these remedial consequences might properly follow from the doctors' disregard for Mr. G's individual right to freedom and the specific judicial declaration of that right. Recall, however, that, at the moment of his conversation with Dr. White, Mr. G was wholly immobile and thus unable either to forestall his death or to hasten it without some other's assistance. Should this circumstance mitigate the penalties imposed by the law if the physicians decide not to release Mr. G to his home because his immediate family was unwilling to accept the painful dilemma (from their perspective) of Mr. G's immobility and expressed wish to die? Should this circumstance mitigate penalties if the physicians decided to attack this dilemma by surgically removing the immobilizing skin grafts from Mr. G's hands, without his consent, so that he might have capacity to kill himself rather than relying on others to perform the fatal act? Are these considerations sufficiently strong either to alter the principle mandating respect for Mr G's individual autonomy or in any degree to justify disobedience of that principle?

Legal institutions can invite the parties to present these questions for advance authoritative resolution, for a declaratory judgment. This is the invitation implicit in existing commitment laws. Or the law can force the parties to resolve this question initially for themselves with only tentative, generalized guidance regarding the law's willingness subsequently to approve or to penalize those resolutions. I propose this latter course. The law should make clear to both Mr. G and the physicians that forced detention or surgery violates an important principle. But adjudication of the specific remedial consequences of any such violation should be postponed until the physicians have decided their course for themselves and acted on that decision in the face of some potential risk of adverse legal consequences.

The law cannot interrupt this dynamic by purporting to take control of relations between doctor and patient. It can only hope to accomplish this by refusing to take control, by forcing both doctors and patients to acknowledge that neither has unquestioned power over the other in order to prod both toward confronting the ultimate reality that neither has unquestioned power over the issues of disease, mortality, and dis-eased thinking that have brought them into relation. The law will only fuel rather than interrupt this destructive dynamic by providing a mechanism for advance review, for declaratory judgments, to decide all specific treatment issues in dispute between patients and physicians.

In a declaratory action, a judge would, in effect, decide whether sufficient conversation had occurred between doctor and patient to justify its termination. It may seem obvious that someone, somewhere, should decide this question. Conversation cannot continue forever: organic disease processes may themselves demand action; physicians have other patients as well as family and friends with legitimate demands on their time. But though the doctor-patient conversation clearly must end at some time, it does not follow that a judge can adequately decide the proper moment for termination.

The judge can address the question of termination only by attempting to stand outside the conversation. But this attempt must inevitably fail. The judge's mind is no more free from the alternating ideas of separateness and self-dissolution, rationality and madness, than anyone's.

The doctor and patient are equally faced with the same judgmental dilemma. This dilemma becomes manageable for them—and they are saved from the self-destructive implications and impulses to destructive actions—only if they can believe that conversation between them and within them is not conclusively ended but has only temporarily abated. This is the role that the judge and the legal system can adequately take. By promising that some subsequent judicial review of the doctor-patient conversation is available, but by withholding that review until the immediate participants have acted on their own disputed or agreed conclusions from that conversation, the law gives both participants a concrete demontion that their conversation has an interminable, and comfortingly indestructible, dimension.

52.
Resolving Doctor-Patient Conflicts   Bernard L. Diamond

The problem posed by Robert Burt is a profound one: Who has, or should have, the power to make critical decisions in the doctor-patient relationship? Does the doctor know best? Perhaps doctors should make all final decisions. Does the patient's right of self-determination override all other considerations? Perhaps we should never tolerate anything short of fully informed consent by the patient. Or should the law intervene in certain difficult situations, making a judge decide what is to be done?

Burt introduces the problem by vividly describing the case of a young man who is horribly mutilated and blinded by an automobile fire and explosion. His treatment is slow, excruciatingly painful, and he will never be restored to a normal condition. Burt uses this case to develop "the proposition that assigning exclusive choice-making authority in one party (whether patient, physician, or judge) and complementary choiceless status to another in an interpersonal transaction readily leads to paradoxically destructive results for all participants." For reasons I will develop below, I am impelled to reply, "Not necessarily!"

Relying almost entirely upon psychoanalytic theories concerning unconscious motives, attitudes, and feelings, the author pursues his theme with vigor and consistency. To mitigate the dangers of unconscious ambivalence and destructive aggressive impulses, Burt proposes that all consent between doctor and patient, for treatment of both physical and mental conditions, be reached only by what he calls "conversation" between them. By "conversation," he really seems to mean a psychotherapeutic interchange, as prolonged as necessary, to resolve completely all unconscious ambivalence, in both the patient and the physician. If such

conversation does not spontaneously resolve all ambivalence, Burt would allow no appeal to the law to make the decision, for the judge, who necessarily suffers from the same ambivalence, will inflict his own brand of unconscious aggression upon the patient and doctor.

Essential to Professor Burt's proposal is the element of uncertainty. The physician must not know in advance the penalty for violating his patient's expressed wishes. Such penalty may be stringent or it may only be symbolic, but

> [t]he principle should remain clear that physicians are obliged to obtain patients' consent in all matters; thus motivation will be established for conversation, for negotiation. But by keeping uncertain the precise consequences of any breach of this principle, the law establishes the motives for intense negotiation, for sustained face-to-face conversation in which each party feels himself personally engaged because each believes in the unavoidability of his own pain and the other's power to inflict pain on him.

If the patient and doctor fail to resolve their conflict, the legal system should tread lightly. Burt's judicial review will not produce a decision as to the correct action in giving or withholding the treatment. Rather, it will only review the adequacy of the conversation, assessing whether the conversation has ended properly or should be carried further. If the physician has acted improperly after an inadequate conversation with the patient, the court will impose a punishment that is appropriate to the wrongdoing but that the physician could not have accurately foretold. The goal is to avoid shifting the responsibility for decision upon the law, and instead to use the authority of the law to force upon the doctor and patient as extensive a negotiation conversation (therapy?) as is necessary.

Many of the inferences and psychoanalytic interpretations that Burt presents as established facts could be disputed: he gives no credit to alternative interpretations of psychological phenomena. His basic writing style expresses an unjustified attitude of certainty, conviction, and enthusiasm. A relevant (apocryphal?) anecdote is told about Sigmund Freud. Freud was an inveterate cigar smoker, and one day a friend asked him, "Doctor Freud, how is it possible that you, who discovered that cigars and similar objects are actually phallic symbols, go around all day with a penis in your mouth?" Freud replied, "Yes, it is true that a cigar is a penis symbol. But do not forget that a good cigar is also a good cigar."

By concentrating on the unconscious dynamics of the participants in the medical-legal-patient relationship and neglecting their conscious and intentional motivations, the author is misled into impractical and perhaps erroneous conclusions. Much of what he says concerning the unconscious destructive dynamics of doctor, patient, and judge may well be true. But it is not the whole story. The unconscious is an important determinant of human behavior, but it is not the sole determinant. Burt seems to give no credence to the possibility that experience, knowledge, and insight might confer sufficient power over one's destructive drives to permit rational actions and relationships, even without prolonged conversations. Professor Burt derives his hypotheses and his solutions from extraordinary and exceptional cases. They well fit what Judge David Bazelon of the District of Columbia Circuit Court of Appeals calls "chamber of horrors cases." Laws and procedures based on such horror cases are not likely to be good. They are the hard cases that can make bad law. It may be that such cases evoke the malicious power of the unconscious. But the rules that govern the millions of everyday interactions of

doctors and patients must be responsive to the conscious egos, and give credibility to the will and intent of the participants. Burt seems to have overlooked the fact that ambivalent feelings do not necessarily give rise to ambivalent decisions and actions. To the contrary, I think that in most ordinary interpersonal situations, one side of the ambivalence is suppressed, for good or bad reasons, and the resultant action is unambivalent. Thus both patient and physician may suppress their mutual hostility and interact with trust and confidence. In the vast majority of simple, direct interchanges between doctor and patient (or between any two persons), it may be best, as Freud says, to pay attention to the cigars and leave the phallic symbols to the psychoanalytic couch.

However, I do agree with Burt that in special cases and special circumstances, this is not likely to be true. These include the chamber of horrors cases of pain, mutilation, and disability as well as the cases of uncooperative, incompetent patients who are involuntarily confined and treated. For some such cases, Burt's extended and extensive conversations motivated by the threat of judicial review may work. But for many of these exceptional problems it cannot be assumed that there is a rational, correct solution. Unfortunately, we cannot assume that every human problem has a proper answer. Sometimes every possible response to a problem will have significant detrimental consequences. Yet to take no action may be much more detrimental. Sometimes the knowledge required for a rational decision does not exist and will not magically appear, no matter how extensive and protracted the conversations between the participants. And in many cases an incorrect decision is better than no decision.

These are the human problems where the issue is not, "Who knows the right answer?" Rather, it is, "Who is accepted by society and the participants as having the *authority* to prescribe an answer?" Such aurority may not necessarily be founded upon superior knowledge or special insights into the human condition. Nor is the responsibility inherent in that authority necessarily a quality of the decision maker. It may well be simply attributed to him by social institutions or customs. Nevertheless, a sort of consensus cloaks the decision with an aura of wisdom and power, action is taken, and everyone can then go about their daily business. Certainly it is possible to demonstrate that the need for such authorities has its roots in the unconscious need for the omnipotent and omniscient father of infancy. But the decision is also a decision that needs to be made, roots or no roots.

Different cultures at different times have used a variety of persons to decide impossible problems. In our society, I believe, judges are admirably suited for this role. They are designated by society as authority figures; their decisions are translated into action. They are surrounded with sufficient mystique and symbols of wisdom and fairness that their decisions can be respected by all concerned. Behind them is the *law*, supposedly the distillation of the moral wisdom of the ages. That all this may be illusory is beside the point. Some illusions are worth retaining. When there is no right answer, when there is no existing wisdom to determine the correct response, when the truth is elusive, yet action must be taken, judges seem to do quite well (unless they suffer from excessive scrupulousness or blind arrogance). When there has been a breakdown in the normal communication between doctor and patient, or when, as with "silent patients," commu-

nication is impossible, Professor Burt would have us avoid the one decision maker in our society peculiarly suited to the task—the judge. Rather than limit his authority, I would extend it. I would reinforce his decisional respectability by establishing, insofar as possible, guidelines (laws?) and precedents that take some of the burden off his shoulders.

I know only too well from my experience as a forensic psychiatrist that judges are not always wise, rational, free from prejudice, or responsible in their decisions. Sometimes I have thought that others would have made better decisions, or that I, personally, could have done better. But neither I nor the others possessed the necessary authority and social ascription of power and respectability to have our decisions accepted. Some judges never make any decisions, let alone difficult or impossible decisions. They pass the problem on to someone else, or they procrastinate, or they rubber-stamp, or they blindly follow what they believe to be precedent. They may do exactly as Burt says—wreak havoc by inflicting their own unconscious aggression on others. But I have more faith than Professor Burt that the law and its representatives, the judges, are the proper instruments for resolving conflict and dispute and for making decisions in all those human situations where no one else has the proper combination of knowledge, experience, wisdom, power, authority, and respectability to do as well.

53.
Tests of Competency to Consent to Treatment
Loren H. Roth   Alan Meisel   Charles W. Lidz

The concept of competency, like the concept of dangerousness, is social and legal and not merely psychiatric or medical.[1] Law and, at times, psychiatry are concerned with an individual's competency to stand trial,

to make a will, and to contract.[2-5] The test of competency varies from one context to another. In general, to be considered competent an individual must be able to comprehend the nature of the particular conduct in

Source: *American Journal of Psychiatry*, vol. 134, p. 3, March 1977.

question and to understand its quality and its consequences.[3,6] A person may be considered competent for some legal purposes and incompetent for others at the same time.[3] An individual is not judged incompetent merely because he or she is mentally ill.[6] Competency plays an important role in determining the validity of a patient's decision to undergo or forego treatment. The decision of a person who is incompetent does not validly authorize a physician to perform medical treatment.[7] Conversely, a physician who withholds treatment from an incompetent patient who refuses treatment may be held liable to that patient if the physician does not take reasonable steps to obtain some other legally valid authorization for treatment.

In psychiatry the entire edifice of involuntary treatment is erected on the supposed incompetency of some people to voluntarily seek and consent to needed treatment.[7] In addition, the acceptability of behavior modification for the patient who is considered dangerous,[8] the resolution of ethical issues in family planning (i.e., sterilization),[9] and the right to refuse psychoactive medications[10]—to cite only a few of the more prominent examples—turn in part on the concept of competency.

In evaluating tests for competency several criteria should be considered. A useful test for competency is one that, first, can be reliably applied, second, is mutually acceptable or at least comprehensible to physicians, lawyers, and judges; and third, is set at a level capable of striking an acceptable balance between preserving individual autonomy and providing needed medical care. Reliability is enhanced to the extent that a competency test depends on manifest and objectively ascertainable patient behavior rather than on inferred and probably unknowable mental status.[6]

Tests for Competency

Several tests for competency have been proposed in the literature; others are readily inferable from judicial commentary. Although there is some overlap, they basically fall into five categories: (1) evidencing a choice, (2) "reasonable" outcome of choice, (3) choice based on "rational" reasons, (4) ability to understand, and (5) actual understanding.

Evidencing a choice. This test for competency is set at a very low level and is the most respectful of the autonomy of patient decision making.[11] Under this test the competent patient is one who evidences a preference for or against treatment. This test focuses not on the quality of the patient's decision but on the presence or absence of a decision. Only the patient who does not evidence a preference either verbally or through his or her behavior is considered incompetent. This test of competency encompasses at a minimum the unconscious patient; in psychiatry it encompasses the mute patient who cannot or will not express an opinion.

Even such arch-defenders of individual autonomy as Szasz have agreed that patients who do not formulate and express a preference as to treatment are incompetent.

The following case illustrates the use of the test of evidencing a choice:

A 41-year-old depressed woman was interviewed in the admission unit. She rarely answered yes or no to direct questions. Admission was proposed; she said and did nothing, but looked apprehensive. When asked about admission, she did not sign herself into the hospital, protest, or walk away. She was guided to the inpatient ward by her husband and her doctor after being given the opportunity to walk the other way.

This test may be what one court had in mind when, with respect to the sterilization of residents of state schools, it ruled that even legally incompetent and possibly noncomprehending residents may not be sterilized unless they have formed a genuine desire to undergo the procedure.

The guidelines proposed by the U.S. Department of Health, Education, and Welfare concerning experimentation with institutionalized mentally ill people also point in this direction by requiring even the legally incompetent person's "assent to such participation . . . when . . . he has sufficient mental capacity to understand what is proposed and to express an opinion as to his or her participation." Although this low test of competency does not fully assure patients' understanding of the nature of what they consent to or what they refuse, it is behavioral in orientation and therefore more reliable in application; it also guards against excessive paternalism.

"Reasonable" outcome of choice. This test of competency entails evaluating the patient's capacity to reach the "reasonable," the "right," or the "responsible" decision.[11] The emphasis in this test is on outcome rather than on the mere fact of decision or how it has been reached. The patient who fails to make a decision that is roughly congruent with the decision that a "reasonable" person in the same circumstances would make is viewed as incompetent.

Judicial decisions to override the desire of patients with certain religious beliefs not to receive blood transfusions may rest in part on the court's view that the patient's decision is not reasonable.[12] When life is at stake and a court believes that the patient's decision is unreasonable, the court may focus on even the smallest ambiguity in the patient's thinking to cast doubt on the patient's competency so that it may issue an order that will preserve life or health. For example, one judge issued an order to allow amputation of the leg of an elderly moribund man even though the man had clearly told his daughter before his condition deteriorated not to permit an amputation.[13, 14]

Mental health laws that allow for involuntary treatment on the basis of "need for care and treatment"[15] without requiring a formal adjudication of incompetency in effect use an unstated reasonable outcome test in abridging the patient's common-law right not to be treated without giving his or her consent. These laws are premised on the following syllogism: the patient needs treatment; the patient has not obtained treatment on his or her own initiative; therefore, the patient's decision is incorrect, which means that he or she is incompetent, thus justifying the involuntary imposition of treatment.

The benefits and costs of this test are that social goals and individual health are promoted at considerable expense to personal autonomy. Ultimately, because the test rests on the congruence between the patient's decision and that of a reasonable person or that of the physician, it is biased in favor of decisions to accept treatment, even when such decisions are made by people who are incapable of weighing the risks and benefits of treatment. In other words, if patients do not decide the "wrong" way, the issue of competency will probably not arise.

Choice based on "rational" reasons. Another test is whether the reasons for the patient's decision are "rational," that is, whether the patient's decision is due to or is a product of mental illness.[11] As in the reasonable outcome test, if the patient decides in favor of treatment, the issue of the patient's competency (in this case, whether the decision is the product of mental illness) seldom if ever arises because of the medical profession's bias toward consent to treatment and against refusal of treatment.

In this test the quality of the patient's thinking is what counts. The following case illustrates the use of the test of rational reasons:

A 70-year-old widow who was living alone in a condemned dilapidated house with no heat was brought against her will to the hospital. Her thinking was tangential and fragmented. Although she did not appear to be hallucinating, she seemed delusional. She refused blood tests, saying, "You just want my blood to spread it all over Pittsburgh. No, I'm not giving it." Her choice was respected. Later in the day, however, when her blood pressure was found to be dangerously elevated (250 over 135 in both arms), blood was withdrawn against her will.

The test of rational reasons, although it has clinical appeal and is probably much in clinical use, poses considerable conceptual problems; as a legal test it is probably defective.[11] The problems include the difficulty of distinguishing rational from irrational reasons and drawing inferences of causation between any irrationality believed present and the valence (yes or no) of the patient's decision. Even if the patient's reasons seem irrational, it is not possible to prove that the patient's actual decision making has been the product of such irrationality. The patient's decision might well be the same even if his or her cognitive processes were less impaired. The emphasis on rational reasons can too easily become a global indictment of the competency of mentally disordered individuals, justifying widespread substitute decision making for this group.

The ability to understand. This test—the ability of the patient to understand the risks, benefits, and alternatives to treatment (including no treatment)—is probably the most consistent with the law of informed consent.[16] Decision making need not be rational in either process or outcome; unwise choices are permitted. Nevertheless, at a minimum the patient must manifest sufficient ability to understand information about treatment, even if in fact he or she weighs this information differently from the attending physician. What matters in this test is that the patient is able to comprehend the elements that are presumed by law to be a part of treatment decision making. How the patient weighs these elements, values them, or puts them together to reach a decision is not important.

The patient's capacity for understanding may be tested by asking the patient a series of questions concerning risks, benefits, and alternatives to treatment.[17] By providing further information or explanation to the patient, the physician may find deficiencies in understanding to be remediable or not. The following cases illustrate the use of the test of the ability to understand:

A 28-year-old woman who was unresponsive to medication was approached for consent to ECT. She initially appeared to be unaware of the examiner. Following an explanation of ECT, she responded to the request to explain its purposes and why it was being recommended in her case

with the statement, "Paul McCartney, nothing to zero." She was shown a consent form for ECT that she signed without reading. Further attempts to educate her were unsuccessful. It was decided not to perform the ECT without seeking approval.

Some of the questions raised by this test of competency are, What is to be done if the patient can understand the risks but not the benefits or vice versa? Alternatively, what if the patient views the risks as the profits? The following case illustrates this problem:

A 49-year-old woman whose understanding of treatment was otherwise intact, when informed that there was a 1 in 3,000 chance of dying from ECT, replied, "I hope I am the one."

Furthermore, how potentially sophisticated must understanding be in order that the patient be viewed as competent? There are considerable barriers, conscious and unconscious and intellectual and emotional,[18] to understanding proposed treatments. Presumably the potential understanding required is only that which would be manifested by a reasonable person provided a similar amount of information. A final problem with this test is that its application depends on unobservable and inferential mental processes rather than on concrete and observable elements of behavior.

Actual understanding. Rather than focusing on competency as a construct or intervening variable in the decision-making process, the test of actual understanding reduces competency to an epiphenomenon of this process.[16] The competent patient is by definition one who has provided a knowledgeable consent to treatment. Under this test the physician has an obligation to educate the patient and directly ascertain whether he or she has in fact understood. If not, according to this test the patient may not have provided informed consent.[16] Depending on how sophisticated a level of understanding is to be required, this test delineates a potentially high level of competency, one that may be difficult to achieve.

The provisional decision of DHEW to mandate the creation of consent committees to oversee the decisions of experimental subjects implicitly adopts this test, as does the California law requiring the review of patient consent to ECT.[19] Controversial as these requirements may be, they require physicians to make reasonable efforts to ascertain that their patients understand what they are told and encourage active patient participation in treatment selection.[20]

What constitutes adequate understanding is vague, and deficient understanding may be attributable in whole or in part to physician behavior as well as to the patient's behavior or character. An advantage that this test has over the ability-to-understand test, assuming the necessary level of understanding can be specified a priori, is its greater reliability. Unlike the ability-to-understand test, in which the patient's comprehension of material of a certain complexity is used as the basis for an assumption of comprehension of other material of equivalent complexity (even if this other material is not actually tested), the actual understanding test makes no such assumption. It tests the very issues central to patient decision making about treatment.

Discussion

It has been our experience that competency is presumed as long as the patient modulates his or her behavior, talks in a comprehensible way, remembers what he or she is told, dresses and acts so as to appear to be in meaningful communication with the environment, and has not been declared legally incompetent. In other words, if patients have their wits about them in a layman's sense[16] it is assumed that they will understand what they are told about treatment, including its risks, benefits, and alternatives. This is the equivalent of saying that the legal presumption is one of competency until found otherwise.

In effect, the test that is actually applied combines elements of all the tests described above. However, the circumstances in which competency becomes an issue determine which elements of which tests are stressed and which are underplayed. Although in theory competency is an independent variable that determines whether or not the patient's decision to accept or refuse treatment is to be honored, in practice it seems to be dependent on the interplay of two other variables, the risk/benefit ratio of treatment and the valence of the patient's decision, i.e., whether he or she consents to or refuses treatment.

When there is a favorable risk/benefit ratio to the proposed treatment in the opinion of the person determining competency and the patient consents to the treatment, there does not seem to be any reason to stand in the way of administering treatment. To accomplish this, a test employing a low threshold of competency may be applied to find even a marginal patient competent so that his or her decision may be honored. This is what happens daily when uncomprehending patients are permitted to sign themselves into the hospital. Similarly, when the risk/benefit ratio is favorable and the patient refuses treatment, a test employing a higher threshold of competency may be applied. Under such a test even a somewhat knowledgeable patient may be found incompetent so that consent may be sought from a substitute decision maker and treatment administered despite the patient's refusal. An example would be the patient withdrawing from alcohol who, although intermittently resistive, is nevertheless administered sedative medication. In both these cases, in which the risk/benefit ratio is favorable, the bias of physicians, other health professionals, and judges is usually skewed toward providing treatment. Therefore, a test of competency is applied that will permit the treatment to be administered irrespective of the patient's actual or potential understanding.

However, there is a growing reluctance on the part of our society to permit patients to undergo treatments that are extremely risky or for which the benefits are highly speculative. Thus if the risk/benefit ratio is unfavorable or questionable and the patient refuses treatment, a test employing a low threshold of competency may be selected so that the patient will be found competent and his or her refusal honored. This is what happens in the area of sterilization of mentally retarded people, in which, at least from the perspective of the retarded individual, the risk/benefit ratio is questionable. On the other hand, when the risk/benefit ratio is unfavorable or questionable and the patient consents to treatment, a test using a higher threshold of competency may be applied, preventing even some fairly knowledgeable patients from undergoing treatment. The judicial opinion in the well-known Kaimowitz psychosurgery case delineated a high test of competency to be employed in that experimental setting.

Of course, some grossly impaired patients cannot be determined to be competent under any conceivable test, nor can most normally functioning people be found incompetent merely by selective application of a test of competency. However, within limits and when the patient's competency is not absolutely clear-cut, a test of competency that will achieve the desired medical or social end despite the actual condition of the patient may be selected. We do not imply that this is done maliciously either by physicians or by the courts; rather, we believe that it occurs as a consequence of the strong societal bias in favor of treating treatable patients so long as it does not expose them to serious risks.

NOTES

1. S.A. Shah, "Dangerousness and Civil Commitment of the Mentally Ill: Some Public Policy Considerations," *American Journal of Psychiatry*, vol. 132, p. 501, 1975.

2. R.C. Allen, E.Z. Ferster, and H. Weihofen, *Mental Impairment and Legal Incompetency*, Prentice-Hall, Englewood Cliffs, N.J., 1968.

3. J.H. Hardesty, "Mental Illness: A Legal Fiction," *Washington Law Review*, vol. 48, p. 735, 1973.

4. G.J. Alexander and T.S. Szasz, "From Contract to Status via Psychiatry, *Santa Clara Lawyers,*

vol. 13, p. 537, 1973.

5. Group for the Advancement of Psychiatry Committee on Psychiatry and Law, Misuse of Psychiatry in the Criminal Courts: Competency to Stand Trial, *Report 89*, New York, 1974.

6. M.D. Green, "Judicial Tests of Mental Incompetency," *Missouri Law Review*, vol. 6, p. 141, 1941.

7. M.A. Peszke, "Is Dangerousness an Issue for Physicians in Emergency Commitment?" *American Journal of Psychiatry*, vol. 132, p. 825, 1975.

8. S.L. Halleck, "Legal and Ethical Aspects of Behavior Control," *American Journal of Psychiatry*, vol. 131, p. 381, 1974.

9. H. Grunebaum and V. Abernethy, "Ethical Issues in Family Planning for Hospitalized Psychiatric Patients," *American Journal of Psychiatry*, vol. 132, p. 326, 1975.

10. R. Michels, "The Right to Refuse Psychoactive Drugs: Case Studies in Bioethics," *Hastings Center Report*, vol. 3, no. 3, p. 10, 1973.

11. P.R. Friedman, "Legal Regulation of Applied Behavior Analysis in Mental Institutions and Prisons," *Arizona Law Review*, vol. 17, p. 39, 1975.

12. N.L. Cantor, "A Patient's Decision to Decline Life-Saving Medical Treatment: Bodily Integrity versus the Preservation of Life," *Rutgers Law Review*, vol. 26, p. 228, 1973.

13. "Judge OKs Amputation of South Sider's Leg," *Pittsburgh Press*, June 4, 1975, p. 1.

14. "Amputation Order More Human than Judicial, Larsen Says," *Pittsburgh Press*, June 8, 1975, p. 1.

15. "Developments in the Law—Civil Commitment of the Mentally Ill," *Harvard Law Review*, vol. 87, p. 1190, 1974.

16. A. Meisel, L.H. Roth, and C.W. Lidz, "Toward a Model of the Legal Doctrine of Informed Consent," *American Journal of Psychiatry*, vol. 134, p. 285, 1977.

17. R. Miller and H.S. Willner, "The Two-Part Consent Form," *New England Journal of Medicine*, vol. 290, p. 964, 1974.

18. J. Katz, *Experimentation with Human Beings*, p. 609, Russell Sage Foundation, New York, 1972.

19. "California Enacts Rigid Shock Therapy Controls," *Psychiatric News*, Feb. 5, 1975, p. 1.

20. R.S. Szasz and M.H. Hollender, "The Basic Models of the Doctor-Patient Relationship," *Archives of Internal Medicine*, vol. 97, p. 585, 1956.

54.

Critical Illness: The Limits of Autonomy
Mark Siegler

Mr. D, a previously healthy sixty-six-year-old black man, came to a university hospital emergency room with his wife and described a three-day history of sore throat, muscle aches, fevers, chills, cough, sputum production, and blood in his urine. The patient was acutely ill with a high fever, shortness of breath, and a limited attention span. A chest x-ray demonstrated a generalized pneumonia in both lungs. The clinical impression was that Mr. D was critically ill, that the cause of his lung disease was obscure, and that a low platelet count and blood in the urine were ominous signs. He was treated aggressively with three antibiotics in an effort to cure his pneumonia.

The next day his condition worsened. After reviewing the available clinical and laboratory data, the physicians caring for this man recommended that two uncomfortable but relatively routine diagnostic procedures be performed: a bronchial brushing to obtain a small sample of lung tissue to determine the cause of the pneumonia and a bone marrow examination to determine whether an infection or cancer was invading the bone marrow. The patient refused these diagnostic procedures. Separately, and together, the intern, resident, attending physician, and chaplain explained that these diagnostic tests were necessary to help the physicians formulate rational treatment plans. Mr. D became angry and agitated by this prolonged pressure, and subsequently began refusing even routine blood tests and x-rays.

A psychiatrist who evaluated Mr. D concluded that although he was obviously ill and had a degree of mental impairment manifested by poor memory, he was not mentally incompetent. The psychiatrist thought that the patient understood the severity of his illness and the reasons the physicians were recommending certain tests, but that he was still making a rational choice in refusing the tests.

The patient's condition deteriorated further and 24 hours later he appeared near death. I was the attending physician, and it was my opinion that the only treatment left was to place Mr. D on a respirator as a stopgap measure that might sustain him for another day or two, during which time the antibiotics and antituberculosis drugs might become effective. Mr. D refused.

The physicians expressed considerable disagreement on whether Mr. D was sufficiently rational to refuse a potentially lifesaving treatment. In an effort to resolve this controversy, I spent two 45 minute periods at his bedside and explained as clearly as I could the reasons for our recommendations. I said that if he survived this crisis he would be able to return to a normal life and would not be an invalid or require chronic supportive care. During these two sessions, Mr. D was breathing rapidly and shallowly, and had trouble talking. But everything he said convinced me that he understood the gravity of his situation. For example, when I told him he was dying, he replied: "Everyone has to die. If I die now, I am ready." When I asked him if he came to the hospital to be helped, he stated: "I want to be helped. I want you to treat me with whatever medicine you think I need. I don't want any more tests and I don't want the breathing machine."

I gradually became convinced that despite the severity of his illness and his high fever, he was making a conscious, rational decision to selectively refuse a particular kind of treatment. In view of the frankness of our discussion, I then asked him

Source: *Hastings Center Report*, vol. 7, October 1977.

whether he would want us to resuscitate him if he had a cardio-respiratory arrest. He turned away and said: "We've been through this before; now leave me alone." I left the bedside.

Throughout this day, despite vigorous attempts by social workers and neighbors, neither his wife nor children could be located.

Mr. D soon became semiconscious and had a cardio-respiratory arrest. Despite the objections of the house officers, I did not attempt to resuscitate him, and he died.

Mr. D's case raised the following questions:

1. Would this critically ill man be permitted to establish diagnostic and therapeutic limits on the care he wished to receive from a health care team in a large university hospital?

2. What were the medically and morally relevant factors that would encourage or permit physicians to respect his wishes? Or, alternatively, on what ground would physicians usurp the patient's presumed rights to liberty, autonomy, and self-determination?

One solution to moral-ethical dilemmas is to establish categorical rules of conduct which obviate the necessity for making agonizing choices in difficult situations. For example, in his writings Robert Veatch has consistently emphasized a commitment to individual freedom and self-determination, and the concomitant need to limit the power and authority of the medical profession. In discussing a patient's right to refuse treatment, Veatch makes the claim that "no competent patients have ever been forced to undergo any medical treatment for their own good no matter how misguided their refusal may have appeared." Veatch concludes that an adult may refuse any treatment as long as he is competent, and the principal determination to be made (in Veatch's view by the courts rather than by physicians) is whether the patient is competent.

In a recent paper entitled "The Function of Medicine," Eric Cassell describes an alternative attitude, and one equally familiar to clinicians. Cassell notes that in cases of acute illness (using pneumococcal meningitis as his example), "It would be a rare hospital where such a patient would not be treated [even] against his will." In such a case, Cassell defends the decision to override a patient's wishes on the grounds that the refusal of treatment in acute illness is tantamount to suicide, that the physician has responsibilities to treat that cannot be relieved by the patient's refusal to accept treatment, that the patient is morally constrained not to prevent the physician from carrying out his responsibilities to treat him, and that in the face of acute illness, the physician does not have sufficient time to assess the patient's motives.

The Veatch and Cassell positions appear not to take into account the medically and morally relevant factors that physicians assess when determining whether to respect the wishes of critically ill patients. Clinical ethics is premised on the particularities of clinical circumstances, and workable clinical guidelines must necessarily take into account and reflect the extraordinary complexity of the medical model.

Factors Influencing the Physician's Decision

The patient's ability to make (rational) choices about his care. Either every critically ill patient in the hospital is incompetent to make choices concerning his care or each case must be assessed separately to determine if there are limits within which the critically ill patient retains some intellectual judgment and is capable of making choices. In the case of Mr. D, as in other critical care cases, the issue confronting conscientious physicians was not simply whether to respect a patient's wishes, but whether it was morally justifiable to accept at face value a critically ill patient's statement of his wishes.

Mr. D's case illustrates the practical difficulties in adhering to any rigid rule (either to defend "radical autonomy" for competent adults or to accept the "doctor's burden to heal" viewpoint) in critical care situations. Mr. D's wishes were forcefully stated and clear. He wished to be helped and to be relieved of his discomfort and pain, and to this end he would permit physicians to treat him with intravenous fluids, oxygen, antibiotics, and other medications. But he was also firm in establishing absolute limits on the diagnostic studies he would permit and in refusing to accept a respirator as a form of treatment. Thus, the perplexing question which continued to trouble his physicians was whether Mr. D was intellectually capable of exercising such a degree of discrimination and choice. Although there was a considerable difference of opinion among the physicians caring for Mr. D—some believed that his illness impaired his thought processes and rendered him incapable of making choices— in my capacity as the attending physician responsible for his care, I decided otherwise and elected to respect Mr. D's wishes. This decision was based upon my subjective clinical judgment that despite the intensity of his illness, Mr. D retained sufficient intellect and rationality to make choices.

The nature of the person making the choice. Rather than assessing the rationality of a particular choice, one can ask an alternative question, whether Mr. D's decisions were consonant with his nature as a person. Who was Mr. D? What were his values? And did his choices in the hospital reflect those he might have made were he not ill? Was the patient acting autonomously— that is, with authenticity and independence? Alternatively, another question to be asked is: in the face of critical illness and within the narrow time-space frame characteristic of acute illness, is it ever possible to determine whether a patient's choices truly reflect his normal personality?

Obviously, if a patient and physician had previously established an ongoing relationship, the physician would be better acquainted with the personality, character, ideas, and beliefs of his patient. Another indicator to assess the validity of a patient's choice is whether it reflects a commitment expressed through time, such as the adher-

ence to a particular religious belief (like a Jehovah's Witness refusing blood transfusions), or the signing and updating of a "living will," or the establishment of certain attitudes and behavior patterns in the course of a chronic illness. In Mr. D's case none of this information was available.

Another valuable insight into the patient as a person might be provided by the family as they describe the personality, character, and beliefs of the patient before the onset of this acute illness. The family could also be asked to offer an opinion on whether a patient is acting as he would normally act, or whether his behavior strikes them as aberrant and unusual. The family then would not be making choices for the patient but would be indicating to physicians the probable validity of the patient's own choices. In Mr. D's case the family was not available and thus could not provide evidence one way or the other.

Many people believe that the rights of individuals are not absolute, but must always be weighed against their responsibilities to social groups like the family or to the community at large. Unfortunately, in Mr. D's case, the absence of family input effectively limited the grounds upon which physicians would accept or reject Mr. D's wishes.

In most clinical circumstances it is possible either from previous knowledge of a patient or from the contributions of his family to assess accurately whether a particular choice made by an ill patient is consistent with his previous behavior and values. In this respect, Mr. D's case represents an extreme example, since none of this background material was available.

In the absence of supporting data, the physician must rely upon his basic skills of communication with the patient and must assess the patient's verbal and nonverbal messages. So much of clinical judgment and clinical decision-making involves the gathering of primary data through talking with patients that this situation should be seen as an extreme variant of the basic clinical model. Further, much of clinical judgment involves "life and death" decisions, and thus this situation is not different in intensity from many others. I assessed Mr. D's personality as intelligent, proud, independent, wary of outsiders, and particularly suspicious of physicians and their motives. It seemed to me that the choices he was making were entirely consistent with his basic personality.

Of anecdotal interest, since it did not influence my decision, was some information that became available only after Mr. D's death which indicated that ten years earlier he had left the hospital "against medical advice" after first refusing to have a bone marrow examination.

Age. Mr. D's age made a difference in my decision. Had he been twenty-six years old, the factors I would use to decide whether to override his wishes would probably have remained essentially the same—competence, the conformity of his choices to his personality, and the medical diagnosis and prognosis—but the standards I would apply to assess these might change. For example, I would have demanded a more perfect "mental status examination" and would have scrupulously checked a younger patient for evidence of a "toxic delirium" or an acute depression. My obvious wavering on this point may have something to do with the notion that wisdom and aging are associated, but more likely has to do with a concept of "natural death." The closer a patient gets to a "normal" life span, the more he has lived, and the more ready I am to "let nature take its course." Even though I appreciate the ambiguities and inconsistencies of taking age into account, I believe that I might have acted differently with a younger patient.

Nature of the illness. In this context, critical illness refers to an acute life-threatening illness. Several subdivisions of critical illness are necessary because physician behavior is premised on (1) whether the illness can be diagnosed or alternatively, whether it is obscure and refractory to diagnosis, and (2) what the prognosis is, whether or not the physician is able to make a diagnosis.

The most straightforward situation is one in which the physician can make a diagnosis that permits him to state with certainty that the prognosis of a particular disease is uniformly fatal if untreated, whereas with appropriate treatment complete recovery is possible. In addition to the infectious diseases such as pneumococcal meningitis which conform to this model, other medical emergencies such as acute respiratory failure, acute pulmonary edema, and diabetic keto-acidosis are also easily diagnosed and treated. It is precisely in such cases where diagnostic uncertainty is at a minimum and where the physician is confident about the probability of success with treatment, and the probability of death without treatment, that the physician will be most likely to usurp an ill patient's desires and treat him even against his wishes. In all other cases, however, the physician will be more inclined but not certain to respect the patient's wishes not to be treated. For example, certain diagnoses, in particular metastatic solid tumors or degenerative neurologic diseases, seem to generate a minimalist approach on the part of physicians and on occasion discourage physicians from aggressively treating patients with such diseases who may develop easily reversible acute conditions such as pneumonia.

The problem of uncertainty of diagnosis or uncertainty of prognosis is particularly disturbing. The absence of a diagnosis is a potential threat to the whole disease-oriented medical system, and generates a very aggressive, no-holds-barred approach to diagnostic testing. Mr. D's refusal to submit to certain routine but uncomfortable diagnostic procedures effectively blocked the efforts of his physicians to name his disease and surely contributed to their frustration. In cases of uncertainty, where the physician and patient are in agreement on pursuing diagnostic and therapeutic procedures, physicians will generally err on the side of diagnostic aggressiveness

in an effort not to overlook a potentially reversible disease process. However, in
cases of uncertainty where physicians
and patients are in disagreement about
diagnostic and therapeutic approaches, physician anxiety is maximized and the need
for a moral-clinical decision is most urgent.
In such cases, and Mr. D's case is a classic
example, physicians must again rely upon
their clinical judgment to assess the likelihood that a particular diagnostic study will
yield a result that may permit a particular
therapy which can change the outcome of
the case. As the probability of a successful
intervention decreases, most physicians can
more easily, but not very easily, conform
to the patient's wishes.

In some cases, however, even if a particular intervention will guarantee success,
the physician may still not usurp a patient's
wishes. A frequent example of this latter
situation arises in Jehovah's Witness cases
where a simple blood transfusion could
forestall a life-threatening emergency but
in which the physician is constrained by
consistent legal precedents not to override
a patient's wishes.

In the case of Mr. D, it soon became
clear to me that whatever the diagnosis of
his obscure illness was, it was fulminant
and aggressive and would probably lead to
his death. Even if we had been able to
make a diagnosis from the bone marrow
and bronchial brushing examinations,
it was likely that no additional therapy
would change his outcome. Even if he had
consented to a respirator, his rapidly progressive deterioration suggested that he was
not going to survive. I readily admit that
my clinical judgment that the disease was
rapidly progressive and almost certainly
fatal further influenced me.

*The attitudes and values of the physician
responsible for the decision.* At every
point in the decision making, the responsible
physician has resorted to value judgment.
The judgments of whether the patient was
rational, of what his baseline personality was, of what importance to ascribe to his
age, and of whether his disease was poten-

tially treatable and reversible, are all determinations that involve subjective value
judgments based upon limited objective
data.

Further, although physicians as a profession may share some general values and
biases, they are not homogeneous in their
basic value orientation. They differ in moral
and religious background, in age, in experience, and in specialty training, to mention
just a few factors. Specifically, what is a
particular physician's attitude toward life
and death? Does a physician view the death
of a patient as a personal defeat, an avoidable tragedy? What is his concept of the role
of the physician in the physician-patient
relationship, that of a technician-scientist, or
an advisor, or a friend, or a party to a
contract? If the responsible physician invokes the doctrine of "do no harm," is
his concept of harm that of omission or
commission?

If all other factors were identical in arriving at a decision to support or override
a patient's wishes not to be treated, we
might discover that two physicians—one
who believed in the primacy of life and
another who believed in "death with dignity"—would reach entirely opposite conclusions. In Mr. D's case, my belief in
the rights of individuals to determine their
own destinies further encouraged me to
support the patient's choices.

The clinical setting. Mr. D's case reflects
some of the special problems of practicing medicine in a large, institutional, teaching
setting. If a physician-patient encounter
similar to the one described here had occurred in a patient's home, or in a nursing
home, or even in many community hospitals
(particularly one without house staff),
there would be little question about acced-
ing to the patient's wishes. There are at
least two reasons. First, the kind of technology and expertise necessary to do many
of these procedures is best represented in
the large teaching hospital.

The second reason is more complex. It
involves the nature of a teaching hospital in
which authority and responsibility are

diffused among the "health care team." Although the attending physician may ultimately be responsible for decisions, he does not care for patients in isolation. Indeed, most of the caring is performed by house staff, students, nurses, and other health care personnel. The house staff are very close to their patients and have very strong feelings about how best to care for them. Despite the house staff's general lack of clinical experience, their views are often very accurate and persuasive. Further, house staff are particularly skilled in the care of acutely ill patients. These young physicians strive diligently to not harm the patients, but when their concept of harm remains obscure, "do no harm" often means "do everything."

One interesting sidelight of this case was the house officers' wish to resuscitate this man after he died. They argued that at no time did the patient state he wanted to die; he did not offer a definitive "no" when asked whether he wished to be resuscitated; and clearly, after his heart and lungs stopped, he was no longer rational

and decisions could then be made for him.

One final observation: this man was extremely strong and dignified in his last days. Despite his illness and fever, he resisted the onslaught of many physicians and consultants and the power of the hospital institution. He established limits for the health care team and would not permit those limits to be transgressed. The intellectual and emotional strength necessary to resist the powers of the medical system to persuade and force him to accept what they wanted to offer must have been enormous. He died a dignified death, and attempts at resuscitation would have violated the position he held while alive. It is unfortunate, and I am sadly moved, that he had to expend his last measures of intellectual and physical energy to engage in ongoing debate with his physicians. But perhaps that is the price the medical system sometimes exacts from those who would assert their independence and preserve their autonomy while suffering from critical illness.

55.

Informed Consent: Why Are Its Goals Imperfectly Realized?

Barrie R. Cassileth   Robert V. Zupkis
Katherine Sutton-Smith   Vicki March

Methods

Procedure and subjects. With the physician's approval, consenting patients completed two paper-and-pencil tests: a test of their recall of information regarding consent, and a questionnaire designed to determine patients' perceptions of the purpose, content, and implications of the material in the form and of oral explanations.

A total of 207 patients were approached consecutively over a 5-month period be-

fore the desired total of 200 participants was obtained.

Two hundred cancer patients at the Hospital of the University of Pennsylvania and at an affiliated Veterans Administration Hospital comprised the study population. Participants ranged in age from 20 to 82 years, with a median age of 59. Each patient's medical status was assessed by the research assistant who administered the questionnaire, with assistance from physicians when necessary, according to Eastern Coopera-

Source: *The New England Journal of Medicine*, vol. 302, no. 16, April 17, 1980.

tive Oncology Group criteria. The status of
the patients was generally good: 60 percent of the patients were fully ambulatory,
18 percent were bedridden less than half
the time, and 22 percent were bedridden
most of the time.

Tests and Scoring Procedures. A test of
recall of written and oral information was
given to each patient. The initial question on
this test was designed to reflect the care
with which patients had read their consent
forms before signing them. They answered
this question by selecting one of four options;
"I read the whole thing very carefully"; "I
just gave it a quick reading"; "I only read
parts of it"; or "I did not read it." The questionnaire went on to test all areas supposedly
covered in patients' consent forms or in
discussions with physicians before signing
consent forms, following Department of
Health, Education, and Welfare guidelines
for informed consent. Test topics included
knowledge of diagnosis or illness, proposed procedure, purpose of the proposed
procedure, possible risks or complications, appropriate alternatives to proposed
procedure, and opportunity to ask additional questions. These items were noted
explicitly on forms giving consent for
chemotherapy and surgery. The form for
radiation therapy contained the statement,
"The effect and nature of this treatment,
possible alternative methods of treatment,
and the risks of injury despite precautions
have been explained to me." Presumably,
these areas were covered by oral explanation.

Results

Consent information-recall test. As a
group, the patients studied had a mean
recall test score of 8.26 ± 2.56 (mean $\pm$ S.D.)
out of a possible maximum score of 12. On-
ly 60 percent of all patients correctly described what their treatment would involve,
59 percent could describe the essential purpose of the treatment, only 55 percent were
able to list even a single major risk or complication, and only 27 percent could name

one alternative treatment. However, 81.5 percent correctly identified their diagnoses.

Factors that contributed to these scores
were identified with the analysis of variance.
No differences were found when test scores
of men and women were compared. Differences in age, race, hospital used (University Hospital versus Veterans Administration
Hospital), and treatment (radiotherapy,
chemotherapy, or surgery) had no effect independent of education. That is, when education was held constant, the effects of age,
race, hospital used, and treatment disappeared. There were no differences between
patients who signed the shorter radiation-
therapy consent forms that relied on oral information and those who signed the more
comprehensive documents. Two factors
proved to have independent effects on test
scores: education and medical status. Bedridden patients gave significantly fewer correct
reponses to each item on the recall test than
did ambulatory patients. Mean scores were
7.03 and 9.00, respectively ($P < 0.01$).

A nondemographic variable that proved
to be related to test score, even after adjustment for education, was the care with
which patients judged themselves to have
read the consent form before signing it. The
mean recall-test score of the 117 patients
who reported reading the entire form either
carefully or cursorily was 8.81, whereas
the mean score of the 64 patients who read
only parts of the form or did not read it
at all was 7.19 ($P < 0.001$). Persons who read
their consent forms carefully tended to be
younger, white, and better educated.

Purpose of consent forms. After the recall test, patients answered a series of questions designed to elicit their understanding
and opinion of consent documents. Given
the opportunity to select one or more
responses to the question: "In your opinion, what are consent forms?" more than
three quarters of the patients circled "legal documents to protect the physician's
rights." Close to half answered that consent
forms were "legal documents to protect the
patient's rights," and 43 percent selected
"explanations of treatment." Because pa-

tients could select more than one response to this item on the questionnaire, it was not possible to evaluate these responses in terms of scores on the recall test.

Need for consent forms. Asked their opinion of consent forms, most patients (80.5 percent) deemed them "necessary." Whether patients believed consent forms to be necessary or unnecessary had no effect on their ability to recall the material. However, the results of an analysis of variance applied to scores on the recall test and the five optional responses to this question were significant ($P<0.01$): patients with no strong opinion (those who answered that consent forms "don't matter one way or another" or "don't know") had lower scores on the recall test. The variation in opinions of consent forms was not related to any demographic or medical characteristic.

Adequacy of explanations on consent. When asked to evaluate the amount of information that they had been given about consent, most patients (76 percent) reported that they had received "just the right amount"; 20 percent thought that the information was inadequate; and 2 percent thought that too much information has been offered. There was a significant relation between response to this question and scores on the test of recall: persons who answered that the explanation offered "just the right amount of information" had higher scores on the recall tests than did patients who selected either of the remaining two responses ($P<0.001$).

Comprehension of information on consent. Patients were asked how much they could understand of the explanatory material about consent. Eighty-five percent said that they could understand "all" or "most" of the information in the explanation; 9.5 percent could understand "only a little," and 3.5 percent "could not understand it." There was a positive relation between the amount of information understood and scores on the recall test ($P<0.001$). As might be anticipated, educational level was also related to responses to this item: the higher the educational level, the greater the percentage of patients who indicated that they could un-

derstand all the information on the form ($P<0.05$ by the Bartholomew test).

Patients' rights to refuse signing. Asked to select one of two statements, 70 percent of respondents answered that "patients have the right not to sign consent forms," and 28 percent believed that "if patients are given consent forms, they must sign them." Responses to this item were not related to any demographic or medical variable, nor did they correlate with scores on the recall test.

Efforts to recall information about consent. The great majority of patients (90.5 percent) said that they would "try to remember most of the information in my consent form explanation." The 6 percent of patients who would "try to forget most of the information" differed from the others only in items of race: 12.5 percent of blacks, but 2.5 percent of whites, said that they wanted to forget ($P<0.01$).

Importance of explanations about consent. No differences in recall-test score, demography, or medical status were found with regard to the final item on the questionnaire, which requested a choice between two statements. Seventy-five percent of the patients thought that "consent form explanations are important, so that I can help decide about my treatment." Most of the remaining 25 percent preferred the alternative statement, "consent form explanations are silly, because I would do what my doctor says anyway."

Discussion

The results of this study corroborate previous work indicating that many patients fail to recall major portions of information on consent. The relation between educational background and patients' ability to describe the information, together with the similar correlation between education and the care with which patients read consent forms, suggests that such communications are too complex and difficult for many patients to grasp, despite the fact that most patients reported understanding all or most of the information.

Bedridden patients were less able to recall this information than were patients in better physical condition. As patients become increasingly ill, their sense of personal control over their own destinies may give way to intensified dependence on their physicians, and this dependence may result in poorer attention to, interest in, and recall of information about consent. Intellectual as well as physical deterioration may have had a role in poorer recall, although the patients studied were competent enough to sign consent documents and participate in this research.

Although most of these patients thought that the information on the consent form was important, comprehensible, worth remembering, and offered appropriate amounts of data, only a few patients actually read their consent forms carefully. It is possible that some patients merely scan the forms because the material has been explained orally by the physician. Reliance on one's doctor as the preferred primary source of information may reduce the personal relevance of the forms and contribute to the idea that they are legal documents. After completion of the questionnaires, 31 patients spontaneously expressed the feeling that official documents seemed out of place and counterproductive in the clinical setting. In addition, 80 percent of the patients studied viewed consent forms as a protection for the physician. The consent form's legalistic, perhaps even adversarial, overtones may appear inconsistent to the patient who has a fundamental orientation to and preference for a doctor-patient relation based on "trust."

The purpose of the consent procedure, to facilitate and ensure informed decisions on the part of the patient, is poorly accomplished and may actually be thwarted by the present procedure. Barriers are imposed by the difficulty of the material and by the legalistic and other negative connotations of the consent document. These barriers need to be removed if consent forms are to achieve their intended objectives and if patients are to function as the informed consumers that many of them wish to become.

NOTES

1. K. Lebacqz and R.J. Levine, "Respect for Persons and Informed Consent to Participate in Research," *Clinical Research*, vol. 25, 1977, p. 101.

2. A.M. Capron, "Informed Consent in Catastrophic Disease, Research and Treatment," *University of Pennsylvania Law Review*, vol. 123, no. 2, 1974, p. 340.

3. A.J. Rosoff, "Informed Consent." In: B.R. Cassileth, ed. *The Cancer Patient: Social and Medical Aspects of Care*, Lea & Febiger, Philadelphia, 1979, pp. 75, 90.

4. G. Robinson and A. Merav, "Informed Consent: Recall by Patients Tested Postoperatively," *Annals of Thoracic Surgery*, vol. 22, 1976, p. 209.

5. A.L. Schultz, G.P. Pardee, and J.W. Ensinck, "Are Research Subjects Really Informed?" *Western Journal of Medicine*, vol. 123, 1975, p. 76.

6. L.C. Epstein and L. Lasagna, "Obtaining Informed Consent: Form or Substance," *Archives of Internal Medicine*, vol. 123, 1969, p. 682.

7. H.B. Muss, D.R. White and R. Michielutte et al. "Written Informed Consent in Patients with Breast Cancer," *Cancer*, vol. 43, 1979, p. 1549.

8. Code of Federal Regulations, "Title 45, Part 46. 103(C)," Government Printing Office, Washington, D.C., November 16, 1978.

9. G. Morrow, J. Gootnick and A. Schmale, "A Simple Technique for Increasing Cancer Patients' Knowledge of Informed Consent to Treatment," *Cancer*, vol. 42, 1978, p. 793.

56.

Beyond Consent: The Ethics of Decision Making in Emergency Medicine

Karen M. Tait   Gerald Winslow

Increasing attention is being given to the problems of informed consent in the practice of medicine. [1-3] Although obtaining informed consent for medical interventions is generally considered imperative, emergency medical care is a widely recognized exception. The ethicist Ramsey[4] defends the right of patients to consent to treatment but acknowledges that in medical emergencies assumed or implied consent is sufficient. Shartel and Plant[5] suggest that it is more appropriate to recognize that the law grants authority to act without reference to an injured person's consent, and that consideration of a "fictitious" consent adds unnecessary confusion. Recently, Johnson and Trimble[6] have discussed the problems encountered in treating a verbally abusive and unwilling patient in an emergency and concluded that physical restraint should be used when necessary and that thorough evaluation and treatment should be carried out regardless of the patient's consent. Only a few discussions[7, 8] have attempted to resolve the many ambiguities of informed consent in an emergency, and these are largely from a legal point of view.

The purpose of the present study is to analyze the *ethical* issues related to the problems of consent and decision making in emergency medicine. The primary concern was for critical emergencies, such as trauma, myocardial infarction, and drug overdose. Some of these patients were unconscious; others were conscious with varying levels of awareness. For simplicity, the word "emergency" is restricted to critical cases in which lives depended on immediate supportive treatment.

Emergency medicine is characterized by the need for rapid intervention, sometimes calling for aggressive measures at a time when pertinent information is inaccessible and medical histories are sketchy. Moreover, if a patient is unconscious or irrational, or an impenetrable language barrier exists, explaining the necessary medical procedures becomes impossible. Other patients at various levels of consciousness or apparent rationality express the desire *not* to be treated in spite of manifestly serious conditions. This predicament is sometimes managed by having a close family member give "proxy" consent in order to satisfy legal requirements. But when the patient is unaccompanied by a family member, even proxy consent is impossible.

If a physician determines that a patient is incapable of making a rational decision, the medicolegal principle of "reasonable therapeutic restraint" may be appropriate. The courts have generally protected physicians who take whatever measures are deemed necessary in a medical emergency.[9] However, whether or not a physician acts, he *may* be legally liable. If he treats the patient without the patient's consent, the physician may be sued on the grounds of assault and battery. If, on the other hand, the physician does not restrain and treat the patient, he may be sued for negligence.[6]

Measures taken contrary to the patient's will require an accurate evaluation of the patient's mental status which, under emergency circumstances, is subject to a wide array of influences. Rational judgment may be affected by such conditions as cerebral hypoperfusion, central nervous system injury, and drug intoxication. Psychological defense mechanisms such as denial and regres-

Source: *Western Journal of Medicine*, vol. 126, no. 2, p. 156, February 1977.

sion[10] may be used by injured patients
and result in a failure to recognize the need
for treatment or a childlike dependency
on others.

Medical advances in resuscitation techniques, especially for trauma victims, have
given impetus to aggressive treatment of
most patients. For example, a 19-year-old-
man was brought to the emergency room with
a stab wound to the chest which penetrated
the right ventricle of the heart. Upon
arrival he was in severe shock and hypo-
thermic (92°F). In earlier years it probably
would have been considered impossible to save
such a patient. However, aggressive resuscitative measures were initiated. In the trauma
room, blood loss from the wound was reduced by thoracotomy before the patient
was taken for emergency surgical operation.
During several weeks in the intensive care
unit, the man failed to respond to verbal
stimuli, although his overall condition
gradually improved. Eventually, he regained
mental alertness and subsequently recovered
to the extent that he was able to return to
work.

In another case, extensive resources, including the services of a large proportion of
the available personnel, were utilized in
the treatment of a 34–year–old woman suffering from a severe upper gastrointestinal hemorrhage. In spite of all efforts
at resuscitation, neurological evidence
of brain death became apparent within
24 hours. Consent was obtained from
the family to remove her kidneys for transplantation. Three days following admission the woman died. From the perspective
of the medical staff this case did not represent an unmitigated failure. The family
was reassured that the obligation to use
all available means to save the patient's
life was fulfilled and, moreover, the donation of the patient's two kidneys benefited two recipients.

The ethical approaches utilized by the
medical personnel when making decisions in
emergency situations seemed consistent
with a predetermined decision to maintain
life in virtually all emergency cases. Sum-

marized as an operating principle, the prevalent attitude appeared to be: Always respond
with whatever measures seem necessary in
order to maintain (or resuscitate) vital functions whether with, without, or against
the patient's expressed will whenever urgent circumstances make attempts to
obtain the patient's informed consent impractical.

In neither of the two cases just cited did
the patients have the opportunity to consent
to treatment. Presumably they would both
have wanted all measures taken that might
have been essential in attempting to preserve their lives. In recent years, however, this
principle of preserving life whenever possible, sometimes called "vitalism," has come
under attack. Fletcher argues that the
"vitalistic ideas that life as such is sancro-
anct, the highest good and somehow
both sacred and untouchable, is obviously
not tenable in actual practice."[11, 12] Mc-
Cormick[13] claims that quality-of-life
decisions must be made; the vitalism which
has characterized much of medical practice is a kind of "idolatry."

Along with criticism of the vitalistic approach, recent years have witnessed an
expanding discussion of the patient's right
to terminate or forgo certain types of
treatment—even essential lifesaving treatment.[14] Commentaries on the well-known
case of Karen Quinlan have indicated a
similar concern.[15] Some patients have written "living wills" which set the conditions
and limits for lifesaving intervention,[16] but
a physician is more likely to encounter the
desire to stop treatment as a verbal expression by the patient.

In commenting on a case in which a
burned patient wished to terminate treatment, Engelhardt argues that the patient's
decision must be honored, yet he also allows
for the notion that *emergency* treatment
might legitimately be forced on a patient in
order to guarantee a later exercise of rational choice. ". . . One can justify treating
a burned patient when first admitted even
if that person protested: One might argue
that the individual was not able to choose

freely because of the pain and serious impact of the circumstances, and that by treating initially one gave the individual a reasonable chance to choose freely in the future."[17]

The making of decisions for another without regard for the involved person's will is often discussed under the heading of "paternalism."[18] Such a practice seems to run counter to the generally held principle of respecting the autonomy of individual persons. Paternalistic decisions are, however, frequently made. Many philosophers have recognized the limited but unmistakable legitimacy of this category of actions in certain situations. Children and even mentally competent adults are guarded against experiences and practices considered detrimental to their well-being, such as the use of street drugs.

It should also be recognized that even when a physician relinquishes the decision-making power, a kind of paternalistic judgment has been made. After initially assessing the patient's competence, the responsible physician provides or withholds the approval necessary to implement a patient's decision. For example, in the hospital studied, two patients under the same doctor's care wished to leave the hospital against medical advice on the same evening. Both patients were in need of observation, one for symptoms of suspected acute appendicitis and the other for complications of a drug overdose. The first man appeared to be rational and cooperative but preferred to watch for developing symptoms at home. The second patient showed his ineptitude during an attempt to get out of bed by upsetting his IV stand and breaking the bottle. The physician in charge released the first man with instructions to call at the first sign of problems but retained the second man against his wishes. Of course, in either case the patient could presumably undertake legal action to challenge the physician's judgment, but the potential for such action in the emergency setting is virtually nil. Furthermore, securing a court's judgment simply

moves the power of paternalistic ratification from the physician to the court.

What is needed is a principle for action which respects the patient's autonomy and takes into account the need to make some paternalistic decisions for the patient. Philosopher John Rawls approaches the problem by asking his readers to imagine a scene in which a group of people have been gathered for the purpose of establishing rules of justice which are as fair as possible. The participants must be rational and self-interested. They must be able to calculate the consequences of their decisions, but they must not know how any of the proposed alternatives will affect their own particular interests. In this so-called "original position" no one is able to act on personal biases. For example, in making rules for just behavior in a medical emergency the rule makers would not know whether in fact they might be patients or physicians. With this perspective in mind, Rawls offers the following principle:

Paternalistic decisions are to be guided by the individual's own settled preferences and interests insofar as they are not irrational. ... As we know less and less about a person, we act for him as we would act for ourselves from the standpoint of the original position. We try to get for him the things he presumably wants whatever else he wants. We mut be able to argue that with the development or the recovery of his rational powers the individual in question will accept our decision on his behalf and agree that we did the best thing for him.[19]

In acting for someone as "we would act for ourselves from the standpoint of the original position," an attempt would be made to make choices with which a rational and prudent person would likely agree. The central concern is *not* the probability that the *actual* person in question will retrospectively agree with the decisions. The crucial point is that the decisions must be justifiable to a theoretical third party—a *reasonable person* in the patient's position.

This ethical principle provides no specific content for decisions, but it does give a basis on which emergency medical decisions can be made. It protects physicians from a patient who, on the basis of idiosyncratic preferences, disagrees with the decisions which have been made. It also protects a patient from a physician who adheres to norms differing from those expected of a representative reasonable person.

Is the established emergency procedure of preserving life whenever possible in harmony with the above principle? In order to assert that it is, we must assume that most reasonable people wish to go on living. Whatever values are maintained, the one "good" which is essential to the realization of nearly all others is life itself. This does not mean that life is the highest good or an absolute good in the "vitalistic" sense. Rather, life is seen as a relative good which is nevertheless basic and precious—a value that ought to be preserved as requisite for other values.

Even if the decision to commit suicide might be deemed rational in some situations, it seems virtually impossible in emergency medicine to take such a consideration into account. One might imagine a case in which a person who had apparently attempted suicide would be accompanied by a family member to the emergency room. The family member might produce a suicide note and show evidence of an overdose of a particular drug. Even if the legal restrictions prohibiting a physician's involvement as an accomplice in a suicide could be set aside, the physician would still find it necessary to decide in favor of the preservation of life. There would be no time to seek answers to absolutely essential questions. The physician could not determine, for example, whether the patient might not actually be the victim of an attempted homicide. Acting on a bias in favor of life would seem to be the most reasonable course under the circumstances.

NOTES

1. A.R. Rosenberg, "Informed Consent—The Latest Threat?" *Journal of Legal Medicine,* vol. 1, p. 17, 1973.

2. D. I. Smith, "Informed Consent and Medical Ethics," *Journal of Pediatrics,* vol. 87, p. 327, 1975.

3. L.B. Jaeckel, "New Trends in Informed Consent?" *Nebraska Law Review,* vol. 54, p. 66, 1975.

4. P. Ramsey, *The Patient as Person,* p. 5, Yale University Press, New Haven, 1970.

5. B. Shartel and M.L. Plant, *The Law of Medical Practice,* p. 15, Charles C. Thomas, Springfield, 1959.

6. R. Johnson and C. Trimble, "The (Expletive Deleted) Shouter," *Journal of the American College of Emergency Physicians,* vol. 4, p. 333, 1975.

7. F.T. Flannery, "Hospital Liability for Emergency Room Services—The Problems of Admission and Consent," *Journal of Legal Medicine,* vol. 3, p. 15, 1975.

8. R.F. Johnson, "Consent in the Emergency Room," *Legal Medicine Annals,* vol. 349, p. 350, 1973.

9. A.R. Holder, *Medical Malpractice Law,* p. 309, John Wiley & Sons, New York, 1975.

10. N. Schnaper, "The Psychological Implications of Severe Trauma: Emotional Sequelae to Unconsciousness," *Journal of Trauma,* vol. 15, p. 94, 1975.

11. J. Fletcher, *The Ethics of Genetic Control: Ending Reproductive Roulette,* p. 83, Anchor Books, Garden City, N.Y., 1974.

12. B. Bard and J. Fletcher, "The Right to Die," *Atlantic Monthly,* April 1968, p. 59.

13. R. McCormick, "To Save or Let Die—The Dilemma of Modern Medicine," *Journal of the American Medical Association,* vol. 229, p. 172, 1974.

14. R.J. Malone, "Is There a Right to a Natural Death?" *New England Law Review,* vol. 9, p. 293, 1974.

15. "The Quinlan Decision: Five Commentaries," *The Hastings Center Report,* vol. 6, p. 8, 1976.

16. W. Modell, "A Will to Live," *New England Journal of Medicine,* vol. 290, p. 907, 1974. (An example of legislative action regarding the "living will" is Assembly Bill 3060 passed by the California Legislature, and signed by the governor, Sept. 30, 1976.)

17. H.T. Engelhardt, Jr., "Case Studies in Bio-

ethics: Case no. 228, a Demand to Die," *The Hastings Center Report,* vol. 5, p. 9, 1975.

18. G. Dworkin, "Paternalism," in R.A. Wasserstrom (ed.), *Morality and the Law,* Wadsworth Publishing Co., Belmont, California, 1971.

19. J. Rawls, *A Theory of Justice,* Harvard University Press, Cambridge, Mass., 1971.

57.
When Consent Is Unbearable: A Case Report
Michael H. Kottow

A 56-year-old man was referred to an orbital tumor clinic because of progressive protrusion of one eyeball. This man worked as a farm laborer in a rural area of an underdeveloped country. He was the father of five children, and his monthly income was approximately equivalent to $40.

The patient's medical history was unremarkable, except that he never had any useful vision in his left eye, because of an uncorrected squint which he had had for quite some time. His present complaint consisted of progressive out and forward displacement of his right eye, with accompanying dull, but not intense, pain of the orbital region, and some loss of vision.

On ophthalmologic examination, a tumor was found, which displaced the right globe and decreased visual acuity to 0.4. The left eye was deviated and amblyopic, with vision of counting fingers.

After a complete medical examination, which was normal, the patient was operated on, and two large, well-encapsulated tumors were removed from his right orbit. On histopathology, the growth was labeled an adenocarcinoma of the lacrimal gland. Although the pathologist was confident of her diagnosis, she expressed some doubts as to its certainty. Nevertheless, she advised the currently recommended treatment of exenteration of the orbit, that is, complete removal of the eye and orbital contents. [1]

The attending physician did not follow the pathologist's advice. The patient was told that a malignant tumor had been removed, and that the patient should come for follow-up visits at regular intervals. After the operation, the patient recovered full vision in his right eye and was discharged without pain or discomfort. He was regularly followed up for two years without any evidence of local recurrence or metastatic spread.

Ethical Considerations

The reasoning behind the attending physician's decisions centers around the evaluation of the circumstances that make moral issues much less clear-cut than standard ethics might wish.

Three ethical problems are apparent in this medical case:

1. Information was withheld from the patient.

2. Medical decisions were taken without his consent.

3. A conservative management was chosen against the recommendations of the pathologist and of current medical thought.

Source: *Journal of Medical Ethics,* vol. 4, p. 78, 1978.

Withholding Information

The patient was not told that the malignant tumors removed from his orbit were, in all probability, of a nature whereby cancerous cells have remained in the orbit or were spread through the bloodstream; that large series of patients with adenocarcinoma of the lacrimal gland report no patient to be alive and free of recurrences and/or metastases, regardless of whether the tumor was cut out or the contents of the orbit remained. In other words, the patient was not informed that he had a fatal, incurable disease.

The pathologist, although confident, was not absolutely certain of her diagnosis, nor of the prognosis, in view of the unusually well-developed fibrous encapsulation of the tumor. Therefore, the patient would receive information, and be required to make decisions, on the basis of a high probability, not a certainty.

Medical experience available was considered to be insufficient to allow clear appraisal of the probabilities involved in making a correct diagnosis and prognosis of the lesion.

The patient, an intelligent and cooperative person, was an unskilled farmhand with little formal education. Although he would have been fully able to grasp the dimensions of his medical problem, he was in no position to change any of the factors which governed his social and economic life. The patient's family was unknown to the physician, and the country where this problem occurred did not offer social, economic, or rehabilitational facilities that might have been effectively used by the patient to adjust to his possibly being handicapped and/or terminally ill.

Finally, it was considered that information could still be offered at the time when the appearance of recurrences or metastases clearly supported the expected fatal outcome.

Informed Consent

Because the patient was not advised of the implications of his illness, informed consent was not possible. The decision made by the physician and not shared with the patient had been reduced from two options: concurring with the current recommendation of exenterating the orbit, which would mean iatrogenically blinding the patient, or leaving the patient with his eye intact and the almost certainty of tumor-induced death. In this alternative pair, the difference between "probable" and "certain" death is statistically insignificant.

The decision to bypass informed consent of the patient in the management of his case was based on two considerations: The options to be offered were equally discouraging (elective blindness and possible death vs. retained vision and possible death) and medical experience was clearly confused as to the current management of these cases; the physician had little in the way of informed arguments to help the patient decide between two similarly cruel alternatives.

The decision to withhold radical treatment was based on doubts about the certainty of the diagnosis, skepticism about the advantages of radical treatment, the particular problem of avoiding blindness in this patient, and the general consideration that restrained treatment was a reversible attitude, avoiding the recognition later that aggressive treatment had been unnecessary (if the histopathologic diagnosis were ever revised) or futile.

In conclusion, this case confronts the physician with the unusual circumstance of choosing to present his patient with two equally hopeless alternatives. Their hopelessness was considered to be sufficient ground to withhold information and to bypass consent for no further treatment. The physician elected to adopt a paternalistic, rather than contractual relationship with his patient.[2] The 2-year favorable follow-up of the patient is certainly satisfying, but can in no way be considered an argument in favor of the original decision.[3]

It should be considered that, had the physician abided by the basic rule that a person is due full information about his disease, there could have been no ethical issue at stake, since the next step, informed consent to institute or withhold treatment, would have been in the hands of the patient. I think this is an important and neglected aspect of medical ethics. If the decision is put in the hands of the patient, the physician is relieved from any ethical dilemma. Medical ethics are applicable only to situations and issues where the physician is fully involved in the act of decision making and affected by its unavoidable ingredients of risk, loss, and responsibility–risk because alternatives can be no more than fragmentary solutions; loss because choosing also implies discarding; and responsibility because deciding must be a process subject to account. Had the physician in this case elected to inform fully the patient of his condi-

tion, and asked him to take the decision of exenteration vs. follow-up, there would have been no further moral issue: The doctor would no longer have any decision to make, and the patient would be confronting a horrifying game of survival probabilities.

NOTES

1. J. W. Henderson, *Orbital Tumors,* W. B. Saunders Co., Philadelphia, 1973.

2. R. M. Veatch, "Models for Ethical Medicine in a Revolutionary Age," *Hastings Center Report,* vol. 2, p. 5, 1972.

3. H. Brody, *Ethical Decisions in Medicine,* Little, Brown & Co., Boston, 1976.

58.
When Consent Is Unbearable: An Alternative Case Analysis
George J. Agich

The decision to bypass informed consent was based upon two considerations, namely, the options (elective blindness and possible death) were equally discouraging and the medical opinion regarding treatment was equivocal. For these reasons the physician chose not to inform his patient. Because the case confronts the physician with the "unusual circumstance" of having to choose between two equally hopeless alternatives, the conclusion is drawn by Dr. Kottow that "had the physician in this case abided by the basic rule that a person is due full information about his disease, there could have been no ethical issue at stake." Corollary to this conclusion is the view that "medical ethics are only applicable to situations and issues where the physician is fully involved in the act of decision making."

I want to disagree with Dr. Kottow's analysis of this case as well as with his conclusion. Unlike Dr. Kottow, my reading of this case indicates that the principle of

informed consent does not rule out ethics for the physician, but precisely emphasizes the relevance of ethical analysis beyond the issue of informed consent.

About what was the patient not informed? The patient was told that a malignant tumor was removed; he was scheduled for regular follow-up visits which persisted for two years. The patient was not told that the malignant tumor removed was likely to metastasize and that in a large series of patients suffering from adenocarcinoma of the lacrimal gland no patient, irrespective of treatment, was alive and free of recurrence and/or metastases. In other words, the patient was not told that he had a fatal, incurable disease.

The values appealed to in this case relate to the economic and material circumstances of the patient. Because the medical information which the physician possessed could not be used in a way which affected the family fortunes, the patient was not informed, the implicit principle being that

Source: *Journal of Medical Ethics,* vol. 5, p. 26, 1979.

there is a direct relationship between the claim which a patient can make to full disclosure of information and the degree of control of the factors governing his economic and social life. But such an alternative to the principle of informed consent is clearly objectionable.

First, it makes the principle of informed consent depend upon a sphere of goods. Values, e.g., of freedom, compassion, and love, are thereby reduced to the domain of material goods.[1] Second, the decision made cannot be justified even on paternalistic grounds. Since the physician did not know the family and its precise circumstances, his decision was premised on ignorance. Thus, he could not be said to be acting in the best interests of the family and his patient, since he did not know those interests.

Not only did the physician not consider (perhaps because he was simply ignorant) the economic, social, and emotional resources of the patient's family, he interpreted these resources in the Western liberal tradition of social services.

The case is said to be difficult because the physician has little to offer except two hopeless alternatives. Kottow argues that the hopelessness was the ground for withholding information and for adopting a "paternalistic" rather than "contractual" relationship. But in making this move, Dr. Kottow seems to confuse two different kinds of physician-patient relationship: treatment relationship and course of treatment relationship.

In the treatment relationship there are three models: activity-passivity, guidance-cooperation, and mutual participation in which the degree of physician autonomy vis à vis patient autonomy changes.[2] The shift from one model to another depends largely upon the nature of the therapy in question. The course of treatment relationship is characterized by two points:

1. The physician chooses the patient's course of treatment until either terminates the relationship.

2. The physician proposes; the patient decides.[3]

Given the importance of informed consent in current medical ethical thought, a point which Kottow readily concedes, it should be clear that the course of treatment relationship now preferred is the second, namely, the physician proposes and the patient decides (i.e., informed consent). The legal and moral justification for this position is well documented throughout the literature. So, if we grant the general validity of the principle of informed consent, namely, that except in emergencies the competent adult patient must decide whether or not he is to accept any proposed treatment (and Dr. Kottow nowhere explicitly challenges this principle), it is inconsistent to sanction a physician's withholding information essential to the patient's forming an intelligent judgment on the question even when the alternatives appear "hopeless."

From our analysis of the values implicit in the interpretation of the facts of this case, it is not clear that this shift in course of treatment relationship is justified. For instance, were the values appealed to fair to the patient and the patient's family? The physician chose not to offer radical surgery (the activity-passivity treatment model), but instead offered a guidance-cooperation treatment model as evidenced by the treatment plan of long-term follow-up. But, the *treatment* model being chosen, guidance-cooperation itself presupposes patient autonomy, autonomy which is denied by the shift from an informed consent *course of treatment* relationship to a paternalistic one.

In other words, by not informing, the physician failed to respect the patient's autonomy; in not respecting patient autonomy, the physician in principle prohibited the patient from participating as a moral and personal agent in the treatment process, while at the same time requiring the patient to so participate (guidance-cooperation). Hence, deception was necessarily required throughout the course of follow-up treat-

ment and constitutes another relevant factor in this case.

Finally, because Dr. Kottow confuses the
course of treatment and the treatment relationship, he draws an unfortunate lesson from
this case, namely, that "if the decision is
put in the hands of the patient, the physician
is relieved from any ethical dilemma."
This conclusion is unfortunate because it
obscures the ethical dimensions of the
course of treatment in which deception is
continuously involved. Rather than presenting a case which justifies withholding
information, the case thus emphasizes
the validity of the principle of informed
consent as a prerequisite to the physician-
patient relationship, and, in doing so, high-

lights poignant value dimensions of that
relationship.

NOTES

1. Max Scheler, *Formalism in Ethics and
Non-Formal Ethics of Value,* Manfred S. Frings
and Roger L. Funk, tr. Northwestern University
Press, Evanston, 1973.
2. Thomas S. Szasz and Mark Hollender, "The
Basic Models of the Doctor-Patient Relationship,"
Archives of Internal Medicine, vol. 97, p. 585,
1956.
3. Alan Donagan, "Informed Consent in Therapy and Experimentation," *Journal of Medicine and
Philosophy,* vol. 2, p. 307, 1977.

59.
Informed Consent by "Well-Nigh Abject Adults"
Drummond Rennie

Society has become increasingly restless
with the paternalistic attitudes of professional experts. The courts, reflecting the values
of society, have increasingly reinforced the
principle of self-determination as enunciated
by Cardozo: "Every human being of adult
years and sound mind has a right to deter
mine what shall be done with his own body."[1]
Physicians are consultants to patients, but
patients, not physicians, must finally decide
for themselves where their best interests
lie. The ordinary patient, whose "dependence
upon the physician for information affecting his well-being, in terms of contemplated
treatment, is well-nigh abject,"[2] cannot
possibly make a reasoned decision without
being told what the physician intends to
do and why, what the alternatives are, and
what the probabilities of success and the
risks may be. It is morally necessary for the
physician to supply this information, and
the physician's moral approach to this mat-

ter may well be spurred on by litigation
involving the issue of consent.[3]

Difficulty arises because of the inevitable
and gross inequality between the two parties
interested in consent to a medical procedure.
One is fit and medically knowledgeable,
the other is sick and medically ignorant. This
inequality has led physicians to assume that
the idea of truly informed consent even for
an ordinary elective procedure is a delusion,[4]
and that it is cruel and even dangerous[5,6]
to reveal all the major hazards to the patient,
who may already be terrified. The courts,
however, concerned that withholding information will make nonsense of the patient's
ability to decide, are reluctant to sanction
any such withholding.[2,7]

Despite anecdotes of catastrophes,[8] studies[9,10] tend to reassure the physician that
patients treated as adults can in fact take the
bad news. Alfidi[9] found, to his surprise,
that "straightforward and perhaps even harsh

Source: *New England Journal of Medicine,* vol. 302, no. 16, p. 917, April 17, 1980.

statements" concerning possible complications of angiography were "accepted and
desired" by patients. More complete information rarely leads to refusal to go through
with the procedure,[11] and one might question whether withholding information really
increases mutual trust.

If efforts to educate patients in order to
obtain their informed consent are, indeed,
not harmful and are morally and legally necessary, how effective are these efforts? Cassileth and her colleagues found that by the
time patients had completed their consent forms, their memory of the information
given to them was inadequate and often
faulty, although they claimed to have understood the forms themselves. This study aug-
ments and confirms what several others[12-15]
have shown: that even when elaborate and
lengthy conversations are held, when demonstrations are given, and when forms are
signed preoperatively, only about half the patients remember the salient points; most
have forgotten factors that would have undermined their decision to go ahead with an
operation once it is over, and some flatly
deny having had any conversations at all.

Grundner also concentrates on the consent form. He points out that the forms
used in the five hospitals that he studied
would be unintelligible to all but the most
legally and technically sophisticated.

Defective forms are signs of a very defective process, but Vaccarino[17] has emphasized that the physician must keep in
mind the difference between substance
(the conversations between physician and
patient) and form (the permission slip or
the detailed book that so many hospitals, but
not the law, require to be signed as evidence
of consent). If consent forms are used, however, they must surely be comprehensible to
the average sick patient laboring under the
usual stress. Whatever their legal purpose,
they should also serve to educate the patient.
It seems astonishing that anyone should
draw up and presumably defend unintelligible, legalistic documents that must inevitably obfuscate, intimidate, and alienate. One
might easily imagine that the courts would

later discount such forms as evidence of informed consent; indeed they might find
them to be evidence that the patient could
not have been informed at all.[18]

Faced by changing societal values, ambivalent courts, the certainty that they will
never be immune to litigation brought by
patients who reject, forget, misinterpret, or
deny their efforts to inform, and by forms
that may be unintelligible to the patient,
what course should prudent physicians follow? I suggest that the physician accept far
more than simply the duty to improve
consent forms. They should accept education of the patient through the process of
consent as a worthwhile therapeutic goal.[19]
To deny the possibility of informed consent is to ensure that it will never be achieved
—an attitude that is immoral and, in hospitals and states that have adopted the Patient's
Bill of Rights, illegal. This means that the
physician must reject the paternalistic role
in favor of the role of counselor and advocate, attempting to give patients equality
in the covenant by educating them to
make informed decisions.

If physicians listen to patients and spend
time with them and their families, if they
speak in a direct, honest, and forthright manner, in layman's terms, and if they avoid
coercion or the building up of unrealistic
expectations, they can scarcely fail to
gain the patient's trust. The physician's integrity is the patient's best guarantee of
fair play.

Physicians should encourage their hospitals to support the Patient's Bill of Rights;
they should ensure that consent forms are
plainly comprehensible to those who must
sign them, and they should also encourage experimentation with booklets,[10] taped
demonstrations,[20] specific forms inviting
further questions,[9] and questionnaires testing understanding.[21]

Such techniques may improve the process. Meanwhile, a trite but reasonable conclusion is that physicians who give plenty of
time and compassion to their patients, helping
them to help themselves, are acting in the best
interests of patients, themselves, and society.

NOTES

1. *Schloendorff v. Society of New York Hospital,* 105 N.E. 92, 93 (N.Y.1914).

2. *Canterbury v. Spence,* 464 F. 2d 772 (1972).

3. *Jones v. Regents of the University of California,* Super. Ct. San Fran. Co., Cal. (1977).

4. E.G. Laforet, "The Fiction of Informed Consent," *Journal of the American Medical Association,* vol. 235, 1976, p. 1579.

5. B.M. Patten and W. Stump, "Death Related to Informed Consent," *Texas Medicine,* vol. 74, 1978, p. 49–50.

6. J.F. Fries and E.E. Loftus, "Informed Consent: Right or Rite?" *CA,* vol. 29, 1979, p. 316.

7. *Cobbs vs. Grant,* 502 P. 2d.1 (Cal. 1972).

8. *Salgo v. Leland Stanford, Jr., University Board of Trustees,* 154 Cal. App 2d 560, 317 P.2d 170 (Dist. Ct. of App. 1957).

9. R.J. Alfidi, "Informed Consent: A Study of Patient Reaction," *Journal of the American Medical Association,* vol. 216, 1971, p. 1325.

10. M.K. Denney, D. Williamson, and R. Penn, "Informed Consent: Emotional Responses of Patients," *Postgraduate Medicine,* vol. 60, 1975, p. 205.

11. A.L. Faden and R.R. Faden, "Informed Consent in Medical Practice: With Particular Reference to Neurology," *Archives of Neurology,* vol. 35, 1978, p. 761.

12. I.A. Priluck, D.M. Robertson, and H. Buettner, "What Patients Recall of the Preoperative Discussion after Retinal Detachment Surgery," *American Journal of Ophthalmology,* vol. 87, 1979, p. 620.

13. D. Leeb, D.G. Bowers, Jr., and J.B. Lynch, "Observations on the Myth of 'Informed Consent'," *Plastic and Reconstructive Surgery,* vol. 58, 1976, p. 280.

14. G. Robinson and A. Merav, "Informed Consent: Recall by Patients Tested Postoperatively," *Annals of Thoracic Surgery,* vol. 22, 1976, p. 209.

15. H.B. Muss, D.R. White, and R. Michielutte, et al. "Written Informed Consent in Patients with Breast Cancer," *Cancer,* vol. 43, 1979, p. 1549.

16. B.H. Gray, R.A. Cooke, and A.S. Tannenbaum, "Research Involving Human Subjects," *Science,* vol. 210, 1978, p. 1094.

17. J.M. Vaccarino, "Consent, Informed Consent and the Consent Form," *New England Journal of Medicine,* vol. 298, 1978, p. 455.

18. R.M. Moore, Jr., "Consent Forms—How, or Whether, They Should be Used," *Mayo Clinic Proceedings,* vol. 53, 1978, p. 393.

19. G.J. Annas, "Avoiding Malpractice Suits through the Use of Informed Consent," *Current Problems in Pediatrics,* vol. 6, 1976, p. 3.

20. G.L. Barbour and M.J. Blumenkrantz, "Videotape Aids Informed Consent Decision," *Journal of the American Medical Association,* vol. 240, 1978, p. 2741–2.

21. R. Miller and H.S. Willner, "The Two-Part Consent Form: A Suggestion for Prompting Free and Informed Consent," *New England Journal of Medicine,* vol. 290, 1974, p. 964.

60.
Informed Consent May Be Hazardous to Health
Elizabeth F. Loftus   James F. Fries

Before human subjects are enrolled in experimental studies, a variety of preliminary rituals are now required. These include an explanation of the nature of the experimental procedure and a specific elaboration of possible adverse reactions. The subjects, in turn, can either withdraw from the experiment or give their "informed consent." These rituals are said to increase the subjects' understanding of the procedures, but perhaps more important, they came into existence because of a strong belief in the fundamental principle that human beings have the right to determine what will be done to their minds and bodies.

Some, on the other hand, consider that the purpose of informed consent is not protection of subjects but rather protection of investigators and sponsoring institutions from lawsuits based on the charge of subject deception should a misadventure result. But lawsuits arise in any case: subjects simply claim that they did not understand the rituals. It is reasonable, then, to ask whether

Source: *Science,* vol. 204, no. 4388, April 6, 1979.

the putative beneficiary, the subject, might be harmed rather than helped by the current informed consent procedure.

A considerable body of psychological evidence indicates that humans are highly suggestible. Information has been found to change people's attitudes, to change their moods and feelings, and even to make them believe they have experienced events that never in fact occurred. This alone would lead one to suspect that adverse reactions might result from information given during an informed consent discussion.

An examination of the medical evidence demonstrates that there is also a dark side to the placebo effect. Not only can positive therapeutic effects be achieved by suggestion, but negative side effects and complications can similarly result. For example, among subjects who participated in a drug study after the usual informed consent procedure, many of those given an injection of a placebo reported physiologically unlikely symptoms such as dizziness, nausea, vomiting, and even mental depression. One subject given the placebo reported that these effects were so strong that they caused an automobile accident. Many other studies provide similar data indicating that to a variable but often scarifying degree, explicit suggestion of possible adverse effects causes subjects to experience these effects. Recent hypotheses that heart attack may follow coronary spasm indicate physiological mechanisms by which explicit suggestions, and the stress that may be produced by them, might prove fatal.

Thus the possible consequences of suggested symptoms range from minor annoyance to, in extreme cases, death.

If protection of the subject is the reason for obtaining informed consent, the possibility of iatrogenic harm to the subject as a direct result of the consent ritual must be considered. This clear cost must be weighed against the potential benefit of giving some people an increased sense of freedom of choice about the use of their bodies. The current legalistic devices, which are designed in part to limit subject recourse, intensify rather than solve a dilemma.

The features of informed consent procedures that do protect subjects should be retained. Experimental procedures should be reviewed by peers and public representatives. A statement to the subject describing the procedure and the general level of risk is reasonable. But detailed information should be reserved for those who request it. Specific slight risks, particularly those resulting from common procedures, should not be routinely disclosed to all subjects. And when a specific risk is disclosed, it should be discussed in the context of placebo effects in general, why they occur, and how to guard against them. A growing literature indicates that just as knowledge of possible symptoms can cause those symptoms, so can knowledge of placebo effects be used to defend against those effects. A move in this direction may ensure that a subject will not be at greater risk from self-appointed guardians than from the experiment itself.

61.

Parental Consent: Its Justification and Limitations
Paul Langham

If there is one principle that is afforded universal assent in writings on medical morals, it is that in the case of children of immature years the parents have a right to be consulted and to decide in matters of medical or sur-

gical procedures. From sterilization to euthanasia, the response seems uniform.

But the uncritical acceptance of the principle of parental consent does stand in need of close scrutiny. There are two rea-

Source: *Clinical Research*, vol. 27, no. 5, December 1979.

sons for this. First, the principle of parental consent may turn out to be a sacred cow; it may be that universal assent is being afforded to a moral maxim of low priority; it may even be that the principle reflects no genuine moral maxim at all, that it is a mere prejudice. In either of such eventualities there might be important consequences, especially in a society in which legal as well as moral sanction is given to the principle.[1] Second, if the principle does deserve the status it is given, it is essential that we discover why this is so and what is its justification. For if there is any obviously valid moral maxim and we can show how it can be justified, we will possess a powerful tool not only for the solution of problems of consent but also for the solution of other moral dilemmas.

The question considered in this paper is: can the negative attitude of the parent count as a crucial moral argument against the physician performing those procedures that his expert diagnosis and prognosis suggest? We will attempt to demonstrate that there are no adequate grounds for believing anything of the sort and that a blanket acceptance of parental consent is inappropriate because it has been derived from some more general principle and thereby contains its own limitations.

In parental consent situations one of the values traditionally prominent in medical moral reasoning is absent, viz., the value placed on the autonomy of the patient. Since the patients as minors are deemed rightly or wrongly to be lacking in some requirement for autonomous action (namely, the ability to make rational decisions), autonomy considerations may disappear.[2] (Whether these situations legitimately replace patient autonomy by parental autonomy or by "proxy" autonomy as a value in consent problems depends upon why parental consent is thought to be appropriate in the first place.) This presents us with an interesting position. The two major rival values appealed to in medical moral arguments are autonomy and well-being, usually reflected in appeals in Kantian and utilitarian theories, respectively. Each of these theories emphasizes a different aspect of personhood:

the person as moral agent on the one hand and as experiencer of pleasures and pains on the other. The difficulties begin when one attempts to determine how these two aspects of personhood are to be balanced one against the other: should we override a person's autonomy in order to alleviate pain or should we allow them to exercise autonomy even when we know that avoidable pain will result? But if considerations of patient autonomy are irrelevant, the difficulties of balancing disappear—unless, of course, some other kind of autonomy is involved. It does not appear strained to allow that for all practical purposes a decision grounded on maximizing the patient's potential for autonomous actions over time will yield the same moral imperatives as obtained from the ethical model that does not stress autonomy as a prime goal.

Both the Kantian and utilitarian moral decision procedures will require the same end, i.e., that the patient be treated in that manner that will best promote physical and mental well-being, since the attainment of such conditions will be seen on the one model as the requirement for later autonomous action and on the other model as good in and of itself. Thus we find that we are dealing with a limiting case where the claims of patient autonomy and patient well-being are no longer in conflict. A discussion of parental consent, therefore, should prove beneficial to any analysis of consent in general, since it will allow for an examination of cases involving simplified parameters.

B is a teen-age girl with leukemia undergoing radiotherapy and chemotherapy. Essential monitoring procedures, bone marrow and spinal taps, are routinely carried out to check on the status of the patient's disease. Spinal taps are necessary to determine changes in the cerebral spinal fluid, an important consideration in determining the activity of the disease and in planning future courses of treatment. B has experienced chronic headaches associated with the spinal tap procedures. During one visit, B clings to her father with tears in her eyes throughout the bone marrow procedure. When the physician prepares for the spinal tap, B refuses; her father concurs with her wishes and refuses to consent.

K is a teen-age girl with osteosarcoma. She has an unresectable tumor that is not susceptible to radiation therapy. The tumor has also proved unresponsive to chemotherapeutic agents and it is considered that there is no longer any hope of saving K's life. The reaction of the patient and her parents to this is primarily that of denial. On asking whether there are any other drugs available, they are told of a "new drug," a phase I chemotherapeutic agent. It is extremely unlikely that the dosages contemplated in the study of the agent would have any effect on K's condition. However, the parents wish to take any possible chance and K, although unhappy about the effects of more drugs, says that she will accept "treatment" so as not to upset her mother. (This is not a case of parental dissent, but of concurrence with the physician's plan of treatment.)

M is a three-day-old baby with signs of Down's syndrome and esophageal atresia, the latter an easily correctable condition. On being informed of the baby's condition and of the intention to perform surgery, the parents decline to sign the consent form. The baby dies.

There are two common responses indicative of some special relationship between parents and children that are given to the question of who should decide for the child: (1) It is *their* child, so they should decide; and (2) the child is *their responsibility*, so they should decide. Notwithstanding their popularity, both of these responses are morally irrelevant and the potential source of great dangers.

We all know, at least in standard cases, whose children are whose. But what does it mean to say that Q is P's child? Actually, it does not mean much at all; it means simply that P is a biological (or adoptive) parent

of Q. But from this nothing follows concerning who should make decisions for Q during Q's minority.

The danger in (1) is that the "my" or "your" or "their" of parenthood may be subtly confused with the "my" or "your" or "their" of possession. This, coupled with certain deep-seated though by no means self-evidently valid societal norms, makes (1) a superficially seductive inference. For in our society we allow, that if this is P's money or that is P's car, then P ought to be the one to say how this money or that car is to be used.

Now, although there may well be something to the claim that possession confers rights of disposition, that claim is clearly irrelevant to our present purpose, for the "my," "your," and "their" of parenthood are obviously not the "my," "your," or "their" of possession: *we do not own our children.* The danger is that if we speak of parental rights instead of parental duties and responsibilities, the confusion of the "my" of parenthood with the "my" of ownership is likely to be aggravated. This can lead to easy capitulation in the face of parental objections, especially when parental "rights" are endorsed by law; after all, the parent is only insisting on what a consideration of pseudoanalogous cases shows to be an obvious moral [and legal] right.

With regard to (2), if a parent hits a child and the child falls and is injured, we would hold the parent responsible for that injury; the injury was the result of the parent's action. However, this is a far cry from what is needed to establish a responsibility, not to mention a right, to make decisions about treatment *for* the child when the child is sick. In the child abuse case, the parent is responsible for the effect and the effect is the child's injury; by analogy, in procreation the parents are also responsible for the effect, but the effect is the existence of the child, not necessarily anything else. Moral obligations to other persons are not grounded in this kind of causal connection; they arise simply because persons are persons. At the very least, some subsidiary argument will be required to establish parental responsibility and parental rights. But even if such a subsidiary argument is forthcoming, unless it resembles the ownership confusion, it will scarcely demonstrate any more than a *duty* on the part of the parents—and that is not enough to justify any talk of rights. Therefore, both responses when taken in conjunction with the rationales cited can be seen as resting primarily on linguistic confusions.

Since parents raise their children in virtual isolation, except for other members of the family, the parents are those, under normal circumstances, who are in a position to render aid to their children. And under normal circumstances the parents also possess the necessary expertise to render that aid. The child is hungry, the parent is there and can provide and prepare food; the child needs psychological support and encouragement, the parent's natural affection can usually supply these; the child needs protection; again, under normal circumstances the parent is well placed and capable of supplying it. Thus, the supposed special moral relationship between parent and child reduces to a simple application of the general moral injunction to render aid as understood and functioning within the limits of a particular socioeconomic framework; the special relationship simply reflects the proximity within that framework of parents to children.

The recognition, even in our own society, that persons other than parents have moral obligations to children is reflected in the provisions that are made for those cases in which parents are unable to render necessary aid or refuse to do so. Thus, society attempts to ensure that all children receive an education, that children of impoverished parents are provided for, that children may be removed from control of parents who might ill-treat them.

It might be stated that nothing has been established except that persons other than parents have obligations to children, or that apart from proximity nothing speaks especially in favor of obligations to close relatives. Nothing has been said vis-à-vis parental *rights.* Even within a social structure in which special obligations fall to parents, there is no justification for inferring any rights on the part of those parents over the treatment of their children. Within the context of our discussion, if the parent is to claim legitimately a priority in performing his duty to his offspring over the physician, then it must be that the physician has, for some reason, a duty to allow the parent that priority. But what those reasons could be can only be elaborated after a consideration of the grounds of the moral obligations of physicians.

A physician's moral responsibility to his patient is derived from the same general rule of aid as that of any person to another. But whereas our society places parents in one apparently special relationship to their children because of their proximity, it is the physician's knowledge and skill that place him in a special relationship to his patient.

When a child is well, the parents may be quite competent to provide all necessary aid. When a child is sick, however, it is the physician who most satisfies the conditions mentioned, not the parent. The moral obligation on the physician is to perform those treatments which will maximize the child's physical and mental welfare. Since the moral obligation on the parents must also be to ensure the maximum benefits for the child, it is difficult even to imagine how any conflict could occur; they would both be obligated to perform actions aimed at the same end.

The only rationales for conflicts are that the parents believe that the child would not consent to the treatment suggested or that they believe that the projected treatment will not be benefit-maximizing. However, since it is already decided that the child is too immature to form a reasoned judgment on matters so important, the first consideration can have no weight. The second can be subdivided into two possibilities: (a) the parents do not agree that the proposed treatment is medically correct, or (b) the treatment involves some feature that the parents believe is harmful in some nonmedical manner. Since the parents do not possess sufficient medical expertise, their disagreement on the first kind of grounds can scarcely be counted for much, although it should, perhaps, not be ruled out completely.

In a society that pays lip-service to pluralism, the second possibility is more plausible. One of the most frequent examples of this is the refusal of Jehovah's Witnesses to permit blood transfusions for themselves and their children. Since the child is deemed too immature to formulate value judgments, it is not the values of the child that are operative, but those of the parent. The child's immediate autonomy is not at stake, only the parents'. But since the ownership thesis is incorrect, the autonomy of the parents, per se, would seem to be irrelevant. If the child's physical and mental well-being are paramount, in and of themselves or as contributing to future autonomy, then the physician's decision, again, is more reliable. Thus the same difficulty arises about breaking a deadlock between persons with different views about what their moral duties are where one has greater expertise than the other.

Arguments in favor of parental control cannot, therefore, rest on claims about moral duties alone; they must also include a justification for one person (the less informed, perhaps) overriding another when conflicts about perceived duties arise. They must go beyond talk of duties to talk about rights; not just the right to determine what shall be done in general, but more specifically to determine when another person shall not be allowed to perform some moral duty.

In the normal course of events, the parents of B and K would be perfectly capable of providing aid to their children; they would satisfy the conditions of both proximity and expertise. However, leukemia and osteosarcoma cannot be regarded as normal. The physician may provide a "mini-medical" education to the parent, but the parent's grasp of the issues can only be as good as the physician allows. The position of the physician is in one respect different from that of the parent. The child is a person; so the physician is under a moral and possibly a professional and legal obligation to render aid. Since the child has been brought to the hospital, the physician also satisfies the condition of proximity. In view of his knowledge and skills, he satisfies both requirements for being morally obliged to provide a special kind of aid. The normal conditions under which the parents were optimally situated to render aid have disappeared.

There is one more factor that makes the physician a more reliable judge of what should be done. Whether the parent is seen as an arbiter of what aid should be given so as to promote the welfare of the child or even if he is seen as a giver of "proxy" consent, in most cases he is not in a frame of mind likely to be conducive to clear thinking. K's parents are blinded by their desire to save their daughter's life—anything must be tried. They refuse to accept a negative prognosis. And in the case of baby M, the parents have been through one stressful experience, the birth of the child, and are now faced with another. The possibility of a rational decision on their part is certainly diminished.

The physician can in one sense detach himself from such consideration and emotions. Thus, both from the point of view of reasoned calculation and from the point of view of rational action, the physician is in a better position to make a decision. However, there are several points that speak in favor of retaining the requirement of parental consent—or, at least, speak against allowing physicians to be the sole arbiters.

The proximity condition, which in our society seems to imply an immediacy of responsibility on the part of the parents, has another side. Since the parents and child are so close, a loving relationship may exist between them that does not exist in other relationships to the same degree. What it does mean is that the parents, normally, will be more concerned about their own children than other people may be. A busy physician may not explore all possible means of treatment or may opt to devote more time to other patients at the expense of a particular child. The bond of love makes the parents appropriate advocates for their child; and parental consent can be seen as a simple safeguard in a system that is open to partiality. But once it has been demonstrated in any concrete case that no such partiality exists, that the physician is totally concerned with the child's well-being, parental consent loses its rationale. Physicians are often swayed by personal judgments that may not be shared either by the parents or even by their colleagues. In a research hospital, for example, such as that attended by K, it is possible that a physician may allow his judgment to be affected by the need for experimental subjects, especially if he believes that his institution is developing a treatment of immense benefit. Here, too, the parents may to some extent serve as advocates for the patient. But, again, once it has been established in any concrete case that such conditions do not exist, parental consent loses its rationale.

In both of these kinds of situations, parental consent exists only as a safeguard in a morally imperfect world. For this reason it would be inappropriate to invest it with too much importance. Specifically, it is essential not to confuse its operation with an exercise of "proxy" consent that might be thought to involve the autonomy of the person giving the consent or the person on whose behalf the consent is given. However, there are two factors that may suggest a legitimate demand for autonomy on the part of the parents.

In the first place, many of the decisions that must be made with respect to the treatment of children (and others) are not medical decisions at all. The decision to abort a fetus or to allow an infant to die when it is known to suffer from Down's syndrome or Tay-Sachs disease, for example, is nonmedical in the sense that all possible

procedures in medicine are known and nondebatable. This being the case, the physician, strictly speaking, is acting outside his professional domain of expertise when he makes suggestions or allows his own bias to surface as to which course of action should be followed.

Arising perhaps from this is a second and more important consideration. The close connection between parents and child makes it impossible to treat the child as a patient "standing alone"; the child must always be viewed as an integral part of a family group. As the people most affected by any decision, they surely should have some input into the decision procedure. Most particularly, the parents often must live with the results of the decision and its effects on the child concerned. This much can be said in favor of parental *input,* but it does not justify a parental right of veto. Against it must be placed the medical ignorance of the parents and their possible emotional state. Even the decision arrived at will affect the parents and may speak against their veto power, since they may be influenced too much by consideration of their own future, e.g., where abortion or passive infanticide questions arise. Neither, for the reasons cited, can the physician's decision be taken as final, even when he and the parents are in agreement.

NOTES

1. It is important not to confuse moral law with societal laws: it may be that a practice or institution endorsed by the laws of some society is immoral. Consider the status of slavery in the nineteenth century or the recent status of abortion.

2. Increasing resistance to this position has manifested itself recently. For example, a U.S. Commission recommends that "assent" of children over seven years of age be required in addition to the "permission" of parents.

62.

The Minor's Consent to Treatment
Angela R. Holder

The Committee on Youth of the American Academy of Pediatrics has written a model act to allow for consent of minors to health services. This act was to be submitted to the legislatures of all states but has thus far not yet been adopted in any. Under the act, a minor who has been separated from his parents, parent, or legal guardian for whatever reason and is supporting himself by whatever means is considered capable of consenting to treatment. Further, a general right to consent to medical treatment under the act would be permitted to those at the age of majority as defined by the state or 18, whichever is lower. The model act suggests that any minor who is found to be pregnant, afflicted with any reportable communicable disease, including venereal disease, or drug or substance abuse has the right to consent to preventive treatment, diagnostic treatment, and treatment of those conditions specified, although the act specifically precludes self-consent of minors to sterilization or abortion. The act provides that any minor who has physical or emotional problems and is capable of making rational decisions and whose relationship with his parents or legal guardians is in such a state that by informing them the minor will fail to seek initial or future help may consent to treatment. The same section of the model act indicates that the professional may thereafter inform the parents or legal guardian unless such action will jeopardize the life of the patient or the favorable result of the treatment.

The act provides that if major surgery, general anesthesia, or a life-threatening procedure has to be undertaken on a minor without parental consent, the physician should obtain approval from another physician for management of the case except in an emergency in a community where it is impossible for the surgeon to contact any other physician within a reasonable time for the purpose of concurrence.

Further, the act provides that any health professional may render nonemergency services to minors for conditions that will endanger the health or life of the minor if services would be delayed by obtaining consent from a spouse, parent, parents, or legal guardian. This would appear to be a very comprehensive act protecting the rights of (1) the minor who needs treatment to obtain it, (2) the parents who are in control of the minor, and (3) the physician who wishes to provide necessary treatment without running substantial risks of being sued.

The Pediatric Bill of Rights, adopted by the board of trustees of the National Association of Children's Hospitals in 1974 as a proposed legislative model, provides even more sweeping guidelines for consent by minors. The bill provides that every person, regardless of age, should have the right to seek and consent to treatment involving contraception, venereal disease, pregnancy including consent to abortion, psychiatric problems, and drug or alcohol abuse and that confidentiality between physician and patient precludes notification of parents without the patient's consent. This confidentiality provision is much broader than the Model Act of the American Academy of Pediatrics.

In addition to the provisions allowing consent to specific types of care, canon 8 of the bill specifies that:

Any person, regardless of age, who is of sufficient intelligence to appreciate the nature and consequences of the proposed medical care and if such medical care is

Source: Angela R. Holder, *Legal Issues in Pediatrics and Adolescent Medicine*, John Wiley & Sons, New York, 1977.

for his own benefit, may effectively consent to such medical care in doctor-patient confidentiality.

Presumably this section would, if adopted by a legislature, entirely preclude an action by parents who were not consulted before treatment, elective or otherwise, was begun unless they contend that the child was incapable of comprehension. The Pediatric Bill of Rights does not, however, deal in any way with a child's right to refuse treatment, which must logically be granted to the same degree that he is allowed the autonomy to consent, and therefore the proposal does not indicate whether the physician would be obliged to maintain confidentiality in a case where he considered the treatment to be necessary but the minor refused it. Any general statute that omits reference to a right to refuse treatment might well create more problems than it solves.

The Mature Minor Rule

No decision can be located within the past 20 years in which a parent recovered damages, even in the absence of a minor treatment statute, for treatment of a child over the age of 15 without parental consent. This is known as the "mature minor rule." Parents were unsuccessful in the few cases in which the issue has been raised.

Although there are very few decisions on the subject, there has been considerable discussion of the issue in legal journals. One authority concludes that parental consent for medical treatment may be omitted if (1) the patient is of the age of discretion, by which is meant 15 or older, and he would appear able to understand the procedure and its risks sufficiently to give a genuinely informed consent; (2) the medical measures are taken for the patient's own benefit, meaning that a minor certainly could not be used as a transplant donor without parental permission (this would be true even if the minor is clearly emancipated, unless the minor is married); (3) the measures can be justified as necessary by conservative med-

ical opinion; and (4) there is some good reason, including simple refusal by the minor to request it, why parental consent cannot be obtained.

Another authority has analyzed the existing cases and arrived at a very similar conclusion. He concludes that from the decisions available, inferences may be drawn about the types of situations in which courts that recognize the mature minor rule would be likely to apply it and dispense with the requirement of parental consent. The cases in which the rule has been applied generally have had the following factors in common:

1. The treatment was undertaken for the benefit of a minor rather than a third party.

2. The particular minor was near majority (or at least in the range of 15 years of age upward) and was considered to have sufficient mental capacity to understand fully the nature and importance of the medical steps proposed.

3. The medical procedures could be characterized by the court as something less than "major" or "serious" in nature.

The mature minor exception to requirements of parental consent would, along with the clear right to treat a child in an emergency, appear to constitute a sensible rule. Apparently, a medical emergency for these purposes does not have to be categorized as a life-threatening situation but rather includes acute illness of any type. A runaway with an acute appendix or fractured leg probably would not die before the parents could be located, but most courts would have no hesitation in concluding that treatment should be given, even if the child refuses to tell the physician how to locate his parents. All the early cases also involved acute illness.

The American Law Institute's *Restatement of the Law of Torts* seems to give substantial support to the mature minor rule. Section 59a provides:

If a child . . . is capable of appreciating the nature, extent and consequences of the invasion (of his body) his assent prevents the invasion from creating liability, though the assent of the parent, guardian, or other person is not obtained or is expressly refused.

Financial liability of parents. It should be noted that parents are liable for necessary expenses for their children. Medical bills are clearly the responsibility of the parents under normal circumstances. Except in an emergency, however, if no effort is made to contact the parents and inform them that the child requests treatment, particularly if the procedure is entirely elective, it is likely that a court would hold that the parent is not liable for payment of the bill. Several decisions in recent years have held that a parent is not liable for the hospital expenses of emancipated minors.

Financial liability of the minor. It is clear, however, that the minor himself is liable for his medical bills if he has the funds to pay for them. Thus the minor himself can be sued. If he has no money, however, such an action is usually not worth the time and trouble required. It thus appears that if consent is not obtained from the parents prior to performance of medical services, if the child is emancipated or claims to be, the parent is not liable for the physician's or hospital's bills. The minor, however, is. Of course, in the treatment of a young child or a child who is clearly not emancipated, the parents are liable for the costs of all necessary treatment.

Informed Consent

Assuming that the minor is one who, under a treatment statute or otherwise, is considered to be capable of consenting to treatment without the notification of his parents, the same standards of informed consent would apply as to an adult patient. The primary reason in fact for requiring parental consent is that children are considered to be fundamentally incapable of giving a truly informed consent. Thus, in the last analysis the child's capacity to understand the risks and benefits of the proposed treatment is the criterion for obtaining his consent to that treatment.

Consent to treatment. The physician-patient relationship is a fiduciary relationship whether the patient is an adult or a minor. A fiduciary relationship in the professional context is one in which one party is considered to be an expert in a field such as law or medicine and the other, the patient or client, is not aware of the intricacies of the field. In a fiduciary relationship, the fiduciary has a positive obligation to disclose fully all relevant facts in an affirmative way, unlike a relationship between presumed equals, such as a car salesman and a customer in which the salesman does not have to reveal negative information about the product unless the prospective purchaser asks him specific questions. Second, under our legal system, a person of sound mind has the right of self-determination and the right to make his own decisions about what becomes of his body.

In any case involving either an adult patient or a minor patient, the doctrine of informed consent may be defined as "the duty to warn a patient of the hazards and possible complications and expected and unexpected results of the treatment." The patient must also be clearly told what alternatives, if any, exist for the proposed treatment. As the probability or severity of risk to the patient increases, so does the duty to inform him of it. There seems to be a common assumption by the courts that where elective treatment is considered, the duty to warn the patient of all risks is virtually absolute. If the patient, adult or minor, does not understand all material facts, any consent that he does give will be held to be legally invalid. If an untoward result occurs of which the patient was not warned and he should have been, he has a cause of action against the physician for failure to obtain a valid consent even though no negligence is shown. The basis of the complaint is not that the procedure has been performed negligently but rather that it has been performed at all.

Although in some cases with an adult patient, the physician does not have to disclose information about risks if he thinks in the use of reasonable medical judgment that the patient will be upset by it and that this distress would interfere with the patient's recovery, this concept of therapeutic privilege presumably does not apply to a minor patient. No physician who is treating a minor without parental knowledge should fail to disclose any risks to the child. If the child's condition is such that therapeutic privilege would be considered justified, the parents should clearly be notified, because under these circumstances the physician is assuming that the child cannot handle the situation sufficiently well to give an informed consent.

In most states, whether or not a disclosure of risks is sufficient is established by the standard of the "reasonably careful medical practitioner in the same or similar community in the same or similar circumstances." Whether the physician has the duty to disclose the facts and if so what facts he is obliged to reveal depends on the normal medical practice in his community. The physician is not usually required to inform his patient of risks that other physicians in his community would not think necessary to disclose.

In an increasing number of states, however, courts have held that the scope of disclosure that the physician must make to a patient is not to be determined by what the reasonable physician would disclose under similar circumstances but by the patient's understanding of what he needs to know.

A 19-year-old young man was paralyzed after a laminectomy. His mother had been contacted by the surgeon and had given permission for the operation but no risk of paralysis was discussed with her or with her son. When the boy was paralyzed, he sued. The court rejected the defendant's claim that there was no practice to disclose the risk of paralysis in that community and upheld the plaintiff's cause of action. The court stated that the patient's right of self-determination shapes the boundaries of the physician's

duty to disclose all material risks, all serious inherent and potential hazards, alternative methods of treatment, and the likely results of nontreatment.

This rule—that the patient's need, not the standard of medical practice, determines what the patient has the right to know—has been adopted in New York, California, and the District of Columbia, and there is every reason to believe that this standard of disclosure will soon become the majority if not the universal rule in this country. Therefore, in dealing with minors it is particularly necessary that they be fully informed.

If the child's capacity for understanding risks, benefits, and alternative methods of treatment is subject to any question, treatment without parental consent should not be attempted except in cases of acute emergency. Furthermore, if the minor's capacity to understand is not questioned, the physician should be extremely careful to disclose all material risks. If the physician thinks that he should not for any reason tell a minor something that he would normally tell an adult patient or the parent of a minor about the proposed procedure, he should immediately conclude as a matter of logic that parental consent or a court order is necessary. The nature of the situation is such that any court would be likely to construe any withholding of information from a minor as a failure of due care in treatment, although there are no cases on this subject to date.

In any situation where a minor has no objection to his parents' knowledge of his condition, the parents should be asked to consent. It is preferable, both in terms of the physician's potential liability and in terms of the family relationships to attempt to involve the parents. Where the minor objects to notification of his family, reasonable efforts to convince him that they are likely to be more understanding and supportive than he expects should be attempted. If the minor remains adamant, however, and appears to be capable of consenting to the proposed treatment, careful documentation of genuine understanding should be made.

If the proposed procedure is one that carries any appreciable degree of risk, including all surgical procedures, in addition to a carefully worded consent form which should include a detailed statement of potential risks, the minor should sign a statement that he has refused to permit notification of his parents. The concept of a two-part consent form should then be employed. A series of written questions based on the information given the minor about the procedure should be answered in the minor's own handwriting. This questionnaire will serve as an immediate indication to the physician of the degree to which the minor has genuine understanding of what he was told and, should any legal problems arise from the parents later, would serve as the best possible evidence that the minor gave a truly informed consent. If the minor is illiterate, he should probably be presumed incapable of consent to a procedure carrying any substantial risk, and if an emergency is presented the physician has no recourse but to obtain a court order if the child refuses to tell him where his parents may be contacted.

It thus appears that if consent is not obtained from the parents prior to performance of medical services, if the child is emancipated or claims to be, the parent is not liable for the physician's or hospital's bills. The minor, however, is. This, of course, does not apply to treatment of a young child or a child who is clearly not emancipated. In that case the parents are liable for the costs of all necessary treatment.

Refusal of treatment. If a minor has the right to consent to treatment, it is probable that he also has the right to refuse treatment. Should the parents wish to have a minor of 14 or over given medical treatment, the child's consent should also be obtained. At this time no decisions can be located in which a minor on reaching the age of majority brought an action against a physician for assault and battery for treating him over his objections but with the consent of his parents. Such a case, however, is not at

all unlikely at some future date, particularly if the treatment is one that causes permanent effects or disfigurement to the child. In a situation where the parents wish to have the child treated but the child refuses, the prudent physician should obtain a court order as he would do if a parent refused to allow a blood transfusion for a dangerously injured child. It is extremely risky as a matter of law to treat a teenager under any circumstance that violates the child's right of self-determination, as was indicated in two cases.

A 16-year-old girl could not be forced to have an abortion over her objection at the request of her mother.

A teenage boy who had been committed by his parents as a "voluntary patient" to a mental institution was entitled to leave the hospital when he wished to do so. The court held that since a statute in that state allowed the child to seek treatment for mental disorders at the age of 16, the child would be held to have the right to refuse that to which he was statutorily entitled to consent.

Therefore, in any case where a child can be treated at his own request and without the consent of his parent, under a minor treatment statute or otherwise, it is quite probable that the same child has the right to refuse treatment at least if the condition is not life-threatening. The two concepts appear to be interlocked: a child who has the right to consent has an equal right to refuse to consent. Thus, it would appear to be extremely unwise to treat any such minor over his objection.

A younger child, however, probably does not have this right. A 7-year-old who needs surgery may take very definite exception to the idea of the operation. Until such time as a court holds that a child does not have the right to refuse treatment which his parents wish him to have, it should be presumed as a matter of practice that the right to consent is equated with the right to refuse, at least where the minor's life is not at stake.

A 7-year-old obviously cannot consent to treatment himself; therefore, equally, he cannot refuse it. A 17-year-old is quite able to do both. In any event, however, for practical purposes of deciding what to do about a sick or injured child who refuses to notify his parent or who refuses to consent to their request that he be treated, the physician should remember that in case of doubt a court will probably uphold the validity of any reasonable medical judgment designed to benefit the child who is the patient. Thus, in case of doubt a sick child should not be turned away because he will not tell his parents of his needs.

As is suggested by the Model Act of the American Academy of Pediatrics, if a minor is to be treated without parental consent and the procedure involves "major surgery, general anesthesia, or a life-threatening procedure," consultation with another physician is advisable. Consultation probably should be requested where there is any material risk of harm, both to obtain corroboration as to the accuracy of the diagnosis to avoid a later charge of unnecessary surgery or treatment and to provide another opinion on the ability of the patient to understand the potential risks.

63.

Commentary on Psychosurgery   Ralph Slovenko

In traditional terms, consent, to be binding, must be made by one having the mental capacity to appreciate the consequences of his choice, while free from duress. In the Detroit psychosurgery case, the subject of Professor Robert A. Burt's reflections ("Why We Should Keep Prisoners from the Doctors," *Hastings Center Report,* February 1975), the concept of consent was used by the court as a means to achieve a desired result. As Burt states it, the court found that "the procedure was highly experimental" and that "institutional coercions deprived confined persons of adequate capacity to consent freely to such a risky operation." Despite his own role in forming the court's opinion, and although he remains "convinced that the court's result was correct," Burt does not, on reflection, find the court's reasons "sufficiently persuasive." On this point Professor Burt and I are in agreement. Burt proceeds to offer a different, and in his view better, rationale for the court's action. Whether that rationale is any more persuasive than the court's original one, I leave to others to decide. My own involvement in the Detroit

psychosurgery case, however, leads me to very different reflections from his about the difficulties inherent in the concept of informed consent.

I was a member of the informed consent review committee established to evaluate the consent given by the confined subjects in Lafayette Clinic's psychosurgery experiment. In September 1972, the principal physician-investigator, whom I had not known previously, asked that I serve on the committee which was a separate entity from the medical committee set up to oversee the soundness of the experimental design. As I was dependent on the clinic for teaching and research opportunities, the appointment of two independent outsiders to the committee—a priest, a man of God, and an accountant, a man of commerce—was welcome.

I have never been an advocate of psychosurgery to control behavior. Indeed, at the time, I was less concerned with psychosurgery than with the issue of whether psychotherapy in general, judging from results, causes more harm than any of the physical, chemi-

Source: *Hastings Center Report,* vol. 5, October 1975.

cal, or behavioral techniques that dominate the discussion on consent. ("If psychoanalysis were a drug," I hear, "the FDA would ban it.")

A few days after the initial meeting of the consent committee, I advised the principal investigator (September 21, 1972) that litigation was pending in Mississippi in connection with psychosurgery performed on young delinquents apparently without consent. I was told that "we will make sure that there is informed consent available from our patient" (October 2, 1972).

I met individually with John Doe (as the subject was known at trial) on six occasions, each session lasting approximately an hour. In addition, with his permission, he was interviewed in my seminar on law and psychiatry. On this occasion the group consisted of approximately thirty persons including some psychiatrists, a judge, and a few staff members from Lafayette Clinic, in particular the principal investigator. Following the interview, after John Doe left the seminar room, the atmosphere was highly critical of the value of the experiment. As is customary, the subject or patient did not hear the discussion of his case.

No one can be sure of another's motives, or even of one's own motives. Some of the group believed John Doe's desire "to do something useful, to atone for my guilt" was a motivating force in his volunteering for the experiment. A few others felt that he was volunteering as a means to obtain release. But there was near unanimity of opinion that his prime motivation was fear—fear that he would explode in the free world as he had done eighteen years earlier, when he had strangled a nurse and performed necrophilia. He insisted that he would seek psychosurgery if it were "the only means of helping my physical problem," even if there were other ways to obtain release. He had little faith in his ability to control himself. (Incidentally, one word he did not know how to spell was "capable," as may hereinafter be noted.) In a conversation with the Director of the State Department of Mental Health I was told that the subject had been informed

that he would be released in a few months, irrespective of the experiment.

Months later the experiment became a matter of public notoriety. At the time I had not filed a report to the principal investigator, though the other two members of the committee, in an individual capacity, had done so and given their approval. If I had been asked for my report, as I later was, I would have said the subject was entering the experiment voluntarily. I suppose I dragged my feet because of my own feelings about psychosurgery.

John Doe was told of the risks. He was issued the *Miranda*-style warnings about the risks. Indeed, he was advised that the procedure might even result in death. There was, actually, a page-one headline in a local paper, "Surgery May Cure—or Kill—Rapist" (*Detroit Free Press,* January 7, 1973). He was made no promises. He was more intelligent and sophisticated than his years of confinement (half of his life) would suggest. He delighted in Joseph Heller's *Catch 22.* To summarize my interviews, I asked John Doe (January 12, 1973) to write his answers to the following questions, which he did:

Q. Would you seek psychosurgery if you were not confined in an institution?

A. Yes, if after testing this showed that it would be of help.

Q. Do you believe that psychosurgery is the way to obtain your release from the institution?

A. No, but it would be a step in obtaining my release. It is like any other therapies or programs to help a person to function again.

Q. Would you seek psychosurgery if there were other ways to obtain your release?

A. Yes, if psychosurgery were the only means of helping my physical problem after a period of testing.

Q. Would you want legal representation to explore whether or not there are ways to obtain your release without psychosurgery?

A. No, because I feel that [the principal

investigator and the Director of the State Department of Mental Health] will release me when I have shown I am a cappable [*sic*] person.

Q. Are you in favor of newspaper and other publicity surrounding your case?

A. It makes no difference, because if the [principal investigator] thinks that by me stating my views in public will be of help to him and the clinic, so be it.

Without consulting the subject, Michigan Legal Services lawyer Gabe Kaimowitz, representing himself and certain individual members of the Medical Committee for Human Rights, filed a taxpayers' suit to halt the state-funded experiment on behalf of John Doe and others similarly situated. Also, without consulting me, he asked the court that the subject be placed under my custody.

John Doe protested the intervention, saying to me: "I was in the institution for seventeen years and no one showed any concern. Now Kaimowitz speaks out for my 'rights' without even talking to me. The doctors came to the institution, gave me a chance, treated me like a man. I have great faith in [the principal investigator]. He'll check out the best treatment. He'll do the best. I did wrong, and perhaps by this experiment something will be learned to help others. I killed a woman. I can't function as I am. I need some kind of treatment."

Shortly after Kaimowitz filed suit, I received a telephone call from Charles Halpern of the Mental Health Law Project in Washington, D.C. At the time I was Chairman of the Committee on Legal Approaches to Mental Health of the American Orthopsychiatric Association, which subsequently cosponsored the Mental Health Law Project. Halpern said that he wanted to join forces with Kaimowitz, who, for reasons known only to him, chose to go it alone.

As I told Halpern, I felt that the experiment could not be tainted because of lack of consent. But, I added, the subject had a great deal of faith in the investigator, the

first person in his seventeen years of confinement to show any interest in him, and a strong relationship had developed between them. The development of such a relationship, de facto though not de jure, causes consent not to be really informed. As the "informed consent" concept has developed at law, "sufficient information must be disclosed to the patient so that he can arrive at an intelligent opinion." But *by whom* is the information to be given? The crucial factor is not the quantity of information given, or even the contents, but rather *who* says it.

The concept of "informed consent" must be redefined to include the source of the information. If consent is to have any real meaning, note has to be taken of transference, one element of which is trance, or hypnosis. The hocus-pocus of being helped is another way of describing suggestibility. An analogy can be made to coach and athlete. The extent of the time that the athlete spends with the coach, and the kind of person he is, determines the ease or the speed with which the athlete explores any new maneuver. Unless the "trance" of the transference is dissipated, the subject or patient will go along with the expressed or implied suggestion.

At the time of the psychosurgery case, a close friend of mine—a potential Davis Cup player—injured his hip. The doctor told him he needed surgery; my friend was reluctant, realizing that it would jeopardize his tennis career. He traveled the country seeking other opinions, and finally obtained a recommendation against surgery. He settled on that opinion, and he is glad he did, for he is now back playing tennis without handicap. He could afford more than one opinion; most people cannot.

Obtaining a statement of alternatives from one experimenter or physician is not the same as obtaining opinions from different parties with whom a relationship has developed. John Doe was advised of the alternatives by the principal investigator. Not until that relationship was diluted by other health professionals did his view change.

(The United Store Workers Union says that it has been able to reduce the amount of surgery performed on its members by having a second doctor review each recommended operation before it is performed. *New York Times,* June 19, 1973, p. 21.)

And so Professor Burt's suggestion that "we should keep prisoners from the doctors" leads to the thought that we ought to keep everyone from the doctors. Indeed, there is an old prayer, "God save us from the doctors." De facto, it is neither age nor confinement that puts consent in question. Indeed, John Doe, not being under pain or stress, made a more valid consent than does the ordinary ill person who calls upon a doctor. The expectations of a patient and the great dependence on a doctor affect mightily the rationality of decision making. When in distress or pain, one regresses to a childlike state. To put it another way, the child in everyone tends to dominate the personality when one is in great stress or pain. We cannot yet quantitate stress to measure the legality of a consent.

Actually, the consent given by John Doe was not before the court. On the first day of the trial, March 12, 1973, the Director of the Department of Mental Health withdrew authorization of the experiment because of adverse public reaction to news reports about it. The court, however, stated that the issues raised were of sufficient public importance to be decided in a declaratory decree. No one, except the state Attorney General, wanted to let go of the case. All of the participating attorneys contended the trial should be continued in order to establish the rights of institutionalized persons.

A panel of three judges listened to three weeks of testimony. As there were no factual issues to be resolved, the proceedings took on the air of a seminar. In a forty-one page opinion, drawing heavily from the briefs submitted by Burt and Halpern, the court concluded that an involuntarily confined individual cannot give a legitimate consent as he is living in "an inherently coercive atmosphere." (The court would allow a prisoner to consent only to low-risk, high-benefit

procedures.) The decision did not foreclose "the performance of psychosurgery on such persons once the procedure has advanced to a level where its benefits clearly outweigh its risk." Given the current state of knowledge about how the brain works, the court judged that presently the benefits do not outweigh the risk.

Historically, the informed consent doctrine has evolved to facilitate proof of cases and the payment of compensation to injured persons. In the usual case of malpractice, the patient must produce an expert to establish that there has been a departure from accepted, proper practice. In contrast, where there is no informed consent, it is not necessary to have expert testimony to prove negligence. Such a case is premised on the theory that had the complainant been informed of the risk and hazards he would not have agreed to the treatment or experiment. The fact that the treatment or experiment was properly performed is immaterial.

In the psychosurgery case, the concept was used not to facilitate proof of the complainant's case but to bar a modality of practice. In any event, to take "informed consent" literally is to miss the point. The use of subterfuge, if you will, is as ancient as history itself. Over 2,000 years ago the Talmud did away with capital punishment, but it could not do so directly for the world was unprepared for it. And so the sages of the Talmud devised regulations which had the quality of religious sanction that made it impossible to carry it out. In the case of psychosurgery, there was no rationalization available to the court in its quest to ban psychosurgery in prisons, with the possible exception of the Eighth Amendment prohibition against cruel and unusual punishment. Those who adhere to the maxim, "call a spade a spade," may be fit only to use one. Assuredly this is not the style of the judicial process.

Informed consent is thus a spurious issue. To apply the time-honored test of consent literally is to expend energy needlessly. Review committees, as they presently look over consent forms, are one example of the waste of time. A more realistic approach would be to provide a subject or patient with different opinions—from different persons over a span of time in which a relationship can develop.

Finally, the information which is disclosed does not now include aftercare. An experimenter sometimes promises a subject that he will receive good care in the event of a poor result. Is he able to make good on that promise? To my knowledge, there has been no systematic study of the subjects of failed experiments. What I have seen is a transfer of them to institutions for the criminally insane. There, they receive the worst of both the hospital and the prison system.

Society, having high stakes in research, must pay the cost of unpredictable results. At a minimum, there should be a "no fault" clinical research insurance plan to provide care for anyone harmed. A guardian *ad experimentem* might be appointed.

The psychosurgery case, like other cases on informed consent, has led us astray.

Aggressiveness of Patient Care

In this section, articles are included on the general topic of aggressiveness of patient care. It is worthwhile to note an important distinction between two different types of situations in which the issue of the termination of medical care is raised, the distinction between terminating care for strictly medical versus nonmedical reasons. The line drawing this distinction is certainly not absolute, and many cases might be seen as borderline situations; however, the distinction is helpful in conceptualizing the issues involved.

One type of situation includes cases in which treatment is thought to be medically not indicated. This estimation can be made on the basis of a number of different indexes (here we are using the indexes set out by the Law and Ethics Working Group of the Harvard School of Public Health). First, the "disease" might be considered "irreversible"; i.e., there are no known therapeutic measures which could be effective in reversing the course of illness. Second, the physiologic status of the patient might be "irreparable"; the course of illness might have progressed beyond the capacity of existing knowledge and technique to stem the process. Third, death might be believed to be "imminent"; i.e., in the ordinary course of events death probably would occur within a stipulated and therefore necessarily arbitrary period not exceeding a specified outer limit.

The second type of situation includes those cases in which treatment can be seen as medically indicated, in that they do not fulfill the criteria listed above against indication and yet arguments can be advanced against such treatment, for "extra"-medical reasons. Such reasons could refer to many factors, including an evaluation of the patient's expected "quality" of life, the economic and psychological burden to the family, the utilization of scarce medical resources or even the pain and suffering intrinsic to the treatment itself, and if competent adult patients are considered, the patient's wishes.

Related to this distinction is the issue of the locus of decision making. It is sometimes argued that for those cases in which treatment is thought to be medically not indicated, the decision to terminate "treatment" or not to initiate any new medical interventions should be seen as a medical decision and consequently the decision maker should be the physician. Alternatively, for those cases in which treatment is medically indicated and yet arguments are advanced against treatment, since the decision to initiate, continue, or terminate medical treatment in such situations is not based on the medical facts alone, it is argued that the physician should not be the sole decision maker.

In line with this description, the articles in this section were chosen to address the issues presented by both of these types of cases, as well as the question of decision-making authority. Specifically, the articles can be seen as examining four different areas of the problem of aggressiveness of patient care: (1) ethical issues in and professional responsibility for the treatment of critically ill hospitalized patients, both young and old; (2) hospital and state policies for making decisions about the above; (3) ethical issues in and professional responsibility for the treatment of defective newborns; and (4) legal issues presented by the above.

The question of how aggressively to treat patients has become one of the central ethical topics in twentieth century medicine. Because of the inevitable importance of the issues of autonomy and the locus of decision making for this question, there is a strong connection between this section and that of informed consent (clinical). Specifically, the primary consent issues raised in this section are the right of a competent adult to refuse medical care and the problem of "proxy" consent or surrogate decision making with regard to both the incompetent adult patient and the young child. In addition, the other sections intimately related to this one are those on the sanctity of life, active and passive euthanasia, the definition of death (Conceptual Foundations), and experimentation and allocation of resources (Issues in Clinical Ethics). When the question of terminal disease is raised, two obvious issues posed are whether to continue so-called treatment given the scarcity of resources and whether to experiment on patients when standard treatment offers little hope of success. (See cases *5, 12, 13, 15*, 17, *19, 20, 23, 26, 27, 32, 33, 38*, 41, *42*, 44, *46*, 50, *51*.)

64.

Optimum Care for Hopelessly Ill Patients
The Critical Care Committee of the Massachusetts General Hospital

When advanced life support and maximum therapeutic efforts are continued in a patient who is judged to be hopelessly ill and the anticipated outcome is death, serious medical, emotional, legal, and economic questions concerning the justification for continued efforts arise.[1-5] The responsible physician and the medical and nursing staff in the intensive-care unit (ICU) as well as the patient's relatives face the dilemma of deciding whether continued maximal efforts constitute a reasonable attempt at prolonging life or whether the patient's illness has reached a stage where further intensive care is, in fact, merely postponing death. Although relatively few such patients are encountered in most intensive-care units, their presence generates medical, moral, and emotional problems out of proportion to their number. Lack of precise knowledge concerning the specifics

of outcome often precludes a satisfactory solution under these circumstances, and the tendency is to persist in heroic measures until death by conventional criteria, cessation of either circulation or cerebral function.[6]

To study the growing issue of how best to manage the hopelessly ill patients, the Critical Care Committee created an ad hoc subcommittee composed of a psychiatrist as chairman, legal counsel, an assistant nursing director in charge of intensive-care nursing, an internist specializing in oncology, a general surgeon and a lay person who herself had been stricken with, and recovered from, serious neoplastic disease.

The subcommittee was charged with a study and recommendation concerning treatment of the hopelessly ill patient and utilization of critical-care facilities.

On the basis of the recommendations of

Source: *The New England Journal of Medicine*, vol. 29, no. 7, August 12, 1976.

the ad hoc subcommittee, the Critical Care Committee submitted a report to the General Executive Committee recommending the formation of a patient-care classification system, which is a modification of that described by Tagge et al.[4] and the establishment of a permanent committee on optimum treatment of the hopelessly ill patient. The classification system and other recommendations from the Critical Care Committee follow:

1. Whenever appropriate, critically ill patients should be classified according to the following system.

   Class A *Maximal therapeutic effort* without reservation.

   Class B *Maximal therapeutic effort* without reservation, but with daily evaluation because probability of survival is questionable.

   Class C *Selective limitation of therapeutic measures.* The criterion which determines every aspect of the therapeutic regimen continues to be the overall welfare of the patient. At this time certain procedures may cease to be justifiable and become contra-indicated. Particular attention must be given to resuscitation measures of all kinds. The therapeutic plan must be clearly detailed to the other members of the care team so that all understand and are united about their caring efforts and responsibilities. As an integral part of caring for the patient, appropriate notes specifically describing the therapeutic plan should be made in the patient's record. The patient's resuscitation status should be similarly recorded in conformance with the policy governing orders limiting full cardio-pulmonary resuscitation.

   A Class C patient is not an appropriate candidate for admission to an Intensive Care Unit. A decision to transfer the patient out of the Intensive Care Unit is based upon the needs of the patient, and transfer is appropriate only after required comfort measures become manageable in a nonintensive care setting. Whatever the patient's location, however, and irrespective of the specific therapeutic measures that have been selectively limited, a Class C patient and his family require and must be given full general support.

   Class D *All therapy can be discontinued.* Any measures which are indicated to insure maximum comfort of the patient may be continued or instituted.

2. (a) The Critical Care Committee recommends the establishment of an advisory committee to be referred to as the Optimum Care Committee. This group should be available to serve *in an advisory capacity* in situations where difficulties arise in deciding the appropriateness of continuing intensive therapy for critically ill patients. Although the ICU Director may *suggest* a review by the committee, *the ultimate request must come from the responsible physician.* When requested by the responsible physician, the Optimum Care Committee will act as expeditiously as possible to review all available information regarding the patient, calling on whatever resources it deems necessary. The committee will then recommend to the responsible physician what it considers to be an appropriate course of action. It should be emphasized that the committee's role is *advisory* and the responsible physician may accept or reject its decision.

   (b) The Optimum Care Committee can most effectively deal with the highly sensitive issues by convening all members of the care team involved, i.e., responsible physician, ICU Director, consultants, nursing staff and committee members, to discuss the care of the patient and mutually explore what the best interest of the patient and his relatives require in the situation. The major aim will be the clarification of the treatment rationale for all concerned.

(c) The ICU Director may have recourse to the chief of service when the responsible physician does not wish to discuss the treatment rationale and the ICU Director feels such discussion is warranted. In the case of a disagreement between an ICU Director and responsible physician, the ICU Director may ask the permission of the chief of service to call the committee. In the event permission is granted and the committee offers a recommendation, the responsible physician nevertheless makes the final decision about treatment.

(d) The services of the Optimum Care Committee should be available to all Intensive Care Units and to individual physicians requesting advice in the management of critically ill patients confined outside the intensive care units.

Assignment and Use of Classifications

On admission to the intensive-care unit, patients will be assumed to be Class A or B. Any patient who is not in Class A must be reassessed daily. It is stressed that the ultimate decision concerning treatment classification rests with the responsible physician. Whenever a question arises about the appropriateness of treatment of a patient with an irreversible illness the situation should be reviewed at unit rounds. Such questions may rise from the patient himself, the family, the responsible physician, the staff of the unit or its director, or consultants called by the responsible physician. If there is a consensus about treatment, no change in classification occurs. If patients or family or someone not at rounds has raised the question, the responsible physician, the director of the unit, or an appropriate designee should explain the treatment rationale to the person who raised the question. If

treatment rationale remains unclear at unit rounds, the patient should be assigned to Class B by the responsible physician. The purpose of assignment to Class B is twofold: to provide opportunity for the responsible physician to obtain further consultation and support in the management of a difficult case; and to ensure dialogue between the primary physician and director and staff of the intensive-care unit through the forum of unit rounds. If the unit nurses and physicians do not understand the reasons for a specific treatment of a patient, or fail to see how a specific treatment may reverse the course of a patient's illness, they are encouraged to request clarification from the responsible physician or unit director, who may relay the request to the primary physician. Since communication failures can cause serious misunderstanding, use of unit rounds to clarify specific treatment considerations is strongly recommended.

When the responsible physician designates a patient for treatment in Class C, it is essential that he receive the support of the unit director, physicians, nursing staff, and his own consultants. Concurrence is probably most conveniently given through discussion at unit rounds, although prior discussion may indicate that such supportive consensus is already clear. If the responsible physician is uncertain whether his clinical reasoning has been properly understood by the unit staff, he is encouraged to review the situation with the director.

Once a patient has been classified in the C category, the guidance of the responsible physician is even more heavily relied upon to specify indications for treatment of hypotension, ventilatory or cardiac failure, acute pulmonary edema, arrhythmias, metabolic intoxication, and other crises heralded by failing organ systems. Nursing and resident staff skilled in use of defibrillators, vasopressors, pacemakers, endotracheal tubes, or other lifesaving treatments feel especially threatened when the responsibility for initiating these efforts is left to their judgment. These decisions must be made by the responsible physician. Efforts to ease the burden of nurses and house staff in this regard will reduce most if not all of the potential for conflict. Nurses and house staff are also encouraged to voice their concerns at rounds so that clarification and guidance can be ensured.

At the transition from Class B to Class C the responsible physician, who must make this difficult decision, should avail himself of any consultation he wishes. Designation of Class C requires judgment entirely independent of the question of whether or not the patient should remain in the intensive-care unit. Because of the high cost of unit beds, considerable pressure may arise to make economic considerations primary in deciding where a particular patient should reside. This committee stresses that economic considerations must never serve as the sole criterion for disposition and treatment of patients.

Although Class C designation implies that death is the probable outcome, it may not necessarily be the case. With improvement, the patient's category may be changed to a more optimistic one. Similarly, with deterioration, therapy may be selectively limited, while the patient remains in Class C without necessarily being assigned to Class D.

Designation of a patient for Class D is to follow the same recommendations as those given for Class C. The definite act of commission, such as turning off a mechanical ventilator, is to be performed only by an appropriate physician after consultation with and concurrence of the family and appropriate hospital committee (or committees) where indicated. Assignment to Class D is generally reserved for patients with brain death, or when there is no reasonable possibility that the patient will return to a cognitive and sapient life.

Clarification of resuscitation status. Unless otherwise stated, full resuscitation will be initiated for all patients. Any limitation on full resuscitative efforts must be stated fully in the patient's record.

Experience with classification system and use of the Optimum Care Committee. The classification system has been in use as a pilot study for 6 months involving 209 admissions to the Respiratory Intensive and Acute Care Unit, an 11-bed multidisciplinary critical-care unit. All patients were classified independently by the charge nurse and the Respiratory Unit staff physician on call upon admission and daily thereafter until discharge. Once all concerned personnel had gained a thorough understanding of the classification there was a remarkable degree of correlation of classification among nurses and physicians.

Requests for Optimum Care Committee consultation have been rare; 15 patients have been reviewed to date. The main benefits of the consultation have been clarification of misunderstanding about the patient's prognosis, reopening of communication, reestablishment of unified treatment objectives and rationale, restoration of the sense of shared responsibility for patient and family, and above all, maximizing support for the responsible physician who makes the medical decision to intensify, maintain, or limit effort at reversing the illness.

NOTES

1. N.H. Cassem, "Confronting the Decision to Let Death Come," *Critical Care Medicine*, vol. 2, p. 113, 1974.

2. N.H. Cassem, "Controversies Surrounding the Hopelessly Ill Patient," *Linacre Quarterly*, vol. 42, no. 3, p. 89, 1975.

3. National Conference Steering Committee, "Standards for Cardiopulmonary Resuscitation (CPR) and Emergency Cardiac Care (ECC)," *Journal of the American Medical Association*, vol. 227, p. 837, 1974.

4. G.F. Tagge, D. Adler, C.W. Bryan-Brown, et al., "Relationship of Therapy to Prognosis in Critically Ill Patients," *Critical Care Medicine*, vol. 2, p. 61, 1974.

5. D.J. Cullen, L.C. Ferrara, B.A. Briggs, et al., "Survival Hospitalization Charges and Follow-up Results in Critically Ill Patients," *New England Journal of Medicine*, vol. 294, p. 982, 1976.

6. Report of the Ad Hoc Committee of the Harvard Medical School to Examine the Definition of Brain Death, "A Definition of Irreversible Coma," *Journal of the American Medical Association*, vol. 205, p. 337, 1968.

65.

Patient Autonomy and "Death with Dignity"
David L. Jackson   Stuart Youngner

The rapid advance in medical technology over the past two decades has raised serious questions about patient autonomy and the right to die with dignity. We will attempt to examine psychologic issues affecting decision making in these areas. Attempts to answer these questions have come from many quarters: legal, ethical and religious, as well as medical. The lay public and press have also participated actively in this dialogue.

Both legislatures and the courts have attempted to clarify these issues. Many states have enacted laws providing for "living wills"—legal documents that give patients the right to refuse heroic measures for their care when in a "terminal" condition.[1] Such laws also protect physicians from legal action by family members when they comply with such "wills." Both the courts and some state legislatures have recently attempted to provide legal definitions of death.[2] The courts have also ruled on who should make the final decisions when patients are not competent. Most recently, in the Saikewicz case,[3,4] the Supreme Court of Massachusetts asserted that all decisions about the institution or termination of life-prolonging measures must be made by the courts if the patient is not legally competent.

Physicians have approached the difficult problem of decision making for critically ill patients in various ways. Attempts have been made to establish reliable clinical criteria for predicting outcome in critically ill patients. This effort has been most successful in defining brain death, where clear-cut clinical criteria can predict with certainty a fatal outcome.[2] Efforts at predicting outcome in "vegetative" brain states and other serious "terminal" conditions have been less successful.

Another approach has been to develop systems for classifying patient-care categories.[5-7] This triage approach is designed to permit direction of maximal effort toward the care of "viable" patients, stressing daily reevaluation of medical status and treatment options and open communication among medical personnel, patient, and family.

Many hospitals have established ethics or "optimal-care" committees that serve in an advisory capacity to physicians, patients, and families when difficult decisions arise about stopping or withholding life-support systems.[8]

Imbus and Zawacki[8] described an approach for patients with "burns so severe that survival is unprecedented." When given a choice between "ordinary" care or "full treatment measures," 21 of 24 patients chose the former. The authors make a strong argument for an aggressive approach to preserve patient autonomy. They ask, "Who is more likely to be totally and lovingly concerned with the patient's best interest than the patient himself?"

Little has been written, however, about the specific clinical and psychologic problems that may complicate the concept of patient autonomy and the right to die with dignity. Cassem[9] has noted that in clinical situations where pain and depression are prominent features, "the physician ethically could proceed against the will of the patient." Rabkin and his colleagues[10] warn that "caution should be exercised that a patient does not unwittingly 'consent' to an ONTR [order not to resuscitate], as a result of temporary distortion (for example, from pain, medication, or metabolic abnormality) in his ability to choose among available alternatives." They go on to say that "it may be inappropriate

Source: *The New England Journal of Medicine*, vol. 301, no. 8, August 23, 1979. Supported in part by a grant (MH 15022–02) from the National Institute of Mental Health.

to introduce the subject of withholding cardiopulmonary resuscitation efforts to certain competent patients when, in the physician's judgment, the patient will probably be unable to cope with them psychologically." Unfortunately, the authors do not develop this concept in a detailed manner and therefore leave it open to criticism.[8]

The issues of patient autonomy and the right to die with dignity are without question important ones that require further discussion and clarification by our society as a whole. However, there is a danger that in certain cases, preoccupation with these dramatic and popular issues may lead physicians and patients to make clinically inappropriate decisions—precisely because sound clinical evaluation and judgment are suspended. This article will attempt to illustrate this concept by use of clinical examples from a medical intensive-care unit. Each case will demonstrate a specific clinical situation where concerns about patient autonomy and the right to die with dignity posed a potential threat to sound decision making and the total clinical (medical, social, and ethical) basis for the "optimal" decision.

Case Reports

Case 1—patient ambivalence. An 80-year-old man was admitted to the Medical Intensive-Care Unit (MICU) with a 3-week history of progressive shortness of breath. He had a long history of chronic obstructive lung disease. He had been admitted to a hospital with similar problems 4 years earlier and had required intubation, mechanical respiratory support, and eventual tracheostomy. The patient remained on the respirator for 2 months before weaning was successfully completed. During the 4 years after discharge, his activity had been progressively restricted because of dyspnea on exertion. He required assistance in most aspects of self-care.

On admission, he was afebrile, and there was no evidence of an acute precipitating event. Maximum attempts at pulmonary toilet, low-flow supplemental oxygen, and treatment of mild right-sided congestive heart

failure and bronchospasm were without effect. After 4 days of continued deterioration, a decision had to be made about whether to intubate and mechanically ventilate the patient. His private physician and the director of the MICU discussed the options with this fully conversant and alert patient. He initially decided against intubation. However, 24 hours later, when he became almost moribund, he changed his mind and requested that respiratory support be initiated. He was unable to be weaned from the respirator and required tracheostomy—a situation reminiscent of his previous admission. Two months later, he had made no progress and it became obvious that he would never be weaned from respiratory support.

Attempts were made to find extended-care facilities that could cope with a patient on a respirator. Extensive discussions with the patient and his family about the appropriate course to follow revealed striking changes of mind on an almost daily basis. The patient often expressed to the MICU staff his wish to be removed from the respirator and said, "If I make it, I make it." However, when his family was present, he would insist that he wanted maximal therapy, even if it meant remaining on the respirator indefinitely. The family showed similar ambivalence. The patient was regularly the center of conversation at the MICU weekly interdisciplinary conference (liaison among medical, nursing, social-work, and psychiatric staff). There was great disagreement among MICU staff members concerning which side of the patient's ambivalence should be honored. Ultimately (after 4½ months on the respirator), the patient contracted a nosocomial pulmonary infection, became hypotensive, and experienced ventricular fibrillation. No efforts were made at cardiopulmonary resuscitation. In this difficult case, the concept of patient "autonomy" became impossible to define.

Case 2—depression. A 54-year-old married man with a 5-year history of lymphosarcoma was admitted to the hospital intensive-care unit for progressive shortness of breath and a 1-week history of nausea and vomiting. Over the past 5 years, he had received three courses of combination-drug chemotherapy, which resulted in remission. His most recent course occurred 4 months before admission. On admission, x-ray examination of the chest showed a diffuse infiltrate, more on the left than on the right. Eight hours after admission, he was transferred to the MICU because of hypotension and increasing dyspnea. Initially, it was not clear whether these findings indicated interstitial spread of lymphosarcoma or asymmetric pulmonary edema. Physical findings were compatible with a diagnosis of congestive heart failure, and he was treated for pulmonary edema, with good response. His neurologic examination was normal, except for a flat, depressed affect. Deep-tendon reflexes were 2+ and symmetric. Laboratory examination revealed only a mildly elevated blood urea nitrogen, with a normal creatinine and a slightly elevated calcium of 11.8 mg per deciliter (2.95 mmol per liter). There were no objective signs of hypercalcemia. His repiratory status improved rapidly.

The patient refused his oncologist's recommendation for additional chemotherapy. Although his cognitive abilities were intact, he steadfastly refused the pleas of his wife and the MICU staff to undergo therapy. Over the first 6 days in the MICU with treatment by rehydration, his calcium became normal, his nausea and vomiting slowly improved, and his affect brightened. At that time, he agreed to chemotherapy, stating that, "Summer's coming and I want to be able to sit in the backyard a little longer." During this course of chemotherapy, the patient discussed his previous refusal of therapy. In his opinion, the nausea and vomiting had made "life not worth living." No amount of reassurance that these symptoms were temporary could convince him that it was worthwhile to continue his fight. Only when this reassurance was confirmed by clinical improvement did the patient overcome his reactive depression and concur with the reinstitution of vigorous therapy.

Case 3—patient who uses a plea for death with dignity to identify a hidden problem.

A 52-year-old married man was admitted to the MICU after an attempt at suicide. He had retired 2 years earlier because of progressive physical disability related to multiple sclerosis during the 15 years before admission. He had successfully adapted to his physical limitations, remaining actively involved in family matters with his wife and two teenage sons. However, during the 3 months before admission, he had become morose and withdrawn but had no vegetative symptoms of depression. On the evening of admission, while alone, he ingested an unknown quantity of diazepam. When his family returned 6 hours later, they found the patient semiconscious. He had left a suicide note.

On admission to the MICU, physical examination showed several neurologic deficits, including spastic paraparesis, right-arm monoparesis, cortical sensory deficits, bilateral ophthalmoplegia, and bilateral cerebellar dysfunction. This picture was unchanged from recent neurologic examinations. The patient was alert and fully conversant. He expressed to the MICU house officers his strong belief in a patient's right to die with dignity. He stressed the "meaningless" aspects of his life related to his loss of function, insisting that he did not want vigorous medical intervention should serious complications develop. This position appeared logically coherent to the MICU staff. However, a consultation with members of the psychiatric liaison service was requested.

During the initial consultation, the patient showed that the onset of his withdrawal and depression coincided with a diagnosis of inoperable cancer in his mother-in-law. His wife had spent more and more time satisfying the needs of her terminally ill mother. In fact, on the night of his suicide attempt, the patient's wife and sons had left him alone for the first time to visit his mother-in-law, who lived in another city. The patient had "too much pride" to complain to his wife about his feelings of abandonment. He was able to recognize that his suicide attempt and insistence on death with dignity were attempts to draw the family's attention to his needs. Discussions with all four family members led to improved communication and acknowledgment of the patient's special emotional needs. After these conversations, the patient explicitly retracted both his suicide threats and his demand that no supportive medical efforts be undertaken. He was discharged to have both neurologic and psychiatric follow-up examinations.

Case 4—patient demands out of fear that treatment be withheld or stopped. An unmarried 18-year-old woman, 24 weeks pregnant and with a history of chronic asthma, was admitted to the hospital with a 2-day history of increasing shortness of breath. She was found to have a left lobar pneumonia and a gram-negative urinary-tract infection. She was transferred to the MICU for worsening shortness of breath and hypoxia resistant to therapy with supplemental oxygen. Despite vigorous pulmonary toilet and antiasthmatic and antibiotic therapy, her condition continued to deteriorate. She was thought to require intubation for positive end-expiratory pressure respiratory therapy. Initially, she refused this modality of treatment. She was alert, oriented, and clearly legally competent. After several discussions with physicians, nurses, family, and friends, she openly verbalized her fears of the imposing and intimidating MICU equipment and environment. She was able to accept reassurance and consented to appropriate medical therapy. She showed slow but progressive improvement and was discharged 8 days later.

Case 5—family's perception differs from patient's previously expressed wishes. A 76-year-old retired man was transferred to the MICU 4 days after laparotomy for diverticulitis. Before hospitalization, he had enjoyed good health and a full and active life-style. He sang regularly in a barbershop quartet until one week before admission. The patient's hospital course was complicated by a urinary-tract infection with sepsis and aspiration pneumonia requiring orthotracheal intubation to control pulmonary secretions. Before intubation, he had emphasized to the medical staff his enjoyment of life and expressed a strong desire to return, if

possible, to his previous state of health. After intubation, he continued to cooperate vigorously with his daily care, including painful procedures (e.g., obtaining samples of arterial-blood gas). However, he contracted sepsis and became delirious, and at this time his wife and daughter expressed strong feelings to the MICU staff that no "heroic" measures be undertaken. Thus, serious disagreement arose concerning the appropriate level of supportive care for this patient. The professional staff of the MICU felt that the medical problems were potentially reversible and that the patient had both explicitly and implicitly expressed a wish to continue the struggle for life. Because this view conflicted with the family's wishes, the MICU visiting physician called a meeting of the Terminal Care Committee (a hospital committee with broad representation that meets at the request of any physician, nurse or family member who would like advice concerning the difficult decision to initiate, continue, stop, or withhold intensive care for critically ill patients). Meeting with the committee were the private physician, the MICU attending physician, as well as representatives from the MICU nursing and house-officer teams. The family was given the opportunity to attend but declined. The committee supported the judgment of the MICU staff that because of the patient's previously expressed wishes and the medical situation, vigorous supportive intervention should be continued. A meeting was then held between medical staff and the patient's family, during which it was agreed by all that appropriate medical intervention should be continued but that the decision would be reviewed on a daily basis. Five days later, the patient contracted a superinfection that did not respond to maximal antibiotic therapy. He became transiently hypotensive and showed progressive renal failure. In the face of a progressing multilobe pneumonia and sepsis caused by a resistant organism, the decision to support the patient with maximum intervention was reviewed. The family concurred with the professional staff's recommendation that cardiopulmonary resuscitation should not be attempted if the patient suffered a cardiopulmonary arrest. On the 18th day in the MICU, the patient died.

Decision making in this case became more difficult because the patient's deteriorating condition made him unable to participate. The advice of the Terminal Care Committee was critically important in this situation, where the family's perception of death with dignity conflicted not only with the patient's own wishes but also with the professional judgment of the MICU staff.

Case 6—misconception by some of MICU staff of patient's concept of death with dignity. A 56-year-old woman was receiving chemotherapy on an outpatient basis for documented bronchogenic carcinoma metastatic to the mediastinal lymph nodes and central nervous sytem when she had a sudden seizure, followed by cardiorespiratory arrest. Resuscitation was accomplished in the outpatient department, and she was transferred to the MICU. She had been undergoing combination-drug chemotherapy as an outpatient for 6 months but continued to work regularly.

In the MICU, her immediate management was complicated by "flail chest" and a tension pneumothorax requiring tube drainage of the chest. She was deeply comatose and hypotensive. Several MICU staff members raised questions about the appropriateness of continued intensive care. After initial medical stabilization, including vasopressor therapy and mechanical respiration, her clinical status was reviewed in detail with the family. Because of the patient's ability to continue working until the day of admission, her excellent response to chemotherapy and her family's perception of her often-stated wish to survive to see the birth of her first grandchild (her daughter was 7 months pregnant), maximal efforts were continued. She remained deeply comatose for 3 days. Her course was complicated by recurrent tension pneumothoraces, gram-negative sepsis caused by a urinary-tract infection and staphylococcal pneumonia. She gradually became more responsive and by the seventh

hospital day was able to nod "yes" or "no" to simple questions. Her hospital course was similar to that of many critically ill patients. As soon as one problem began to improve, a major setback occurred in another organ system. With each setback, there was growing dissension among the MICU staff about the appropriate level of supportive care. The vast majority of the MICU staff felt strongly that continued maximum intervention was neither warranted nor humane. A smaller group of staff, supported by the patient's daughter and (once she was able to communicate) the patient herself, felt that as long as there was any chance for the patient to return to the quality of life she had enjoyed before cardiorespiratory arrest, maximum therapy was indicated.

The patient was the subject of many hours of debate and was a regular topic of conversation at the weekly interdisciplinary conference. She survived all her medical complications and was discharged home after 7 weeks in the MICU, awake, alert, and able to walk and engage in daily activities around her home without limitation. She saw the birth of her granddaughter, and spent Thanksgiving, Christmas, and New Year's Day at home with her family. She died suddenly at home 11 weeks after discharge.

Discussion

Our purpose is not to refute the importance of patient autonomy or discredit the more complex concept of death with dignity. Rather, we have attempted to provide a specific clinical perspective that may help to clarify the difficult and often conflicting factors underlying the decisions made daily at the bedsides of critically ill patients.

Veatch[11] has effectively argued that many of the decisions regarding the withholding or stopping of life-support systems are ethical, not medical, and therefore not the exclusive responsibility of the physician. Capron and Kass[12] state, "Physicians *qua* physicians are not expert on these philosophic questions, nor are they experts on the question of which physiological functions decisively identify the 'living human organism.'" However, careful examination of the legal guidelines suggested by these authors or the living-will statutes enacted by several states reveals vague terms, such as "irreversible,"[11, 12] "hopeless,"[13] and "terminal condition."[14] As Cassem has pointed out,[9] "In most cases in intensive care units, the confidence with which these label(s) [sic] can be applied depends entirely on the clinical judgment of the primary doctor, along with the best consultations he is able to acquire." Public policy can establish useful guidelines when medical evidence is clear, when exact physiologic measurement is possible, and when disease outcome is accurately predictable (e.g., criteria for brain death[2] or Imbus and Zawacki's burn patients[9]). But rigid guidelines are not useful in most clinical situations, where separation of medical from social or ethical responsibility is difficult or artificial.

We heartily support the plea by Imbus and Zawacki[8] for "more and earlier communication with the patient." However, their question, "Who is more likely to be totally and lovingly concerned with the patient's best interest than the patient himself?" may be somewhat naive and, in certain clinical situations, potentially dangerous. Physicians must not use "professional responsibility" as a cloak for paternalism, but they must be alert not to let the possibility of abuse keep them from the appropriate exercise of professional judgment. Physicians who are uncomfortable or inexperienced in dealing with the complex psychosocial issues facing critically ill patients may ignore an important aspect of their professional responsibility by taking a patient's or family's statement at face value without further exploration or clarification.

The cases presented in this article illustrate specific situations in which superficial preoccupation with the issues of patient autonomy and death with dignity could have led to inappropriate clinical and ethical decisions. They suggest a checklist that may aid the clinician in evaluating such difficult situations.

Case 1—patient ambivalence. One must be cautious not to act precipitously on the side of the patient's ambivalence with which one agrees, while piously claiming to be following the principle of patient autonomy. Ambivalence may not be detected if communication is not a continuing feature of the situation or if the physician makes clear to the patient the answer he expects to hear. Ideally, one hopes for resolution of the ambivalence through clarification of the issues or changes in the course of the illness. However, in some instances, ambivalence may not resolve despite a protracted course and maximal communicative efforts.

Case 2—depression. A patient's refusal or request for cessation of treatment may be influenced by depression. If the depression is adequately treated or, as is more frequently encountered, is reactive to physical discomfort that can be relieved, the patient may well change his or her mind. The astute clinician must be alert for a history of endogenous depression, vegetative signs of depression, and any acute conditions to which the patient may be reacting. Vigorous attempts to treat the causes of the depression should be made before automatically acquiescing to the patient's wishes.

Case 3—patient who uses a plea for death with dignity to identify a hidden problem. As demands for autonomy and death with dignity become acceptable and even popular, patients may use them to mask other less "acceptable" problems or complaints. As case 3 illustrates, a thorough psychosocial history and clinical interview with the patient and family may identify the real problem. If the MICU team can deal effectively with the underlying "real" problems, the plea for death with dignity may radically change.

Case 4—patient demands out of fear that treatment be withheld or stopped. Situations do exist in which fear is rational, unshakable, and ultimately a reasonable basis for refusing treatment. On the other hand, fear is often transient and based on misperception or misinformation. When a patient refuses treatment, the physician should try to identify any fears that may underlie the refusal of therapy. The physician can attempt to overcome the fear by means of honest, open explanation and reassurance and by efforts from family, friends, and members of the health-care team.

Case 5—family's perception differs from patient's previously expressed wishes. Case 5 illustrates this difficult problem. In the absence of a legal document specifically expressing the patient's wishes, who has the right to decide? Clearly, the family represents the interest of the patient, but must a physician comply if both his medical judgment and his assessment of the patient's wishes conflict with the family's view? Of course, the issue could be decided in court. Fortunately, in this case, consultation with the ethics committee of the hospital led to a compromise satisfactory to both family and the MICU staff.

Case 6—misconception by some of MICU staff of patient's concept of death with dignity. In case 6, some of the MICU staff assumed that a comatose patient with metastatic cancer would not want intensive "heroic" treatment. They were mistaken. This patient's will to live was revealed in her desire to see her grandchild born. In such cases, efforts must be made to ascertain the patient's wishes, rather than to make assumptions by the test "what would I want." Questioning family or waiting until the patient can communicate are methods of discovering the wishes of the patient. Supportive therapy must be continued until this information can be gathered.

This checklist describes six patients we have seen in a busy MICU. It is by no means complete, but we hope it will help to clarify situations in which superficial and automatic acquiescence to the concepts of patient autonomy and death with dignity threaten sound clinical judgment. As physicians, we strongly support the principles of patient autonomy and death with dignity and welcome any dialogue that promotes them. Spencer[15] highlighted the importance of judiciously balancing the role of patient and family input into these often difficult decisions with the exercise of sound professional judgment. We must continue to emphasize our professional responsibility for thorough clinical investigation and the exercise of

sound judgment. Living up to this responsibility can only enhance the true autonomy and dignity of our patients.

NOTES

1. K.W. Zucker, "Legislatures Provide for Death with Dignity," *Journal of Legal Medicine,* vol. 5, no. 8, p. 21, 1977.

2. P.M. Black, "Brain Death," *New England Journal of Medicine,* vol. 299, p. 338, 1978.

3. W.J. Curran, "The Saikewicz Decision," *New England Journal of Medicine,* vol. 298, p. 499, 1978.

4. A.S.Relman, "The Saikewicz Decision: Judges as Physicians," *New England Journal of Medicine,* vol. 298, p. 508, 1978.

5. A. Grenvik, D.J. Powner, J.V.Snyder, et al., "Cessation of Therapy in Terminal Illness and Brain Death," *Critical Care Medicine,* vol. 6, p. 284, 1978.

6. G.F. Tagge, D. Adler, C.W. Bryan-Brown, et al., "Relationship of Therapy to Prognosis in Critically Ill Patients," *Critical Care Medicine,* vol. 2, p. 61, 1974.

7. Critical Care Committee of the Massachusetts General Hospital, "Optimum Care for Hopelessly Ill Patients," *New England Journal of Medicine,* vol. 295, p. 362, 1976.

8. S.H. Imbus, and B.E. Zawacki, "Autonomy for Burned Patients When Survival Is Unprecedented," *New England Journal of Medicine,* vol. 297, p. 308, 1977.

9. N. Cassem, "When to Disconnect the Respirator," *Psychiatric Annals,* vol. 9, p. 84, 1979.

10. M.T.Rabkin, G. Gillerman, and N.R. Rice, "Orders Not to Resuscitate," *New England Journal of Medicine,* vol. 295, p. 364, 1976.

11. R.M. Veatch, *Death, Dying, and the Biological Revolution,* Yale University Press, New Haven, 1976.

12. A.M. Capron, and L.R. Kass, "A Statutory Definition of the Standards for Determining Human Death: An Appraisal and a Proposal, *University of Pennsylvania Law Review,* vol. 121, p. 87, 1972.

13. L.F. Taylor, "A Statutory Definition of Death in Kansas, *Journal of the American Medical Association,* vol. 215, p. 296, 1971.

14. West's Annotated California Codes: Health and Safety Code. Section SS7185, Vol 39A. Accumulated pocket part for use in 1979, p. 46.

15. S.S Spencer, "'Code' or 'No Code': A Nonlegal Opinion," *New England Journal of Medicine,* vol. 300, p. 138, 1979.

66.

Death with Dignity
Bruce E. Zawacki and Others

Bruce E. Zawacki and Sharon H. Imbus

To the Editor: "Ethics is like breathing; we do it all the time,"[1] although we are usually unaware of it. When it is pointed out to us that our clinical decisions are almost invariably also ethical, many of us try self-consciously to hold our breath and pretend that we can practice value-free medicine.[2] In their recent special article,[3] Jackson and Youngner admirably avoid this very common self-deception. They are in error, however, when they imply that our approach to burned patients with little hope for survival[4] is naive and gives "superficial and automatic acquiescence to the concepts of patient autonomy" without full consideration of the unique physical and psychosocial circumstances of each case.

Diagnostic and therapeutic thoroughness and skill are our first ethical responsibilities to our patients.[5] Just as we recognize that carbon monoxide or morphine intoxication, untreated shock, or psychologic denial may affect the judgment and competence of burned patients,[3] so do Jackson and Youngner recognize in their patients the similar effects of hypoxia (case 4), hypercalcemia (case 2), ambivalence (case 1), and depression (cases 2 and 3). Their case 5 illustrates our experience that turning to the family for decision making when death seems imminent is rarely satisfactory,[3] and along with their case 6 illustrates the great value of learning and giving primacy to the wishes of a competent patient.

Every patient is different; it is naive to apply any medical or ethical principle rigidly and independently of circumstances. As so well illustrated by Jackson and Youngner, however, the principle of patient autonomy has validity in certain cases, and seeking and giving due weight to the opinion of a competent patient often clears the air and allows us to "breathe easier" in managing many difficult medical-ethical problems.

NOTES

1. D.C. Maguire, *The Moral Choice,* Doubleday, New York, 1978.
2. W. Carlton, *In Our Professional Opinion . . . the Primacy of Clinical Judgment over Moral Choice,* University of Notre Dame Press, Notre Dame, Ind., 1978.
3. D.L. Jackson and S. Youngner, "Patient Autonomy and 'Death with Dignity': Some Clinical Caveats," *New England Journal of Medicine,* vol. 301, p. 404, 1979.
4. S.H. Imbus and B.E. Zawacki, "Autonomy for Burned Patients When Survival Is Unprecedented," *New England Journal of Medicine,* vol. 297, p. 308, 1977.
5. E.D. Pellegrino, "Toward a Reconstruction of Medical Morality: The Primacy of the Act of Profession and the Fact of Illness," *Journal of Medical Philosophy,* vol. 4, p. 32, 1979.

Paul Benzaquin

To the Editor: We nonphysicians who interpret medical events for the media find that one of the thorniest issues for us to deal with is informed consent relative to death with dignity. We are inclined to hold the physician not only responsible but reprehensible in cases of protracted agony.

But all of us must reconsider that view after reading the brilliant if troubling report by Drs. Jackson and Youngner. They have shown us that the choice between life and death may be a moment-to-moment matter, not to be decided at any given time by the patient, the next of kin, or the court.

Source: *New England Journal of Medicine*, vol. 302, no. 2, Jan. 10, 1980.

Most particularly, the responsibility is not to be placed with physicians alone. They are enough concerned with available therapy and changing prognoses that they ought to be freed from serving as the fulcrum for the weight of the choice.

We have often accused the medical profession of regarding death and the waging of war against it as a matter of professional defense. If all that can be done has been done, we are quick to conclude, the physician's conscience is clean, regardless of the patient's pain or the relatives' remorse. Jackson and Youngner's report on patient autonomy disabuses us of that. Part of pain is the wish to end it. Death surely does that but deprives good doctoring of its try.

I congratulate the authors for their sensitivity, although their findings involve more of us in this still unanswered problem. At least they have shown us that judgment of the judges is to no avail. The extension of life is not the same as the postponement of death, but they are often too intimately entwined to separate.

Thomas A. Shannon

To the Editor: Drs. Jackson and Youngner are to be commended for their perceptive and sensitive article. They provide an excellent model of how a sensitive and concerned staff can practice a high standard of scientifically correct and ethically appropriate medicine. If more physicians and staff members were as concerned as those represented in these case studies, the number of such medical-ethical dilemmas would decrease dramatically.

I am concerned, however, about the relation between clinically appropriate decisions and the patient's values. The authors seem to imply that professional judgments and clinical decisions are to be normative in resolving the problem. At least, I think that the authors suggest that the medical dimensions of the situation should count for more than the values of the patient. Such an orientation does not help answer the question of Imbus and Zawacki: "Who is more likely to be totally and lovingly concerned with the pa-

tient's best interest than the patient himself?" It does not come to terms with the admittedly difficult situation of a competent adult Jehovah's Witness who refuses a clinically appropriate blood transfusion on the basis of religious commitment.

Frank Guerra

To the Editor: The importance of deciding what conditions might be operative in a patient's decision with regard to critical care cannot be stressed enough. Unfortunately, such decisions are often not made with the kind of knowledge that the authors deem important. The lot of the internist and particularly of the specialist in intensive care is a busy one, and often the time is not available for the physician to sit down with a patient and family and unravel all the details of the psychosocial history that might reveal why the patient has made a certain choice.

As Jackson and Youngner intimate, decision making cannot occur in a vacuum. Most large medical institutions have psychiatric-liaison divisions with psychiatrists who devote themselves to psychologic issues as they affect medical practice. Because of his or her special skill and training, the psychiatrist is often in a position to explore and evaluate in great detail issues that might otherwise be hidden. I would encourage internists to seek help from their psychiatric colleagues in the hospital in the decision-making process.

Alan A. Stone

To the Editor: The psychology of the patient and the dynamics of the family, which complicate decisions to accept death with dignity, are only half the problem. The other half is the psychology of the physician and the dynamics of the treatment team. Another checklist that parallels the one provided by the authors is needed. It might include the following.

Projection: The physician or the staff, or both, impose their own values and religious beliefs on the patient. These may conflict with the patient's beliefs, and often the staff are in conflict with each other.

Insensibility: Physicians can become inured and hardened to the suffering of patients. Deadening of sensibilities can be an occupational hazard.

Professional agenda: The training needs of physicians and staff in the intensive-care unit can lead to emergency measures that are otherwise meaningless and that interfere with death with dignity.

Fear: The wish to keep alive a patient who has suffered an iatrogenic mishap may lead physicians to put their own fears of family and peer reactions ahead of the patient's dignity in death.

After many discussions of the legal and ethical implications of death with dignity, I find that physicians, ironically, are at the deepest level concerned with their own loss of autonomy. But if we are to be concerned about the psychologic factors that complicate our patients' decisions, we must be equally concerned about the psychologic factors that complicate our own decisions. Unilateral psychologizing will only lead back to unexamined paternalism, and we must go beyond that.

Stuart Youngner and David L. Jackson

The above letters were referred to the authors of the article in question, who offer the following reply:

To the Editor: We think that the efforts of Zawacki and Imbus to communicate and share decision making with critically burned patients are both innovative and commendable. In no way did we intend to imply that such an overall approach to patients with severe burns is naive. However, their question, "Who is more likely to be totally and lovingly concerned with the patient's best interest than the patient himself?" concerns us. The acceptance of this noble phrase may lead physicians to overlook or ignore situations in which depression, fear, ambivalence, or misunderstanding of clinical reality can interfere with a patient's judgment.

Benzaquin stresses the rapidly changing nature of the decision process associated with the care of critically or terminally ill patients. Although we agree with his formulation of these issues and believe that such decisions should not be made by physicians acting alone, we are not convinced that physicians should be "freed from serving as the fulcrum" for this choice. We also hope that our paper does not show that "judgment of the judges is to no avail." Judicial involvement can be counterproductive or of limited usefulness in many clinical situations, but the judiciary is a critically important force organizing and articulating the basic values of our democratic society. We support the rule of law, not the rule of professional judgment applied randomly or on an ad hoc basis.

We would be troubled, as would Dr. Shannon, if our paper were taken to imply that the medical dimensions of the situation should count for more than the values of the patient. Rather, we attempted to cite examples in which an accurate determination of the patient's values was made much more difficult by confounding influences.

Guerra emphasizes the value of a psychiatrist on a critical-care team. We obviously agree; the interaction between internist, nurse, and psychiatrist on our own team continues to be a major positive influence on both patient care and staff morale. We would only add that the active involvement of a skilled social worker should also be considered, since that brings a different but equally important dimension to the team approach to critical-care medicine.

Stone's checklist for reviewing the psychologic and dynamic aspects of physician and treatment-team attitudes can provide a useful addition to the one proposed in our article. We emphasized the danger of projection of the staff's values onto the patient in our own case 6. The multidisciplinary team approach can help to minimize the danger from deadening of sensibilities. It is vital for appropriate role models to be present in intensive-care units, to minimize the dangers of the unthinking performance of any "professional agenda" or continuation of therapy out of fear of the consequences of an iatrogenic mishap.

67.

"Code" or "No Code": A Nonlegal Opinion

Steven S. Spencer

The widespread familiarity with cardio-pulmonary-resuscitation techniques and the prompt availability of portable defibrillators and "crash carts" in most modern hospitals have made it possible to attempt resuscitation in virtually all in-hospital deaths. The policy in many hospitals is that a resuscitative effort is made on all patients in the event of death unless the physician has written a "no-code" order. Although making decisions about resuscitating patients is certainly not a new responsibility for physicians, the current state of affairs has introduced some new complexities into this decision-making process.

The new complexities concern the timing of such decisions and the question of who should be involved in making them. Not only must the physician now consider the question of code or no code virtually at the time of admission to the hospital rather than at the time of crisis, but he must also record it in writing if he arrives at a "no-code" decision. Furthermore, in this litigation-conscious era physicians are looking to the courts and the legal profession for guidance and protection and are also asking families of patients to share the burden of responsibility for such decisions to a degree unthinkable a few years ago. The recent article in the *Journal* by attorneys Schram et al.[1] was an interesting effort to provide physicians with guidance about what they legally can or should do in matters pertaining to "no-code" orders, with respect to current laws in Massachusetts. Although helpful in some respects, it also served to illustrate the complexity and diffusion of responsibility that has recently characterized decision making involving life-or-death issues. Careful consideration and recollection of numerous examples by an experienced physician will show that dilution and sharing of responsibility and relying upon current legal guidelines is often detrimental to the welfare of both the patient and the family.

Resuscitation is a traumatic event for the patient and for any family and friends who may be present. It is a violent intrusion into what otherwise may be the peaceful final stage of life or early stage of death. A decision not to undertake such efforts may therefore be at least as important, in terms of the patient's welfare, as a decision to attempt resuscitation.

Our unwritten contract is with the patient, and we try to involve the patient in major decisions about hospitalization, diagnostic procedures, and therapy. A mentally competent patient always has the right to say, "No," to us, and his word is final. The "living will" is an effort on the part of the patient to extend his authority to say, "No," to therapeutic measures attending his death when he may not be capable of entering into decision making.

The wishes of the family clearly should not guide the physician when they are in conflict with those of a mentally competent patient. When the patient is not competent, the family members should be involved in major decision making, but their opinions should not, it seems to me, carry the same weight as those of a competent patient—the contract is still between physician and patient, not physician and family.

In either case two very important considerations are operative. The first is that the patient (competent or not) and the family place a trust in the physicians to act in the patient's best interest. This is a very great, and at times, very difficult responsibility for the physician to carry, but he must be willing to shoulder it, often alone. The second consideration is that the physician is the one in possession of most of the knowledge on which major decisions must be based—i.e., the med-

Source: *The New England Journal of Medicine,* vol. 300, no. 3, Jan. 18, 1979.

ical knowledge. This situation means that, for the patient and family to enter intelligently into decision making, the physician must educate them carefully with an objective presentation of the essential medical facts, alternatives, and expected outcomes. Many patients and families do not want this amount of education and participation, find it confusing, and recognize their inherent lack of objectivity in decisions so close to themselves or their loved ones. Families often, and understandably, fear the responsibility and possible guilt connected with such decisions as "code or no code." It is far easier and safer for them simply to say, "We want you to do everything possible." If the physician has gone to the family for help in deciding whether resuscitation should be attempted, he is now left with the instruction from the family to "code" the patient even if that action is contrary to his judgment and to the welfare of the patient and possibly even contrary to the true feelings of the family.

In cases in which the physician has firmly decided that a "no code" order is the proper course, it usually works out better for him to explain to family members why resuscitation will not be attempted than to ask them whether or not they want it attempted. They will rarely disagree if they have placed their trust in the physician. Such explanations to the patient, on the other hand, are thoughtless to the point of being cruel, unless the patient inquires, which he is extremely unlikely to do. The patient ordinarily trusts his physician not only to act in his best interest during his life but also to help see that his death is as comfortable, decent, and peaceful an event as possible. This is an implied trust that he may not want to verbalize or discuss. As in most matters concerning the life and death of the patient, it is wise for the physician to follow the lead of the patient about what he wants to know or discuss. In any event, it devolves upon the physician to guide the patient and family through these difficult decision areas, to give them the benefit of his recommendations, and to be willing to assume responsibility for major decisions. This can never be a strictly "objective" process

because it is based on nonquantifiable human data as well as laboratory results. That is what makes it difficult, and that is why it is important for the physician to know and understand his patient and the family as well as possible.

There is general agreement that people who experience sudden death in the setting of good health or a reversible medical condition should be resuscitated, and that patients whose underlying condition is one of rapid and inevitable progression to death should not be resuscitated when that event finally occurs. The chances of successful resuscitative efforts parallel these two extremes. The middle ground between these two extremes is the difficult area where wisdom and judgment are required, where we may want the help of a more knowledgeable or experienced colleague, and where we may make mistakes. However, as Gorovitz points out,[2] the question of who should decide is a moral question involving considerations that cannot be resolved by an appeal to the law (nor, I would add, to the patient's family), and the physician is in a position where there is no escape from making such decisions.

As physicians, we have an obligation to keep our priorities straight, to do always what we consider to be in the best interests of our patients and in keeping with our moral and ethical precepts. This task is not always simple or easy, but we nevertheless must have the courage to do it and even to risk censure or litigation, rather than to depend on third parties for guidance or leadership. Experienced physicians have a further obligation to guide their younger colleagues and house staff down this difficult path in these times of increasing societal involvement in questions of life and death.

NOTES

1. R.B. Schram, J.C. Kane, Jr., and D.T. Roble, "'No Code' Orders: Clarification in the Aftermath of *Saikewicz*," *New England Journal of Medicine*, vol. 299, p. 875, 1978.

2. S. Gorovitz, "Ethical Dilemmas in Medicine: Who Should Decide?" *National Forum, Phi Kappa Phi Journal*, vol. 58, no. 2, p. 3, 1978.

68.

Orders Not to Resuscitate

Mitchell T. Rabkin Gerald Gillerman Nancy R. Rice

Medical opinions on the inappropriateness of cardiopulmonary resuscitation of certain patients are now openly discussed, as acknowledged by the New Jersey Supreme Court in its recent Quinlan decision. As early as 1974 the AMA proposed that decisions not to resuscitate be formally entered in patients' progress notes and communicated to all attending staff.[1] There has been little open discussion, however, of the process by which a decision not to resusciate is formulated. Within a single institution, practices may vary among physicians, in part from the lack of a clearly articulated hospital policy.

An apparent need for hospital definitions of the process by which decisions not to resuscitate should be made led to the development of the following statement, which is proposed as a policy statement for hospitals concerned with regulating the process whereby Orders Not to Resuscitate may be considered and then implemented. It was developed by us out of discussions held over the past 6 months in the Law and Ethics Working Group of the Faculty Seminar on the Analysis of Health and Medical Practices of the Harvard School of Public Health. We are indebted to the other members of the Working Group for their useful and constructive criticism.

Both as a standard of medical care and as a statement of philosophy, it is the general policy of hospitals to act affirmatively to preserve the life of all patients, including persons who suffer from irreversible terminal illness. It is essential that all hospital staff understand this policy and act accordingly.

As a matter of policy, hospitals also respect the competent patient's informed acceptance or rejection of treatment, including cardiopulmonary resuscitation, and recognize that in certain cases, the unwanted use of heroic measures on a patient irreversibly and irreparably terminally ill might be both medically unsound and so contrary to the patient's wishes or expectations as not to be justified.

To ensure adherence to each of these policies, we have prepared this statement to guide a hospital in the process of decision making regarding the use of cardiopulmonary resuscitation.

Notwithstanding the hospital's pro-life policy, the right of a patient to decline available medical procedures must be respected. For example, if a competent patient who is not irreversibly and irreparably ill issues instructions that under stated circumstances, he is opposed to the use of certain procedures, the following guidelines should be observed. The physician should explore thoroughly with the patient the types of circumstances that might arise, and warn that the consequences of a generalized prohibition may be to allow an unintended termination of life. If after a careful disclosure the patient persists in some form of order declining use of certain medical procedures when otherwise applicable, the physician is legally required to respect such instructions. Such situations are not unknown to hospitals that have treated Jehovah's Witnesses and other persons with fixed opinions unlikely to be affected by unforeseen medical exigencies. If the physician finds the medical program as ordered by the patient so inconsistent with his own medical judgment as to be incompatible with his continuing as the responsible physician, he may attempt to transfer the care of the patient to another physician more sympathetic to the patient's desires.

The specific issue of the appropriateness of cardiopulmonary resuscitation arises frequently with the irreversibly, irreparably ill patient whose death is imminent. We refer to the medical circumstance in which the disease is "irreversible" in the sense

Source: *New England Journal of Medicine*, vol. 295, no. 7, Aug. 12, 1979.

that no known therapeutic measures can be effective in reversing the course of illness; the physiologic status of the patient is "irreparable" in the sense that the course of illness has progressed beyond the capacity of existing knowledge and technique to stem the process; and when death is "imminent" in the sense that in the ordinary course of events, death probably will occur within a period not exceeding 2 weeks.

When it appears that a patient is irreversibly and irreparably ill, and that death is imminent, the question of the appropriateness of cardiopulmonary resuscitation in the event of sudden cessation of vital functions may be considered by the patient's physician, if not already raised by the patient, to avoid an unnecessary abuse of the patient's presumed reliance on the physician and hospital for continued life-supporting care. The initial medical judgment on such question should be made by the primarily responsible physician for the patient after discussion with an ad hoc committee consisting not only of the other physicians attending the patient and the nurses and others directly active in the care of the patient, but at least one other senior staff physician not previously involved in the patient's care. The inquiry should focus on whether the patient's death is so certain and so imminent that resuscitation in the event of sudden cessation of vital functions would serve no purpose. Although the unanimous opinion of the ad hoc committee in support of the decision of the responsible physician is not necessarily required (for some may be uncertain), a strongly held dissenting view not negated by other staff members should generally dissuade the responsible physician from his or her initial judgment on the appropriateness of resuscitation efforts.

Even if a medical judgment is reached that a patient is faced with such an illness and imminence of death that resuscitation is medically inappropriate, the decision to withhold resuscitation (Orders Not to Resuscitate, ONTR) will become effective only upon the informed choice of a competent patient or, with an incompetent patient, by

strict adherence to the guidelines discussed below, and then only to the extent that all appropriate family members are in agreement with the views of the involved staff. In this context, "appropriate" means at least the family members who would be consulted for permission to perform a post-morten if the patient died.

"Competence" in this context is not to be restricted to the legal and medical tests to determine competence to stand trial or to form a criminal intent. For the purpose of making an informed choice of medical treatment, "competence" is understood to rest on the test of whether the patient understands the relevant risks and alternatives, and whether the resulting decision reflects a deliberate choice by the patient. Caution should be exercised that a patient does not unwittingly "consent" to an ONTR, as a result of temporary distortion (for example, from pain, medication, or metabolic abnormality) in his ability to choose among available alternatives.

It is recognized that it may be inappropriate to introduce the subject of withholding cardiopulmonary resuscitation efforts to certain competent patients when, in the physician's judgment, the patient will probably be unable to cope with it psychologically. In such event, Orders Not to Resuscitate may not be directed because of the absence of an informed choice. Appropriate family members should be so informed, and the physician should explain the course that will thus follow in the event of sudden cessation of the patient's vital functions. This discussion with the family should be noted by the physician in the medical record. If, however, the physician is able to discuss the essential elements of the case with a competent patient without violating the principles of reasonable and humane medical practice, a valid consent may follow.

If the competent patient thus chooses the ONTR alternative, this is his choice, and it may not be overridden by contrary views of family members. Nevertheless, it is important to inform the family members of the patient's decision (with the patient's permission and in accordance with his directions) so that the failure to resuscitate or to take other heroic measures is not unanticipated. In any event, the decision should be documented by the responsible physician and at least one witness. Such decisions shall remain in effect if the patient subsequently becomes incompetent and if the clinical circumstances for Orders Not to Resuscitate otherwise remain in existence.

Minors who are not emancipated by state law will be deemed incompetent to make a decision not to resuscitate. Such persons, however, will be kept informed if such a communication is appropriate, and have the right to reject a decision not to resuscitate, despite their presumed incompetence.

If a patient is incompetent, he should not be denied the benefits of the evaluation process described above. The physician and the ad hoc committee will consider initially whether the conditions of irreversibility, irreparability, and imminence of death are satisfied in their opinion. The basis for a final decision for Orders Not to Resuscitate must be concern from the patient's point of view, and not that of some other person who might present what he regards as sufficient reasons for not resuscitating the patient. It is only the clinical interest of the patient that must be considered; consideration of other factors would violate the fundamental policy of the hospital. An additional condition for the issuance of Orders Not to Resuscitate for an incompetent patient is approval of at least the same family members who are required to consent to post-mortem examination. Failure to obtain and record family approval of Orders Not to Resuscitate may expose those involved to charges of negligent or unlawful conduct. Thus, the failure to obtain such approval would foreclose further consideration of Orders Not to Resuscitate in cases in which the patient is incompetent.

To prevent any uncertainty or confusion over the status of a patient's treatment, the decision for Orders Not to Resuscitate and its accompanying consent by the competent patient or the appropriate family members

should be recorded promptly in the medical chart. In addition to the formal consent, the written and dated record must include the following: a summary of the staff discussion and decision; the disclosures to the patient, which must include the elements of informed consent, the patient's response, the responsible physician's documentation of the patient's competence, the patient's decision to inform appropriate family members, and the resulting discussion with them that may then follow. Each hospital must specify what it deems to be the elements of informed consent and the formats in which consent must be witnessed and documented. Whether or not the patient's signature must be required invariably should also be decided; the signature removes ambiguity, but the physical act of signing may be deemed unpalatable by certain patients and therefore unacceptable to them as a necessary or appropriate formalization of the meaningful discussion and their resulting verbal consent.

It is the responsiblity of the physician to convey the meaning of the Orders Not to Resuscitate to all medical, nursing, and other staff as appropriate and, simultaneously, to insist upon being notified immediately if the patient's condition should change so that the orders seem no longer applicable. If the circumstances described to such a patient do not change, a subsequent resuscitation would constitute treatment without consent.

After the issuing of Orders Not to Resuscitate, the patient's course, including continued evaluation of competence and consent, must be reviewed by the responsible physician at least daily, or at more frequent intervals, if appropriate, and documentation made in the medical chart to determine the continued applicability of such orders. If the patient's condition alters in such a way that the orders are no longer deemed applicable, the Orders Not to Resuscitate must be revoked, and the revocation communicated without delay.

Nothing in the entire procedure leading to Orders Not to Resuscitate, nor the ONTR itself, should indicate to the medical and nursing staff or to the patient and family any intention to diminish the appropriate medical and nursing attention to be received by the patient. It is the responsibility of the physician in charge to be certain that no diminution of necessary and appropriate measures for the patient's care and comfort follows from this decision.

When the incompetent patient is sufficiently alert to appreciate at least some aspects of the care he is receiving (the benefit of doubt must always assign to the patient the likelihood of at least partial alertness or receptivity to verbal stimuli), and especially with a child, whose "incompetence" by legal definition may not be supported by clinical observation, every effort must be made to provide the comfort and reassurance appropriate to the patient's state of consciousness and emotional condition regardless of the designation of incompetence.

In every case in which Orders Not to Resuscitate are issued, the hospital shall make available to the greatest extent practicable resources to provide counseling, reassurance, consolation, and other emotional support as appropriate, for the patient's family and for all involved hospital staff, as well as for the patient.

Occasionally, a proposal for Orders Not to Resuscitate may be initiated by family members. It is essential to recognize that a family member's instructions not to resuscitate are not to be viewed as the choice of the patient. Thus, the attending physician and the ad hoc committee must not simply concur in the Orders Not to Resuscitate suggested by the family, but such concurrences shall be forthcoming only upon the timing and conditions described above.

NOTE

1. "Standards for Cardiopulmonary Resuscitation (CPR) and Emergency Cardiac Care (ECC), V, Medicolegal Considerations and Recommendations," *Journal of the American Medical Association*, vol. 227, suppl., p. 864, 1974.

69.

The Specter of Joseph Saikewicz: Mental Incompetence and the Law

Richard A. McCormick   Andre E. Hellegers

Joseph Saikewicz, aged 67 in 1976, was profoundly mentally retarded. He had an IQ of 10 and a mental age of approximately 2 years and 8 months. He could communicate only by gestures and grunts, and was deeply disoriented when out of his familiar environment. Mr. Saikewicz had lived in state institutions since 1923, and in Belchertown State School since 1928.

On April 19, 1976, Saikewicz was diagnosed as suffering from acute myeloblastic monocytic leukemia. This blood disease results from the body's production of excessive white blood cells, and is associated with

Source: *America*, April 1, 1978.

enlargement of organs (spleen, lymph glands, bone marrow), internal bleeding and, in acute stages, with severe anemia and vulnerability to infection. The disease is unavoidably and invariably fatal.

Chemotherapy can produce remission of the disease (temporary return to normal) in around 30 to 50 percent of cases, but this remission lasts typically between 2 and 13 months. With some patients over 60 the prognosis is somewhat poorer. If left untreated, Saikewicz would die within a matter of several weeks or months. Should he receive the chemotherapy? The authorities at

Belchertown thought so and, on April 26, 1976, petitioned the Probate Court of Hampshire County, Mass., for the appointment of a guardian *ad litem* with authority to make medical decisions. The guardian *ad litem* was appointed on May 5. The very next day the guardian filed a report that "not treating Mr. Saikewicz would be in his best interests." At the hearing on May 13, 1976, the probate court agreed in essence with that recommendation. Chemotherapy was not administered. On Sept. 4, 1976, Joseph Saikewicz died at the Belchertown State School hospital from complications of bronchial pneumonia, a complication of leukemia.

The "no chemotherapy" decision of the probate judge was referred to the Massachusetts Supreme Court. Two questions were put for appellate review: (1) Does the probate court have the authority to order in certain circumstances the withholding of treatment, when withholding may lead to a shortening of life? (2) Was its judgment correct in the Saikewicz case? On July 9, 1976, the Supreme Court of Massachusetts answered both questions in the affirmative and said that its opinion would follow. That opinion was issued Nov. 28, 1977.

We think the decision of the Massachusetts Supreme Court to be of enormous importance to all of us. Therefore, we propose to review the reasoning of the decision, its implications, and our objections to that decision.

The court first admits that human dignity requires that individuals have a general right to self-determination where medical decisions are involved. We say "general right" because there are certain state interests that can take precedence over this right. The court mentions four state interests that may override the right: (1) preservation of life; (2) the protection of the interests of innocent third parties (e.g., where children would suffer "abandonment" by the death of the parent if the parent refused treatment, as in the case of a Jehovah's Witness): (3) prevention of suicide; and (4) maintaining the integrity of the medical profession. When one of these interests competes with the individual's

right of self-determination, the court must engage in a balancing process to determine which is more important. The most important of these interests (and the one on which all others depend) is the preservation of life. Here the court is sensitive and balanced. It states: "Recognition of such an interest, however, does not necessarily resolve the problem where the affliction of disease clearly indicates that life will soon, and inevitably, be extinguished. The interest of the State in prolonging a life must be reconciled with the interest of the individual to reject the traumatic cost of that prolongation."

Applying these considerations to Saikewicz, the court concluded that two state interests (prevention of suicide, protection of innocent third parties) had no relevance. The other two did not override the right to decline treatment because Saikewicz was a dying patient whose life could be only "briefly extended" (hence the *preservation* of life is not precisely the issue) and because it is fully within accepted medical standards to withhold treatment when the expected outcome is merely prolongation of dying.

The Massachusetts Supreme Court developed its analysis in terms of the rights of the competent patient. But since Saikewicz was incompetent, it next turned to this factor. Does a choice to refuse treatment exist even if the person is incompetent, or must the court always order life-prolonging treatment? If a choice exists, what considerations enter the decision-making process? The court agreed that a choice does exist, because the best interests of the incompetents are not always served by imposing on them what competent persons may rightfully choose to omit. "To presume that the incompetent person must always be subjected to what rational and intelligent persons may decline is to downgrade the status of the incompetent person by placing a lower value on his intrinsic worth and vitality." Rather, incompetent persons have the same rights here as competent persons: that is, they may at times refuse treatment.

But how are incompetents to exercise this

right? Here the court explicitly accepts the doctrine of substituted judgment. In short, with an eye to the patient's best interests and preferences, "the decisions in cases such as this should be those which would be made by the incompetent person if that person were competent. . . ."

What, then, would Saikewicz himself choose? Weighing the factors both for and against chemotherapy, the Massachusetts Supreme Court concluded that Saikewicz would reject chemotherapy, for such a decision best serves "his actual interests and preferences."

Thus far, we agree with this conclusion and analysis. Saikewicz was a dying patient in the court's opinion—though it is not always that easy to determine who should be said to be dying and who is not. He had a terminal disease; an optimistic prognosis would extend his life from 2 to 13 months at most. Furthermore, any extension of life he gained would be associated with continuing painful and distressing side effects of disorientations due to chemotherapy. Therefore, we believe with the court that his overall best interests would not be served by this treatment, and hence that he would not choose to undergo it.

In arriving at this same judgment, the court was careful to distinguish a factor adduced by the lower court: "the quality of life available to him even if the treatment does bring about remission." If this phrase ("quality of life") is taken to refer to Saikewicz's retardation, the court stated that "we firmly reject it." If, however, it refers to the continuing state of pain and disorientation associated with chemotherapy, the court accepts it. We agree and strongly underline this distinction. Substituted judgments about acceptance or rejection of treatment should not be made merely on the basis of the retarded condition. This is not to say, however, that quality-of-life considerations have no place in such judgments.

But here our agreement with the court ends and profound misgivings arise. For the court then turned to the procedures appro-

priate for decision making in cases of using or withholding life-prolonging treatment for a "person allegedly incompetent." In the Karen Ann Quinlan case, the New Jersey Supreme Court entrusted the decision whether to continue artificial life support to the patient's guardian (her father, Joseph Quinlan), in consultation with physicians and a badly named "Ethics Committee" (as its functions were described by the court, it was really a prognosis committee). The Massachusetts court rejected "the approach adopted by the New Jersey Supreme Court in the *Quinlan* case." Rather, the questions of life and death require a "detached but passionate investigation and decision that form the ideal on which the judicial branch of government was created." Achievement of this ideal is the responsibility of the courts and "is not to be entrusted to any other group." Briefly, the proper and only tribunal for determining the best interests of all incompetent persons is the courts.

The implications of this are enormous, and, we think, highly questionable. What are the immediate implications? As Richard A. Knox wrote in the *Washington Post* (Feb. 18, 1978): "The new Massachusetts ruling essentially holds that issues of both withholding and terminating critical care—for elderly stroke victims or cancer patients, as well as for severely ill newborns—are matters for the probate courts to decide, not for the families, doctors, nurses, social workers, priests, committees or anyone else."

Why are these the implications of the decision? For two reasons. First, the term "incompetent" includes the mentally retarded, insane, comatose, unconscious, infants, etc. Second, the court made it clear that it regarded Saikewicz as a *dying* incompetent patient. Therefore, its ruling extends in principle to all dying incompetents. This is of crucial importance. Thus, the court distinguished preserving life from prolonging life. It stated: "There is a substantial distinction in the State's insistence that human life be saved when the affliction is curable, as opposed to the State interest where, *as here* [emphasis ours], the issue is not whether, but when, for how long and at what cost to the individual that life may be briefly extended." Furthermore, the court referred to the Saikewicz case with the following phrases: "a brief and uncertain delay in the natural process of death"; "life-saving treatment is available—a situation unfortunately not presented by this case"; "treatment which . . . may increase suffering in exchange for a possible yet brief prolongation of life." And finally: "Nor was this a case in which life-saving, as distinguished from life-prolonging, procedures were available."

In support of the court's decision, George Annas, assistant professor of law and medicine at the Boston University School of Medicine, has argued in *The Hastings Report* (February 1978) that a correct resolution of the case of the incompetent "is more likely to come from a judicial decision after an adversary proceeding in which all interested parties have fully participated . . . than from the individual decisions of the patient's family, the attending physician, an ethics committee or all of these combined."

We disagree. Indeed, we find this intolerable. It is one thing to recognize that the cases of certain incompetent persons are doubtful, agonizingly ambiguous, extremely difficult, and vulnerable to abusive decision. These cases-in-dispute might appropriately call for judicial overview. But it is something else to say that all cases of life-prolonging treatment or withholding of treatment from the incompetent must be routinely decided in probate court.

Our disagreement with Professor Annas and the Massachusetts Supreme Court is rooted in several considerations. First, we disagree with the contention that it is "only by using the admittedly difficult machinery of a legal proceeding" that the best interests of the incompetent can be promoted. This contention assumes that the ordinary consultative process involving family, physicians, nurses, and so-called ethics committees is insufficient or is likely to be widely abused. We know of no such evidence to justify Mr. Annas's implied assertion. Furthermore, a careful and conscientious consultation by

the concerned parties will contain the very virtues and cautions he attributes to an adversary procedure. We have seen this happen repeatedly. To say that a more correct decision is likely to come from a judicial proceeding (after all the interested parties have been consulted) denies to concerned people the very discernment, wisdom, and prudence attributed to the probate judge. This is contrary to our experience. For example, we agree with the decision of the probate judge and the Massachusetts Supreme Court in the Saikewicz case; but we think that conclusion was not terribly difficult to arrive at in the light of the pros and cons that went into its making.

At some point, then, there is an unintentional but undesirable arrogance in the court's assumption that a probate judge can determine, better than anyone else, the best interests of desperately ill patients. We do not deny the wisdom of appeal to the courts when concerned parties are in dispute about these interests. But when such appeal becomes a mandatory routinized procedure, it makes a new priesthood of the judiciary. Treatment and management decisions are not mere medical decisions; nor are they mere legal decisions. They are above all human decisions. To shift them routinely to the courts tends to undermine this fact. What evidence is there to support the idea that probate judges are the only persons who can safely make such decisions? Indeed, the assumption that the courts do a better job is challenged by some recent history. In the Quinlan case, for example, Judge Muir and the New Jersey Supreme Court came to diametrically opposite conclusions on the same facts. We agree with the court that these questions of life and death demand a "detached but passionate investigation," but we believe that families, physicians, nurses, and moral advisors consulting together should not be presumed incapable of such investigation and decision.

Second, the ruling and its language mean that everybody must be resuscitated, and that all incompetents must be kept on respirators until the probate judge decides otherwise. For the court's language ("Life may be briefly extended . . . a brief and uncertain delay in the natural process of death . . . a possible yet brief prolongation of life") encompasses these cases. What we have in mind is that the physician is now forced to start the treatment in order to find out from the probate court whether he should have started it. Therefore, the procedural requirements of the court force the initiation of therapies that the court itself might deem unnecessary and would indeed countermand.

This is highly problematic. For instance, what is to happen to the incompetent patient (baby, elderly, retarded, etc.) while this "admittedly difficult machinery of a legal proceeding" is grinding into action? Do we simply continue life supports in the interim, a perhaps long, drawn-out interim? Or do we withhold them pending judicial intervention? Much that is at best inappropriate, at worst abusive, could happen to a patient as the adversary procedure unfolds. The result is that patients are now to be made to suffer, often needlessly, for the purposes of the court's procedures.

Moreover, in the sometimes long process of dying, conditions and prognoses change. The intent of the court could be met only if physicians and family returned to the probate court on several occasions. The Massachusetts Supreme Court seems to be ignorant of the fact that therapies are often started on a trial basis, only to be discontinued if a desired effect is not obtained or adverse results are obtained. The idea is intolerable and absurd that, as prognoses change, all should have to return to the probate court. This is to set up the court as cophysician. We do not see the physician as the master of the patient, but neither do we see judges as masters of physicians who can decide which therapies should be tried and which not, which stopped and which not.

The immediate impact of this ruling, then, will inevitably be a renewed vitalism, a never-say-die policy. This is threatening in itself, because it is at odds with the cherished convictions of many people about the meaning of life and death. But it is also subtly threatening in its implications. For the prospect of such end-stage treatment will all but force us to support legislation that recognizes living wills. We have already stated our serious misgivings about such legislation (*America,* March 12, 1977). One of the major objections is that legislated living wills are a reinforcement of the idea that physicians (or the medical system) are masters of the patient, who must then extract himself by making such a will. Embedded in this notion is a subtle shift from the medicomoral axiom *primum non nocere* (first do no harm) to *primum non nocere societati* (first do no harm to society).

The practical consequence of all this may well be a policy that leads to what we call the "undertreatment-overtreatment syndrome"—a kind of safe policy. That is, foreseeing the demand of a legal procedure, some hospitals will prevent the cumbersome problem from arising by failing to resuscitate where perhaps the patient is resuscitable. Other hospitals, from fear of malpractice suits or criminal liability, will keep incompetents on life-prolonging equipment when such treatment is not indicated.

Third and finally, the Massachusetts Supreme Court seems to have no idea about the number of cases of incompetence that occur each day. These cases (involving what the court called "a brief and uncertain delay in the natural process of dying") are not simply occasional. They occur by the hundreds on a daily basis. The courts will be simply incapable of dealing with the problem. Hospital personnel, aware of this sheer impracticality, will quietly ignore the ruling—a practice that not only undermines the integrity of the legal system but intensifies the liability and malpractice atmosphere that already plagues American hospitals. Or, if they do not ignore it, they will keep every incompetent person alive, regardless of the condition, prospects, and circumstances of that individual.

There is a long and honored moral and legal tradition that medical treatment decisions are the prerogative of the patient (which the court admits when the patient is competent) or of those who presumably have the best interests of the patient at heart (e.g., the family) when the patient is incompetent. This is as it should be, always saving the right of appeal where abuses are judged to be present or very likely. We could accept the court's solution for wards of the state or patients restricted to institutions even before their dying had begun (e.g., prisoners, the mentally retarded in state institutions). In brief, if the court had restricted its decision to the abandoned, where it could not be assumed that anyone had their interest at heart, we could have thought of the decision as a prudential one, designed for the protection of a small segment of the population. But to apply it to all incompetents is to fail to understand the process of dying in an age of high technology and to misconceive the court's role as *parens patriae.*

Treatment decisions are utterly personal. They must be made in terms of the individual's history, aspirations, achievements, age, family, beliefs, etc. They are a glove fitting an individual hand. For this reason they have been appropriately made within the patient-family-physician context of health care. When these decisions are routinely (*all* incompetents) removed from this matrix, they are handed over to two impersonal forces, technology and the law. Individual and personal decisions begin to be made by impersonal forces. That is a threat to our well-being. If technology and the law were largely to usurp the patient-family-physician prerogatives in management decisions, we would all be worse off. Impersonal considerations would too easily replace personal ones and preprogram our treatment. That is always the root of oppression and depersonalization, in medicine as well as in other areas. That is why the case of Joseph Saikewicz remains not simply an individual case, but a threatening specter.

70.

Quinlan, Saikewicz, and Now Brother Fox
George J. Annas

When a judge decides to play legislator on issues like the termination of treatment, in which there are strong and competing social values and case law is embryonic, the result is likely to be very unsatisfactory indeed. Nevertheless, judges do not seem to be able to resist the temptation to make final pronouncements in this interesting area of the law.

The Brother Fox case shows what happens when judges attempt not only to decide the specific case before them, but also to decide how all future cases like it should be dealt with. And even though the Brother Fox case hasn't provided "final answers," its seventy-three pages do provide a fruitful field on which to begin discussion. The decision of the intermediate appeals court (*In the Matter of Eichner*, N.Y. App. Div., 2d Dept., March 27, 1980) is a philosopher's dream, and should find its greatest use as a discussion-provoker—much like its predecessors: *Quinlan* and *Saikewicz.*

Brother Fox's Story

Brother Joseph Charles Fox joined the Catholic Order of the Society of Mary in 1912 when he was 16 years old. At the age of 57 he met Father Philip Eichner and remained his close friend for the remainder of his life. In August 1979, at the age of 83, he sustained an inguinal hernia while gardening. During otherwise uneventful

Source: *Hastings Center Report*, vol. 10, June 1980.

corrective surgery, Brother Fox suffered a heart attack. He sustained substantial brain damage, slipped into a coma, and was placed on a respirator in an intensive care unit.

Father Eichner called in two neurosurgeons to examine Brother Fox. Both agreed that there was no reasonable possibility he would ever regain consciousness. Father Eichner accordingly asked the hospital authorities to discontinue the respirator. Had they agreed, the case would have ended at this point. But they refused, saying they would comply only if a court order was obtained. Father Eichner then went to court to seek appointment as Brother Fox's committee (New York's term for a guardian) with authority to discontinue life-support systems.

At trial Father Eichner testified that Brother Fox had discussed both the Quinlan case and Pope Pius XII's *allocutio* with him, and had stated that he wanted no "extraordinary means" used to sustain him if he were ever in a condition similar to that of Karen Quinlan. The surgeon who operated on him testified that Brother Fox was in an "irreversible" and "permanent" coma, and "would remain a vegetable." A neurosurgeon testified similarly. The District Attorney, who was invited to intervene by the Court, called two physicians, who testified that it was possible that his condition had not "absolutely stabilized." One case in the medical literature reported a patient recovering from a similar coma.

The trial court concluded from the testimony that there was "no reasonable possibility" that Brother Fox would ever return to a "cognitive and sapient" state; and that were he himself competent, he would "order a termination of the life-supporting respirator." On December 6, 1979, it accordingly granted the petition. The District Attorney appealed. On January 24, 1980, while the panel was considering the case, Brother Fox died.

The Appeals Court, which issued its ruling on March 27, began by reaffirming "the undeniable right of a terminally ill but competent individual to refuse medical care, even if it will inexorably result in his death." The problem, as in *Quinlan,* was how to make decisions for an *incompetent* patient in a chronic, persistent vegetative state. The court saw three issues: (1) medical, (2) legal, and (3) procedural. The medical issue is prognosis, and the court determined that the medical prognosis should be proved *in court* using a "clear and convincing" standard of proof.

The legal issue is substituted judgment, and the court insisted that life support should not be discontinued, even on patients in a chronic vegetative state, *unless* it could be demonstrated that they themselves would make such a decision if they could. On this issue the court opined that a "living will" executed at a time "when the patient contemplated the catastrophic medical possibility that actually befell him" would make the decision easy because all could be sure they were just "carrying out the stated wishes of the patient and, therefore, face no moral dilemma." The court further found that Brother Fox's express statements were "highly probative of his choice" and "entitled to great weight." It accordingly affirmed the lower court's decision.

Instead of concluding the opinion at this point, however, the court decided to set up a procedure for deciding all future cases involving individuals in chronic vegetative states. The court determined that before life-sustaining treatment could be removed, *both* the medical prognosis test and the legal substituted judgment test must be met, and these tests *must* be reviewed by a court "on an *individual,* patient-to-patient basis," similar to the requirement that requests to transfuse blood to a child against the wishes of his parents routinely go to court.

The "Brother Fox" Procedure

1. The physicians attending the patient *must* first certify that he is (1) terminally ill; and (2) in an irreversible, permanent, or chronic vegetative coma; and (3) that the

prospects of his regaining cognitive brain function are extremely remote.

2. Thereafter, the person to whom such a certification is made (family member, friend, or hospital official) *may* present this prognosis to an appropriate hospital *prognosis committee* of no fewer than three physicians with specialties relevant to the patient's case.

3. The committee *shall* either confirm or reject the prognosis by majority vote of the members.

4. Upon confirmation of the prognosis, the person who secured it *may* commence a court action for appointment as the committee of the incompetent, and for permission to have life-sustaining measures withdrawn.

5. The attorney general and appropriate district attorney *shall* be notified and given an opportunity to intervene and arrange examinations by their own physicians if they so desire.

6. A guardian *ad litem shall* be appointed to represent the best interests of the patient.

7. The court *shall* determine that the prognosis is accurate by "clear and convincing" evidence.

8. The court *shall* determine that the patient would decide to terminate extraordinary life-support measures if he were able to make this decision himself (apparently by preponderance of the evidence).

9. An appropriate order for the discontinuation of extraordinary measures *shall* be entered and no participant shall be subject to criminal or civil liability in the event death follows the termination of these measures.

The court acknowledges that such a procedure "may appear cumbersome and too time-consuming to accommodate the need for speedy determinations in cases where termination of treatment is proposed." Nevertheless, the court believes such procedures are necessary to protect the terminally ill patient involved. The mixing of "musts" and "mays" will confuse many, but the court seems to be saying that the procedure is required *only if* one wants to terminate treatment, and not that the procedure itself is optional (even though there is no crime of "not going to court" and no new sanctions).

The Price of Progress

It is important to stress the positive in novel areas of the law where courts are attempting to reconcile conflicting values. Tragic choices will never be happily made. The decision can be seen as a step forward: first, hospital officials would not have permitted the removal of life-support systems without it. There is now a mechanism to implement the wishes of a patient in a condition like Brother Fox's. Second, the committee used to confirm the prognosis is now clearly termed a "prognosis committee" (and not an "ethics committee" as in *Quinlan*) and is composed entirely of physicians. Third, a clearer-than-usual distinction is drawn between medical prognosis questions and legal questions of substituted judgment. Fourth, a written "living will," and prior oral statements of preference, are given strong judicial weight. And fifth, the decision is a very narrow one—applying only to patients like Brother Fox (and Karen Quinlan) in a "permanent or chronic vegetative coma" from whom "extraordinary" means of care can be removed.

Unfortunately, these advances are purchased at a very high price. Questions of medical prognosis and substituted judgment are treated as if they are fundamentally similar, whereas they are fundamentally different. While both arguably mix fact and value positions, it seems appropriate to permit physicians to make decisions based primarily on scientific fact as long as the *criteria* on which these decisions are made are socially approved. For example, we routinely permit physicians to pronounce people dead, based on criteria set by the courts and the legislatures. Similarly, the Quinlan court essentially permitted families and physicians to apply a prognosis criteria without court intervention. I think this is sound, and as long as society finds prognosis a relevant variable, we should permit physicians to determine it themselves.

The will of the patient is something quite different. The court acknowledges that the patient is the best source of information, and the "best solution" may be to get all competent individuals to express their preferences regarding treatment in such circumstances. Without this, we are left to the speculation of the patient's family and friends. It seems appropriate that this speculation be subjected to court review in cases where there are real choices to be made concerning the patient. On the other hand, judicial review is unnecessary when, according to medical criteria, the patient is terminally ill, and in an "irreversible, permanent or chronic vegetative coma" from which recovery is "extremely remote."

In such cases I would permit the patient's legal guardian to decide the issue without further court review (requiring the guardian to use the substituted-judgment standard if possible, and the best-interests standard if he were unable to determine the patient's actual preferences). It *is* appropriate for the court to set the ground rules, but it does not seem either desirable or necessary for the court routinely to review medical prognosis before the fact. And in the narrow medical confines of this case, it does not seem to add sufficient protection for the patient to require review of the guardian's determination either. On the other hand, where—as in cases like *Saikewicz*—there is a real choice between painful treatment with a chance of remission, and no treatment with a "peaceful" death, court review seems perfectly appropriate.

The reintroduction of the notion of "extraordinary" technologies is also unfortunate. The concept surfaces here only because Brother Fox, a devout Catholic, discussed *his own* views on treatment in the terms utilized by Pope Pius XII. But many will overlook this point, and assume that courts are willing to make a legally meaningful distinction between ordinary and extraordinary. In this case the court had to use this language in order to carry out Brother Fox's desires; but unless adopted by the patient himself, such a distintion is legally irrelevant.

Philosophers will likely enjoy an examination of some of the court's language about patients in a permanent vegetative coma, for example, the possible call for a new definition of death: "As a matter of established fact, such a patient has *no* health and, in a true sense, no life, for the State to protect." The court follows this by calling up the specter of a "slippery slope": ". . . the State's interest in preservation of the life of the fetus would appear to be *greater* than any possible interest the State may have in maintaining the continued life of a terminally ill comatose patient . . . [their] claim to personhood is certainly no greater than that of the fetus." These statements are simply wrong as a matter of law: the fetus is *not* a person for the purposes of the United States Constitution; the person in a coma—permanent or not—is. The court's own opinion acknowledges this implicitly by setting up a much more elaborate (although not constitutionally mandated) scheme to terminate the life of a comatose person than is needed to terminate the life of a fetus.

The Brother Fox case is under appeal, and New York's highest court, the Court of Appeals, has the opportunity to take a giant step forward by taking a step back from the intermediate appeals court decision. Judges should permit the law to develop on a case-by-case basis in this area. This case is like the Quinlan case, and should not be confused and conflated with *Saikewicz*. By deciding it on its facts and leaving it at that, the Court of Appeals will do us all a service.

71.
Autonomy for Burned Patients When Survival Is Unprecedented

Sharon H. Imbus   Bruce E. Zawacki

No burn is certainly fatal until the patient dies; the most severely burned patient may speak of hope with his last breath. Unable to prophesy, and unwilling to strip the patient of any hope he may cherish, we therefore prefer to diagnose burns as "fatal" or "hopeless" only in retrospect. Every year, however, several patients are admitted to our burn center with injuries so severe that survival is not only unexpected but, to our knowledge, unprecedented. Although difficult to face, the problems that these patients present must be anticipated and not simply ignored.

The surgical literature gives little attention to these patients except for brief phrases allowing an occasional glimpse into a particular surgeon's philosphy.[1-3] The literature on death and dying, voluminous since Kubler-Ross's work,[4] offers rich background but says little about the unique situation of our patients, who, after their injury, often have only a few hours of mental clarity in which to respond to their predicament. Several recent articles about withholding intensive care seem to ignore or incompletely answer the problem of obtaining the patient's informed consent. In some of these discussions, the authors simply assign to the physician what we believe to be the patient's ultimate right to decide whether he will or will not receive a particular form of therapy.[5-7] One suggests, perhaps unconstitutionally, that "certain competent patients" may be excluded from such decision making "when, in the physician's judgment, the patient will probably be unable to cope with it psychologically."[8] Still others, who recognize patient primacy in such decision making, offer no practical suggestion how it is best honored in practice.[9]

Our approach, developed empirically over several years, is based on our conviction that the decision to begin or to withhold maximal therapeutic effort is more of an ethical than a medical judgment. The physician and his colleagues on the burn-care team present to the patient the appropriate medical and statistical facts together with authoritative medical opinion about the available therapeutic alternatives and their consequences. Thus informed, the patient may give or withhold his consent to receive a particular form of therapy, but it is his own decision based on his value system, and it is arrived at before communication and competence are seriously impaired by intubation or altered states of consciousness.

Definitions and Methods

The patient whose management this paper addresses is characterized by some combination of massive burns, severe smoke inhalation, or advanced age. Such a patient's condition is designated by "1" on the Bull Mortality Probability Chart[10] and "0" in the National Burn Information Exchange Survival Analysis Diagrams,[11] both indicating nonsurvival from the indexes of age and percentage of body-surface area burned. Furthermore our staff members cannot, from their own experience, our burn unit statistics, or references from the literature, recall survival in a similar patient.

To allow the patient maximal clarity of thought in decision-making, several points must be communicated to the paramedic

Source: *The New England Journal of Medicine*, vol. 297, no. 6, Aug. 11, 1977.

teams in the field and to local hospitals who transfer burned patients to our burn center immediately after injury: no administration of morphine or other narcotics before arrival; prompt fluid resuscitation; oxygen administration in treatment of possible carbon monoxide intoxication; avoidance of tracheostomy or endotracheal-tube insertion unless absolutely necessary to preserve the airway and maintain ventilation; and rapid transportation to the burn center.

Upon admission of a patient for whom survival seems in doubt, the burn center's most experienced physician is consulted, day or night, to evaluate the patient. His assessment, combined with a social and family history, is presented to all involved team members. Standard works are rechecked to determine if there has ever been a precedent for survival.

When the diagnosis is confirmed, the physician and other team members enter the room. Family members are not invited into the room, to ensure that the decision of the patient is specifically his own. In an attempt to establish a relation with the patient, the attending physician or resident under his guidance tries to assume the role of a compassionate friend who is willing to listen. Hands are often held, and an effort is made to look deeply into the patient's eyes to perceive the unspoken questions that may lie there. Nonverbal cues are watched for closely. The presence of the burn team serves to witness and validate the patient's desires and requests, gives consensus to the gravity of the situation and supports the physician member of the team in this delicate, painful task.

At times, when the question of impending death does not spontaneously arise, suggestions such as "You are seriously ill," "You are sicker than you have ever been," or "Your life is in immediate danger" may be made, always in a caring, gentle way.

Some patients will not respond because of coma or mental incompetency. In those circumstances, the burn team and the family confer, again in a compassionate, concerned relation. All attempts are made to determine and do what the patient would be most likely to want if he were able to communicate.

A few patients will hear but not listen because of a need to deny their predicament. In general, such denials, if persistent, are considered an expression of a strong desire to live, and the patients are treated accordingly with maximal therapeutic effort.

A large majority of patients, however, understand the gravity of their situation and make further inquiries. The very frequent question—"Am I going to die?"—is answered truthfully by the statement, "We cannot predict the future. We can only say that, to our knowledge, no one in the past of your age and with your size of burn has ever survived this injury, either with or without maximal treatment." At this point, those who interpret this diagnosis of a burn without precedent of survival as an indication to avoid heroic measures, typically become quite peaceful. Regularly, they then try to live their lives completely and fully to the end, saying things that they must say to those important to them, making proper plans, reparations and apologies and, in general, obtaining what Kavanaugh refers to as "permission to die."[12] These patients receive only ordinary medical measures and sufficient amounts of pain medication to assure comfort after their choice is made explicit. Fluid resuscitation is discontinued, they are admitted to a private room, and visiting hours become unlimited. An experienced nurse and, frequently, a chaplain are in constant attendance, using their expertise to comfort and sustain the patient and his family, chiefly by their continued presence and willingness to listen.

The patients who understand that survival is unprecedented in their case but, nevertheless, choose a maximal therapeutic effort are admitted to the burn intensive-care unit. Fluid resuscitation is continued, and full treatment measures are instituted, as with any other patient in the unit. As with those who choose only ordinary care, however, they may change their minds at any time; their decision is reviewed with them on a daily basis.

In general, when patients are mentally in-competent on admission because of head injury or inhalation injury or some other in-jury and may reasonably be expected to remain so indefinitely, the socially designated next of kin or other relatives are allowed to speak for the patient.[13] With children who are legally incompetent because of age, how-ever, we have for the past five years been unwilling to declare any burn as being with-out precedent of survival, chiefly because mortality rates for very large burns in pediat-ric patients appear to be improving more rapidly than can be reported.

After interviewing the patient or his fam-ily, the physician is responsible for record-ing the salient points and decision in the patient's chart. Accurate documentation serves to clarify communication with other team members and avoids legal ambiguity.

"Postvention," described by Shneidman as "those activities which serve to reduce the aftereffects of a traumatic event in the lives of survivors,"[14] is now being evolved on our unit. Nurses are learning how to help survivors comfort each other and, together with the chaplain and social worker, are ar-ranging for safe transportation of the be-reaved to their homes, counseling families on the difficult matters of explaining death to children and explaining such points as legal necessity of an unwanted autopsy. Our hospital chaplain is available to conduct the funeral services if the family does not have its own pastor. He gets in touch with families on the first anniversary of their loved one's death to answer any unfinished ques-tions that may have been bothering them. The social worker also offers her continuing services to the bereaved.

Results

During 1975 and 1976 there were 748 dis-positions from our burn center, excluding readmissions, transfers, and nonthermal in-juries. Of these patients 126 died, 18 children and 108 adults. Of the adults who died, 24, or 22 percent, were diagnosed on admission as having injury without precedent of sur-vival. Twenty-one of these patients or their families chose nonheroic or ordinary med-ical care. Only three chose full treatment mea-sures, and their desires were fulfilled.

The following case histories illustrate our approach.

Cases 1 and 2. Two sisters, 68 and 70 years of age, and their husbands were search-ing for a schizophrenic daughter who had disappeared after her discharge from a psychi-atric hospital. While their car waited for a stoplight, a nearby construction machine hit a gasoline line. The spraying gas exploded, leveling a city block and igniting the car.

The sisters arrived in our burn center two hours later. The younger sister had 91 per-cent full-thickness, 92 percent total-body burn, with moderate smoke inhalation; the older had 94.5 percent full-thickness, 95.5 percent total-body burn, with severe smoke inhalation. The burn team agreed that survival was unprecedented in both cases. Both women were alert and interviewed separately.

The younger sister asked about death di-rectly, looking intently into the physician's eyes. When he answered, she replied matter-of-factly, "Well, I never dreamed that life would end like this, but since we all have to go sometime, I'd like to go quietly and comfortably. I don't know what to do about my daughter . . . "

After she was made comfortable, the nurse obtained a description of the missing daugh-ter and possible whereabouts. The social worker alerted the police to look for her, and telephoned relatives, informing them of the accident as gently as could be conveyed by telephone. The husbands were located at another burn unit. An attempt was made to arrange a final spousal conversation, but both husbands were intubated.

Meanwhile, the older sister doubted whether her injuries were as serious as re-ported. "I feel so good, wouldn't I be hurting horribly if I were going to die?" The effect of full-thickness burns on nerve end-ings was explained. The physician reiterated that we wished to do what she thought was best for her. She hedged, "What did my sister say? I'll go along with her decision." Since the patient seemed unsure of her decision, she was offered full therapy in the room with her sister. She then refused the therapy adamantly but denied that she was dying.

The sisters' beds were placed next to each other so that they could see and touch each other easily. They discussed funeral arrangements and then joked, in the next breath, about the damage done to their hair. The hospital chaplain prayed with them. By active listening, he was able to convey to the older that her husband was not to blame for the accident as she had thought. "It's good to go out not cursing him after all our years together," she said. The younger sister died several hours later after her sister lapsed into a coma; the older died the next day. The daughter was not located.

Case 3. A 58-year-old man was cleaning his kitchen with an aerosol when the fumes were ignited by the stove pilot. He arrived at the hospital one hour later with a 97 percent full-thickness burn, severe smoke inhalation and corneal abrasions. The team consensus that survival was unprecedented was unanimous. When the physicians talked with him, the man replied that he preferred his wife and his mother-in-law to decide for him. His wife and her mother, stunned and horrified by the accident, refused. Further conversation with the patient revealed that he wished to live by any and all means "until God is ready for me." In the burn intensive-care unit he required a tracheostomy and respirator. He continued to communicate, although imperfectly, by "writing" letters in the air. Despite an armamentarium of intensive nursing care, a cardiac out-put monitor, silver nitrate dressings, Swan-Ganz catheter, and intravenous dopamine, he died three days later in septic shock.

Discussion

Unlike diseases such as uncontrolled cancer, the prognosis of burns without precedent of survival is evident almost immediately at the time of admission, because the extent and severity of burn are easily recognized and rapidly quantifiable, and mortality statistics are more detailed and complete than for most other pathologic processes. Although severe burns are rapid and even violent in onset, the patient is usually alert and mentally competent on admission and may remain so for hours to a day after the burn—longer if aggressive fluid resuscitation is given. There is no way to predict the length of this lucid interval for a particular patient, but certainly there is little time for the patient to gain a gradual awareness of his condition or for the burn team suddenly to acquire insight into the ethical issues involved.

The California Natural Death Act requires a 14-day waiting period after a "terminal" condition is diagnosed and the appropriate document is signed and witnessed before a person's wish for nonheroic measures is legally binding. It is not applicable to these patients because death almost always occurs before the waiting period has lapsed. The lack of specific legal guidelines, however, does not negate the desirability of a planned and efficient approach.

The approach described above evolved slowly and unevenly through experience, interdisciplinary conferences and informal debate. Although medical factors were always involved, the final issues invariably proved to be primarily ethical and could be stated approximately by the question "Which is better for this patient, maximal therapy or ordinary care, and upon whose value system should the judgment be based?

As pointed out by Kubler-Ross, when a patient is severely ill, he is often treated like a person with no right to an opinion.[4] Yet it is the patient's life and rights that are at stake. Statistics may describe past experience with a given type of injury receiving maximal therapy or ordinary care; physicians may cite such an experience and are experts in carrying out programs of maximal therapy or ordinary care, but only the patient may choose between them, because only he has the right to consent to one or the other.

Just as Lincoln stated that "No man is good enough to govern another man without that other's consent,"[15] so no physician is so skilled that he may treat another without the other's consent.[16] If asked, the physician may offer his opinion about the choice, but it will be merely his personal, inexpert opinion about whether it is better to accept death or fight to make history as the first survivor in such an injury.

It took many months before we could shed a "we-know-best" defense and actually ask the patient what he wanted on admission when he was most competent to decide. Our approach seems obvious and right to us now; the first few times were agonizing. Our words seemed clumsy and awkward. If we had acted individually, without colleague support, the plan would probably have reverted rapidly to denial or, even worse, to a paternalistic decision-making for the patient. Our patients and their families were able to see the human concern behind our first faltering phrases. Their warmth, gratitude, and peace confirmed what we later read: that what we say to the patient, the exact words, matters less than how we say it in an atmosphere of honesty, caring, and constant human presence.[18]

Turning to the family for decision-making when death seems imminent for an incompetent patient is rarely satisfactory; guilt-ridden families often find it very difficult to be objective and unselfish in their decision-making. The more voiceless and vulnerable the patient, the more easily we have found ourselves slipping into a paternalistic role, using terms such as "hopeless," which we realize now are so obviously prejudicial (literally, judging before the fact). Yet our experience continues to convince us that "truth is the greatest kindness." It seems inevitable that more and earlier communication with the patient will prove to be the most honest and compassionate answer to many of the remaining problems of ethical decision-making in the intensive-care unit.

NOTES

1. D.M. Jackson, "The Psychological Effects of Burns," *Burns,* vol. 1, p. 70, 1974.

2. I.F.K. Muir, T.L. Barclay, *Burns and Their Treatment,* second edition. Year Book Medical Publishers, Chicago, 1974, p. 110.

3. H.H. Stone, "The Composite Burn Solution," in H.C. Polk, Jr., and H.H. Stone (eds.), *Contemporary Burn Management,* Little, Brown, Boston, 1971, p. 96.

4. E. Kubler-Ross, *On Death and Dying,* Macmillan, New York, 1969.

5. Critical Care Committee of the Massachusetts General Hospital, "Optimum Care of Hopelessly Ill Patients," *New England Journal of Medicine,* vol. 295, p. 362, 1976.

6. G.F. Tagge, D. Adler, C.W. Bryan-Brown, et al., "Relationship of Therapy to Prognosis in Critically Ill Patients," *Critical Care Medicine,* vol. 2, p. 61, 1974.

7. J.J. Skillman, *Intensive Care,* Little, Brown, Boston, 1975, p. 21.

8. M.T. Rabkin, G. Gillerman, N.R. Rice, "Orders Not to Resuscitate, *New England Journal of Medicine,* vol. 295, p. 364, 1976.

9. N.H. Cassem, "Confronting the Decision to Let Death Come," *Critical Care Medicine,* vol. 2, p. 113, 1974.

10. J.P. Bull, "Revised Analysis of Mortality due to Burns," *Lancet,* vol. 2, p. 1133, 1971.

11. I. Feller, C. Archembeault, *Nursing the Burned Patient,* Institute for Burn Medicine, Ann Arbor, 1973, p. 10.

12. R.E. Kavanaugh, *Facing Death,* Nash, Los Angeles, 1972, p. 67.

13. H. Brody, *Ethical Decisions in Medicine,* Little, Brown, Boston, 1976, p. 98.

14. E. Shneidman, *Death of Man,* New York Times Book Co., New York, 1973, p. 33.

15. A. Lincoln, "In Peoria, Illinois during Lincoln-Douglas Debate on Oct. 16, 1854," quoted in *Bartlett's Familiar Quotations,* Little, Brown, Boston, 1968, p. 635a.

16. P. Ramsey, *The Patient as Person,* Yale University Press, New Haven, 1970, p. 7.

17. J.W. Robb, "The Joseph Fletcher/Paul Ramsey Debate in Bioethics and the Christian Ethical Tradition," *Religion in Life* (in press).

18. H. Feifel, "Attitudes toward Death in Some Normal and Mentally Ill Populations," in H. Feifel (ed.), *The Meaning of Death.* McGraw-Hill, New York, 1959, p. 124.

19. A.D. Weisman, *On Dying and Denying: A Psychiatric Study of Terminality,* Behavioral Publications, New York, 1972.

72.

Terminal Care in Patients with Chronic Lung Disease
John J. Skillman

Life begins at birth and extends in a continuum to death; or does it? Is there a point when it may be said that death is beginning? Does it not seem that in caring for a seriously ill patient there is a point when almost every physician and nurse of experience can say to himself or herself (even though one may not outwardly express it) that the patient is beginning to die? At times there is considerable doubt when this point has been reached, for it is clearly less precise than the moment of birth or the time of death. Those who would agree that a point of beginning death can never be defined are likely to be the same ones who argue most strongly against the discontinuation of life support systems. For them the uncertainty is too great ever to give up seeking a cure. Their sensitivity to the time of beginning death is muted by an overpowering desire to continue the fight—the eyes look but do not see, the hands touch but do not feel, the ears hear but do not listen. To the experienced physician and nurse, the clues are there; all that remains is to face them squarely.

The seriously ill patient with chronic lung disease represents an extremely difficult problem. These individuals frequently exist under severe physical limitations. It may be difficult for the patient to do the daily housework, to walk to a store for groceries, to drive to a friend's house for a visit, or to get up and walk to the bathroom. Even a prolonged conversation may be a physical effort that is exhausting and pushes such a patient to the limits of endurance. As time goes on and the lung disease progresses, even a simple cold may add a physical burden that cannot be tolerated, and the patients's ability to ventilate himself without the aid of a machine nears an end. Such individuals are often brought to the hospital by ambulance in a semicomatose state. At the hospital, the emergency room staff rapidly evaluates the condition of the gasping patient. They search for causes of the episode of acute respiratory decompensation. Is the patient in heart failure? Has an acute infection occurred that has further decreased the spontaneous ventilatory efforts by increasing the dead space and metabolic rate? Both these factors increase the minute ventilation required to maintian sufficient alveolar ventilation, to prevent CSF acidosis and coma. Or has the patient forgotten to take his digitalis or diuretic medication? Is there any evidence for pulmonary embolism?

Soon, we reach the first major therapeutic decision. Should we intubate the patient and give him assistance with a ventilator? If the patient has a respiratory or cardiac arrest, the staff almost always carries out endotracheal intubation and resuscitation. But before an arrest occurs, a small dose of oxygen may forestall the need for intubation if the patient is still conscious. There may be time to give a rapidly acting diuretic, which could relieve pulmonary edema; or an antibiotic could be employed to treat the infection; or heparin might be administered to treat pulmonary embolization. If a correctable condition can be diagnosed, its specific treatment may save the patient from the need for a respirator.

Frequently, the patient is admitted directly from the emergency room to the intensive care unit for close observation, monitoring, and intensive chest physical therapy. Gradually the patient's ventilation and oxygenation may improve and endotracheal intubation may be avoided. The intensive care unit

Source: *Archives of Internal Medicine*, vol. 139, August 1979.

staff carefully monitors the patient's condition and practices a form of justifiable "brinksmanship," in which the goal is to avoid intubation and artificial ventilation of the patient if at all possible. Even when intubation seems absolutely necessary, placement of a Swan-Ganz catheter may frequently indicate that congestive failure has occurred, even though physical examination and the chest roentgenogram have not pointed to this diagnosis as the reason for the acute respiratory decompensation. Treatment of congestive heart failure under these circumstances may obviate endotracheal intubation. Although these diagnostic possibilities and their specific therapeutic solutions are always sought for, in some patients no discernible reason for the episode of acute decompensation may be found. For such patients, the chronic lung disease has entered a terminal phase and the point of beginning death has been reached. They will require endotracheal intubation and artificial ventilation.

Efforts at weaning these patients from the assistance of the ventilator are pursued vigorously. All permutations of the weaning process are tried, i.e., short periods of spontaneous ventilation interspersed with return to the ventilator, intermittent mandatory ventilation, or change from a constant-volume ventilator to a patient-triggered pressure ventilator. Eventually, the caring physicians and nurses become frustrated in their attempts to wean the patient from the respirator.

Anxiety and frustration, anger, and despair—these emotions are felt by the patient, his family, and the staff. Discussions about the lack of progress are held with the family by the staff caring for the patient. All too often, the patient is not included in these discussions, because it is extremely difficult to tell a critically ill patient that all is not going well. I am frequently guilty of this lack of consideration. However, the messages are given to the patient by nonverbal means—worried looks of staff, or the anguish on the face of the chest therapist who gives a painful treatment to the patient. These communications, though perhaps more distressing to the patient because they are indirect, are felt by the patient. I now believe that both the patient and his family should be kept informed about the patient's progress or the lack of it.

The second crossroad is now reached. Even though the ventilator can be gradually removed, while keeping the patient comfortable with medication for pain and air hunger, the physician may be unable to make this decision. What should be done now? He may choose to continue with the ventilator. Other staff members, particularly the nurses who spend their hours caring for the patient's needs, may wish that the ordeal, which is theirs, the family's, and the patient's, would end. In my opinion, it is the physician's own unresolved fears and needs, and rarely those of the family, that force him to continue therapy when all seems lost. Certainly the patient's wishes about discontinuation of therapy should be honored, even if they are different from the wishes of the family.

When such a terminal point has been reached, when the likelihood of getting back to the previous minimal, dismal existence, without a respirator, has disappeared, I do not support the continuation of ventilation. The difficulty is in being certain that the point of terminal irreversible illness has been reached. I suggest that it is not impossible to know when that point has been almost certainly reached. The caring staff of nurses and physicians need to talk together openly about this difficult issue, for doubts and fears always exist. Since care should not be discontinued without a unanimous decision from all concerned, sometimes a strong difference of opinion (usually by a physician who cannot "let go") forces a confrontation that may ultimately result in the patient's transfer from the intensive care unit to a medical ward. There, the ventilator care is usually continued. Unfortunately, this is often regarded by a new set of house officers and nurses as "dumping" the patient on them. In part, their feelings are justified. Anxiety and frustration, anger, and despair begin all over again because the patient's problems must be completely discussed and faced by the new group, who cannot do otherwise than try to find some solution to the medical crisis. In rare instances, they temporarily succeed. The patient, meanwhile, is subjected again to more weaning trials, more drugs, and more painful chest physical therapy, until resistant organisms finally cause an intractable infection and the patient dies.

What is our obligation in such cases? I suggest it is one of caring for the human being in the broadest sense, not in a restricted or mechanical way. The physician should learn to handle his guilt and frustration to avoid a withdrawal of emotional support and a dehumanization of the patient. I believe we need to use all our love and human sensitivity to do the best that we can for these patients. Sometimes the very best we can do is to avoid prolonging death by continuing treatments that may lead to a cruel, slow, and painful end.

NOTE

1. E.W.D. Young, "Reflections on Life and Death," *Stanford MD*, vol. 15, p. 20, 1975.

73.

Responsibility of the Physician in the Preservation of Life
Franklin H. Epstein

The Physician is Not Omniscient

Physicians are fallible. Their wisdom tends to be greatly exaggerated by the popular press and, too often, by physicians themselves. Patients have an enormous need to feel that their physicians can prognosticate with great accuracy, but the kindest, best-intentioned physician is often wrong. Moreover, a physician's prognosis tends to be weighted toward pessimism, because patients who do badly claim most of his time and attention and remain in his memory longer than those who do well.

Physicians who are in charge of intensive care units have a special problem to overcome in that their training and experience are often heavily weighted toward the care of acute emergency illness rather than that of chronically ill patients. When an elderly person with chronic cardiopulmonary disease and acute bronchitis is assisted by a respirator, the expectations of the nurses and physicians may be attuned to the usual prompt recovery of a young post-operative patient with respiratory failure rather than the slow convalescence of a chronic pulmonary cripple.

It is tragic to see life support withdrawn because of a mixture of impatience and ignorance. Equally tragic is the assumption that an incurable but indolent illness is causing new symptoms when in fact a co-incidental curable disease is at fault. The best way to ensure that a cure is not overlooked is to make it very hard for the physician to give up.

The Physician is an Interested Party

Psychological pressures on the physician in caring for terminally ill patients conspire against his impartiality. The physician suffers when the patient doesn't get well and

Source: *Archives of Internal Medicine*, vol. 139, August 1979.

his suffering ends when the patient dies. It's hard to appreciate how difficult it is to attempt to support a dying patient day after day with condolence and hope; how frustrating it is to contemplate months of decline, of weary and anxious relatives, of no treatment working. Physicians and nurses know the overwhelming sense of relief that comes when, on hurrying to the patient's room, steeling yourself to face the ordeal of a patient who is not getting better, you learn that death has arrived, unexpectedly, an hour earlier. The sense of relief can be so intense that it is hard to remember that the patient cannot share it.

The Physician's Contract

Our obligation to assuage the pain of our patients is sometimes discussed as if it involved an equal obligation to minimize suffering of relatives, friends, and other onlookers. In fact, much of the "suffering" of terminally ill patients from nasal oxygen tubes and intravenous drips exists only in the imagination of shocked relatives, who are sickened and frightened by unfamiliar procedures and apparatus. The physician must remember that he has only one client—the patient. He is the advocate of the patient—not the family, or the welfare agency, or the kindly clergyman, squeamish at the sight of tracheostomy.

Useless Treatments

If we are indeed obligated to do everything we can to preserve our patient's lives, then we have a special and balancing obligation to evaluate our expensive methods of treatment in impartial, prospective studies, so that resources will not be unnecessarily squandered. It should be clear that when life is irretrievable, useless treatments should not be employed. But ad hoc judgments about the "quality of life" should be discouraged as a major factor in such decisions.

In the best hospitals, the principle that human life itself has dignity and worth will affect all the actions in every department. To maintain that attitude is the unique responsibility of the medical profession. In the last analysis, that attitude of the profession may be as important for society as any miracle that modern technical medicine can perform. Death always comes at last, despite our best efforts. But what little we can do carries a message to our patients and to the world: Human beings are important. Humanity is to be preserved.

74.
Decisions Regarding the Provision or Withholding of Therapy
Philip E. Cryer

Dr. Gerald Perkoff: Two patients presented difficult problems during their care. The first patient, an 86-year-old woman, had been essentially well except for poor memory; she had assigned legal responsibility for her affairs to a guardian. However, she was able to communicate well with her physician and to give an accurate history. She was found to have an asymptomatic abdominal aortic aneurysm. After initial eval-

Source: *The American Journal of Medicine,* vol. 61, December 1976.

uation and consultation, it was decided
that the patient's age and her history of hypertension made the surgical risks of elective aneurysm replacement too high, and it
was decided not to perform surgery. Although this decision was discussed with the
guardian, it was not discussed with the patient.

Approximately 6 months later the aneurysm ruptured. Hypotension responded
initially to the intravenous administration
of saline solution, and the patient was
alert and mentally clear when a different
surgeon discussed the problem with her,
pointing out the low probability of surgical
success. Despite the risks, the patient desired surgery. The guardian was not available.
The patient died 30 hours after surgery.

The second patient was a 90-year-old man
who had poor vision due to cataracts and
who was nearly deaf due to chronic otitis.
He had anorexia with a 20-pound weight
loss and was found to have a bladder neck
obstruction due to prostatic hypertrophy.
A transurethral prostatectomy was planned
but was never performed. Following cystoscopy, the patient had fever, chest pain,
hypoxemia, pulmonary infiltrates, and
abnormal ventilation-perfusion lung scans,
and he was treated with heparin for pulmonary emboli. Because of the history of
a bowel mass, a barium enema was performed; it revealed only diverticulosis. The
barium was not expelled and produced
obstipation with increasingly severe abdominal pain for which he required narcotics.
The patient refused further diagnostic procedures and stated repeatedly that he
wanted no additional therapy, that he wished
to die. When pneumonia developed, a minimal course of therapy with penicillin was
chosen. When he had a retroperitoneal
hemorrhage, he continued to refuse therapy.
It was decided not to give him blood transfusions. He became obtunded, then comatose, and after several days, died.

I would like to begin our discussion with
the first patient. Dr. Jaffe, what is the
prognosis in patients with a recognized ab-

dominal aortic aneurysm who are not
operated upon?

Dr. Bernard Jaffe: It is quite difficult to
get good current data because the great
majority of patients are now treated. In the
mid-1950s a series of 68 cases was published in which it was shown that patients
with untreated abdominal aortic aneurysms had a 5-year life expectancy of only
5 percent and that 60 percent of patients
died within one year of diagnosis. Since the
first patient had a 7- to 8-cm aneurysm,
her 5-year life expectancy, based on nothing
else but the aneurysm, was about 5 percent without an operation.

Dr. Perkoff: The life expectancy of anyone at 76 or 87 years probably averages
about 6 years; so this risk is greater than
the risk of death from other causes. In
general, then, do you believe 86-year-old
people with aortic aneurysms should
be operated upon? Our patient was asymptomatic; she had a murmur, mild hypertension, and memory loss at the time the
decision was made not to operate.

Dr. Jaffe: I think that any patient with a
large abdominal aortic aneurysm whose
general medical condition or coronary disease is not so severe as to preclude long-
term survival should be operated upon. In
this hospital, the operative mortality rate
in patients undergoing elective aneurysm re-
section is 3 percent, and there are a number of 80-plus-year-old survivors.

Dr. Perkoff: What is the expected mortality rate when such a patient is operated upon after aneurysm rupture with
shock?

Dr. Jaffe: In otherwise healthy people,
the mortality in patients with a ruptured abdominal aneurysm is 50 percent.
In an 86-year-old patient, the mortality
rate would be significantly greater.

Dr. Perkoff: Dr. Vavra, what should we
make of the fact that this woman had
given a third party the authority to make
major decisions? How does the guardian figure into this?

Dr. John Vavra: It sounds to me that this

woman did not want to make any foolish mistakes with her estate and, because of memory loss, sought power of attorney to protect her from some bad decisions. It does not sound as though she was unable to make certain kinds of decisions for herself, or that she was incapable of understanding medical problems.

The decision not to perform the elective operation was made with the knowledge and approval of the guardian, but without the patient's knowledge. On the other hand, the emergency operation was performed with the patient's consent, but without the guardian's consent. This brings up a problem now being debated—what is a physician's responsibility to his patient? There are three views. The physician's primary responsibility to the patient is (1) to keep "the contract," or to keep promises, which means to involve the patient in all-important information obtained during the medical workup and to permit the patient to be involved in decisions about what ought to be done; (2) the duty not to harm the patient; and (3) the duty to protect other people who are involved. If we are not to harm a patient, then when medical decisions are made complicated information must be interpreted to the patient. He cannot just be given all the data as raw facts. The obligation to protect implies that other people may be involved who need to be protected in the course of the medical workup. Other personal relationships and factors, such as the family finances, need to be considered. If you ask a patient what the primary responsibility of the physician is, he will state that the primary responsibility of the physician is to keep promises, to keep the contract, and to provide information. If you ask a physician what his primary responsibility is, he is likely to emphasize to be sure not to harm the patient and to protect all people involved. In the case of the first patient, the decision not to operate was made on the physician's promise not to harm. The guardian and the

physician discussed the medical problem, and the decision was made without involving the patient. There is no reason to believe that the patient was unable to understand or that she could not have been involved in the decision about surgery; she probably should have been consulted. Very interestingly, when the patient returned with her aneurysm bleeding, the opposite decision was made. The patient was supplied with information, and gave her consent to surgery. The guardian was not involved; there obviously was a disparity in the way the physician's obligation was formulated during the course of the patient's illness.

Dr. Perkoff: Dr. LeFrak, would you comment on this patient? In this instance there was a certain diagnosis, sound knowledge about the prognosis, and a specific form of therapy with a known outcome was available.

Dr. Stephen LeFrak: I believe that the elderly make up the group that is most discriminated against in hospitals. Many health professionals are willing to say, "this patient is very old and has lived a full life; let him die in peace." I think we owe the elderly a great deal more than that. We must not invoke age alone as a rationale for not providing intensive care, surgery, or other treatment modalities for them. Because of their age, the elderly deserve the best of modern medicine, humanistically and technically.

I think every physician ought to take a look at the Metropolitan Life actuarial tables. An 86-year-old woman is expected to live a little over 5 years, a fairly long time. Medical decisions should be based on that life expectancy. If an aneurysm ruptures, we have heard that mortality exceeds 50 percent. Since age is not a contraindication to aneurysmectomy, medical judgment would seem to dictate that this woman should have undergone an elective surgical procedure before her aneurysm ruptured.

Dr. Perkoff: Basically, the question I asked

myself when the issue was presented to us and subsequently, is, "Can a physician do other than treat a patient if the patient is completely informed and desires treatment?" The answer I gave was that there is no other choice but to treat such a patient. I think the qualifications I stated before I asked Dr. LeFrak to comment are of some importance here. This woman presented a much simpler problem than the second patient. We knew exactly what was wrong with her, we knew the diagnosis early and a standard form of therapy was available with a known outcome. Whether the patient was 50 or 90 years of age mattered less than that the outcome could be predicted in a reasonable way and that a logical decision could be made about therapy. That being the case, it was appropriate to operate even when the risks were the highest. By the same token, it was a mistake not to have operated earlier when she was well. Further, a telephone consultation is not the appropriate way to confront anyone with a patient. Had this patient interacted personally with the surgeon at the time of her first visit, it clearly would have been preferable. All of us wish to make decisions under the best possible circumstances; these were not provided to this patient at the time. Either the internist or the surgeon, or both, should have insisted upon a consultation visit.

The second patient is much more complex. He was too ill to receive definitive surgical treatment for his primary problem, prostatic hypertrophy. He literally had complications of every diagnostic and therapeutic procedure which was carried out. Until he became comatose, he was actively involved in discussions about his problems and clearly stated that he did not wish to receive treatment; he wished to die. At best, successful aggressive therapy would have left him chronically bedridden and unacceptable for surgery. These facts were clearly involved in the course followed by his physicians, of whom I was one. Dr. Vavra, two major views have been developed in this situation;

would you outline them and expand upon them for us?

Dr. Vavra: Let me start by saying that one of the important aspects of this protocol was that the patient was given information, and he made fairly definite statements that he did not want to be treated and that he wanted to die. Is that correct?

Dr. Perkoff: Yes.

Dr. Vavra: He was also informed, as complications arose, that if he did survive he would likely end up in a nursing home, with a catheter, and of the problems likely to ensue?

Dr. Perkoff: No, I do not believe I ever told him that. You did not either, did you Dr. Rudnick?

Dr. Seth Rudnick: No, he did not know that, or if he knew it, he knew it on his own and not from us.

Dr. Paula Clayton: Did he come in wanting to die or was it only as complications arose that he expressed this idea?

Dr. Perkoff: It was only as the complications occurred that he said he wanted to die. However, he was brought to MCG much in the same manner as many patients are brought to the emergency room of a hospital and left there. He had no family; an elderly friend, who believed he could no longer care for himself in his apartment, had helped him get to MCG and then had left. He did not seek medical attention of his own free will.

Dr. Vavra: Before commenting on how to deal with dying patients, I would like to indicate that at times it is very difficult to understand why a patient asks a physician to discontinue treatment and to do nothing more. It is not usually clear, particularly when the physician has not seen the man before, whether the patient is really speaking out of some sense of violation of his dignity, whether it is the "disease" speaking, or whether he is depressed and has had enough of procedures and manipulation.

The two different points of view in the medical and ethical debate as to the physician's responsibility to the dying patient have been best articulated by Robert Morison and Leon Kass.[2] Leon Kass states that the physician's responsibility is to the patient and to the patient alone. Robert Morison states that patients cannot be abstracted from the community to which they belong and the environment in which they live; so that it is not possible to talk about them either alive or dead without seeing them in relation to other people and to the environment. Robert Morison has a broader focus than Leon Kass.

From Kass' point of view it is the physician's responsibility to use his medical skills to the utmost to save the life of the patient, to keep his pain and suffering to a minimum, and to continue to treat him until it is quire clear that his pain and suffering cannot be alleviated and that there is almost nothing else to offer in terms of useful therapy. Patients may make statements that life is not worth living and that they should be permitted to die, but after treatment is instituted they are usually glad that things were done and that they are still alive. There is always the anticipation that disorders not treatable now may be controllable in the very near future, as we all know from the very rapid recent advances in medical science. From Kass's point of view everything possible should be done for sick people, and the physician has no right to withhold therapy unless he is certain it would not be successful.

Morison states the obligation differently. Morison says that physicians obviously have to be sensitive to the dying patient but when the patient is on the downward projectory of his life, he and his family may indicate clearly that important relationships are being compromised and that the patient's dignity is being violated much as Jonathan Swift's was; Swift was kept alive by his doctors for several years despite his wishes to be permitted to die. Morison states that the cost of maintaining life with dignity for the person or for the family includes an appreciation not only of medical factors but also of social and eco-nomic factors within the larger contextual framework. Kass rejects outright the view that economic and social factors are important and that physicians have a right to force their decisions to stop therapy upon them. In the second patient it was decided not to give him antibiotics other than penicillin and not to give him blood transfusions. Morison says that if physicians are allowed to make decisions of this type, they need to find a way to talk about these decisions rather than following their "conscience." The two points of view revolve on whom the physician is responsible to; the patient alone, or the patient in the larger context of his environment. With regard to the second patient, it is very difficult to tell what the proper decision should have been. The patient's statements were made when he was seriously ill and there were valid reasons for treating him vigorously. We believe that he was a person with a fairly strong sense of his integrity who earlier had refused surgery out of a sense of his own dignity.

Once patients are in the hospital, it is very hard for physicians not to do something. It is much easier to make these decisions outside the hospital environment. Once a patient is admitted to the hospital, a lot of people are involved in their care and physicians very frequently will do more then than they might have if they knew the patient better or if he were still at home.

Dr. Perkoff: This man was treated with penicillin but he was not given any transfusions. This difference in decision making is an example of both the emotional and factual confusion with which we approached this particular patient.

Dr. LeFrak, I know that the Kass view is the one you hold over the Morison view. Would you comment?

Dr. LeFrak: I think that it is fallacious to contrast the physician's responsibility to his patient with his responsibility to society. This is a false distinction. The only way we fulfill our responsibility to society is by fulfilling our responsibility to the individual patient. Once society becomes "more important than the individual" and once "cost-benefit analysis" becomes more important than the individual, our whole society as we have known it changes. So, to contrast the interests of the individual with that of "society as a whole" is not only wrong but also has far-reaching consequences. Although I do not think that Kass and Morison are opposed in quite this way, this is not a simple distinction to make, nor one that should be made.

It is very difficult to define dying in the dying patient. It appears that the second patient was not dying when he came to the hospital. He started to die while he was in the hospital. Very few people bring themselves to the hospital to die or wanting to die. If they want to die, they do not come to the hospital. So, by the very act of presenting themselves at the hospital, they have already made a decision, "I want to live, I want to get better, do the most you can for me." I think we have the obligation to do all we can. There is always time to allow the patient to die with dignity tomorrow. To allow someone to die one day too soon is a mistake that cannot be rectified.

Dr. Vavra: Being sensitive to the relativistic ethic of Morison, I think it is very important to keep the patient's needs in primary view, but it is also important to be cognizant of the consequences to other people. To overemphasize unlikely consequences is the camel's nose or slippery slope argument; i.e., if you let a camel get his nose into a tent then the rest of the camel will go in, or if you do not plant your feet firmly on the ice you will slide to the bottom. I think it unlikely that patients will be denied good medical care if the physician considers the social and economic consequences as well as the important medical and psychologic problems of dying patients.

Dr. Clayton: I think that when you talk about this patient you have to consider that he certainly was a very independent man. He was 90 years old, had no family, lived by himself, and had a great deal of

pride in his independence. He made a decision years earlier not to undergo surgery that had been recommended. When you talk about responsibility to the patient, you should consider that if he then sees himself as losing his independence in the hospital and this leads him to want to die, a part of your responsibility may be to let him die.

Dr. Perkoff: As Dr. Vavra mentioned earlier, a physician who is faced with a situation in which there is no reasonable likelihood of success has a difficult time. One of the things that impressed us was that everything that had been done to this man made his condition worse rather than better. In fact, other than choosing a more potent group of antibiotics or giving him a transfusion, we really had no therapy to offer him. That may not be adequate justification for the course that was followed, but recognition of those feelings surely influenced the decisions which were made. Dr. Rudnick, you were directly involved with this man. I know there was a great difference of opinion and much concern on the part of the house staff about the care of this patient. Would you comment, please?

Dr. Rudnick: I think that, in a sense, it is a bit easier for a house officer to approach the problem of the patient who is critically and probably terminally ill. The house officer's prime concern is to the patient. The societal concern that intrudes upon him is limited to the family. I think I am less concerned than the patient's primary physician with cost effectiveness or a general consideration of what the patient will do when he returns to society.

However, we are faced with life and death decisions daily. Our entire training is to prolong life, to do everything we can to improve the patient's care. I do not think any of us ever consciously consider doing anything that would allow the patient's life to be shortened. Yet there is a conflict for all of us, and it usually occurs in a case like that of the second patient. The patient or the family make certain demands on us. Those demands can be quite divergent, either to do everything for the patient or to do nothing for the patient. We are never quite sure what "nothing" or "everything" is. We are confronted with critical questions and decisions. Am I doing this for the patient's benefit? Am I killing him by not performing some procedure or by performing it? Active or passive euthanasia is almost a useless distinction for us. We are quite aware of the potentially fatal consequence of withholding an antibiotic. Conversely if we put the patient through innumerable procedures and therapies, and all the complications of heparinization or of a barium enema develop, we also know we have contributed to his death. Recently, another complication has been presented, "Am I going to be sued if I do not do exactly what the patient and/or his family desires?"

A final element of our quandary, one that crosses our minds all the time, is if we know that the patient is going to die, do we back off a little bit? Do we say, "I am not going to do quite everything I can, I am not going to remain awake until 5 o'clock in the morning with this one patient, because I know no matter what I do he will die?" Nowhere in this decision-making process are there formal guidelines. We perform in this situation on the basis of our knowledge, intuition, and occasionally, prayer.

NOTES

1. I.S.Wright, E. Urdaneta, and B. Wright, "Reopening the Case of the Abdominal Aortic Aneurysm," *Circulation,* vol. 13, p. 754, 1956.

2. R. S. Morison, and L. R. Kass, "Death: Process and Event," *Science,* vol. 173, p. 694, 1971.

75.

Medicine, Ethics, and the Elderly   Sally Gadow

It is evident to those in gerontology that social views are part of the basis for understanding social issues. This is because social problems often derive directly from the prevalence of certain views. Issues involving the elderly are a graphic example of this. In the discussion that follows, some ethical problems in the health care of the elderly and suggestions as to how these might be addressed in the light of different social/medical views of aging and different principles of medical ethics are discussed.

First, what are some of the ethical problems in the medical care of the elderly? The following three examples are useful by way of illustration:

- Mr. A, age 85, was treated 5 years earlier for carcinoma. At that time he was depressed about his condition, seemed to

respond negatively to the information given him about his situation, and wondered aloud repeatedly, "Why should this happen to an old man who just wants to live out his last years in peace?" Now, metastatic lesions have been discovered upon a visit to his physician for a routine examination. The physician chooses not to tell him of the findings or to treat him, believing that it would be more than he could bear. "At his age," reasons the physician, "he doesn't have much time left even if we arrested the disease. Why make his last months miserable with futile treatments or with the knowledge that he is dying?"

- Mrs. S, age 80, has developed gangrene of the right foot, requiring amputation to prevent further deterioration. The prognosis with or without amputation is uncertain. Two physicians agree that surgery would not

Source: *The Gerontologist,* vol. 20, no. 6, 1980.

be viewed as a lifesaving measure and might not even arrest the deterioration. However, the sons of Mrs. S demand that she be treated, and another physician maintains that her condition *is* a life-and-death matter. All agree that Mrs. S herself is not capable of making an informed judgment, although they acknowledge that she is aware of her bodily integrity and wants no amputation of any part of her.[1]

At age 90, Mrs. E is bedridden, blind, and never has fully recovered her mental faculties after striking her head in a fall. She is cared for in a comparatively inadequate nursing home. Except for an occasional respiratory infection and arthritic pain, she seems in no distress. She sometimes recognizes her husband, but her attempts to speak to him are usually unintelligible. Six years ago, Mrs. E gave a talk on the miseries of prolonging the life of the dying elderly, particularly in nursing homes, and made an eloquent plea for "a dignified and simple way to choose death." Now her husband and physician face the problem of determining whether her present situation is a violation of the concept of "death with dignity" that she seemed to advocate.[1]

Views of Aging

Contemporary views of aging are complex and varied. The social and moral value of the elderly patient and the resolution of ethical problems such as the three above will differ according to the view of aging a medical practitioner holds. A glance at the spectrum of views is helpful in pointing out that despite seeming progress, we have yet to devise a genuinely positive valuation of dying or of elderly persons. We have undoubtedly advanced beyond a strictly negative view but may have come only as far as a "false positive."

What does this spectrum look like at present?

(1) At the negative extreme, aging is viewed as the antithesis of health and vigor. This negative valence toward aging finds expression in medicine in a decep-

tively "objective" form in the designation of clinical changes in aging as *deterioration, disorganization,* and *disintegration,* from the level of psyche to the level of cells. To the truly objective observer, however, there is nothing a priori degenerative about the changes in aging unless one uncritically accepts as the only ideal of health the condition that younger individuals manifest. Using that ideal, of course, aging by definition is a profound deviation.[2]

(2) A less axiomatic but still negative view is that aging is an unwelcome reminder of our mortality. Death is a more common occurrence among older than among younger individuals. As if to ameliorate this assumed tragedy of human finitude, death is thought to be more natural an outcome because it is more common and, moreover, more acceptable because it is thought more natural. The effect of this view is that the more natural and acceptable mortality is thought to be for the elderly, the more unthinkable it is for the nonelderly, and the more the aged are avoided as symbols of the unthinkable.

(3) A more charitable view has emerged in which the elderly are elevated from outcasts to underprivileged citizens. On this view, although their age in itself has no intrinsic value for society, they are brought out of the closet to become recipients of our benevolence toward the oppressed. This benevolence, in the form of social and medical services, may indeed be so great as to constitute a form of reverse discrimination, that is, compensatory justice as atonement for past discrimination. The danger in this view is the danger in all designation of "handicapped" individuals as special groups needing services: the beneficiary remains subordinate to the benefactor.

(4) An auspicious development seen in the rise of geriatric medicine is the view of aging as a clinical entity in its own right. According to this view, aging is a unique human phenomenon, worthy of a practitioner's or a researcher's full attention. The aged are not health deviants; on the

contrary, they are the "biologically elite." As an elite, they present special problems as well as special strengths that other patients do not manifest. As positive as this development is, it too carries a risk, the possibility that subspecialty medicine would become the model for a broader social approach to the aged. This would mean that aging would be of interest as a highly specific class of unusual phenomena, bearing little relation to the more general features of experience shared by persons of all ages. This trend already is evident in attempts to identify sociological and psychological features of aging that distinguish it from the rest of human experience.

(5) Perhaps the most positive of all attitudes so far is the once venerable view that the aged are a cultural treasure, a repository of wisdom, an embodiment of history. The growing interest in oral history regards the elderly as an irreplaceable historical elite. Interestingly, the assumption underlying this regard for the aged is one of modern society's most unquestioned beliefs, that is, the belief that the *value* of time is proportional to the *amount* of time. For the elderly, the amounts of time already lived far outweighs *in quantity* the time remaining; consequently, the past experience of the aged is of greater social interest and value than the experiences still ahead of them. The positive direction of this view cannot be denied; it brings the elderly into the center of efforts to understand our world in terms of history. But it leaves little room for the 74-year-old woman who insisted to her psychotherapist, "But doctor, all I have left is my future."

This then is the spectrum of views, from extremely negative to relatively positive, that characterize this culture's approach to the elderly. One view not described above belongs near the negative end of the spectrum. It is the "false positive" view that aging is a time in which, barring a few extra maladies, nothing changes. One continues to work, to be active, independent, maintain-

ing the same scope and intensity of social and professional involvement. This ostensibly positive view is more accurately a neutralization of the negative value of aging, achieved by means of omitting, ignoring, or bypassing aging. It amounts to a false positive because "it assumes that the only way of making aging human is to make it as nearly like youth or mid-life as possible."[4]

Medical views of aging reflect all the diversity of the spectrum just outlined. Focusing upon only the two ends of the spectrum, one can identify two conflicting views of aging in medicine. These are, on one hand, the philosophy that the elderly have *less* social and moral value than other individuals and, on the other hand, the view that they have *greater* value than other persons. Probably most health professionals fall between these extremes; however, it is important to recognize that both philosophies inform clinical decisions and for that reason to recognize current expressions of these two positions.

The belief that the aged are less valuable than other persons is based on the determination that the elderly contribute less either to the attainment of general social goals or to the happiness of the individuals around them.

This frankly utilitarian position would perhaps be thought obsolete, with emergence of the patients' rights movement, the political significance of advocacy groups, and the general reluctance to assign personal value as a function of social worth. But it is a philosophy that survives in one important respect in medicine, as the degree-of-benefit rationale for allocating professional care to the elderly patient. The degree-of-benefit rationale is of special importance because it is ususally not recognized as a value judgment. According to this allegedly neutral principle, patients are preferred who show greatest promise of responding to treatment, regardless of status, race, or other nonmedical variables. While the intent is not to discriminate, the effect *is* discriminatory, because from a clinical view, 15 years of additional life or improvement is a greater benefit than 15 months. In effect, the older the person, the less likely that he or she will benefit "as much" (as long) as a younger person. Clearly, the definition of benefit in terms of time cannot be a subjective sense of benefit, since no one possibly could judge *for* an older person that 15 months is worth less to that person than 15 years to a younger individual. In this most basic clinical criterion, then, lies an implicit devaluing of the aged.

In the alternative view, the aged have *greater* value rather than less, relative to other persons. It may be that neither medicine nor society is likely to subscribe soon to such a view. Yet, it would seem that there already is a precedent by analogy in the hospice movement, where it must be the case that hospice staff value dying persons more than other persons and are concerned more with enhancing the dying person's care than with the care of other types of patients. If hospice care is possible in the face of still overwhelming cultural negativity toward death, perhaps a comparable revaluing of elderly persons by health professionals is possible. Geriatric medicine is one indication of such a revaluing.

Principles of Medical Ethics

Social and medical views of aging are important contexts in which to elucidate ethical issues in medicine. But in resolving specific clinical problems, more is required. A practitioner's tendency to value or to devalue the elderly does not yet indicate whether Mr. A should be told his prognosis, Mrs. S should have her leg amputated, or in Mrs. E's case "death with dignity" requires euthanasia. As an expression of (or perhaps in spite of) the view of aging that a professional holds, the additional application of moral principles is necessary. The use of moral principles may of course be only implicit in a clinician's decision making, but I shall assume that even if applied unconsciously, some value or set of values operates in resolving situations such as the three cases described. The principles of benefi-

cence and autonomy are discussed below and the outcomes compared when each of them is applied to the cases described.

The principle of beneficence. The principle that requires, broadly speaking, "doing good" in medicine entails actions toward patients to (1) prevent harm to them, (2) benefit them, (3) permit harm only when the harm is unavoidable and when it is significantly outweighed by the benefit.

The basic maxim of medicine, "Above all, do no harm" (*primum non nocere*), can be considered part of the beneficence principle. In itself, "do no harm" cannot stand alone, for there are so few instances in which medical intervention is wholly without harm that a principle forbidding harm would virtually condemn practioners to standing by helplessly while most diseases take their natural course. Thus, the admonition "do no harm" must be viewed in light of the primary concern of medicine, namely, the intent to benefit patients. The beneficence principle places the prohibition against harm in the context of doing good. Doing harm is not forbidden absolutely, but only that harm which is unnecessary and is not balanced by a greater good. Even the abhorrence of many physicians to euthanasia is based not so much on the belief that killing violates an absolute prohibition as on the belief that the harm of killing relative to its possible benefit to most patients is too great to be justified.

The difficulty in applying the principle of beneficence lies in the determination of benefit. This is evident in all three cases. In order to apply the principle in Mr. A's situation, the clinician must determine whether the benefit to Mr. A of not knowing his terminal prognosis outweighs the harm of being deceived. Notice that, using the beneficence principle alone, there is no a priori obligation of truth telling. Truth may be judged a benefit in some cases; in others, a harm. However, in order to determine whether disclosure is a harm or a benefit, some ethical standard or norm must be applied. In medicine the criteria for defining benefit relate to the alleviation of suffering and the preservation of life. Alternative criteria could be imagined, of course, which might designate deception to be a greater harm than suffering and truthfulness a greater good than prolonging life.

In the case of Mrs. S, the balance of benefit over harm is more involved because she has expressed her own feelings about the benefit of the amputation. Thus the harm to her of an otherwise beneficial, even life-saving, treatment may outweigh the good of prolonging life. That is the difficulty I indicated. Patients and physicians may disagree on definitions of benefit. Clinicians themselves may disagree.

The problem becomes more serious as the degree of possible harm increases. In Mrs. E's case, the issue of "death with dignity" seems insoluble with the benefit principle alone. The reason is the recognition in medicine that the possible infliction of great harm, such as allowing a patient to die whose life might have been prolonged, is justified, if at all, only when that patient herself judges the good to outweigh the harm. Despite Mrs. E's past opinions, it is not known whether she now actually experiences the maintaining of her life as such a great harm that ending it would by comparison be a benefit. Here the best one can do, using only the principle of beneficence, is to balance benefit against *risk* of harm, since actual harm cannot be ascertained without discussion with Mrs. E. Because her present wishes are not known, the risk of harm in mistakenly judging death to be a benefit for her is greater than the possible benefit. That is, if an error in judgment is made and she is allowed to die when she has no wish to die, the harm to her is greater than if she is kept alive when in fact she wishes to die. Indeed, the harm of the first error is irreparable.

In Mrs. E's case it was suggested that the principle of beneficence is by itself inconclusive. In issues as important as withdrawing treatment to allow or hasten death, a central moral consideration is the patient's desire. When the harm of a possible error is

irreparable, it becomes imperative to verify with the patient the way in which harm and benefit are to be defined. That concern with the patient's view is based on the value of autonomy.

The principle of autonomy. When the value of patient self-determination is the *primary* consideration in clinical determinations, the ethical principle that is being applied is no longer the principle of beneficence but that of autonomy. At times the two will converge. If the exercise of autonomy is subsumed under the category of benefit, the principles even become identical. But it must be acknowledged that at times, autonomous patient decisions defy medical definitions of benefit, just as professional decisions can violate patient autonomy. In those cases it is necessary to recognize that distinct principles are in conflict and a choice must be made; both cannot be satisfied at once.

The principle of autonomy requires respect for the freedom of self-determination of those affected directly by a decision—that is, patients. (The autonomy of the professional is not addressed by this principle, though professional freedom is sometimes raised as an objection to patient autonomy. Similarly, the principle of beneficence does not address the good of the professional, mandating that practitioners benefit themselves.)

The exercise of personal autonomy involves two levels: (1) *agency,* the freedom to decide among all the options available, and (2) *action,* the freedom to carry out the course of action that is chosen. Freedom of action is protected in medicine by formal consent requirements; forced medication of a patient who refuses treatment with drugs is an example of infringing that freedom. Patient agency is more involved. It requires allowing patients to participate, fully and freely, in determinations about their care. This entails access to information about one's condition and options, as well as freedom from coercion in making one's choice. (In addition to these safeguards, I have argued elsewhere that respect for autonomy also entails active *assistance* to patients in both developing and exercising their self-determination.)[5]

Applying the principle of autonomy in Mrs. E's case is the most difficult of the three. However, the reason for that may be that no one involved with Mrs. E has yet *attempted* to apply it. There is no indication that her present feelings about her situation have been ascertained, or that such a determination is impossible. The facile assumption of incompetence in many elderly patients often reflects only the lack of professional energy, interest, or imagination needed to communicate with persons of different mentation than "normal."

In the case of Mrs. S, incompetence is the justification offered for infringement of her autonomy, yet unlike Mrs. E, she has clearly expressed her desire to refuse the amputation. If the desire could *not* have been ascertained, then the consideration of irreparable harm discussed earlier would seem to justify the amputation. Similarly, if the desires of Mrs. E cannot be ascertained, maintaining her life can be justified. Faced with patients who are not, for whatever reason, self-determining, the principle of autonomy requires the course of action that has the greatest possibility of facilitating or restoring autonomy, or the least possibility of permanently precluding it. When there is no way of ascertaining a patient's wishes in a situation, the principles of autonomy and benefit converge in prescribing the action which has the greatest balance of benefit over harm in standard terms, alleviation of suffering and preservation of life. This requirement is based on the belief that the possibility of autonomy depends upon preservation of health and life. (It is not based upon absolute sanctity of life, for life is not assumed here to be an end in itself; according to the autonomy principle, life is valued and preserved because it is the essential grounds for the possibility of autonomy.) But as soon as a case involves a patient like Mrs. S who wishes to participate in a decision, it cannot be assumed that regard for au-

tonomy and concern for health and life will have the same outcome.

In the case of Mr. A, regard for health and for autonomy produce two clearly different medical judgments. The physician's concern for Mr. A's peace of mind and body in the last years of life result in the decision to value benefit over autonomy and to ignore the patient's metastases. Alternatively, a concern primarily for Mr. A's autonomy would dictate allowing him, first, access (which he may waive) to all information about his condition and options, and second, access to any treatment program the physician legally and morally can provide.

The principle of autonomy does not force patients to participate in treatment decisions. Rather, it ensures them the possibility and the assistance needed for participation if they so choose. It is an unfortunate assumption that elderly patients, who have lived their "appointed lifespan," are ready to relinquish life and would not desire aggressive treatment. This gives too much weight to the sheer number of years one has lived. On the other hand, the expectation that older persons who, out of personal choice or social necessity, may have long accepted a minimum of autonomy, will readily participate in treatment decisions when invited to do so is a view that places too little importance on the reality of one's history and the integrity of one's character.

If the principle of beneficence is difficult to apply because of problems in determining benefit, the principle of autonomy is difficult because not only does it require engaging with patients of diverse cultural and educational backgrounds and often with complex health problems to assist in their decisions about care. It also requires that patients be allowed to waive their autonomy and to acquiesce in the clinician's determinations on their behalf. However, it is crucial for the principle of autonomy that the waiver be consciously and freely given, neither assumed nor coerced.

Is there some way of reconciling these two

moral principles of medicine? Is either of them more appropriate than the other as the primary principle in the care of the elderly?

In keeping with the traditional medical ideal of service, we can ask which of the principles is likely to yield the highest return to those medicine serves? Which of the two is more encompassing, the less restricting?

The principle of autonomy, it is suggested, meets the criteria. It entails the fundamental requirement of benefiting patients, but with the qualification that "benefit" be defined by patients with their physicians rather than by physicians for their patients. The converse is not true: the benefit principle does not entail regard for autonomy, except perhaps when autonomy is subsumed under the category of benefit and is respected only when the professional deems it therapeutic; in theory, the benefit principle assumes the waiving of autonomy.

Patients thus lose nothing and gain significantly when the autonomy principle is primary in medicine. They still have the benefit of professional expertise and judgment, which they can make the basis for their decisions if they choose. In addition, they have the freedom to exercise personal judgment and "expertise" regarding the uniqueness of their situation and values.

It may be objected that medicine need not be this generous, that it is sufficient to strive to help patients, simply using the professional's concept of benefit. Patients who prefer their own notions about care can seek care elsewhere. One argument for such a view is based on the principle of justice, requiring fair and equitable distribution of services. Medicine based upon the principle of autonomy might appear wasteful of costly health resources.

In the care of elderly patients, however, it may be that we prefer the principle from which the patient has the most to gain, even if it be too demanding and costly an ideal for all of health care. The suggestion that older patients have a special moral claim on medicine is based on the possibility that life, health, and autonomy are more precious to older persons as they perceive that the time in which to enjoy those values is significantly diminished. The values that the principle of autonomy expresses may thus have greater moral relevance—though perhaps also more difficult application—in the care of elderly patients.

NOTES

1. R. M. Veatch, *Case Studies in Medical Ethics,* Harvard University Press, Cambridge, Mass. 1977.

2. E. Leach, "Society's Expectations of Health," *Journal of Medical Ethics,* vol. 1, p. 85, 1975.

3. J. Jernigan, *The Biologically Elite,* Third Annual Medical Aspects of Aging, University of Florida, Gainesville, Nov. 30, 1979.

4. G. Berg and S. Gadow, "Toward More Human Meanings of Aging—Ideals and Images from Philosophy and Art," In S. Spicker et al. (eds.), *Aging and the Elderly: Humanistic Perspectives in Gerontology,* Humanities Press, New York, 1978.

5. S. Gadow, "An Ethical Model for Advocacy: Assisting Patients with Treatment Decisions," In J. Swazey (ed.), *Dilemmas of Dying: Policies and Procedures for Decisions Not to Treat,* G. K. Hall, Boston, 1980.

76.

Dying Right in California: The Natural Death Act
Albert R. Jonsen

The right to die with dignity has been much proclaimed, discussed, and analyzed in recent years.[1] The issue has worked itself from the hospital room to the courts and the legislative halls. Discussion surrounding "the right to die" is often confused. Technical complexities such as the definition of "brain death" intertwine with painstaking philosophical investigations of "rights" and "euthanasia" as well as with cries of moral outrage voiced in condemnations of "mercy killing." At the center of the confused and complex discussion lies the question, "Should a dying person be kept alive by medical treatment?" Behind this question is the accusation, sometimes tacit, but often loudly asserted: doctors keep dying persons alive for no purpose—or worse, for their own purposes. Physicians are criticized for their insensitivity to the dying, for their failure to understand death, and for their inability to let go. Unlike their predecessors who honestly acknowledged the arrival of the blessed relief of death, it is said that modern doctors crowd death away from the bedside with a bevy of breathing, beating machines.

Even before the Karen Ann Quinlan case made headlines of these questions, a young California legislator, Assemblyman Barry Keene, sensed the public concern over "prolonging death." In 1974, he authored a bill which declared quite starkly, "Every person has the right to die without prolongation of life by medical means."[2] Using this unadorned proclamation as the basis for hearings, debates, and consultations, Keene finally produced a highly nuanced piece of legislation, The Natural Death Act. It won the enthusiastic endorsement of many interested parties, the cautious approval of the California Medical Association, and the eventual "nonopposition" of the Roman Catholic hierarchy of California. After some hesitation, the bill was passed by the legislature and signed by Governor Brown. It became a part of the Health and Safety Code of California on January 1, 1977. By July 1977, seven more states had passed similar legislation (Arkansas, Idaho, Nevada, New Mexico, North Carolina, Oregon, and Texas); bills are pending in 16 states. Physicians throughout the country will soon find themselves obliged to acknowledge their patient's "right to die." The purpose of this article is to review the California legislation and to anticipate the issues which it, and perhaps its emulators in other states, will present to physicians. They will find a few advantages and many perplexities in the notion of "natural death."

The Natural Death Act

The Natural Death Act[3] is a complex piece of legislation. In essence it declares that:

> The laws of the State of California shall recognize the right of an adult person to make a written directive instructing his physician to withhold or withdraw life-sustaining procedures in the event of a terminal condition.

Life-sustaining procedures are defined as:

> Any medical procedure or intervention which utilizes mechanical or other artificial means to sustain, restore, or supplant a vital function, which, when applied to a qualified patient, would serve only to artificially prolong the moment of death and, where, in the judgment of the attending physician, death is imminent whether or not such procedures are utilized.

Source: *Clinical Research*, vol. 26, no. 2, February 1978.

Pain medication is expressly excluded from this definition. A terminal condition is defined as:

An incurable condition caused by injury, disease, or illness, which, regardless of the application of life-sustaining procedures, would, within reasonable medical judgment, produce death, and where the application of life-sustaining procedures serves only to postpone the moment of death.

While any adult may execute the directive at any time in anticipation of future incapacity, those persons who are diagnosed by two physicians as having a "terminal condition" may execute or reexecute the directive after waiting 14 days. They are then designated as "qualified patients." As will be mentioned further, the physician has stricter obligations relative to qualified patients. These are the principal provisions of the Natural Death Act.[3,4]

The law is applicable only when mentally competent adults state (and do not revoke) their intent in a written and witnessed document. It does not apply to many other cases such as those involving children or adolescents, nor does it apply to cases where no written and witnessed directive exists. Thus, it would not deal with a case like that of Karen Ann Quinlan. Termination of treatment for children or for those whose wishes are undeclared in a document remains as problematic as it was before the enactment of the Natural Death Act.

The law has several principal effects. It makes clear for the first time that a physician or health care facility, acting in accord with a valid directive of a patient, will not be subject to either civil or criminal liability or charges of unprofessional conduct. It also makes clear that the death of a person who has signed a valid directive does not constitute suicide for purposes of the law. Insurance policies and the ability to purchase them shall not be jeopardized by the existence of such a directive.

Physicians whose patients have executed directives have certain obligations. They

must determine that the directive accords with the law, i.e., it is worded as the law specifies, properly witnessed by persons not related to or in a position to gain by the death of the patient, and is executed by a mentally competent person. If the patient has executed the directive in good health and subsequently becomes incompetent during the course of a terminal illness, the physician may "give weight to the directive as evidence of the patient's directions" but may also consider other factors such as information from the family or the nature of the illness, "in determining whether the totality of circumstances justify effectuating the directive." The physician has a stricter duty to a "qualified patient," i.e., one who has executed the directive after having been diagnosed by two physicians as suffering from a terminal condition. In this case, the "Directive shall be conclusively presumed, unless revoked, to be the directions of the patient." Should the physician refuse to honor the directive, he or she is obliged to "take the necessary steps to effect the transfer of the qualified patient to another physician who will effectuate the directive . . ." Failure to do so constitutes unprofessional conduct.

Among many other provisions about conditions for validity, recording, revocation, penalties for falsification, and special protections for those in nursing homes, two are particularly important. The first states that this law does not impair or supersede any legal right or responsibility which any person may have to effect withdrawal of life-sustaining procedures in any lawful manner; i.e., reasonable medical judgments about termination of care for those who have not executed a directive are not, by virtue of this legislation, to be cast into legal doubt.

Second, the law states, "nothing in this chapter shall be construed to condone, authorize or approve mercy killing, or to permit any affirmative act or omission to end life other than to permit the natural process of dying." In other words, these two provisions make it obvious that two ma-

jor areas of legal understanding are untouched by this legislation: the broad and
often quite unclear problems surrounding termination of medical care for those
who do not execute directives, and the
clearer but sometimes still cloudy positions
on "active and positive" medical interventions to terminate life.

In sum, the Natural Death Act establishes
only one previously questionable point: an
anticipatory refusal of care when expressed
in a certain way and under certain circumstances can be honored without fear of criminal or civil liability.

Ethical Problems

For the first time in the United States the
Natural Death Act establishes a statutory
right to die or, more properly, a right to be
allowed to die. The existence of this right
will probably relieve the anxiety of many potential patients, the legal qualms of many
attending physicians, and, it is to be hoped,
the suffering of many persons in their last
hours. However, the existence of a right imposes a duty, e.g., the right to die imposes
on attending physicians the duty to desist
from medical care or at least from medical
care of a certain kind. While the patient's
right to die clarifies some legal obscurities,
the physician's duty to desist creates some
ethical perplexities.

The problems begin to appear in the central words of the legislation. The physician
is directed to refrain from "life-sustaining
procedures" when the patient is in an

> incurable condition caused by injury, dis-
> ease or illness which, regardless of the
> application of life-sustaining procedures
> would, within reasonable medical judg-
> ment, produce death and where the appli-
> cation of life-sustaining procedures
> would serve only to postpone the moment
> of death.

In another place, the text reads,

> where, in the judgment of the attending
> physician, death is imminent whether
> or not such procedures are utilized.

This language was dictated by an attempt,
under strong political pressures, to draw
the legislation very tightly. Indeed, its tight-
ness assured its passage since many other
legislative initiatives in this area had failed
due to obscure and ambiguous language.
Language such as the traditional "ordinary
vs. extraordinary" is so obscure as to frus-
trate the law's purpose in endless argument.
Language referring to "quality of life"
might raise the threat of serious abuses from
"mercy killing" to "systematic extermina-
tion of the useless." The language was chosen
in hope of finding an expression which
would satisfy very divergent objections. Yet,
when applied to the situations where the
law might be pertinent, the language is extremely puzzling.

It is obvious that the legislation affirms the
right of a patient to refuse medical treatment in anticipation of the moment when
he or she is, on the one hand, under the
care of a physician for life-threatening illness and, on the other, incapable of enun-
ciating the refusal. However, the refusal
incorporated in the Natural Death Directive
appears to differ from that which has already achieved some status in law and ethics.
If patients refuse to be treated because
they consider the treatment immoral, as a
Jehovah's Witness would consider blood
transfusion, or because they believe it ineffective, as a chiropractor might consider
cortisone, or merely because they do not like
the physician or do not wish to spend the
time or the money—if these and many other
reasons for refusal obtain—the physician
must usually step back. Being no longer
wanted by the patient, the physician should
retreat even when a retreat is anguishing
or seems foolish. Unless special circumstances
prevail such as harm to others, the refusal
of a competent patient is a necessary and sufficient condition for the creation of the
physician's duty to desist.

However, persons who sign a Natural
Death Directive are not refusing care. If they
read the small print they will find they are
refusing useless care, i.e., care which even if it
is provided will not restore health. Pre-

sumably, patients who sign the Natural Death Directive are persons who would accept treatment for illness or injury if they had some assurance that the treatment would restore them to partial or complete health. The directive is designed for the moment when the patient can no longer say "stop." The physician alone, with directive in hand, must judge whether what he or she is doing is merely "prolonging death." In all such cases the patient's refusal of care is no longer a necessary and sufficient condition but only a necessary condition. To it must be added the physician's judgment of the imminence of death with or without treatment.

The imminence of death, with or without treatment, is a perplexing clinical judgment. It involves problems of prediction, empirical observation, and definition. However, there are times when a physician can say with great assurance that a person is about to die. These are the times when a cascade of deterioration destroys vital functions one by one and when many clinical signs and laboratory tests affirm the collapse of the integration of the organism. The patient is "in extremis." However, this sort of imminence of death, which is easiest to declare, seems to bypass the ultimate purpose of the law and the wishes of the patient who has signed a directive. It is already common practice contradicted only by the most frantic or fearful physicians to remove therapeutic devices, discontinue medications, and transfer the patient from the intensive care unit to the ward. The curtain is drawn. Paradoxically, where the clinical judgment required by the law can be made most readily there is little need for the law; yet, the law seems written only to apply to such cases.

On the other hand, the situation that the legislators certainly intended to remedy requires a clinical judgment which is extremely difficult and perhaps impossible to make. Since patients who avail themselves of the law apparently hope to prevent long, distressing, painful, expensive, and ultimately useless courses of treatment,

the judgment of imminence must be made before such courses are initiated or at least in their earliest stages. At this point physicians will be concerned whether patients are "salvageable" or not. A number of diagnostic procedures will be performed, therapeutic efforts will be undertaken, and supportive and palliative measures will be instituted. If a critical unexpected event interrupts an apparently successful therapy, it will be vigorously countered; or if complications of the therapy appear, they will be combated. The scenario is familiar to anyone—patient, professional, or relative—who has experienced the intensive care unit. Many a poignant tale is told of the exhausted patient not allowed to die. These tales inspired the Natural Death Act. But, again paradoxically, where need for the law is most felt, it is least possible to make the judgment of imminence which the law requires. At what point in the course of events surrounding critical care can it be said with moral certitude, "death is imminent, whether or not treatment is provided"?[5-7]

Professor Diana Crane, after studying the criteria that physicians invoke in making decisions about the medical treatment of seriously ill patients, concludes that "salvageability" is the dominant norm. She writes:

> These findings suggest that the dimensions of prognosis and type of deficit are of primary importance in the physician's decision to use or withhold treatment. Within this framework, the patient who wants active treatment is likely to receive it, but withdrawal of treatment by the physician depends less upon the consent of the patient or his agent than on the physician's assessment of the patient's prognosis and type of deficit.[8]

Even if the Natural Death Directive pushes the "consent of the patient" to the forefront of consideration and even if a physician is extremely sensitive to the patient's expressed desire, the judgment of "salvageability" will be made. The duty to desist depends on it as well as upon the patient's orders. Yet it is not a judgment readily or lightly made.[9]

A third situation presents yet another paradox. Many patients suffering from a serious chronic disease may benefit from medical treatment over a long period of time. They may come to find their treatment burdensome and their lives increasingly difficult and futile. They tell their physician that, at the next crisis, they would prefer to be allowed to die as painlessly as possible. A Natural Death Directive is prepared in order to attest to this wish. When the next serious myocardial infarction occurs, the physician does not try to resuscitate; when the dialysis shunt clots, no revision is attempted. It seems impossible to interpret the law to fit this situation, desirable as it may seem to some patients and their physicians. Certainly, cardiac resuscitation will "prolong life"; a shunt revision and dialysis will prevent the imminence of death. These procedures may "salvage" the patient and restore him or her to their former life, burdensome as it was. It is likely this sort of case will represent the most frequent application of the Natural Death Act, despite the awkwardness, indeed, the impossibility of its fit. These cases, of course, will never stand on their own; they will, in the end, come to the attention of the physician in the guise of the first two sorts of cases we have described. It is best for those who seriously wish to die that they never come to the attention of physicians at all!

Discussion

The California Natural Death Act is young. How it will be interpreted by the courts and used by the public and the medical profession remains to be seen. However, at the beginning of its tenure, it poses a difficult problem. The essence of the problem is this: where its application is clearest, it is least relevant; where it is most relevant, it seems most difficult to apply. However, its problematic nature does not render it a useless piece of legislation. In my judgment, it is useful precisely for the problems it creates.

The problem can be put quite directly: the law creates a duty to desist from medical care when two conditions are verified, evidence of a valid refusal of care on the part of the patient, and a judgment of imminence of death on the part of the physician. The law spells out the manner in which a valid refusal of care is effected; it is silent on how a judgment of imminence of death is to be made. This silence is, of course, understandable. It is the task of medical science, not law, to explain how a physician should judge the imminence of death. However, modern medicine has little to say about the imminence of death. That is the problem. The distinguished medical philosopher, Dr. Otto Guttentag,[10] has written, "Textbooks of physiology do not list the subject of death in their indices."

Long before the emergence of patients' rights," physicians recognized their duty to desist was created by the fact that none of their skills could be effectively employed to reverse the course of a disease toward death. "There is nothing more I can do," was the acknowledgment of that duty. To continue treating, after that judgment, was unethical because it was simply dishonest. As more "things to do" became available and even more existed around the next research corner, this aspect of the duty to desist seemed to fade. The duty to treat engulfed it. In order to correct the extreme manifestations of the duty to treat, ethics and law, exemplified in this legislation, stressed the patient's right to refuse. This emphasis must not be allowed to obscure the earlier and essential component—the judgment to be made about the futility of care in the face of imminent death.[11] This judgment must be learned and taught in clinical medicine.

To some extent that judgment might be learned and taught in the intensive care unit. At present, the growing realization that a patient is shifting from an "acute" to a "chronic" case generates considerable anxiety. The anxiety is sometimes manifested by a *furor therapeuticus,* a flurry of new drugs and manipulations. Awareness of the problem of prolonging death may slowly inspire more caution and circumspection. More explicit orders for management may reveal more about the futility of certain procedures under certain circumstances.[12, 13] Scrutiny of the "other than medical reasons" which prompt some actions may make clearer the complex motivations that urge vigorous intervention in some cases and benign neglect in others.[14] The day of the clinical-pathological-ethical conference is at hand.

However, much more can be learned outside the intensive care unit. In one sense, the judgment of the "imminence of death" can often be made years before death comes. Oncologists and neurologists often make it on the occasion of the first diagnostic visit. Death hangs over their patient in a way quite unlike the shadow of death which lurks behind us all.

The management of the patient through the intervening treatment ought to acknowledge this imminence or proximity of death. Early plans must be laid by patient and physician to avoid the ultimate ethical perplexities of emergency and intensive care. The emergence of an honest and ethical approach to terminal illness and of forms of excellent medicine devoted to the easing of death rather than its defeat may make such planning more possible than ever before.[15-17]

A cloud of particular problems—psychological, medical, legal, economic, cultural—surrounds the ultimate human problem, death. It will certainly always be so. The California Natural Death Act will hardly solve them. Indeed, it may create more. It is probably impossible to write legislation which can deal with them. However, the importance of this legislation transcends the literal interpretation of its words and provisions. Even if it has but a narrow application for literalists, it should inspire physicians and educators of physicians to look again at a vital element in medical ethics, the duty to desist from medical care, not only when the patient refuses one's service, but when that service does not, in fact, serve the end of medicine, the correction of disease,

and the repair of injury. Often one hears, "let's try it, it probably won't hurt," which is an echo of the ancient maxim of medicine, "do no harm." But the harm done by useless treatment should remind physicians of a modification of that maxim: Thomas Sydenham,[18] the father of modern clinical medicine, said, "When I perceive my remedies really will do no good, I consider it is better I do nothing at all."

NOTES

1. R.M. Veatch, *Death, Dying and the Biological Revolution,* Yale University Press, New Haven and London, 1976.

2. California Assembly Bill 3060.

3. California Health and Safety Code. Part 1, division 7, chapter 3.9, sections 7185–7195.

4. M. Garland, "The Right to Die in California," *Hastings Center Report,* vol. 6, p. 5, October 1976.

5. F. Epstein, "The Role of the Physician in the Prolongation of Life," in Ingelfinger et al. (eds.): *Controversy in Internal Medicine,* II, p. 103, W. B Saunders Co., Philadelphia, 1974.

6. N. Caroline, "Dying in Academe," *New Physician,* vol. 21, p. 665, November 1972.

7. M.G. Netsky, "Dying in a System of "Good Care": Case Report and Analysis," *Pharos,* vol. 39, p. 57, April 1976.

8. D. Crane, "Physician Attitudes toward Ill Patients," in J. Behnke and S. Bok (eds.), *The Dilemmas of Euthanasia,* p. 114, Anchor Press-Doubleday, New York, 1975.

9. R. Glaser, "A Time to Live and a Time to Die: The Implications of Negative Euthanasia," in J. Behnke and S. Bok (eds.), *The Dilemmas of Euthanasia,* p. 133, Anchor Books-Doubleday, 1975.

10. O. Guttentag, "On the Clinical Entity," *Annals of Internal Medicine,* vol. 31, p. 484, 1949.

11. K. Lebacqz, "Against the California Natural Death Act," *Hastings Center Report,* vol. 7, p. 14, April 1977.

12. Critical Care Committee of the Massachusetts General Hospital, "Optimum Care for Hopelessly Ill Patients," *New England Journal of Medicine,* vol. 295, p. 362, 1975.

13. S. Imbus and B. Zawacki, "Autonomy for Burned Patients When Survival Is Unprecedented," *New England Journal of Medicine,* vol. 297, p. 308, 1977.

14. D. Crane, *The Sanctity of Social Life: A*

Study of Doctors' Decisions to Treat Critically Ill Patients, Russell Sage Foundation, New York, 1975.

15. C. Saunders, "A Therapeutic Community—St. Christopher's Hospice," in *Psychological Aspects of Terminal Care,* Colorado University Press, Denver, 1972.

16. E. Cassell, "Permission to Die," in J. Behnke and S. Bok (eds.), *The Dilemmas of Euthanasia,*

p. 121, Anchor Press-Doubleday, New York, 1975.

17. Swiss Academy of Medicine, "Guidelines on Care of the Dying," *Hastings Center Report,* vol. 7, p. 30, June 1977.

18. T. Sydenham, Epistolary Dissertation 134, in R.G. Latham (ed.), *The Works of Thomas Sydenham,* vol. II, p. 115, The Sydenham Society, London, 1850.

77.

The Deformed Newborn: Medical Aspects
Angela R. Holder

Newborn babies unfortunately are not always perfect human beings. Many of them have serious defects. One in 600 has Down's disease. Down's babies do not die of being mongoloid, and the question of allowing such a child to die arises because these children also have a very high rate of physical anomalies such as heart problems or intestinal obstructions. Other newborns, however, have serious conditions that may cause mental retardation and/or serious physical handicaps that will usually result in their death without surgical intervention. In this category fall, for example, infants with myelomeningocele. Until recently children in both groups rarely survived the first few days of life. As neonatal surgery has improved, however, these children can be kept alive after surgery to grow up with serious handicaps.

Nineteen percent of the children in one study who were born with myelomeningocele but who were not treated survived for a year; thus, they were likely to remain alive indefinitely. Where active treatment is given, including several operations shortly after birth, most survive, but of that number virtually all are totally paralyzed from the waist down and incontinent with no present hope for improvement. As a result of the accompanying hydrocephalus, at best 40 per-

cent of these children will be intellectually normal. Of the other 60 percent, the degree of retardation may vary from moderate to so severe that the child is in effect properly termed "a vegetable." In typical cases by the time a child of normal intelligence with myelomeningocele reaches his ninth birthday, he will have had 18 major operations to maintain his life, not to allow him to walk.

As one pediatric surgeon writes:

All pediatric surgeons, including myself, have "triumphs"—infants who, if they had been born 25 or even five years ago, would not have been salvageable. Now with our team approaches we can wind up with "viable" children three and four years old, well below the 3rd percentile in height and weight, propped up on a pillow, marginally tolerating an oral diet of sugar and amino acids and looking forward to another operation.

The increasing efficiency of pediatric surgery has created the dilemma in which a pediatrician finds himself, because prior to the early 1960s the question was irrelevant, since there was nothing that could be done for the children even if treatment was desired.

Some persons argue that a child should not be declared to be a "person" at all

Source: Angela R. Holder, *Legal Issues in Pediatrics and Adolescent Medicine,* John Wiley and Sons, Inc., New York, 1977.

for some stated time after birth. For example, one writer has argued, in determining what to do about a defective child, "It may be that two or three days or weeks of probationary life should be accepted as a period during which doctors could check for defects and parents could decide whether or not they wanted to keep and rear a damaged baby."

We must first look to the law for a determination of when a "person" becomes a person. Legally, a human being is entitled to all the rights and statuses possessed by all other human beings from the time he is born. Prior to that moment, as has been indicated in the earlier chapters in this book, it is at least highly debatable that our legal system recognizes the fetus as a human person in terms of protection of his rights. Once his first breath is drawn, however, and he signifies that he is alive, even if such a period of viability is a very short one and he dies in a few minutes, that baby in the eyes of the law has joined the human race and is entitled to the protection of our legal system.

A legal system of any type, including ours, is obliged to deal with status questions on a mass basis. Individual variances normally cannot be accommodated because in many status situations it is more important that the law be certain and easily ascertainable than that it be correct. Thus, an unusually mature 12-year-old has no claim to a variance in order to obtain a driver's license, which, by statute, is restricted to those 16 and over. Whether one is married de facto may be subject to a discussion of human covenants and/or ethical obligations; de jure one is either married or one is not. Whether one is "alive" for legal purposes is also not amenable to individual variances because of the enormous implications of the status. Therefore, the legal system quite sensibly has chosen the moment of birth as the moment of being alive. It is an easily ascertainable moment, understood by all, and it can be universally applied to the population. Thus, for administrative convenience, if for no better reason, legally one cannot be a little bit alive. The question of nontreatment thus arises quite clearly in the legal context that to fail to treat a deformed baby and allow him to die is indisputably allowing a living person to die.

The argument that no treatment should be given to a severely deformed newborn is predicated on the theory that the long-term physical suffering and mental anguish of the child, his parents, and perhaps his other siblings, their economic losses, their future prospects, and their other human interests, make it more merciful for both child and parents if the child dies within the first few hours or days of life.

One noted pediatric neurosurgeon has written of babies with myelomeningocele:

> There are large numbers who are so severely handicapped at birth that those who survive are bound to suffer from a combination of major physical defects. In addition, many will be retarded in spite of everything that can be done for them. It is necessary to enumerate all that this means to the patient, the family and the community in terms of suffering, deprivation, anxiety, frustration, family stress and financial cost. The large majority surviving at present have yet to reach the most difficult period of adolescence and young adult life and the problems of love, marriage and employment. . . . It is unlikely that many would wish to save a life which will consist of a long succession of operations, hospital admissions and other deprivations, or if the end result will be a combination of gross physical defects with retarded intellectual development.

Others who argue that medical ethics allows or perhaps requires nontreatment maintain that the harm done to the baby's family by his life outweigh the benefits of allowing that life to continue. In their view the minimal benefit of treatment of a person incapable of full development does not justify the burden that care of the defective infant imposes on parents, siblings, and others. Caring for such a child is far more difficult and the costs are greater

than for any normal child. The rewards
common with parenthood of a normal pre-
schooler do not exist. It is not at all uncommon for parents of a handicapped child
to get a divorce when economic and emotional resources are exhausted to the breaking
point and either the husband or the wife
just runs away.

It is not seriously questioned that pediatricians everywhere are willing to allow
these children to die. There is simply no open
admission of the practice.

Raymond Duff and A. G. M. Campbell of
Yale Medical School published an article
in 1973 in the *New England Journal of Medicine* in which they discussed the fact that
43 newborn babies died from deliberate withholding of treatment in the Yale-New Haven
Hospital after consultation between parents
and physicians. All these children would
have been seriously defective. Their report
raised the issue that no one else had been
willing to discuss openly. Their thesis was
that the parent has the right to decide
whether or not the child should be treated
if the handicap is sufficiently serious so
that physicians conclude that treatment cannot give the child a normal life. It is generally conceded, as the authors wrote, that
there are limits on vigorous applications
of treatment to extend life for deformed
newborns, but the limits largely depend on
the ethical view of the physician in charge.

As has been demonstrated in many studies,
initial parental response to the knowledge
that a newborn child is seriously defective is
usually one of rejection of the child. John
Fletcher writes:

Despite a readiness in modern consciousness to accept a scientific explanation
of congenital defects, both literature
about and experience with parents
of defective newborns in the United
States and Great Britain shows almost
a universally negative initial reaction
to the child and a personal assumption
of guilt on the part of the parents.
Grief and anger are almost universal
responses.

Unfortunately, at the very moment when
the parents are overwhelmed with feelings
of rejection of the child, they are called on to
consent or to withhold consent to life-
saving treatment. The mother has just been
through labor and delivery and is usually
exhausted, since most of these decisions have
to be made within the first few hours after
birth. A normal and common response in the
first moments or hours of being presented
with this situation is anger at the baby for
putting the parent in this position, a purely irrational response but one that is perfectly
understandable. Fletcher points out:

The parental response to the newborn defective usually represents an initial rejection based upon disappointed hope, and
the rejection may be conditioned by
two factors, one, the nature of the defect
and two, the social status of the parents. They feel disgusted, grieved, helpless, full of rage, and it is very common
in handicapped children who obviously will not die for parents to wish first to
get rid of the child, and this feeling is
followed by intense guilt, blame and intense anxiety.

Where the decision for or against surgery
has to be made at a time before the parents have worked through their wish to "get
rid of" the child, they may make a decision not to treat, which could very easily fill
them with guilt and horror later, thus raising serious problems in the physician-parent
relationship.

Because of the peculiar vulnerability of
the parents at this moment, the physician,
whether he wants to or not, plays an extremely important role in helping them make
a determination of what to do, but he
does so as an ethicist, not as a treating physician. An editorial in the same issue of the
New England Journal as Duff and Campbell's
article, entitled "Bedside Ethics for the
Hopeless Case," indicates that the physician
is and should be the one to decide to live
with that decision. The author states:

So when Duff and Campbell ask "who decides for the child" the answer is you:

you, the child's doctor, for who else is in a similarly pivotal position to make sure that the proper medical consultation has been obtained in ascertaining the hopeless condition of the patient, that the parents receive sympathetic and thorough explanation, that they are exposed to broadly based advice? Who else can lead all those involved to a decision and who else is more responsible for consoling after the decision has been reached? Social ethics, institutional attitudes and committees can provide the broad guidelines but the onus of decision-making ultimately falls on the doctor in whose care the child has been put.

This may be a much more honest view than any writers' attempts in this context to argue for the possibility of meaningful parental consent. If the physician raises the issue of nontreatment with the parents at all, it may be assumed that by so doing he is indicating the parents do have a choice. Presumably he would not make such a choice available if he thought there were any indications that the child could be given a near-normal life. Duff clearly stated that any physician would get a court order for surgery on a defective newborn if the child's condition was not one in which the physician thought a failure to treat was medically justifiable. Where, for example, the defect was cosmetic, such as a club foot, the author indicated that he would not hesitate to get a court order consenting to surgery and in fact has done so. Thus, the medical context within which the decision to treat or not to treat is made is that the physician offers the parent the option only if he thinks the child should not be treated. If parents initiate discussion of allowing the child to die under circumstances in which the physician thinks treatment is indicated, he is not bound by their desires. It is obvious that the parents are doing what the physician thinks best, no matter how conscientiously the physician attempts to make them aware that the right of decision is theirs and not his.

It may be hypocritical not to say so. Some pediatricians, unlike Duff and Campbell, simply make a unilateral decision not to treat the child, do not discuss it with the parents, and announce either at the time of delivery or shortly thereafter that the child was born dead. This may lead to a malpractice suit, but in many ways, unless one believes that there is a duty to apply vigorous treatment in all cases, this seems to be more honest than maintaining that the parents made the choice. On any rational basis the choice should be the parents', but it may be logically impossible that the choice can ever genuinely be the parents'. As one neurosurgeon writes:

> Parents should obviously be part of such a decision, but their decision can hardly be an informed one. Despite the best efforts of the physician to educate parents, such education and full understanding of the consequences cannot take place in the short time before a decision should be made.

Under the circumstances, when the parents are in shock and feeling enraged by the child and wish to reject him, they cannot make the same type of rational decision they would make in calmer contexts, and the physician obviously has assumed more influence over what that decision will be than he does in most other treatment situations by his presentation of a choice at all. In this context the ethics of a physician-patient relationship are quite different from the one in which a physician sits in his office and discusses the merits and demerits of surgery for a rational, adult patient. Even if he must tell a patient that a life-threatening condition exists and radical surgery is necessary, the patient rarely must decide to have treatment or to forgo it within the few minutes within which the decision to treat a newborn frequently must be made.

In terms of the aspects of this situation, the physician should realize that he is probably making the decision. If a physician can console himself with the idea that it was really the parents' choice and that he himself did not decide not to treat a child, he could become less sensitive to the medical needs of his patients. As an editorial in the *Journal of Pediatrics* has pointed out, "It is not the patient or the problem that goes away—it is the physician who goes away from the problem, leaving the family and the patient to suffer."

None of the commentators who have written on this subject doubts that the primary motivation for refusing to treat a defective newborn is unwillingness to struggle with the problems of life as the parent of a retarded child, and the retardation is the primary factor in the decision not to treat in most cases.

Several years ago there was a great deal of comment about a case at Johns Hopkins Hospital where parents refused permission to operate on a mongoloid baby who took 15 days to starve to death. Nearly everyone who has commented on this case has disagreed with the decision, and most objection has centered on the fact that the child took so long to die.

Only one trial court decision exists on this subject.

Baby Houle was born on February 9, 1974, in the Maine Medical Center. His entire left side was malformed, he had no left eye, he was practically without a left ear, he had a deformed left hand and some of his vertebra were not fused. He also had a tracheal fistula and could not be fed by mouth. Surgery for repair of the fistula, the only immediate threat to his survival, could have been performed easily, but the parents refused to consent. Several physicians at the medical center, including the pediatric surgeon who was to operate, felt differently and took a neglect case to the Superior Court. The trial judge ordered the surgery to be performed and stated in his Order: "At the moment of live birth there does exist a human being entitled to the fullest protection of the law. The most basic right enjoyed by every human being is the right to

life itself." The child died the day after the surgery was performed.

At the time Baby Houle was born, there was no suspicion of brain damage, but as a result of either heart or lung abnormalities his blood transmitted insufficient oxygen and his brain was quickly damaged. His reflexes deteriorated, and prior to the last day of his life he had ceased to kick when his knee and ankle were touched. One physician said that the six-day delay between his birth and the surgery ordered by the court had caused a gradual deterioration and that if he had been operated on at once he could have been saved.

Apparently the defects were primarily cosmetic and yet the parents elected not to treat. From all reports of this case, the child was not paralyzed and, with extensive treatment, could have enjoyed all the activities that anyone with one eye can lead.

Peter Rickham, a pediatric surgeon in England, has written an article in which he divides infants into five categories: (1) infants who are likely to be completely cured by surgery, (2) infants who after treatment will be handicapped to some extent but still may be able to lead a relatively normal life, (3) infants who after treatment will have a severe physical handicap and will have to lead a more or less sheltered life, (4) infants in classes 1 to 3 who in addition are of subnormal intelligence but who can be trained to some extent, (5) infants in classes 1 to 3 who in addition are idiots, leading a vegetable existence. Rickham points out that these classes denote different degrees of "living as human beings" and continues, "One might ask whether the class five can be regarded as being humanly alive in the sense in which we usually understand those words" and would allow nontreatment only for that group.

My own ethical views differ markedly from those of any ethicists who have written on this question. It seems to be legally mandatory for treatment to be instituted if it can cure the condition for which it is performed. If a Down's baby has an intestinal obstruction or, as in Baby Houle's case, an infant has a fistula, either one of which can be cured by relatively simple surgical procedures *and if* those procedures would clearly be performed by court order if necessary on an otherwise normal newborn, then it is arguable that treatment is legally required.

On the other hand, neurosurgery for a paralyzed newborn is by no means "ordinary care," since normal babies do not require it. Second, the condition for which surgery might be performed is not curable, and thus the operation may be regarded as both futile and one that would subject the baby to more pain than he would have felt if left alone. Third, if the child survives he may well have sufficient self-awareness to suffer the agonies of knowing his limitations and to be tormented by them. Thus, it may be possible to justify as good medical practice a determination that a child whose condition is incurable should not be subjected to surgery for that condition solely to keep him alive.

78.

Ethical Problems in the Management of Myelomeningocele and Hydrocephalus
John Lorber

Within the last generation the application of major advances in drug therapy, intensive care, transfusion techniques, surgery, anesthesia, and radiotherapy, together with a vast expansion of knowledge due to increased investigative facilities, have led to an unprecedented, dramatic, and beneficial increase in the number of persons who would previously have died or lived with severe handicaps but can now be cured.

Techniques have also been developed to prolong the lives of many people who are now able to enjoy several extra years of productive and meaningful existence, and to alleviate and improve the quality of life of many seriously handicapped persons, enabling them to become integrated as useful and contented members of the community.

Choosing from numerous examples of pediatric experience, it is notable that many more extremely premature infants now survive without physical or intellectual damage; infection can almost always be cured, including neonatal and all other forms of pyogenic meningitis and the now rare cases of tuberculous meningitis and miliary tuberculosis.

The few remaining new cases of Rh-hemolytic disease are also readily cured. There are outstanding successes in the treatment of childhood malignancy. Pediatric surgery has made great strides. The prognosis of congenital heart disease, of obstructions of the alimentary canal, and many other conditions has improved beyond recognition.

Unfortunately, the indiscriminate use of advanced techniques of all types has also kept alive those who would have died but now live with distressing physical or mental handicaps or both, often for many years, without hope of ever having an independent existence compatible with human dignity. There are many examples, including those who have sustained major brain or spinal cord injuries.

Source: *Nursing Times*, February 26, 1976.

Spina Bifida and Hydrocephalus

These modern techniques have been used on a massive scale for the treatment of infants born with spina bifida and hydrocephalus. There are many who have benefited greatly and more will continue to benefit in the future but, unfortunately, there are also large numbers who have suffered from the uncritical application of technological advances. It is to be hoped that with the knowledge of this experience, further unnecessary disasters will be avoided.

Spina bifida has existed throughout human history. Ferembach showed that malformations of the lumbosacral vertebrae were common in 12,000-year-old skeletons. Hippocrates was aware of the condition. It was Tulpius, the teacher in Rembrandt's *The Anatomy Lesson,* who described and illustrated it in 1652, and who first called the condition spina bifida. In 1714, von Ruysch distinguished between the paralytic and nonparalytic forms, and later, Morgagni (1761) first associated hydrocephalus with spina bifida, and described hydrocephalus which was not associated with spina bifida. It was in 1883 that Cleland first described the almost constant anatomical malformation of the hind brain, now called Arnold-Chiari malformation, as well as the now well recognized associated lacunar skull.

Treatment of Myelomeningocele

The treatment of simple meningocele, without neurological involvement, will not be discussed here because the indications and techniques are not controversial, the results are good, and the subject raises no ethical or moral issues. An infant born with myelomeningocele, however, is very different because treatment raises complex surgical, medical, and ethical problems.

There are five phases in the history of the treatment of myelomeningocele. The first phase lasted from the beginning of mankind until the late nineteenth century. No treatment was possible, and the majority of the sufferers died early in infancy, although a few less severely affected may have survived with variable degrees of handicap.

The second phase was a brief period in the late nineteenth century, when Morton (1877), a Glasgow surgeon, injected a solution of iodine in glycerin into the spina bifida sac and claimed success. Others followed him, but the method was soon forgotten, no doubt because it was impossible to treat the many other aspects of spina bifida. At about the same time Mayo-Robson (1885) attempted surgical excision and closure of the lesion, but his technique gained no acceptance and was abandoned. Nothing further happened until the middle of the twentieth century.

The third phase lasted some 20 years, up to 1958. There was more interest in treatment and an appreciable minority of patients were operated on at some centers. Treatment was highly selective. By now there was no difficulty in closing the spinal lesion, but there was little enthusiasm for such surgery because there was no adequate treatment for the associated hydrocephalus. Most infants were still left untreated and allowed to die, including some who might have had a reasonable prognosis.

Even in the most advanced neurosurgical center in Boston, Ingraham and his colleagues (1944) operated on infants only if they had no serious neurological lesions and had survived for at least a year or 18 months from birth, and if their general condition was then good. Most infants died of meningitis or of hydrocephalus or of other illnesses long before then. Matson (1969) adhered to a highly selective policy throughout his career.

In England more and more infants were treated during the early 1950s. Zachary, in Sheffield, and McNab, in London, were among the more active, and Naish (1956), also in London, was one of the first to carry out ileocutaneous urelerostomy on children with neurogenic incontinence of the bladder, with the object of reducing their handicap. During this third phase very few were operated on early in infancy, and those who were selected themselves as milder cases, often without significant hydrocephalus, by the fact that they had survived long enough to be treated. The results were nevertheless disappointing and far less satisfactory than might have been achieved in the same children had they had the total care known to be necessary and available for them today.

In Sheffield a more aggressive surgical policy was adopted in the early 1950s, and though the mortality was high, in 1974 it was possible to review the condition of 100 young survivors who were born before 1959. Although few of those born before 1957 had significant hydrocephalus, the condition of this initially favorable group was disappointing. About half were retarded, most had major physical sequelae, and very few were able to obtain or hold a job.

The fourth phase lasted from the late 1950s to the early 1970s. It was characterized by the vast increase in the number of infants treated and was brought about by a new shunt system developed by Holter, an American engineer. It was used by Spitz, for the first time, on Holter's own child. This shunt incorporated two unidirectional valves which opened at a predetermined pressure. With it, for the first time, it was possible to treat hydrocephalus adequately.

There had been many other forms of surgical treatment before this development, but none was satisfactory for this purpose. A little later, Pudenz introduced a slightly different shunt, using only one valve. Since then there have been many modifications and different types have been introduced in an attempt to avoid the many late complications of shunt therapy.

As hydrocephalus is present in over 80 percent of cases of myelomeningocele, and as untreated hydrocephalus is an important cause of mortality and morbidity, it is easy to see that a new technique that makes it possible for the child's head to grow at a normal rate and allows him a chance of developing with normal intelligence could lead to uncritical enthusiasm

to treat all infants with myelomeningocele, irrespective of the severity of their condition at birth. This was the policy adopted in Sheffield and Liverpool and later, largely through moral pressure from these units, that was adopted all over the western world.

By the 1960s it was difficult for any doctor not to refer babies for surgery and for a surgeon not to operate, for fear of adverse criticism. The parents were hardly ever adequately consulted or informed. They usually understood that their baby had to be operated on and that they had to sign a document signifying their agreement, although most had very little idea what this signature meant for the future of their infant or for their family life.

Untreated severe cases. Nevertheless, not all units followed this pattern of treating all infants, even during this period. In Oxford, Edinburgh, and Melbourne the more severely affected newborn infants were not treated, though exact criteria for selective treatment were not laid down. In these series 2 to 10 percent survived for 2 years and the survivors were not necessarily in a worse condition than they would have been had they been treated. Every patient who was referred to the Liverpool unit was treated, but in 1960–1962 56 infants born in Liverpool were not referred to hospital; presumably they were the more severe cases. None survived for 6 months.

These results fit in with Laurence's experience in South Wales where between 1956 and 1962 all infants were left largely untreated. By 1972, 11 percent of 272 myelomeningocele cases were still alive. These must have included many initially mild cases, as 9 of the 31 survivors walked unaided and were continent. This series does not show that 11 percent of unoperated severe cases would have survived in the absence of early operation and full treatment.

Long-term results in Sheffield. In Sheffield, treatment was carried out on a wide scale. No patient was refused admission or full treatment and we accepted all the most difficult cases from a wide area. A combined team of pediatric and orthopedic surgeons, pediatricians, and all supporting services was set up in 1959. It was soon established that the best results were obtained if the infant's spina bifida was closed on the first day, and more and more of well over 1,000 patients treated during a 10-year period were admitted on the first day of life.

During this time we carried out much basic research and several therapeutic trials that would not have been possible without such large numbers. A sound neurological basis was established for the orthopedic care of our patients, and many ingenious orthopedic procedures were developed. The urological aspects received increasing attention. We were supported magnificently by the laboratory and our radiological colleagues, not to mention the parents and the parents' associations. We established a thriving research fund.

Between 1959 and 1968 we treated 848 infants with myelomeningocele from the first day of life. In spite of all the care, all the innumerable operations and medical treatment, only 50 percent survived. Most of the deaths occurred during the first year, but a quarter occurred later and there is a steady annual mortality of 2 percent. The commonest causes of the later deaths were shunt complications and progressive renal disease. Twenty percent of our shunt-treated children died as a direct result of shunt complications. It was much harder for parents to lose their child after several years of devoted care and after many operations than it would have been had they lost their child soon after birth.

Only 6 survivors (1.4 percent) have no handicaps, and a further 73 (17.2 percent) have what might be termed moderate handicap in a spina bifida context, though the combination of incontinence with partial paraplegic deformities and a well-controlled hydrocephalus may not be considered moderate by the patients or their parents.

Of the survivors, 345, or over 80 percent, have severe multisystem physical defects consisting of at least two but usually many more, of the following, in combination:

1. Incontinence of urine, or a urinary bypass, with frequent infections, hydronephrosis, or hypertension or impending renal failure. Incontinence of the bowel.

2. (a) Considerable paraplegia, often with gross deformities of the legs and feet. They require calipers, elbow sticks, or rollators and wheelchair. Many can only take a few laborious steps and others are fully chair-bound.
(b) Gross kyphosis, scoliosis, or lordosis, alone or in combination. A lot of these have undergone heroic surgery with improvement, but the relapse rate is very high.
(c) Repeated fractures, unreduced or recurrent dislocated hip joints. Many children had had well over 10 orthopedic operations by the time they reached secondary school.
(d) Recurrent trophic ulcers that may take months to heal.

3. Shunt-treated hydrocephalus requiring several revisions. The child with the largest number of revisions has had 17, so far.

4. Blindness, fits, sexual precocity, gross obesity, and other less common defects.

Intellectual development: Employment. Almost all the moderately handicapped and 59 percent of the physically severely handicapped children are of normal intelligence with an IQ of 80 or more. There are, however, 144, or 41 percent of the physically handicapped who are retarded, and 51 of these (14 percent) are profoundly retarded, chair-bound, or bedridden, and a few even have an abnormally large head. If we had a similar number of severely handicapped children who had not been treated, we would rightly be horrified and justifiably be criticized by others. Yet, for every such untreated child who was referred to us in later life, we have at least 30 such children in spite of all the effort we have made on their behalf.

No person with severe handicaps is likely to be able to earn his living in competitive employment, unless his IQ is at least 100. This statement is borne out by the experience of our patients in the earlier series who have now left school. Yet we have very few with an IQ of over 100. It is unlikely that more than 5 percent of the 848 admitted during this 10-year period will be able to earn their living: fewer will have a chance to marry.

Lessons of the fourth phase. It became more and more obvious that the pendulum, which was at one extreme in the first three phases in the history of the treatment of myelomeningocele, had swung to the other extreme in the fourth. In spite of a progressively increasing survival rate to some 60 percent, the problems we created were greater than those we solved.

With increasing technical experience we could save more and more badly handicapped children, without increasing the proportion of the less severely affected. Treating all babies, without selection, resulted in much suffering for large numbers, in spite of the massive effort of large and devoted teams. The cost of the medical care and of the special education of each severely handicapped child exceeded £50,000 by the time they had reached 16 years of age.

The problems created by a severely affected child often have disastrous effects on family life. A large proportion of the mothers are on tranquilizing drugs and more need them. Young parents age prematurely through constant anxiety and recurrent crises. The upbringing of brothers and sisters suffers. Some families break up. Perhaps worst of all, because severely affected infants were "saved," many more potentially normal lives never started because their parents did not dare to have other children.

Selection for Treatment

Five years ago a detailed analysis of a group of 524 patients was presented to the Society for Research in Hydrocephalus and Spina Bifida in Freiburg. In this analysis an attempt was made to find, if possible, suitable criteria for selective treatment. It was essential to find such criteria so that no infant should be denied good treatment if he had a chance of surviving with only moderate handicaps. This meant that some infants who would end up with severe handicaps would still be treated because, after a complete neurological examination, it is easy to forecast, on the first day of life, the minimum handicap any patient will have later on, but not what complications or deterioration will occur later, and the actual eventual handicap is often more severe than anticipated.

Fortunately, it was possible to find criteria that could be readily detected by an expert in this field, without wasting time and without recourse to elaborate or costly investigations.

No child who had any one or a combination of the following physical signs survived with less than severe handicaps:

1. A large thoraco-lumbar or thoraco-lumbo-sacral lesion.
2. Severe paraplegia with no innervation below the L3 segment.
3. Kyphosis or scoliosis clinically evident at birth.
4. Gross hydrocephalus, as shown by a head circumference exceeding the 90th centile by at least 2 cm.
5. Other gross congenital defects, for example, congenital heart disease.
6. Severe cerebral birth injury or intracranial hemorrhage.

In addition, if an infant whose spinal lesion is closed and who already has hydrocephalus develops meningitis, this infant should be treated only with analgesics.

Finally, the infant's social condition should be considered in detail. The fate of an abandoned or unwanted child is very grave, even if his physical condition is a little better than those with major adverse criteria. These criteria were subsequently adopted as a basis for selection.

The main object of selection is not to

avoid treating those who would die early in spite of treatment, but to avoid treating those who would survive with severe handicaps. Therefore, it is essential that the criteria against treatment should not be any less severe than those suggested above.

Admittedly, it is difficult to forecast future intelligence for any individual baby with certainty, though the presence and the degree of hydrocephalus are important pointers. Stein and his colleagues in Philadelphia claim that there is close correlation between the presence of lacunar skull in early infancy and later intellectual development. The mean IQ of 85 survivors who had lacunar skull was 63.8 in contrast with 95.8 in those 71 who did not have lacunar skull. They propose that babies with craniolacunia should not be treated.

Unfortunately, our experience on a similar number born between 1967 and 1969 did not confirm these findings. Using our criteria, some children who would have survived with normal intelligence will be excluded from treatment and will die. Nevertheless, it is my experience, as it is that of psychologists, social workers, teachers,

and parents, that those young people who are severely handicapped by multisystem defects suffer far more if they have normal intelligence than if they are retarded. Only the intelligent realize fully what they have been through, what they have missed and will miss. Only the intelligent will worry about the frustrations of employment, loneliness, lack of opportunity and of normal family life. Only they will worry about their future and who will look after them when their parents are too old or are no longer alive.

Had we not treated any infant who had adverse criteria at birth we would not have lost a single child who now survives with only moderate handicaps. In other words, all those who had one of these criteria and survive are permanently and severely handicapped.

The case and indications for selective treatment were overwhelming. Such a conclusion could not have been reached without the vast experience gathered during the nonselective approach in the preceding 10 years.

79.
The Duty to Prolong Life   Angela R. Holder

A legal issue may arise when a normal child develops a terminal illness in which treatment to prolong life is available but would leave the child severely handicapped for his remaining life, as the following example illustrates: A school-age child who has developed normally and who is of normal or above-normal intelligence (i.e., is unquestionably consciously aware of his situation) becomes ill and a brain tumor is diagnosed. There is no possibility that the child can be cured, but surgery is available that will prolong life for some considerable time, perhaps a year or more, during which it is conceivable that new procedures to save the child's

life will be developed. The surgery will leave the child's intelligence, perceptions, and awareness unimpaired, but will utterly destroy his sight. Suppose that the parents decide that since the child will die rather quickly without surgery but will be able to lead a more normal life until almost the very end without being blind, they will refuse to consent to surgery. Are either the surgeon or the parents guilty of any criminal offense? It would appear that in this case they are not.

Given proper treatment, the child would not make a full recovery. It would appear that a refusal to permit treatment that

Source: Angela R. Holder, *Legal Issues in Pediatrics and Adolescent Medicine,* John Wiley and Sons, Inc., New York, 1977.

would allow the child to swallow, digest food, and breathe and when in its absence the child is condemned to die an agonized and painful death would constitute clear abuse, but as long as the effects of the surgery would be devastating to the child and cause him physical and mental pain, it is highly improbable that any court would hold that such an operation was necessary medical care. Thus, it would seem that a child in this situation, given such ordinary therapy as is reasonably available without undue discomfort to him and who thus dies months or perhaps a year before he would have with surgery has received treatment that has met the requirements of the law.

In this situation reasonable parental decisions, it would seem, should control. Unlike the case of a defective newborn, where the mother has not yet recovered from the effects of childbirth and where the diagnosis is a tremendous shock in addition to her physical exhaustion, the diagnosis of an older child as having a malignancy or some other disease does not present a situation in which a decision must be made within a few minutes or hours by at least one exhausted parent. Thus, the ethical dilemma of obtaining a genuinely informed consent is not presented.

It is clear that a mentally competent adult patient has the right to refuse on his own behalf lifesaving treatment that will prolong a miserable and painful existence. No ethicist, theologically inclined or otherwise, has argued that a terminally ill patient has any moral or ethical obligation to God, his family, or himself to consent to heroic measures that will only prolong his suffering or in fact increase it without offering any hope of recovery. In fact, the entire concept of "death with dignity," on which many books and articles have recently been written by eminent ethicists, reflects a growing concern with the refusal of many members of the medical profession to desist from extraordinary treatment when it is arguably inhumane to pursue it. [1]

It would seem, in this case, that a parent should be able to make the same decision for death with dignity for his child. As long

as ordinary care is provided, it would appear that the parents have a legal right to refuse extraordinary care.

Quite a different situation, however, would be presented by disagreeable but nonmaiming treatment. For example, children with leukemia are given drugs with severe side effects, including hair loss and nausea. They also must spend long periods of time in hospitals. If a parent refused to allow treatment on the ground that the child would suffer anguish from baldness or would get homesick in the hospital, it is presumable that any judge would rule that such chemotherapy is now "ordinary treatment" and that failure to provide it would constitute neglect. Furthermore, as research continues, the child in remission with leukemia and living a normal life may well eventually survive the disease. Where recovery even with a handicap is probable, there is probably an arguable ethical duty to treat a child, but whether a court would order brain surgery that would blind or paralyze a child but which could completely remove a tumor would undoubtedly depend less on strict adherence to common law than on the judge's personal philosphy. A decision either way could be based on the existing jurisprudence.

One pediatric hematologist has written about prolonged treatment of children with leukemia: "Personally, I will fight for every day if I have even the slightest chance of doing more than just gaining one more day. . . . I do not believe in throwing the towel in if there is any chance of even a small and temporary victory, but when defeat is completely certain with the medical armamentarium we have presently available, then we are entitled to use supportive care only and not overdo it." [2] This would appear not only to constitute good medical practice but also to comply with any requirements the legal system, civil or criminal, may demand.

The Child's Right to Die

Only one article can be located discussing a case of an adolescent who decided to refuse lifesaving treatment.

A 16-year-old girl with acute kidney problems received a transplanted kidney from her father. The transplant, however, failed and the girl was placed on hemodialysis. She tolerated this poorly, vomited constantly, and about 8 months after she began dialysis she announced following a lengthy period of acute illness that she no longer wanted to be maintained on hemodialysis. The parents concurred. Treatment was stopped and she died quickly.[3]

This child was evaluated by several psychiatrists, none of whom found any evidence of psychosis and all of whom were convinced that the girl had carefully thought out her decision and grasped its implications. The issue is whether the legal system should accept such a decision by a minor or whether the physician should ask the court to order treatment.

Most literature on the subject of the dying child indicates that prior to 14 or 15 years of age most children do not understand the real implications of death.[4] In numerous discussions of proper medical management of the emotional needs of a terminally ill child, most of which have involved children with acute leukemia, it becomes clear that even a very young child is aware of some terminal "events" which happen to other children in the hospital, at least that they disappear permanently, but it also seems clear that prior to adolescence it is extremely unlikely that a child has a serious concept of the meaning of death.[3]

The report of the girl with kidney disease indicated that it is rare that children who have not reached adolescence decide to die, but the statistics on children's suicides (probably before they fully comprehend the finality of their act) would appear to argue against that conclusion. It might be reasonable to argue the principle that prior to adolescence a child's rejection of lifesaving treatment should not be considered as being an informed consent and that the child prior to that time is incapable of comprehending the meaning of what he has decided.

If a 12-year-old child with bone cancer declined to consent to amputation of his leg because he would sincerely rather die than

live with one leg (which many boys at that age might very well believe), it is unlikely that a wise physician would accede to the child's request even if the parents agreed to be bound by the child's decision. The handicap would not be an overwhelming one. By contrast, if a younger child wished to discontinue hemodialysis, it would seem that a refusal by the parents to continue the treatment, even if instigated by the child's request, would probably be a valid and legal determination since there is no hope of normal life.

Assume, however, that a competent adolescent, aged 16 or 17, wishes to refuse treatment and the parents do *not* concur. The parents wish the child to be treated as completely as possible with life prolonged as long as possible. It would appear in this case that the physician is legally bound to abide by the judgment of the parents who are responsible for the child legally, morally, and economically.

It should be remembered that adolescents are generally consulted about a petition for court-ordered treatment if their parents refuse permission.

> In one case parents refused for religious reasons to allow surgery for a harelip and a cleft palate and the child was very vehement in his agreement with their views. The court held that ordering major surgery over the objection of the patient would diminish its success, since his full cooperation in postoperative therapy would be essential. The petition of the welfare department was therefore denied.

> A 17-year-old boy's parents refused for religious reasons to permit orthopedic surgery for a severe curvature of the spine if blood transfusions were to be used. Medical testimony indicated that the transfusions were vital. The appellate court remanded the case for the trial judge's determination of the boy's wishes and implied that those wishes would control and an order would issue if he wanted surgery.

It is perfectly sound logic and law to conclude that if a terminally ill child wants treatment and his parents do not, a physician is entitled to abide by a wish to preserve life and, if necessary, do so by court petition. The same principle should apply if one or both parents want to have the treatment given and the child does not.

Only two decisions can be located that have held that an adolescent has a right to refuse treatment if his parents wish him or her to have it, and in neither situation was the child in danger of death.

A 16-year-old pregnant girl wanted to marry her boyfriend and raise their child. Her mother wanted her to have an abortion, and the gynecologist asked the court to decide the issue. The trial court held, and the Maryland supreme court agreed, that the child could not be aborted against her will.

The Supreme Court of Connecticut held that a teenage boy had the right to be released from a mental hospital over his parents' objections since an adult would have had the right to leave at will and no claim was made that the boy was dangerous to himself or others.

In neither case would the issue appear at all analogous to that of an adolescent with a serious, intractable disease who wishes to refuse treatment, since neither child was in any serious danger of death.

In most cases involving conflicts between parents and children the legal system automatically assumes that the parent is correct. While this assumption may be seriously questioned in cases involving commitments of children by parents to mental hospitals or juvenile institutions as unmanageable and in some other contexts, it does seem that where the child life is at stake, a conflict between the parents and the child should be resolved in favor of preservation of the child's life, even if treatment is given over the child's objection. Only when all three agree or the one parent who is available concurs with the child and it is also clear the child understands the meaning of a decision to die

should life-prolonging treatment that cannot restore the child to health be terminated.

If an emancipated child, either de facto (such as a runaway) or de jure, should refuse treatment for a condition that could be terminal without the full consent of the parent, who may not be available, it would appear to be extremely unwise as a matter of law for a physician to accede to an unmarried adolescent's "right to die" in the absence of clear and convincing proof that (1) reasonably normal function cannot be restored in any case and (2) the parents cannot possibly be located. Unless the parents are notified, come to the scene if they wish, and fully concur in the child's right to die, it would seem to be extremely unwise to allow an adolescent to make that decision on his own. A married minor whose spouse is an adult presumably should be requested and probably required to give consent before treatment is terminated. If both are minors, prudence would dictate parental consultation where a life is at stake.

NOTES

1. E.g., Paul Ramsey, *The Patient as Person.* Yale University Press, New Haven, Conn., 1970; "Facing Death," symposium, *Hastings Center Studies*, vol. 2, no. 2, May 1974; Jay Katz, *Experimentation with Human Beings,* Russell Sage Foundation, New York, 1972.

2. Rudolph Toch, "Management of the Child with a Fatal Disease," *Clinical Pediatrics*, vol. 3, no. 7, p. 423.

3. John Schowalter, Julian Ferholt, and Nancy Mann, "The Adolescent Patient's Decision to Die," *Pediatrics*, vol. 51, no. 1, p. 97, January 1973.

4. E.g., Albert J. Solnit and Morris Green, "Pediatric Management of the Dying Child: Part II, The Child's Reaction to the Fear of Dying," in *Modern Perspectives in Child Development*, International Universities Press, New York, 1963; Toch, footnote 2 at 2; Joel Vernick and Myron Karon, "Who's Afraid of Death on a Leukemia Ward?" *American Journal of Diseases of Children*, vol. 109, p. 393, May 1965.

80.

Passive Euthanasia of Defective Newborn Infants: Legal Considerations

John A. Robertson   Norman Fost

Parents and physicians now face a dilemma when infants with Down syndrome, myelomeningocele, and other birth defects require medical or surgical attention merely to stay alive. If parents withhold consent for medical care and the physician acquiesces, the infant may die. To provide the appropriate medical care, however, may maintain the existence of a being with only minimal capacity for personal development and human interaction.

Withholding treatment seems to have become a widespread, if not frequent, event. Widely publicized cases have arisen in Maine,[1] Arizona,[2] New York,[3] Denver,[4] and Los Angeles.[5] Duff and Campbell[6] reported 43 instances over a 2-year period in the newborn unit of a university medical center. A number of eminent physicians recently appeared before the Senate Subcommittee on Health and at that time justified the practice.[7] Leading textbooks and journals discuss indications for withholding treatment.[8,9]

Although the growing visibility of the practice has generated much ethical debate, discussion of the legality of the practice and the appropriateness of current law has been minimal. This absence is unfortunate for several reasons. The first and most important is that parents, physicians, and nurses may be risking criminal liability without awareness of the legal ramifications of their decisions. Physicians can hardly assist parents to reach an informed choice concerning treatment if they do not also disclose that their choice may have serious legal consequences. Also, analysis of the law may expose inconsistencies or inadequacies, and thus point the way to changes that will enhance the certitude and security of future decision making. Finally, the traditional legal concern with procedures for balancing conflicting interests may point the way to a reasonable solution to a perplexing dilemma of modern medicine.

This article briefly reviews the potential criminal liability of parents, physicians, and nurses involved in the decision to withhold ordinary care from defective newborn infants. Finding that any or all of them may be subject to criminal prosecution for murder, manslaughter, neglect, child abuse, or conspiracy, we then discuss some issues relevant to an evaluation of these policies. Finally, we propose an approach to the problem which avoids the excesses of present law and present practices. *The authors do not contend that the criminal liability here enumerated should necessarily be pursued*, nor is it clear as a practical matter that this would occur. Rather, we are concerned with elucidating the legal issues so that participants in such decisions can be fully informed, and legal policy, where desirable, altered.

Liability of Parents

Generally, homicide by omission occurs when a person's failure to discharge a *legal* duty to another person causes that person's death.[10] If the required action is intentionally withheld, the crime is either first- or second-degree murder, depending on the extent of premeditation and deliberation.[10] When the omission occurs through gross carelessness or disregard of the consequences of failing to act, the crime is involuntary manslaughter.[10]

In the case of a defective infant the with-

Source: Reproduced with permission from *Journal of Pediatrics*, vol. 88, p. 883, 1976, copyrighted by The C. V. Mosby Company, St. Louis, Missouri.

holding of essential care would appear to present a possible case of homicide by omission on the part of parents, physicians, and nurses, with the degree of homicide depending on the extent of premeditation. Following a live birth, the law generally presumes that personhood exists and that there is entitlement to the usual legal protections, whatever the specific physical and mental characteristics of the infant may be.[11] Every state imposes on parents a legal duty to provide necessary medical assistance to a helpless minor child. If they withhold such care and the child dies, they may be prosecuted for manslaughter or murder, as has frequently occurred when parents have refused or neglected to obtain medical care for nondefective children. Although no parent has yet been prosecuted for withholding care from defective neonates, the well-recognized rule would appear equally applicable to non-treatment of defective infants. Defenses based on religious grounds, or even on poverty, if public assistance is available, have been specifically rejected, and other legal defenses, such as the defense of necessity, may not apply.[12] While care may be omitted as "extraordinary" if there is only a minimal chance of survival, when survival is likely, treatment cannot be withheld simply because of cost or the future social disutility of the infant.[12]

In addition to homicide, parents may also be liable under statutes that make it criminal for a parent to neglect to support or to provide necessities, to furnish medical attention, to maltreat, to be cruel to, or to endanger the child's life or health.[12]

Liability of Attending Physician

The attending physician who counsels the parents to withhold treatment, or who merely acquiesces in their decision and takes no steps to save the child's life, may also incur criminal liability. Since withholding needed medical care by the parents would in many states constitute child abuse or neglect, the physician who knows of the situation and fails to report the case to proper authorities

would commit a crime in the 20 or so states where failure to report child abuse is a crime. While failure to report is only a misdemeanor, under the common law "misdemeanor-manslaughter rule" a person whose misdemeanor causes the death of another is guilty of manslaughter. Since reporting might have led to appointment of a guardian and thus saved the child's life, the physician who fails to report could be guilty of manslaughter.

The physician may also be guilty of homicide by omission (by the same reasoning discussed under Liability of Parents), because he has breached a legal duty to care for the child and thereby caused the child's death. The legal duty of the physician would be to intervene directly by carrying out the procedure, or at least to report the case to public or judicial authorities who may then intervene to save the child. The sources of this duty are several. One is the child abuse-reporting statutes, which impose a legal duty to report instances of parental neglect even in those states where failure to report is not criminal.

The duty may also derive from the physician's initial undertaking of care of the child. Although it may appear that by refusing consent the parents have terminated the physician's legal duty to care for the child, there are at least three possible grounds for arguing that the parents are not able to terminate the physician's obligations to the infant-patient, once the doctor-patient relationship has begun, if the patient will be substantially harmed by his withdrawal.

1. The first argument is based on the law of contract. The attending physician has contracted with the parents to provide care for a third party, the infant. Ordinarily the contract for services will be made with an obstetrician, a general practitioner, and/or a pediatrician before or at birth to provide all necessary medical care. When the child is born, this contractual obligation to provide services begins. Under the law of third-party beneficiary contracts, the parties contracting for services to another cannot terminate the obligation to a minor, if the minor would be thereby substantially harmed.[12] Since

the parents are powerless to terminate the physician's obligation to care for the child, the physician would have a legal duty to take such steps as are necessary to protect the interests of the child. If emergency treatment were required, the physician would be privileged to proceed without parental consent. In most cases and where feasible, the physician's duty would be better fulfilled by seeking the appointment of a guardian who could then consent to treatment.

The attending physician's contractual duty to care for the child despite parental denial of consent would not exist if the physician clearly agreed to treat the child only if normal or if the parents in engaging the physician made their agreement subject to modification in case of a defective birth. However, neither parents nor physicians are likely in prenatal consultations to be so specific. Prosecution could, of course, change prevailing practices.

2. Even if the contract theory were rejected, physicians would still have a legal duty to care for the child on the traditional tort doctrine that one who assumes the care of another, whether gratuitously or not, cannot terminate such care if the third person would be hurt thereby.[10] This rule is based on the idea that one who undertakes care prevents others who might have come to the infant's aid from doing so.[10] Again, the physician could withdraw or not treat only if he has taken steps to notify public or hospital authorities, which would protect the child by leading to the appointment of a guardian.

3. It could be argued that the physician would have a legal duty to protect the child on the ground that he has placed the child in peril through his role as a source of information for the parents. A person who puts another in peril, even innocently and without malice, incurs a legal duty to act to protect the imperiled person.[10] By giving the parents adverse prognostic information regarding the infant's handicaps, the economic and psychologic burdens to be faced by the parents, and so on, he may be the immediate cause of nontreatment of the infant, by leading the parents to a decision they would

not have made or perhaps even considered. Under this theory even a consultant might be liable if he communicated information which led to a nontreatment decision and death, particularly if the information was incorrect or unfairly presented and then he took no action to save the child.[12]

In addition to liability for homicide by omission or under the misdemeanor-manslaughter rule, the physician may also be subject to homicide liability as an accessory; an accessory is one who "counsels, encourages or aids or abets another to commit a felony."[10] This would be clearest in a case in which the physician counseled or encouraged the parents to withhold treatment. If the omission of care by the parent is criminal, then the physician's liability as an accessory follows. If the physician were indifferent to the child's fate, or preferred that it would live but felt obligated to provide the parents with all the facts, it is less likely he would be culpable, since the requisite intent would be lacking.[12]

The attending physician may be guilty of conspiracy to commit homicide or violate the child abuse or neglect laws. Conspiracy is an agreement between two or more parties to achieve an unlawful objective, with (in most jurisdictions) an overt action toward that end.[10] If parents and physician agree that a defective newborn infant should die, and take any action toward that end, conspiracy could exist. Similarly, a staff conference on a particular case could amount to conspiracy, if the attending physican and others agreed that medical or surgical procedures should be withheld from the child.[12]

Liability of Other Physicians and Nurses

Physicians other than the attending physician, such as consultants, house officers, and administrative personnel, might also incur criminal liability under the statutes and common-law principles reviewed above.

Nurses who participate or acquiesce in parental decisions to withhold treatment may also be at risk. While a nurse's care is subordinate to the orders of a physician, her legal duty is not fulfilled simply by carrying out physician orders with requisite skill and judgment. In some cases she is required to act independently or directly counter to the physician, if protection of the patient requires it. At the very least, she might be obligated to inform her supervisor. A finding consistent with this view was reached in *Goff* v. *Doctors Hospital of San Jose* where two nurses, the attending physician, and the hospital were held civilly liable when a patient died from postpartum cervical hemorrhage. The nurses were aware the mother was in peril but did not contact the attending physician, because they thought he would not come. The court found that they had a duty to report the situation to a superior.

The Possibility of Prosecution

The existence of potential criminal liability is no guarantee that parents, physicians, nurses, and hospitals will in fact be prosecuted, not that any prosecution will be successful. Parents who have actively killed defective children have often been acquitted (though not always), [13] and no parent has been prosecuted for withholding care from, as opposed to actively killing, a defective newborn infant. [13] Similarly, the only physicians prosecuted for homicide in euthanasia situations involved terminally ill patients, and both were acquitted. [13-15] No doctor has yet been prosecuted for passive euthanasia of a defective newborn infant.

The infrequency of past criminal prosecutions, however, may not be a reliable guide for the future. As the practice becomes more openly acknowledged, pressure may build to prosecute and some prosecution is likely, if only to clarify the law. The manslaughter conviction of a Boston physician for allegedly killing a viable fetus after removal from the uterus during a lawfully performed hysterotomy illustrates the dangers of ignoring the legal issues, and the politics of the process by which a prosecution might be initiated. Physicians, parents, and others may decide that they are willing to risk prosecu-

tion, or believe that the law should be broken. Such a position entails risks, and one cannot safely predict from past experience that criminal liability will never in practice be imposed.

Practical Implications for Physicians and and Hospitals

Parents and health professionals with experience in the complex and heart-wrenching decisions involving defective newborn infants might justifiably react to this legal synopsis with shock and rage. Such decisions are made by people trying to do what they think is best under extremely difficult circumstances. The suggestion that such sincere and well-intended decisions might be criminal is offensive.

The authors do not intend to suggest, in this review, that such criminal charges should be made, nor do we intend to comment, pro or con, on the ethical issues involved in such decisions. Our primary purpose is to suggest that criminal charges *could* be brought, given a susceptible case and a prosecutor willing to pursue it. Some legal scholars might reasonably disagree with the validity of such charges, and we would not predict that such proceedings would necessarily end in conviction. Many would have moral objections to the initiation of such a trial, whatever the law. But few would dispute that such a case could be brought to court and, conceivably, to conviction. The experiences of Dr. Edelin and the participants in the Quinlan cases demonstrate dramatically how parents and physicians involved in medical decisions which have occurred countless times without judicial interference can find themselves unexpectedly at the center of a raging controversy.

What are the implications of these possibilities for physicians and hospitals caring for such infants and desirous of avoiding prosecution? First, physicians could consider informing parents that criminal liability might attach to a nontreatment decision, so that parents could be sufficiently informed of the risk to seek legal advice. In addition, such parents might be informed that even if they do not wish to keep the child, they are legally obligated, at least until parental rights are formally terminated, to provide it with needed medical care. If the parents insist on risking prosecution, the physician might then inform them that he is legally obligated to take steps toward saving the infant's life. In some jurisdictions it would be sufficient to report the matter to the child welfare or other authorities prescribed in the child abuse-reporting laws; in others the physician or the hospital might have to initiate neglect proceedings. The parents cannot terminate the physician's legal duties by withholding consent or even by discharging him. The law does not permit a physician to avoid criminal liability by submitting to the wishes of the parents and doing nothing, if this will lead to injury or death of the infant.

To avoid liability, hospitals could adopt rules prohibiting medical staff from not treating defective newborn infants, or, at least, for following certain procedures when faced with those decisions. The procedure could include reporting such cases to hospital authorities who would then seek a judicial ruling authorizing treatment. Resort to judicial approval, however burdensome and painful in this situation, could perform several useful functions. It would shield parents, physicians, nurses, and hospitals from criminal liability, pass the burden of a difficult decision to a more impartial process, and provide an opportunity to test or challenge the law before rather than after criminal prosecution. If a court ruled for or against treatment, the decision could be appealed to state appellate courts, which could define more precisely the duties involved and, conceivably, permit nontreatment in specific cases. While time would not permit appellate review of most cases, such issues of broad public policy which are sure to recur can be reviewed even though the specific controversy has been resolved by death or treatment.

Evaluation of Legal Policy

Many persons who have experienced the dilemma of caring for defective newborn infants would disagree with current law. Duff and Campbell,[6] for instance, argue that "if working out these dilemmas in ways we suggest is in violation of the law . . . the law should be changed." They would grant parents and their physicians the final discretion to decide whether a defective infant should be treated, and hence live or die:[6]

We believe the burdens of decision making must be borne by families and their professional advisors because they are most familiar with the respective situations. Since families primarily must live with and are most affected by the decision, it therefore appears that society and the health professions should provide only general guidelines for decision making. Moreover, since variations between situations are so great, and the situations themselves so complex, it follows that much latitude in decision making should be expected and tolerated.

What law, if any, should govern this situation? Ideally, the law should provide clear rules and predictable enforcement while resolving conflicting interests in a way consistent with prevailing moral, personal, professional, and economic values. Satisfactory law in respect to the defective-infant dilemma depends on the answers to two questions. First, is there a definable class of human offspring from whom, under prevailing moral standards, ordinary medical care may be withheld without their consent? If withholding care can never be justified, the sole policy question is whether the existing legal structures best implement that goal or whether a new offense and penalty structure should be created. The second question arises after one concludes that withholding care in some instances may be morally justified or socially desirable, and asks who among parents, physicians, and other decision makers is best equipped to decide when care is to be withheld? Here policy will focus on criteria, procedures, and decision-making processes for implementing a social policy of involuntary passive euthanasia.

It is the first question over which moral and policy issue is most keenly joined and which is therefore most crucial. Supporters of present law argue that there is no reasonable basis for allocating the right to life among human offspring on the basis of physical and mental characteristics, or social contribution— that all are persons and all deserve the legal protections and rights accorded persons. [12, 16] Many defective newborn infants in fact are capable of achieving some meaningful existence; even if they are not, the social and other costs of maintaining them is but a minute portion of health expenditures. [12] State assistance may be available to parents of modest means, and, in any event, parents who do not wish to keep a defective child are free to terminate their legal obligations. Furthermore, a policy of allocating rights according to personal characteristics, capacity, or social utility requires an arbitrary choice among personal and social characteristics reflective of social, cultural, or racial bias which is easily abused and inconsistent with a democratic society. [17] Determining the right to life by the net social utility of a person's future pitches one onto a slippery slope, the bottom of which holds no person or value sacred as against social utility.

Opponents of the law argue that not only may we reasonably and carefully distinguish between human offspring by their capacities, but we can draw narrow boundaries which do not set us onto the slippery slope where all values are subject to social worth assessments. Given high social and personal costs in keeping alive human beings with only marginal ability for personal development or interaction, the delineation of such a class is justified. Proponents of this view need not hold that every child with Down syndrome or myelomeningocele should be treated, only that in some cases, such as anencephaly or myelomeningocele with an extremely unfavorable prognosis, [9] the defects are so extensive that nontreatment is morally and socially justified.

Due Process and Decision Making

A choice between these two positions depends ultimately on deeply held philosophical and religious views and is only partially susceptible to rational argument and mar-

shaling of evidence. Rather than attempt to persuade the reader to any one personal view or analyze the ethical issues of specific cases, we suggest that even if after reflection one decides that there is a class of defective newborn infants from whom treatment can be justifiably withheld, it does not follow that parents and physicians should be the sole judge in each case of who shall survive.

The question of specifying the class of defectives and circumstances in which treatment may be justifiably withheld remains. The claim is not that treatment may be withheld from any infant, or even from all infants with some defect, but rather that in some circumstances infants with certain kinds of anomalies should or need not be treated. [18] How then are that class and those circumstances to be identified? What checks or safeguards should exist to be sure that an infant meets those criteria?

The position offered by Duff and Campbell [6]—that parents and physicians should have absolute discretion to decide whether an infant should live or die—appears to go too far. Simply because nontreatment decisions are acceptable in some circumstances of extreme defect, it does not follow that parents and physicians should *always* be free to decide whether all defective infants should live or die. Otherwise they may decide not to treat infants with less extensive defects, whom few persons would agree should die. Indeed, there is no reason to think that parents and physicians would always consider all the factors relevant to a nontreatment decision and reach a socially justified choice. (1) The emotional trauma and conflict of giving birth to a defective newborn infant may make the parents incapable of careful consideration of the issues. [19, 20] (2) Given their own, often conflicting interests, parents and physicians might not scrutinize all factors or balance them out in a fair way. [12] Thus, many parents might decide against treating a baby with Down syndrome, and the physician might agree, even though neither social, financial, nor psychic cost in a particular instance would justify nontreatment. (3) Neither parents nor physicians can claim the special expertise in making complex ethical-social judgments which warrant giving them such broad authority.[21]

What is needed, then, is either a set of authoritative criteria describing the limited circumstances in which ordinary care may be withheld from defective newborn infants, or a process of decision making which minimizes the risk of abuses or mistakes. We do not here attempt to articulate those criteria, other than to point out that if nontreatment is ever justified, it is because the nature of the defect, developmental potential, cost to parent and society, etc., seems overwhelmingly to argue against treatment. Such criteria could be set forth for assessment by the medical and lay community and would have to be revised frequently to incorporate changing medical and social facts. Only in scrutinizing our reasons can we be sure that these decisions are in fact morally defensible. This would reduce the risk of arbitrary decision making and assure that infants are not being allowed to die for specious reasons. One problem concerns the process by which criteria would be formulated. Would a national commission, a legislature, or professional bodies be convened for this purpose? A second major difficulty with specific criteria is the almost limitless and unpredictable complexity of individual cases. Also, defining or articulating criteria in an open public way does lend legitimacy to the practice of taking life on grounds of social utility.

An alternative to the articulation of specific criteria would be a requirement for a better *process* of decision making. A concern with process demonstrates the solemnity of the commitment to life, and the exceptional nature of any deviation from that commitment. In addition, process can assure that criteria are being accurately applied, that limits exist, and that the possibilities of conflicts of interest are minimized.

The essence of due process is to maximize the probability that decisions will be made impartially after full consideration of all relevant facts and interests, rather than on the uncontested perceptions and self-interest of one party.[12,22] Such a process can be helpful, even if only advisory to parents and phy-

sicians, by exposing or sensitizing them to considerations which they might have ignored on their own. A legal conception of due process would entail turning over decision making to someone more likely to be disinterested than the parents or their private physician and assuring that the interests of the child are fully represented in that forum.[12] Alternative decision makers might include one or a group of physicians, a judge, or a mixed lay and medical committee: they could consider the need for decisions and reasons to be stated in writing, and in some cases, judicial review.[12] Although the notion of a "God committee" has been much maligned,[23] experience with institutional "human subjects" committees in recent years suggests that groups can be formed which will improve the ethical acceptability of controversial and complex medical decisions. One last alternative would be a strictly post hoc institutional review process of specific decisions, within the limits of confidentiality, similar to review of other hospital practices as occurs with tissue committees, clinico-pathologic conferences, and the like. One objection to this approach is that whatever change it produces is slow, and unjustified deaths might result in the interim.

A crucial theoretical problem in requiring due process would be the setting of limits within which the process must be invoked. If no defective infant can be allowed to die without due process, why should any nonconsenting patient be allowed to die? A requirement for inclusion of all such cases would involve a *reductio ad absurdum,* namely, review of every pediatric patient who dies under the care of a physician, since life can almost always be extended to some degree. The public concern over the defective newborn infant, however, does not seem to extend to patients who are teminally ill and allowed to die.

Judicialization of medical decision making is often inappropriate, but where long life is at stake, the forms and procedure of due process may serve to focus the precise issues and increase impartiality. Such process would limit the cases of passive euthanasia to the clearest ones, and thereby limit the precedent-expanding signifance of nontreatment.

Unless those who favor nontreatment are willing to subject their selection criteria to critical scrutiny, the practice could be presumed unjustified, and present legal policy countinued. If, as Duff and Campbell[6] say, the law needs to be changed, this should not be done unofficially in newborn nurseries but in the traditional open forums, such as legislatures or courtrooms. By claiming the right to act in ignorance or defiance of existing legal principles and statutes, the physician, parent, nurse, or hospital administrator claims a right which he would not ascribe to others.

We believe that resolution of this controversy by a criminal proceeding would not be desirable. We also believe that public opinion would be supportive of such decisions being made outside the courts, provided the public could be assured that the possibility of abuse is minimal. Such reassurance would at the least depend on a process of institutional or professional review. Alternatively, test cases could be brought anonymously through the legal system. Whatever the mechanism, public scrutiny and involvement is unlikely to disappear and the medical community can probably help patients best by actively participating in the structuring of a resolution, rather than responding to thrusts initiated by others.

NOTES

1. *Boston Globe,* Feb. 25, 1974, p. 1, col. 1.
2. *New York Times,* Jan. 18, 1974, p. 32, col. 8.
3. *Newark Star Ledger,* Oct. 3, 1973, p. 32, col. 8.
4. *Time,* March 25, 1974, p. 84.
5. R. Trubo, *An Act of Mercy: Euthanasia Today,* Nash, Los Angeles; 1973.
6. R.S. Duff and A.G.M. Campbell, "Moral and Ethical Dilemmas in the Special-Care Nursery," *New England Journal of Medicine,* vol. 289, p. 890, 1973.
7. *New York Times,* June 12, 1974, p. 18, col. 4.
8. F.D. Ingraham and D.D. Maton, *Neurosurgery of Infancy and Childhood,* p. 35, Charles C. Thomas, Publisher, Springfield, Ill., 1954.
9. J. Lorber, "Results of Treatment of Myelomenigocele," *Developmental Medicine and Child Neurology,* vol. 13, p. 279, 1971.
10. W. LaFave and A. Scott, *Handbook of Criminal Law,* p. 182, West Publishing Company, St. Paul, 1972.
11. J.A. Robertson, "Medical Ethics in the Courtroom," *Hastings Center Report,* vol. 4, p. 1, 1974.
12. J.A. Robertson, "Involuntary Euthanasia of Defective Newborns: A Legal Analysis," *Stanford Law Review,* vol. 27, p. 213, 1975.
13. J. Sanders, "Euthanasia: None Dare Call It Murder," *Journal of Criminal Law, Criminology and Political Science,* vol. 60, p. 351, 1969.
14. *New York Times,* Jan. 13, 1974, p. 44, col. 4.
15. *New York Times,* Feb. 10, 1974, p. 98, col. 3.
16. F. Grunberg, "Who Lives and Dies?" *New York Times,* April 22, 1974, p. 35, col. 2.
17. S. Bok, "Ethical Problems of Abortion," *Hastings Center Studies,* vol. 2, p. 33, 1974.
18. R.A. McCormick, "To Save or Let Die—The Dilemma of Modern Medicine," *Journal of the American Medical Association,* vol. 229, p. 172, 1974.
19. J. Fletcher, "Attitudes toward Defective Newborns," *Hastings Center Studies,* vol. 2, p. 21, 1974.
20. A. Mandelbaum and M.E. Wheeler, "The Meaning of a Defective Child to Parents," *Social Casework,* vol. 41, p. 360, 1960.
21. R. Potter, "The Paradoxical Preservation of Principle," *Villanova Law Review,* vol. 13, p. 784, 1968.
22. N. Fost, "How Decisions Are Made: A Physician's View," *Proceedings of the Skytop Conference on Ethical Issues in Spinal Bifida* (in press).
23. E. Freeman, The "God Committee," *New York Times Magazine,* May 21, 1972.

Clinical Treatment and Procedures

Seven different clinical areas were selected for this section—issues concerning psychiatry, transplantation, placebos, abortion, genetic screening and counseling, reproductive technologies, and gender identity and sex assignment. Obviously, many other topics might have been included, but we believe that these topics are the most significant special clinical areas in contemporary medicine which pose ethical problems.

Under the heading of psychiatric issues, three articles focus on the general question of involuntary commitment, Thomas Szasz arguing in two pieces against the validity of psychiatric categorization and hence against commitment for this reason and Paul Chodoff arguing in favor of at least a more moderate position. Another piece in this section is on psychosurgery. By focusing on the National Commission's report on this topic, Annas critically evaluates some of the ethical issues posed by the procedure itself as well as the role of IRBs. The piece by Stone raises the controversial issue of sexual activity between a psychiatrist and patient, and while it focuses primarily on the legal implications of such a relationship, it implicitly highlights the ethical concerns as well. (See cases 2, 14, 21, 31, 34, 59, 69.)

The section on transplantation includes three pieces. Culliton's brief selection presents the issue of good samaritanism with regard to transplants and raises the question of an individual's obligation to help another. Fost's piece discusses the use of children as renal donors, and rejects the general presumption against their use. The third piece on transplants, by Perry, discusses alternative policies for obtaining human organs and, after criticizing the three policies of donating, salvaging, and trading organs, argues in favor of a market mechanism for distribution—the selling of human organs for medical purposes. (See cases 6, 32.)

Two articles address the use of placebos. Schindel's piece focuses on the dilemma of using placebos in evaluating drug efficacy, but many of his comments can be extrapolated to other clinical procedures. Brody's piece focuses more on the "placebo effect" of medical care in general and on what Brody calls "the meaning model" or the patient's own explanatory model for his disease state. His main argument is that physicians should become more aware of the meaning of illness for their patients and in this way will be able to elicit the placebo effect, without the use of deception. (See cases 45, 57.)

Two pieces were selected for the section on abortion. Thomson's well-known article focuses on the question of whether abortion can be shown to be permissible, even if the fetus is a person with protectable rights, including the right to life. Annas' piece discusses and criticizes the Supreme Court's decision not to provide federal funding for abortion. Although only these two articles appear in the abortion section, two other articles in the text are directly relevant. The excerpt from Feinberg's piece on abortion in the Conceptual Foundations section focuses on the concept of a person and Fletcher's piece in the section on Genetic Counseling and Screening discusses selective abortion for genetic reasons. (See cases *28, 30, 43, 48, 53,* 60, *61, 70, 74.*)

In addition to Fletcher's piece on the ethics of prenatal diagnosis, we include another piece by him on genetic screening for sex identification. Here Fletcher argues that the Supreme Court's ruling on abortion necessarily implies the right of a woman to undergo amniocentesis for sex identification. Steinfels argues, however, that there is nothing in the *Roe v. Wade* decision to support Fletcher's conclusion. The pieces by Redmon and Macklin focus on the ethical issues presented by genetic counseling, specifically the question of the possibility of nondirective counseling, counseling for sex assignment for an intersex child, and the justifiability of ever withholding information from parents. The recently developed technology of selective births is discussed in the piece from the *New England Journal of Medicine* raising the whole question of risking the life of the individual to secure the abortion of another. The last piece, by Rowley, discusses public programs for genetic screening and emphasizes the responsibility of the personal physician. (See cases 43, *48,* 53, *74.*)

Three different reproductive technologies are discussed in the next three articles. Annas' first piece questions current practices with regard to donor screening and record keeping for artificial insemination; Ramsey's piece presents a strong argument against in vitro fertilization, even if it is successful; and Annas' last piece discusses the ethical and legal issues in surrogate parenting. (See cases *39,* 40.)

The final issue under Clinical Treatment and Procedures is that of gender identity and sex assignment. The piece included is a panel discussion of some of the clinical issues raised by this procedure. The primary issues presented, whether explicitly or implicitly, are the following: the definition of gender identity; the professional responsibility of physicians in dealing with patients requesting sex-change operations; the question of whether such procedures should be viewed as experimentation and what that would imply; the possibilities of informed consent; the difference between surgical vs. nonsurgical interventions; and the question of funding for such procedures. (See case *25.*)

Psychiatric Issues

81. The Illogic and Immorality of Involuntary Psychiatric Interventions: A Personal Restatement   Thomas S. Szasz

Involuntary mental hospitalization—or compulsory admission to hospital, as it is called in England—is the paradigmatic policy of psychiatry. Whenever and wherever psychiatry has been recognized and practiced as the medical specialty dealing with the treatment of insanity, madness, or mental disease, then and there persons have been incarcerated in insane asylums, madhouses, or mental hospitals. [1]

In recent years, this deprivation of liberty has been justified on two different grounds, one more popular in America, the other in England. In the United States, the defenders of involuntary psychiatry claim that mental health is more important than personal freedom and that the well-being of the individual and the nation justify certain psychiatric infringements on individual liberty. In England, its defenders, sidestepping the dilemma of such a rank-order of values, claim that the civil-liberties problem inherent in compulsory mental hospitalization is now so small as to be insignificant. [2]

In the American view, then, compulsory psychiatric confinement is a sort of limited martial law; while in the British view, it is a sort of dead-letter law. But mental patients do not menace society so gravely as to justify suppressing them by extralegal measures, nor are they suppressed so rarely as to justify our regarding the measures used against them as moribund.

Because involuntary mental hospitalization continues to be the paradigmatic practice of coercive or institutional psychiatry, it seems to me worthwhile to recapitulate briefly the justifications for its legitimacy advanced by its supporters and the justifications for its illegitimacy that I have advanced.

The coercion and restraint of the mental patient by the psychiatrist—or, better, of the madman by the alienist, as these protagonists were first called—is coeval with the origin and development of psychiatry. As a discrete discipline, psychiatry began in the seventeenth century with the building of insane asylums, first in France, then throughout the civilized world. These institutions were of course prisons in which were confined not only so-called madmen but all of society's undesirables—abandoned children, prostitutes, incurably sick persons, the aged and indigent. [3]

How did people in general, and those directly responsible for these confinements—the legislators and jurists, the physicians and the victim's relatives—in particular justify such incarceration of persons not guilty of criminal offenses? The answer is: by means of the imagery and rhetoric of madness, insanity, psychosis, schizophrenia, mental illness—call it what you will—which transformed the inmate into a patient, his prison into a hospital, and his warden into a doctor. Characteristically, the first official proposition of the Association of Medical Superintendents of American Institutions for the Insane, the organization that

Source: Thomas S. Szasz, *The Theology of Medicine,* Harper & Row, New York, 1977.

became in 1921 the American Psychiatric Association, was, "Resolved, that it is the unanimous sense of this convention that the attempt to abandon entirely the use of all means of personal restraint is not sanctioned by the true interests of the insane."[4]

Ever since then, this paternalistic justification of psychiatric coercion has been a prominent theme in psychiatry, not only in America but throughout the world. Thus, in 1967— 123 years after the drafting of its first resolution—the American Psychiatric Association reaffirmed it support of psychiatric coercion and restraint. In its "Position Statement on the Question of the Adequacy of Treatment," the association declared that "restraints may be imposed [on the patient] from within by pharmacologic means or by locking the door of a ward. Either imposition may be a legitimate component of a treatment program."[5]

The British Mental Health Act of 1959 provides medicolegal measures for both civil and criminal commitment virtually identical to those of the various American states. Part IV of the act, entitled "Compulsory Admission to Hospital and Guardianship," articulates the criteria for civil commitment as follows: "An application for admission for observation may be made in respect of a patient on the grounds (*a*) that he is suffering from mental disorder of a nature or degree which warrants the detention of the patient in a hospital under observation . . . (*b*) that he ought to be so detained in the interests of his own health or safety or with a view to the protection of other persons."

Justifications for involuntary psychiatric interventions of all kinds—and especially for involuntary mental hospitalization—similar to those accepted in the United States and the United Kingdom are, of course, advanced in other countries. In short, just as involuntary servitude had been accepted for millennia as a proper economic and social arrangement, so involuntary psychiatry has been accepted for centuries as a proper medical and therapeutic arrangement.

It is this entire system of interlocking psychiatric ideas and in-situations, justifications, and practices, that for some twenty years I have analyzed and attacked. I have described and documented the precise legal status of the mental-hospital patient—as an innocent person incarcerated in a psychiatric prison; articulated my objections to institutional psychiatry—as an extralegal system of penology and punishments; and demonstrated what seems to me, in a free society, our only morally proper option with respect to the problem of so-called psychiatric abuses—namely, the complete abolition of all involuntary psychiatric interventions.

My objections to the principles and practices upon which involuntary psychiatric interventions rest may be summarized as follows:

The term *mental illness* is a metaphor. More particularly, as this term is used in mental-hygiene legislation, *mental illness* is not the name of a medical disease or disorder but is a quasi-medical label whose purpose is to conceal conflict as illness and to justify coercion as treatment.

If mental illness is a bona fide illness—"like any other," as official medical, psychiatric, and mental-health organizations such as the World Health Organization, the American and British medical associations, and the American Psychiatric Association maintain—then it follows, logically and linguistically, that it must be treated like any other illness. Hence, mental-hygiene laws must be repealed. There are no special laws for patients with peptic ulcer or pneumonia; why then should there be special laws for patients with depression or schizophrenia?

If, on the other hand, mental illness is, as I contend, a metaphor and a myth, then it also follows that mental-hygiene laws should be repealed.

Further, if there were no mental-hygiene laws—which create a category of individuals who, though officially labeled as mentally ill, would prefer not to be subjected to involuntary psychiatric interventions—then the misdeeds now committed by those who care for mental patients could not arise or endure.

In short, all those who draft and administer laws pertaining to involuntary psychiatric interventions should be regarded as the adversaries, not the allies, of the so-called mental patient. Civil libertarians, and indeed all men and women who believe that no one may be justly deprived of liberty except upon conviction for a crime, should oppose all forms of involuntary psychiatric interventions.

What, then, are some of the most important objections to my contention that mental disorders are not bona fide diseases and to my claim that imprisonment for insanity, as opposed to lawbreaking, is incompatible with the moral principles of a free society?

First, some of my critics say that I am wrong because what we now call mental diseases may yet be shown to be caused, at least in some cases, by subtle pathophysiological processes in the body—in particular, by disorders in the molecular chemistry of the brain—that we do not yet know how to measure or record. Nevertheless, such processes, like those responsible for the psychoses associated with paresis or pellagra, exist (so runs this argument), and it is only because of the present state of our knowledge, or rather ignorance, that we cannot yet properly diagnose them. But such an advance in the science and technology of medical diagnosis would only add to the list of literal diseases and would not in the slightest impair the validity of my argument that when we call certain kinds of disapproved behaviors mental diseases, we create a category of metaphorical diseases. This type of objection to my views, which actually represents just another instance of biological reductionism, misses the point I try to make; to uphold it would be like upholding the view that because certain canvases thought to be forged Renoirs or Cézannes prove to be, on closer study, genuine, all forged masterpieces are genuine. If there are real or literal diseases, there must also be others that are fake or metaphorical.

Second, other critics say that I am wrong, not because I say that mental illnesses are unlike bodily illnesses (an assertion with which they claim to agree), nor because I say that involuntary hospitalization or treatment is no more justified for so-called mental illness than it is for bodily illness (a moral principle with which they also claim to be in sympathy), but because the term *mental illness* often designates a phenomenologically identifiable and hence valid category of conduct. But I do not deny that. I have never maintained that the conduct of a depressed or elated person is the same as that of a person who is contented and even-tempered or that the conduct of a person who claims to be Jesus or Napoleon is the same as that of one who makes no such false claims. I object to psychiatric diagnostic terms not because they are meaningless, but because they are used to stigmatize, dehumanize, imprison, and torture those to whom they are applied. To put it somewhat differently, I oppose involuntary psychiatry, or the rape of the patient by the psychiatrist; but I do not oppose voluntary psychiatry, or psychiatric activities between consenting adults.

The idea that a person accused of crime is innocent until proven guilty is not shared by people everywhere but is, as I need hardly belabor, characteristically English in its historical origin and singularly Anglo-American in its consistent social application. And so is its corollary—that an individual has an inalienable right to personal liberty unless he has been duly convicted in court of an offense punishable by imprisonment. Because this magnificent edifice of dignity and liberty is undermined by psychiatry, I consider the abolition of involuntary psychiatric interventions to be an especially important link in the chain I have tried to forge for restraining this mortal enemy of individualism and self-determination. I hope that my work will help people to discriminate between two types of physicians: those who heal, not so much because they are saints but because *that is their job;* and those who harm, not so much because they are sinners but because *that is their job.* And if some doctors harm—torture rather than treat, murder the soul rather than minister to the body—that is, in part, because society, through the state, asks them, and pays them, to do so.

We saw it happen in Nazi Germany, and we hanged many of the doctors. We see it happen in the Soviet Union, and we denounce the doctors with righteous indignation. But when will we see that the same things are happening in the so-called free societies? When will we recognize—and publicly identify—the medical criminals among us? Or is the very possibility of perceiving many of our leading psychiatrists and psychiatric institutions in that way precluded by the fact that they represent the officially correct views and practices; by the fact that they have the ears of our lawyers and legislators, journalists and judges; and by the fact that they control the vast funds, collected by the state through taxing citizens, that finance an enterprise whose basic moral legitimacy I have called into question?

NOTES

1. See my (ed.) *The Age of Madness: The History of Involuntary Mental Hospitalization Presented in Selected Texts,* Doubleday, Anchor Press, Garden City, N.Y., 1973.

2. See my "The ACLU's 'Mental Illness' Cop-Out," *Reason,* vol. 5, p. 4, 1974; and Preface to the British Edition, *The Age of Madness,* Routledge & Kegan Paul, London, 1975.

3. See my *The Manufacture of Madness: A Comparative Study of the Inquisition and the Mental Health Movement,* Harper & Row, New York, 1970.

4. Quoted in N. Ridenour, *Mental Health in the United States: A Fifty-Year History,* Harvard University Press, Cambridge, Mass., 1961.

5. Council of the American Psychiatric Association, "Position Statement on the Question of the Adequacy of Treatment," *American Journal of Psychiatry,* vol. 123, p. 1459, May 1967.

82. *The Case for Involuntary Hospitalization of the Mentally Ill*
Paul Chodoff

I will begin this paper with a series of vignettes designed to illustrate graphically the question that is my focus: under what conditions, if any, does society have the right to apply coercion to an individual to hospitalize him against his will, by reason of mental illness?

Case 1. A woman in her mid 50s, with no previous overt behavioral difficulties, comes to believe that she is worthless and insignificant. She is completely preoccupied with her guilt and is increasingly unavailable for the ordinary demands of life. She eats very little because of her conviction that the food should go to others whose need is greater than hers, and her physical condition progressively deteriorates. Although she will talk to others about herself, she insists that she is not sick, only bad. She refuses medication, and when hospitaliza-

Source: Reprinted with permission of the author and the publisher from *American Journal of Psychiatry,* vol. 133, no. 5, p. 496, May 1976. Copyright 1976, the American Psychiatric Association.

tion is suggested she also refuses that, on the grounds that she would be taking up space that otherwise could be occupied by those who merit treatment more than she.

Case 2. For the past 6 years the behavior of a 42-year-old woman has been disturbed for periods of 3 months of longer. After recovery from her most recent episode she has been at home, functioning at a borderline level. A month ago she again started to withdraw from her environment. She pays increasingly less attention to her bodily needs, talks very little, and does not respond to questions or attention from those about her. She lapses into a mute state and lies in her bed in a totally passive fashion. She does not respond to other people, does not eat, and does not void. When her arm is raised from the bed it remains for several minutes in the position in which it is left. Her medical history and a physical examination reveal no evidence of primary physical illness.

Case 3. A man with a history of alcoholism has been on a binge for several weeks. He remains at home doing little else than drinking. He eats very little. He becomes tremulous and misinterprets spots on the wall as animals about to attack him, and he complains of "creeping" sensations in his body, which he attributes to infestation by insects. He does not seek help voluntarily, insists there is nothing wrong with him, and despite his wife's entreaties he continues to drink.

Case 4. Passersby and station personnel observe that a young woman has been spending several days at Union Station in Washington, D.C. Her behavior appears strange to others. She is finally befriended by a newspaper reporter who becomes aware that her perception of her situation is profoundly unrealistic and that she is, in fact, delusional. He persuades her to accompany him to St. Elizabeths Hospital, where she is examined by a psychiatrist who recommends admission. She refuses hospitalization and the psychiatrist allows her to leave. She returns to Union Station. A few days later she is found dead, murdered, on one of the surrounding streets.

Case 5. A government attorney in his late 30s begins to display pressured speech and hyperactivity. He is too busy to sleep and eats very little. He talks rapidly, becomes irritable when interrupted, and makes phone calls all over the country in furtherance of his political ambitions, which are to begin a campaign for the Presidency of the United States. He makes many purchases, some very expensive, thus running through a great deal of money. He is rude and tactless to his friends, who are offended by his behavior, and his job is in jeopardy. In spite of his wife's pleas he insists that he does not have the time to seek or accept treatment, and he refuses hospitalization. This is not the first such disturbance for this individual; in fact, very similar episodes have been occurring at roughly 2-year intervals since he was 18 years old.

Case 6. Passersby in a campus area observe two young women standing together, staring at each other, for over an hour. Their behavior attracts attention, and eventually the police take the pair to a nearby precinct station for questioning. They refuse to answer questions and sit mutely, staring into space. The police request some type of psychiatric examination but are informed by the city attorney's office that state law (Michigan) allows persons to be held for observation only if they appear obviously dangerous to themselves or others. In this case, since the women do not seem homicidal or suicidal, they do not qualify for observation and are released.

Less than 30 hours later the two women are found on the floor of their campus apartment, screaming and writhing in pain with their clothes ablaze from a self-made pyre. One woman recovers; the other dies. There is no conclusive evidence that drugs were involved.[1]

Most, if not all, people would agree that the behavior described in these vignettes deviates significantly from even elastic definitions of normality. However, it is clear that there would not be a similar consensus on how to react to this kind of behavior and that there is a considerable and increasing ferment about what attitude the organized elements of our society should take toward such individuals. Everyone has a stake in this important issue, but the debate about it takes place principally among psychiatrists, lawyers, the courts, and law enforcement agencies.

Points of view about the question of involuntary hospitalization fall into the following three principal groups: the "abolitionists," medical model psychiatrists, and civil liberties lawyers.

The Abolitionists

Those holding this position would assert that in none of the cases I have described should involuntary hospitalization be a viable option because, quite simply, it should never be resorted to under any circumstances. As Szasz[2] has put it, "we should value liberty more highly than mental health no matter how defined" and "no one should be deprived of his freedom for the sake of his mental health." Ennis[3] has said that the goal "is nothing less than the abolition of involuntary hospitalization."

Prominent among the abolitionists are the "anti-psychiatrists," who, somewhat suprisingly, count in their ranks a number of well-known psychiatrists. For them mental illness simply does not exist in the field of psychiatry.[4] They reject entirely the medical model of mental illness and insist that acceptance of it relies on a fiction accepted jointly by the state and by psychiatrists as a device for exerting social control over annoying or unconventional people. The anti-psychiatrists hold that these people ought to be afforded the dignity of being held responsible for their behavior and required to accept its consequences. In addition, some members of this group believe that the phenomena of "mental illness" often represent essentially a tortured protest against the insanities of an irrational society.[5] They maintain that society should not be encouraged in its oppressive course by affixing a pejorative label to its victims.

Among the abolitionists are some civil liberties lawyers who both assert their passionate support of the magisterial importance of individual liberty and react with repugnance and impatience to what they see as the abuses of psychiatric practice in this field—the commitment of some individuals for flimsy and possibly self-serving reasons and their inhuman warehousing in penal institutions wrongly called "hospitals."

The abolitionists do not oppose psychiatric treatment when it is conducted with the agreement of those being treated. I have no doubt that they would try to gain the consent of the individuals described earlier to undergo treatment, including hospitalization. The psychiatrists in this group would be very likely to confine their treatment methods to psychotherapeutic efforts to influence the aberrant behavior. They would be unlikely to use drugs and would certainly eschew such somatic therapies as electroconvulsive therapy (ECT). If efforts to enlist voluntary compliance with treatment failed, the abolitionists would not employ any means of coercion. Instead, they would step aside and allow social, legal, and community sanctions to take their course. If a human being should be jailed or a human life lost as a result of this attitude, they would accept it as a necessary evil to be tolerated in order to avoid the greater evil of unjustified loss of liberty for others.[6]

The Medical Model Psychiatrists

I use this admittedly awkward and not entirely accurate label to designate the position of a substantial number of psychiatrists. They believe that mental illness is a meaningful concept and that under certain conditions its existence justifies the state's exercise, under the doctrine of *parens patriae,* of its right and obligation to arrange for the hospitalization of the sick individual even though coercion is involved and he is deprived of his liberty. I believe that these psychiatrists would recommend involuntary hospitalization for all six of the patients described earlier.

There was a time, before they were considered to be ill, when individuals who displayed the kind of behavior I described earlier were put in "ships of fools" to wander the seas or were left to the mercies, sometimes tender but often savage, of uncomprehending communities that regarded them as either possessed or bad. During the Enlightenment and the early nineteenth century, however, these individuals gradually came to be regarded as sick people to be included under the humane and caring umbrella of the Judeo-Christian attitude toward illness. This attitude, which may have reached its height during the era of moral treatment in the early nineteenth century, has had unexpected and ambiguous consequences. It became overextended and partially perverted, and these excesses led to the reaction that is so strong a current in today's attitude toward mental illness.

However, reaction itself can go too far, and I believe that this is already happening. Witness the disastrous consequences of the precipitate dehospitalization that is occurring all over the country. To remove the protective mantle of illness from these disturbed people is to expose them, their families, and their communities to consequences that are certainly maladaptive and possibly irreparable. Are we really acting in accordance with their best interests when we allow them to "die with their rights on"[1] or when we condemn them to a "preservation of liberty which is actually so destructive as to constitute another form of imprisonment"?[7] Will they not suffer "if [a] liberty they cannot enjoy is made superior to a health that must sometimes be forced on them"?[8]

Many of those who reject the medical model out of hand as inapplicable to so-called "mental illness" have tended to oversimplify its meaning and have, in fact, equated it almost entirely with organic disease. It is necessary to recognize that it is a complex concept and that there is a lack of agreement about its meaning. Sophisticated definitions of the medical model do not require only the demonstration of unequivocal organic pathology. A broader formulation, put forward by sociologists and deriving largely from Talcott Parsons' description of the sick role,[9] extends the domain of illness to encompass certain forms of social deviance as well as biological disorders. According to this definition, the medical model is characterized not only by organicity but also by being negatively valued by society, by "nonvoluntariness," thus exempting its exemplars from blame, and by the understanding that physicians are the technically competent experts to deal with its effects.[10]

Except for the question of organic disease, the patients I described earlier conform well to this broader conception of the medical model. They are all suffering both emotionally and physically, they are incapable by an effort of will of stopping or changing their destructive behavior, and those around them consider them to be in an undesirable sick state and to require medical attention.

Categorizing the behavior of these patients as involuntary may be criticized as evidence of an intolerably paternalistic and antitherapeutic attitude that fosters the very failure to take responsibility for their lives and behavior that the therapist should uncover rather than encourage. However, it must also be acknowledged that these severely ill people are not capable at a conscious level of deciding what is best for themselves and that in order to help them examine their behavior and motivation, it is necessary that they be alive and available for treatment. Their verbal message that they will not accept treatment may at the same time be conveying other more covert messages—that they are desperate and want help even though they cannot ask for it.[11]

Although organic pathology may not be the only determinant of the medical model, it is of course an important one, and it should not be avoided in any discussion of mental illness. There would be no question that the previously described patient with delirium tremens is suffering from a toxic form of brain disease. There are a significant number of other patients who require involuntary hospitalization because of organic brain syndrome due to various causes. Among those who are not overtly organically ill, most of the candidates for involuntary hospitalization suffer from schizophrenia or one of the major affective disorders. A growing and increasingly impressive body of evidence points to the presence of an important genetic-biological factor in these conditions; thus, many of them qualify on these grounds as illnesses.

Despite the revisionist efforts of the anti-psychiatrists, mental illness *does* exist. It does not by any means include all the people being treated by psychiatrists (or by nonpsychiatrist physicians), but it does encompass those few desperately sick people for whom involuntary commitment must be considered. In the words of a recent article, "The problem is that mental illness is not a myth. It is not some palpable falsehood propagated among the populace by power-mad psychiatrists, but a cruel and bitter reality that has been with the human race since antiquity."[12]

CRITERIA FOR INVOLUNTARY HOSPITALIZATION

Procedures for involuntary hospitalization should be instituted for individuals who require care and treatment because of diagnosable mental illness that produces symptoms, including marked impairment in judgment, that disrupt their intrapsychic and interpersonal functioning. All three of these criteria must be met before involuntary hospitalization can be instituted.

Mental illness. This concept has already been discussed, but it should be repeated that only a belief in the existence of illness justifies involuntary commitment. It is a fundamental assumption that makes aberrant behavior a medical matter and its care the concern of physicians.

Disruption of functioning. This involves combinations of serious and often obvious disturbances that are both intrapsychic (for example, the suffering of severe depression) and interpersonal (for example, withdrawal from others because of depression). It does not include minor peccadilloes or eccentricities. Furthermore, the behavior in question must represent symptoms of the mental illness from which the patient is suffering. Among these symptoms are actions that are imminently or potentially dangerous in a physical sense to self or others, as well as other manifestations of mental illness such as those in the cases I have described. This is not to ignore dangerousness as a criterion for commitment but rather to put it in its proper place as one of a number of symptoms of the illness. A further manifestation of the illness, and indeed, the one that makes involuntary rather than voluntary hospitalization necessary, is impairment of the patient's judgment to such a degree that he is unable to consider his condition and make decisions about it in his own interests.

Need for care and treatment. The goal of physicians is to treat and cure their patients; however, sometimes they can only ameliorate the suffering of their patients and sometimes all they can offer is care. It is not possible to predict whether someone will respond to treatment; nevertheless, the need for treatment and the availability of facilities to carry it out constitute essential preconditions that must be met to justify requiring anyone to give up his freedom. If mental hospital patients have a right to treatment, then psychiatrists have a right to ask for treatability as a front-door as well as a back-door criterion for commitment. [7]

All of the six individuals I described earlier could have been treated with a reasonable expectation of returning to a more normal state of functioning.

I believe that the objections to this formulation can be summarized as follows:

1. The whole structure founders for those who maintain that mental illness is a fiction.

2. These criteria are also untenable to those who hold liberty to be such a supreme value that the presence of mental illness per se does not constitute justification for depriving an individual of his freedom; only when such illness is manifested by clearly dangerous behavior may commitment be considered. For reasons to be discussed later, I agree with those psychiatrists [13, 14] who do not believe that dangerousness should be elevated to primacy above other manifestations of mental illness as a sine qua non for involuntary hospitalization.

3. The medical model criteria are "soft" and subjective and depend on the fallible judgment of psychiatrists. This is a valid objection. There is no reliable blood test for schizophrenia and no method for injecting gray cells into psychiatrists. A relatively small number of cases will always fall within a gray area that will be difficult to judge. In those extreme cases in which the question of commitment arises, competent and ethical psychiatrists should be able to use these criteria without doing violence to individual liberties and with the expectation of good results. Furthermore, the possible "fuzziness" of some aspects of the medical model approach is certainly no greater than that of the supposedly "objective" criteria for dangerousness, and there is little reason to believe that lawyers and judges are any less fallible than psychiatrists.

4. Commitment procedures in the hands of psychiatrists are subject to intolerable abuses. Here, as Peszke said, "It is imperative that we differentiate between the principle of the process of civil commitment and the practice itself. [13] Abuses can contaminate both the medical and the dangerousness approaches, and I believe that the abuses stemming from the abolitionist view of no commitment at all are even greater. Measures to abate abuses of the medical approach include judicial review and the abandonment of indeterminate commitment. In the course of commitment proceedings and thereafter, patients should have access to competent and compassionate legal counsel. However, this latter safeguard may itself be subject to abuse if the legal counsel acts solely in the adversary tradition and undertakes to carry out the patient's wishes even when they may be destructive.

COMMENT

The criteria and procedures outlined will apply most appropriately to initial episodes and recurrent attacks of mental illness. To put it simply, it is necessary to find a way to satisfy legal and humanitarian considerations and yet allow psychiatrists access to initially or acutely ill patients in order to do the best they can for them. However, there are some involuntary patients who have received adequate and active treatment but have not responded satisfactorily. An irreducible minimum of such cases, principally among those with brain disorders and process schizophrenia, will not improve sufficiently to be able to adapt to even a tolerant society.

The decision of what to do at this point is not an easy one, and it should certainly not be in the hands of psychiatrists alone. With some justification they can state that they have been given the thankless job of caring, often with inadequate facilities, for badly damaged people and that they are now being subjected to criticism for keeping these patients locked up. No one really knows what to do with these patients. It may be that when treatment has failed they exchange their sick role for what has been called the impaired role,[15] which implies a permanent negative evaluation of them coupled with a somewhat less benign societal attitude. At this point, perhaps a case can be made for giving greater importance to the criteria for dangerousness and releasing such patients if they do not pose a threat to others. However, I do not believe that the release into the community of these severely malfunctioning individuals will serve their interests even though it may satisfy formal notions of right and wrong.

It should be emphasized that the number of individuals for whom involuntary commitment must be considered is small (although, under the influence of current pressures, it may be smaller than it should be). Even severe mental illness can often be handled by securing the cooperation of the patient, and certainly one of the favorable efforts. However, the distinction between voluntary and involuntary hospitalization is sometimes more formal than meaningful. How "voluntary" are the actions of an individual who is being buffeted by the threats, entreaties, and tears of his family?

I believe, however, that we are at a point (at least in some jurisdictions) where, having rebounded from an era in which involuntary commitment was too easy and employed too often, we are now entering one in which it is becoming very difficult to commit anyone, even in urgent cases. Faced with the moral obloquy that has come to pervade the atmosphere in which the decision to involuntarily hospitalize is considered, some psychiatrists, especially younger ones, have become, as Stone[16] put it, "soft as grapes" when faced with the prospect of committing anyone under any circumstances.

The Civil Liberties Lawyers

I use this admittedly inexact label to designate those members of the legal profession who do not in principle reject the necessity for involuntary hospitalization but who do reject or wish to diminish the importance of medical model criteria in the hands of psychiatrists. Accordingly, the civil liberties lawyers, in dealing with the problem of involuntary hospitalization, have enlisted themselves under the standard of dangerousness, which they hold to be more objective and capable of being dealt with in a sounder evidentiary manner than the medical model criteria. For them the question is not whether mental illness, even of disabling degree, is present, but only whether it has resulted in the probability of behavior dangerous to others or to self. Thus they would scrutinize the cases previously described for evidence of such dangerousness and would make the decision about involuntary hospitalization accordingly. They would probably feel that commitment is not indicated in most of these cases, since they were selected as illustrative of severe mental illness in which outstanding evidence of physical dangerousness was not present.

The dangerousness standard is being used increasingly not only to supplement criteria for mental illness but, in fact, to replace them entirely. The recent Supreme Court decision in *O'Connor v. Donaldson* is certainly a long step in this direction. In addition, "dangerousness" is increasingly being understood to refer to the probability that the individual will inflict harm on himself or others in a specific physical manner rather than in other ways. This tendency has perhaps been carried to its ultimate in the *Lessard v. Schmidt* case in Wisconsin, which restricted suitability for commitment to the "extreme likelihood that if the person is not confined, he will do immediate harm to himself or others." (This decision was set aside by the U.S. Supreme Court in 1974.) In a recent Washington, D.C., Superior Court case the instructions to the jury stated that the government must prove that the defendant was likely to cause "substantial physical harm to himself or others in the reasonably foreseeable future."

For the following reasons, the dangerousness standard is an inappropriate and dangerous indicator to use in judging the conditions under which someone should be involuntarily hospitalized. Dangerousness is being taken out of its proper context as one among other symptoms of the presence of severe mental illness that should be the determining factor.

1. To concentrate on dangerousness (especially to others) as the sole criterion for involuntary hospitalization deprives many mentally ill persons of the protection and treatment that they urgently require. A psychiatrist under the constraints of the dangerousness rule, faced with an out-of-control manic individual whose frantic behavior the psychiatrist truly believes to be a disguised call for help, would have to say, "Sorry, I would like to help you but I can't because you haven't threatened anybody and you are not suicidal." Since psychiatrists are admittedly not very good at accurately predicting dangerousness to others, the evidentiary standards for commitment will be very stringent. This will result in mental hospitals becoming prisons for a small population of volatile, highly assaultive, and untreatable patients.[14]

2. The attempt to differentiate rigidly (especially in regard to danger to self) between physical and other kinds of self-destructive behavior is artificial, unrealistic, and unworkable. It will tend to confront psychiatrists who want to help their patients with the same kind of dilemma they were faced with when justification for therapeutic abortion on psychiatric grounds depended on evidence of suicidal intent. The advocates of the dangerousness standard seem to be more comfortable with and pay more attention to the factor of dangerousness to others even though it is a much less frequent and much less significant consequence of mental illness than is danger to self.

3. The emphasis on dangerousness (again, especially to others) is a real obstacle to the right-to-treatment movement since it prevents the hospitalization and therefore the treatment of the population most amenable to various kinds of therapy.

4. Emphasis on the criterion of dangerousness to others moves involuntary commitment from a civil to a criminal procedure, thus, as Stone[14] put it, imposing the procedures of one terrible system on another. Involuntary commitment on these grounds becomes a form of preventive detention and makes the psychiatrist a kind of glorified policeman.

5. Emphasis on dangerousness rather than mental disability and helplessness will hasten the process of deinstitutionalization. Recent reports[17, 18] have shown that these patients are not being rehabilitated and reintegrated into the community, but rather that the burden of custodialism has been shifted from the hospital to the community.

6. As previously mentioned, emphasis on the dangerousness criterion may be a tactic of some of the abolitionists among the civil liberties lawyers[19] to end involuntary hospitalization by reducing it to an unworkable absurdity.

DISCUSSION

It is obvious that it is good to be at liberty and that it is good to be free from the consequences of disabling and dehumanizing illness. Sometimes these two values are incompatible, and in the heat of the passions that are often aroused by opposing views of right and wrong, the partisans of each view may tend to minimize the importance of the other. Both sides can present their horror stories—the psychiatrists, their dead victims of the failure of the involuntary hospitalization process, and the lawyers, their Donaldsons. There is a real danger that instead of acknowledging the difficulty of the problem, the two camps will become polarized, with a consequent rush toward extreme and untenable solutions rather than working toward reasonable ones.

The path taken by those whom I have labeled the abolitionists is an example of the barren results that ensue when an absolute solution is imposed on a complex problem. There are human beings who will suffer greatly if the abolitionists succeed in elevating an abstract principle into an unbreakable law with no exceptions. I find myself oppressed and repelled by their position, which seems to stem from an ideological rigidity which ignores that element of the contingent immanent in the structure of human existence. It is devoid of compassion.

The positions of those who espouse the medical model and the dangerousness approaches to commitment are, one hopes, not completely irreconcilable. To some extent these differences are a result of the vantage points from which lawyers and psychiatrists view mental illness and commitment. The lawyers see and are concerned with the failures and abuses of the process. Furthermore, as a result of their training, they tend to apply principles to classes of people rather than to take each instance as unique. The psychiatrists, on the other hand, are required to deal practically with the singular needs of individuals. They approach the problem from a clinical rather than a deductive stance. As physicians, they want to be in a position to take care of and to help suffering people whom they regard as sick patients. They sometimes become impatient with the rules that prevent them from doing this.

I believe we are now witnessing a pendular swing in which the rights of the mentally ill to be treated and protected are being set aside in the rush to give them their freedom at whatever cost. But is freedom defined only by the absence of external constraints? Internal physiological or psychological processes can contribute to a throttling of the spirit that is as painful as any applied from the outside. The "wild" manic individual without his lithium, the panicky hallucinator without his injection of fluphenazine hydrochloride and the understanding support of a concerned staff, the sodden alcoholic—are they free? Sometimes, as Woody Guthrie said, "Freedom means no place to go."

Today the civil liberties lawyers are in the ascendancy and the psychiatrists on the defensive to a degree that is harmful to individual needs and the public welfare. Redress and a more balanced position will not come from further extension of the dangerousness doctrine. I favor a return to the use of medical criteria by psychiatrists—psychiatrists, however, who have been chastened by the buffeting they have received and are quite willing to go along with even strict legal safeguards as long as they are constructive and not tyrannical.

NOTES

1. D. A. Treffert, "The Practical Limits of Patients' Rights," *Psychiatric Annals*, vol. 5, no. 4, p. 91, 1971.

2. T. Szasz, *Law, Liberty and Psychiatry*, Macmillan Co., New York, 1963.

3. B. Ennis, *Prisoners of Psychiatry*, Harcourt Brace Jovanovich, New York, 1972.

4. T. Szasz, *The Myth of Mental Illness*, Harper & Row, New York, 1961.

5. R. Laing, *The Politics of Experience*, Ballantine Books, New York, 1967.

6. B. Ennis, "Ennis on 'Donaldson'," *Psychiatric*

News, Dec. 3, 1975, p. 4.

7. R. Peele, P. Chodoff, and N. Taub, "Involuntary Hospitalization and Treatability. Observations from the DC Experience," *Catholic University Law Review,* vol. 23, p. 744, 1974.

8. R. Michels, "The Right to Refuse Psychotropic Drugs," *Hastings Center Report,* Hastings-on-Hudson, N.Y., 1973.

9. T. Parsons, *The Social System,* Free Press, New York, 1951.

10. R. M. Veatch, "The Medical Model: Its Nature and Problems," *Hastings Center Studies,* vol. 1, no. 3, p. 59, 1973.

11. J. Katz, "The Right to Treatment—An Enchanting Legal Fiction?" *University of Chicago Law Review,* vol. 36, p. 755, 1969.

12. M. S. Moore, "Some Myths about Mental Illness," *Archives of General Psychiatry,* vol. 32, p. 1483, 1975.

13. M. A. Peszke, "Is Dangerousness an Issue for Physicians in Emergency Commitment?" *American Journal of Psychiatry,* vol. 132, p. 825, 1975.

14. A. A. Stone, "Comment on Peszke, M. A.: Is Dangerousness an Issue for Physicians in Emergency Commitment?" Ibid., p. 829.

15. M. Siegler, and H. Osmond, *Models of Madness, Models of Medicine,* Macmillan Co., New York, 1974.

16. A. Stone, Lecture for course on The Law, Litigation, and Mental Health Services, Mental Health Study Center, Adelphi, Md., September 1974.

17. S. Rachlin, A. Pam, and J. Milton, "Civil Liberties versus Involuntary Hospitalization," *American Journal of Psychiatry,* vol. 132, p. 189, 1975.

18. S. A. Kirk, and M. E. Therrien, "Community Mental Health Myths and the Fate of Former Hospitalized Patients," *Psychiatry,* vol. 38, p. 209, 1975.

19. A. A. Dershowitz, "Dangerousness as a Criterion for Confinement," *Bulletin of the American Academy of Psychiatry and the Law,* vol. 2, p. 172, 1974.

83. *Reagan Should Let the Jurors Judge Hinckley*
Thomas S. Szasz

With the dramatic unfolding of events after the attempted assassination of President Reagan, even his bitterest critics were forced to concede that his behavior under fire was courageous and inspiring. Veritably, Reagan seemed to possess all the virtues of the Western hero he had portrayed so often and so well on the screen. Unfortunately, on April 22, in the first interview he gave the press since the shooting, he fell off his horse and didn't even seem to know it. Quite unwittingly, Reagan offered some comments about John W. Hinckley, Jr., that were, in my opinion, unfounded and misguided and that have gravely prejudiced his trial.

What President Reagan said was this: "I hope, indeed I pray, that he can find an answer to his problem. He seems to be a very disturbed young man. He comes from a fine family. They must be devastated by this. And I hope he'll get well, too."

I believe that these remarks are important enough to justify my taking them one sentence at a time.

"I hope, indeed I pray, that he can find an answer to his problem," In the old Westerns, if memory doesn't deceive me, the good men first hanged the bad men and only then did they pray for their souls. Elsewhere in the same interview Reagan also said that he prays daily for Brady's recovery. As I do not pray, I grant that my views on prayer may be impious and "incorrect." Nevertheless, I believe that the dignity of prayer is cheapened when it is bestowed as indiscriminately as this. Is there anyone for whom Reagan would not pray? Would he pray for Brezhnev's health? For Stalin's soul? If not, then why for Hinckley? Surely,

Source: *The Washington Post,* May 6, 1981, p. A-19.

Solzhenitsyn is no less pious than Reagan, but I do not recall Solzhenitsyn's ever mentioning that he prays for communist murderers. Perhaps capitalist would-be murderers who fail to kill anyone and succeed only in lobotomizing a press secretary are more deserving.

One more comment on this brief but psychiatrically significant sentence needs to be added here. President Reagan's statement implies that Hinckley has a "problem" and is looking to "find an answer" to it. But I think Reagan (and the conventional psychiatric mind-set he so naively displays) may have got this backward. Hinckley had a *problem* before the assassination attempt. The criminal act was his *solution* to it. Now other people, especially poor Jim Brady and his family, have got a problem. I, for one, find the compassion for Hinckley premature. Like the men Reagan used to impersonate, I believe that Hinckley deserves punishment first, compassion and forgiveness later, if ever.

"He [Hinckley] seems to be a very disturbed young man." Anyone with any respect for language—and without such respect there can be neither truth nor justice—must realize that while this may be a piece of received psychiatric truth, it is a big lie nevertheless. Hinckley is not disturbed, he is disturbing. He is not sick, he is sickening.

"He [Hinckley] comes from a fine family." How does Reagan know this? All we were told so far is that Hinckley comes from a wealthy family.

There is one more thing we know, and I cannot emphasize its importance enough: namely, that Hinckley has not been allowed to speak for himself. In effect, he has been muzzled, he has been silenced, while everyone, including the president of the United States, is busy explaining that he is "disturbed." For all we know, Hinckley may now feel quite undisturbed.

"They [Hinckley's family] must be devastated by this." That is likely and is probably one of the reasons for Hinckley's dastardly deed. But this is a speculation. And so is the possibility that the Hinckley family might have preferred George Bush for president. But that is heresy. We treasure our received psychiatric truths about mentally ill assassins precisely in order to banish such thoughts from our collective consciousness. In America, political motives for the murder of the high and mighty exist only in the half-forgotten pages of Shakespeare's tragedies.

"And I hope he'll get well, too." By thus acknowledging that Hinckley is ill, Reagan here implicitly supports an insanity defense for him. Should Hinckley plead insanity his lawyers would be able to appeal to the "expert testimony" of the president of the United States to support the contention that Hinckley is innocent because he was insane when he wounded Reagan instead of killing him.

President Reagan made a mistake in answering any questions about Hinckley at all. Respect for the law should have made him say, quite simply, that Hinckley's fate—and in particular the question of whether he is disturbed or depraved—will be for the jury to determine. The fact is that the distinction between disturbance and depravity—between madness and badness, between mental illness and criminality, call it what you will—is not a specialized or technical judgment doctors can make because they possess an M.D. degree; or psychiatrists can make because they possess training in diagnosing and treating mental illness; or the president of the United States can make because he occupies a lofty office. That distinction is a *moral judgment,* which is why a jury, and no one else, is supposed to make it. If we forget that, we might as well forget about America.

84. *Psychosurgery: Procedural Safeguards*   George J. Annas

Psychosurgery, the selective destruction of brain tissue to alter behavior, and fetal research were the only types of human experimentation that Congress specifically required the National Commission for the Protection of Human Subjects of Behavioral and Biomedical Research to review.[1] Neither the tone nor the content of the Commission's initial report on psychosurgery in August 1976 was anticipated. Headlines in *Science* noted, "National Commission Issues Surprisingly Favorable Report" (October 15, 1976), and in the *Nation*, "Congress [sic] Endorses Psychosurgery" (October 23, 1976). Since an endorsement of psychosurgical procedures was not what the commissioners had in mind, the report was reconsidered at subsequent meetings, and has undergone significant revisions during the past six months. The Commission's final report on the subject was issued on March 14, 1977. Certain provisions are unlikely to please either avid promoters of psychosurgery or those favoring a complete ban; nonetheless, it is a reasonable response to a highly complex problem, and its basic approach is likely to gain general acceptance.

Briefly, the Commission found that psychosurgery is an experimental procedure, that in certain cases it could have a therapeutic effect, that a potential subject's status should not de facto prohibit him from undergoing psychosurgery, and that procedural safeguards could and should be set up to ensure that psychosurgery is performed only when it is both medically indicated and when the subject has given informed consent. The Commission's primary recommendation is:

> (1) Until the safety and efficacy of any psychosurgical procedure have been demonstrated, such procedure should be performed only at an institution with an institutional review board (IRB) approved by DHEW specifically for reviewing proposed psychosurgery, and only after such IRB has determined that: (A) the surgeon has the competence to perform the procedure; (B) it is appropriate, based upon sufficient assessment of the patient, to perform the procedure on that patient; (C) adequate pre- and postoperative evaluations will be performed; and (D) the patient has given informed consent. . . .

If there is any reason to call the patient's consent into question, more elaborate procedural safeguards—including a court hearing for prisoners, involuntarily committed mental patients, and children—are also required.

A system of elaborate procedural safeguards is the only viable alternative to a complete prohibition of psychosurgery. Like any such safeguards, however, their implementation will demand both a philosophical and an economic commitment if they are to be carried out in a manner which will protect the rights of potential subjects. What are the implementation problems as they relate to the protection of subjects?

Potential Future Abuses

Since the recommendations deal only with experimental surgery, they apply only until the "safety and efficacy" of a particular psychosurgical procedure are demonstrated. This leads to at least two major problems. The first is one that was arguably not within the Commission's mandate to consider: the potential danger that once safety and efficacy have

Source: Hastings Center Report, vol. 7, April, 1977, pp. 11–13.

been demonstrated, psychosurgery may be used to modify the behavior of prisoners, dissidents, minorities, and other deviant groups. An "approved" procedure is likely to take on a technological imperative of its own, with unpredictable results. I would submit that psychosurgery that "works" poses a greater danger to society than psychosurgery that doesn't, and that this issue demands attention to such things as deviance and violence *before* "safety and efficacy" are demonstrated. Upon full consideration of the potential dangers involved, a decision to either prohibit psychosurgery for certain "indications" (like violence) or to require court review for certain populations (like prisoners and children) may well be in order, even after safety and efficacy have been established.

Inadequate Data

The second danger is illustrated by the Commission's own report—the possibility that "safety and efficacy" may be determined on grossly inadequate data. On the basis of two "pilot" studies conducted by researchers at Boston University and MIT of four different psychosurgical procedures on sixty-one adults, the Commission concluded that there is "at least tentative evidence that some forms of psychosurgery can be of significant therapeutic value in the treatment of certain disorders or in the relief of certain symptoms." (Comment to Recommendation 1). While this statement is not an overly enthusiastic endorsement, I would argue that it cannot be supported by the Commission's evidence. First, the Commission neglects to identify which forms of psychosurgery it finds might be of value and for what symptoms. This omission is especially troubling since the Commission expanded the term "psychosurgery" as contained in its legislative mandate to include operations to relieve the emotional responses to pain, and that if the pain patients were excluded from the sixty-one studied (fifteen such patients with eleven "successes"), the overall success rate would drop from a majority to about 43 percent. Moreover, of the remaining forty-six patients, twenty, or almost half, had more than one psychosurgical procedure. If the first operation (and the second in those cases that had three procedures) had been counted as a failure by the Commission, as it reasonably could have, the overall success rate in the nonpain group would have dropped to under 30 percent—less than the surgical placebo success rate identified by Henry Beecher.[2]

Since the placebo effect may be especially high in a behavior-altering procedure done by a surgeon who is a true believer and has a strong rapport with his patients, the Commission could just as logically have concluded from these studies that the only evidence it had was that psychosurgery "worked" only for pain patients, but that for any other indication it was less effective than a placebo. The Commission's own statistics indicated that during the years 1971–1973, about 500 psychosurgical procedures were performed annually in the United States by about 140 neurosurgeons. The Commission looked only at sixty-one cases of four surgeons who volunteered their cases for study. Most forms of psychosurgery were not seen at all; and since, in the present malpractice climate, surgeons cannot be expected to volunteer their failures or worst cases for study, one is skeptical of those that were seen. In fact, given the built-in bias in the selection process, the very limited sampling, and problems in testing and comparability, I would argue that *no* conclusions about psychosurgery in general can be drawn from the Commission's data. The point is not who is right in interpreting the data; the data can be interpreted in many different ways. The critical issue is *who* decides what is "safe and effective," and on what basis. It would seem essential that, in addition to adequate public representation, at least one highly respected biostatistician or epidemiologist be made a member of the Commission's proposed "National Psychosurgery Advisory Board" to help prevent any overly enthusiastic reading of reported results.

Confusing Confidentiality and Privilege

A third danger is that the IRB review process might act simply as a rubber stamp, legitimizing an otherwise questionable procedure. Experience at the Boston City Hospital and in Oregon indicates that this is unlikely to happen if the psychosurgery review committee actually discusses the procedure with the subject. The Commission's recommendation makes such a face-to-face meeting optional for the subject, noting the patient's right to confidentiality. Here the Commission seems to be confusing three concepts: privacy, confidentiality, and privilege. As to privacy, the Commission seems to be saying at a number of points that there might be a constitutional right to be the subject of a psychosurgical procedure, and that it would be morally wrong (if not illegal) to deny certain populations (like prisoners and children) "access to potentially beneficial therapy." Since this premise implies that there may not be categorical exclusions from the pool of potential research subjects, such an argument strikes at the essence of almost all the Commission's deliberations. If the Commission is making policy recommendations on this premise, Congress deserves an open and well-articulated statement of its rationale.

As to privilege and confidentiality, the Commission states (when discussing the California statute that requires review by a committee of three physicians): "Because the committee is composed only of physicians, its proceedings are clearly covered by the physician/patient privilege." In its recommendation on IRB hearings with the subject present, the Commission says that the IRB "should maintain confidentiality, unless the patient waives this privilege." The confusion between privilege, a concept which applies only to testimony in a legal proceeding, and confidentiality, which may be established in *any* relationship, is common. The confusion seemingly results here, however, in a Commission conclusion that HEW cannot compel appearance of the subject before the IRB's psychosurgical subcommittee (either because all its members are not physicians or because the subject has a "right" to psychosurgery). This conclusion is neither persuasive nor legally accurate. The privilege applies to physicians *only* if they are in a doctor-patient relationship with the subject, and confidentiality can be made to apply to all members of a review committee by contract. A change in the regulations to require a personal appearance by the potential subject before the review committee on the issue of informed consent would be both appropriate and enforceable.

Informed Consent

A number of additional points merit attention. Adult prisoners and mental patients are rightfully given the absolute right to refuse psychosurgery. Proxy consent is, however, permissible under the regulations for children. I would submit that this is unjustified in that the Commission found *no* evidence of psychosurgery ever being beneficial for children.

The Commission's dismissal of the holding of *Kaimowitz* v. *Michigan Department of Mental Health*—the Detroit psychosurgery case—regarding informed consent is highly superficial and cavalier. The case is attacked on its constitutional arguments, after which its much stronger arguments on informed consent are simply dismissed by a comment that to exclude proxy consent for involuntarily committed mental patients and prisoners "seems unfair." One might reasonably ask "unfair to whom?"—the Commission, the prisoner, the surgeon, or society? The *Kaimowitz* opinion presents problems, but I would submit that it is not persuasively refuted by the Commission, which studied *no* actual cases involving either involuntarily committed mental patients or amygdalotomies for violence—the facts at issue in *Kaimowitz.*

Finally, the Commission's recommendation that the Secretary of HEW "conduct and support studies to evaluate the safety of specific psychosurgical procedures and the efficacy of such procedures in relieving specific psychiatric symptoms and disorders" is inappropriate. It is outside the Commission's Congressional mandate and unsupported by the evidence available to the Commission. Nothing in the Commission's report supports the concept that psychosurgery research should be on HEW's priority list, or that studies of the multiple types of procedures being used and the multiple "indications" for surgery employed by the more than 140 surgeons in this field would be fruitful. The Commission was set up to protect subjects, and not to promote research. While these two activities are certainly compatible, emphasis on the latter tends to detract from the former.

In summary, the Commission's final recommendations on psychosurgery are a reasonable attempt to establish procedural safeguards for potential subjects of this controversial method of behavior modification. Following a few refinements, perhaps along the lines mentioned, they are likely to be generally accepted and adopted by HEW following their formal rule-making procedures. While such regulations should do much to help protect potential subjects of psychosurgery, they should not be used as an excuse for not exploring the much more difficult question: what do we do if it "works?" While an outright ban may be unnecessary, there may be some "accepted" medical or surgical treatments that should never be used for some "indications," or should be performed on certain populations only following review procedures generally reserved for experimental treatments.

Whatever Happened to John Doe?

The case of Louis Smith, known as "John Doe" in the Detroit psychosurgery case, keeps taking bizarre turns. In 1955, while a mental patient at Kalamazoo State Hospital, Smith was accused of raping and murdering a student nurse. Instead of being brought to trial, Smith was committed to Ionia State Hospital under Michigan's Criminal Sexual Psychopath statute. In 1972, he was transferred to the Lafayette Clinic in Detroit as the prime candidate for an experimental psychosurgery project.

When the project was brought to public attention, a lawsuit was instituted to stop the procedure from being performed. The court that heard the case ruled that the statute under which Smith had been committed was unconstitutional, and that he was being held illegally. He subsequently withdrew his consent for the psychosurgery.

After his release in March 1973, Smith worked for a few months as a silk-screener in Detroit, and then returned to his home town of Kalamazoo, where he enrolled at Valley College. Shortly thereafter he was apprehended stealing a woman's girdle from a local department store. After he was booked, he was searched and found to be wearing nineteen pairs of women's underpants and ten slips. He entered a plea of guilty to the shoplifting charge and was sentenced for thirty-two months to four years.

While in custody, Smith confessed to the crime that had occurred more than twenty-one years earlier. At the trial held early in 1976, Smith pleaded innocent, with a defense of insanity. The jury, however, did not accept the defense, and found him guilty of murder in the second degree. Now in his mid-40s, he was sentenced in April 1976 to life imprisonment, with credit for the eighteen years he had already spent in institutions.

Smith is now serving his sentence at the Southern Michigan Prison at Jackson. His case is being appealed to the Michigan Supreme Court.

NOTES

1. Psychosurgery regulation is discussed in detail in a chapter in *Informed Consent and Human Experimentation: The Subject's Dilemma* by the author and health lawyers Leonard H. Glantz and Barbara F. Katz.

2. "Surgery as Placebo," *Journal of the American Medical Association,* vol. 176, p. 1102, 1961.

85. *The Legal Implications of Sexual Activity between Psychiatrist and Patient*   Alan A. Stone

Last year at the APA meeting in Anaheim, Calif., Dr. William Masters suggested that any therapist who exploits the power and position of his or her professional status to have sexual intercourse with a patient should be charged with rape. He and Virginia Johnson stated,

> We feel that when sexual seduction of patients can be firmly established by due legal process, regardless of whether the seduction was initiated by the patient or the therapist, the therapist should initially be sued for rape rather than for malpractice, i.e., the legal process should be criminal rather than civil. Few psychotherapists would be willing to appear in court on behalf of a colleague and testify that the sexually dysfunctional patient's facility for decision making could be considered normally objective when he or she accepts sexual submission after developing extreme emotional dependence on the therapist.[1]

In this paper I will examine the gap between Masters and Johnson's moral indignation and the existing sanctions in law. There are three specific limitations in the scope of this paper. First, I shall for convenience assume that the problem is one of male therapists being involved with female patients, although the legal ramifications are by no means confined to this assumption; indeed, one of the most well-known criminal cases involved homosexual activities between a male physician and his male adolescent patients.[2] Second, I have omitted any discussion of the legal problems of using sexual surrogates other than the psychotherapist in sexual treatment; that would require another paper. Third, I have elected as a matter of personal judgment not to use the names of psychotherapists or patients despite the fact that the records are in most instances in the public domain.

There are three possible legal sanctions against sex between therapist and patient. First there are the various statutes of the criminal law, including rape and rape by fraud or coercion. The latter at least theoretically might be applicable to the situations Masters and Johnson had in mind. Second, there are tort actions, including malpractice, in the civil courts. Third, there is revocation of license to practice by the medical board of licensure. Beyond

Source: *American Journal of Psychiatry,* vol. 133, no. 10, p. 1138, October 1976. Copyright 1976, the American Psychiatric Association. Reprinted by permission.

these legal approaches there are the ethical sanctions of professional associations, societies, and institutions that might potentially have teeth by limiting career opportunities, patient referrals, and staff privileges at various institutional facilities.

Criminal Law

My review of the legal literature suggests that the criminal courts have been extremely reluctant to adopt Masters and Johnson's suggestion. Rape charges apparently are rarely brought, and, when they are, rarely do they stick. The few reported cases involved some element of physical coercion or force rather than the kind of psychological coercion Masters and Johnson referred to. In fact, in cases in which psychiatrists have been convicted of rape or sexual assault, their behavior has been egregious by almost any moral or legal standard.

Thus an East Coast psychiatrist who gave his patients ECT and/or injections of hypnotic drugs and then had intercourse with them was convicted and served time in prison. Similarly, a West Coast psychiatrist who had intercourse with a 16-year-old girl who was referred for therapy for promiscuity was prosecuted for and convicted of statutory rape.

In contrast to these cases, when a legally competent patient is told that sexual intercourse is to be administered as therapy and the patient consents, the presiding judicial opinions are that there is no rape because there has been neither force nor fraud.[3] However, a few states have passed statutes that specifically encompass Masters and Johnson's moral judgment. The clearest example is Michigan, which has adopted the following statutory language defining coercion in rape: "When the actor engages in the medical treatment or examination of the victim in a manner or for purposes which are medically recognized as unethical or unacceptable." Under this statute sex as therapy might be construed as rape. The implications of this statute are quite novel in that the definition of rape is placed in the hands of the expert witnesses.

Ohio has adopted even broader statutory language, which would inculpate psychotherapists for the lesser offense of sexual battery. The Ohio statute reads as follows: "The offender knowingly coerces the other person to submit by any means that would prevent resistance by a person of ordinary resolution."

Although the criminal law has been invoked almost not at all when a psychotherapist exploits the transference for sexual gratification but does not claim that the sexual activity is treatment, this Ohio statute might be applicable if prosecutors and juries believed that transference creates a coercive relationship.

Summing up, unless new criminal statutes are enacted, criminal charges of rape or related sexual offenses against psychotherapists who exploit their patients are a remote possibility at best.

Civil Law

Let me then turn to the civil area, which involves suits for damages and particularly malpractice. Although it may be an unimportant professional distinction, it is important in these legal cases whether the sexual activity is designated as therapy or not. If a therapist induces a patient to engage in sexual activity on the basis that it is treatment, it will more readily be considered under the rubric of malpractice. If the therapist has an affair with a patient separate from the treatment, no legal cause of action may be available. This legal distinction becomes apparent when suits are brought by husbands whose wives have been seduced by their therapists. In this context the courts seem unwilling to allow the husband's claim of malpractice; indeed, most suits of this sort have failed.

However, this legal distinction is somewhat muddied because there are cases in which judges have held that misuse of the transference is a basis for psychiatric malpractice. One southern psychotherapist who told his patient that he was going to divorce his wife and wanted to marry her was said by the court to have engaged in "conduct below acceptable psychiatric and medical standards." The husband was allowed to recover the cost of his wife's hospitalization and treatment. All the experts in this case agreed that the psychiatrist had acted out his countertransference and that his profession of love was inappropriate.

Presumably, all the experts would a fortiori agree with the testimony given in a recent case by Dr. Willard Gaylin that "there are absolutely no circumstances which permit a psychiatrist to engage in sex with his patient." All such instances constitute misuse of the transference.

Unfortunately, there are more legal complications to a civil suit of this sort than one might imagine. Many states have passed so-called heart balm statutes that bar civil liability for sexual activity, e.g., seduction, alienation of affections, or criminal conversation. It is the heart balm act that prevents husbands from collecting. In a recent case an East Coast psychotherapist claimed that the heart balm act meant there could be no basis for a malpractice suit by the patient. However, the court held to the contrary that the relationship of a psychotherapist to a patient was a "fiduciary relationship" analogous to that between a guardian and his ward. Further, the court stated that "there is a public policy to protect a patient from the deliberate and malicious abuse of power and breach of trust by a psychiatrist when that patient entrusts to him her body and mind."

The judicial decision that analogized the therapist-patient relationship to the guardian-ward relationship not only undercuts the heart balm act but also does away with the difficult problem of consent.

The facts alleged in this case were that a patient with homosexual predispositions and heterosexual anxiety was induced to have repeated sex with her psychiatrist as a form of therapy. There is in this case, as in all sexual situations that take place in private, the problem of corroborating evidence for the patient's testimony. Ordinarily in such cases testimony as to similar conduct by the psychiatrist could be excluded, but the psychiatrist in this case claimed to be impotent. Therefore, the patient was able to offer the testimony of three other women patients, two of whom reported similar sexual experiences with the psychiatrist and one of whom described blatant and inappropriate sexual behavior and attempted seduction by him. Some of this testimony was stricken from the record as not relevant to the time period during which the psychiatrist claimed impotence. The psychiatrist claimed that the two patients whose testimony was admissible were both suffering from erotomania. The jury, after a lengthy trial, awarded the patient $250,000 compensatory damages and $100,000 punitive damages. However, these huge awards did not remain in effect.

The reasons for the revocation of the amount of damages are quite complex; I will summarize and highlight what I take to be important. First, the therapist's malpractice insurer refused to defend him, leaving the therapist to support three years of litigation on his own. However, after the damage judgment was awarded, the patient sued the insurance company for part of the damages and settled for $50,000. The therapist pursued his own legal appeals, and in a subsequent decision a higher court dismissed the punitive damages of $100,000 and reduced the compensation award to no more than $25,000. At most, therefore, the patient will receive $75,000, less legal fees.

Furthermore, despite the important holdings in this case, the decision does not clarify the malpractice implications of sex between therapist and patient because there were two lines of defense that this therapist did not assert: (1) that the patient had freely consented to an affair and had known it was not therapy; (2) that the therapist believed sex between the doctor and patient was therapeutic, the patient had been told in advance that sexual activity would be part of the therapy—that is, she had been given full disclosure before the transference developed. Instead, the therapist insisted that the patient had a psychotic transference.

Both of these defenses, although unacceptable to American psychiatry, may still be appropriate defenses in a court of law. Nonetheless, insurers have responded as if sex between therapist and patient is a clear instance of malpractice. The APA insurers have been quick to settle claims. The result is that malpractice rates for all of us will escalate while the offending therapists are protected from the adversities concomitant to a trial.

The American Psychological Association has pursued an alternate avenue: they have obtained insurance that excludes liability for sexual activity. Whether the adverse effects of sex between therapist and patient should be compensable by an insurance policy is, I think, a debatable question.

The problem of estimating the damages suffered in these malpractice suits was reflected in the appellate decision in the case I have been discussing. The court reduced the $350,000 award to $25,000. There was one dissenting judge who was prepared to argue that there was no malpractice and no damages. He argued that the civil courts were not the place for dealing with the problems of sex therapy or sex between doctor and patient. As he put it, "Although the plaintiff was suffering from a number of emotional problems, her competency was never placed in issue." Thus he rejected the fiduciary theory, insisting that the patient was legally competent to consent to have intercourse. He went on,

> Is it not fair to infer therefore that she was capable of giving a knowing and meaningful consent? For almost one and a half years while this "meaningful relationship" continued the plaintiff was not heard to complain. Upon the defendant terminating the relationship this law suit evolves.

Although the judge made it clear that he believed the jury finding that the psychiatrist had had intercourse with his patient and that the psychiatrist "obviously did not help his cause by denying what the jury found to be the fact. . . . Nevertheless, however ill-advised or ill-conceived was the choice of his defense, in my view this did not constitute malpractice." He also stated,

> I neither condone the defendant's reprehensible conduct, nor maintain that it was not violative of his professional ethics and Hippocratic oath. . . . For violation of his Hippocratic oath, if there be any, let him suffer the sanctions of the medical ethics board or other appropriate medical authority.

In this disposition of turning the case over to the medical licensing board and the profession for appropriate action, the dissent was in fact joined by the majority, who stated,

> Sex under cloak of treatment is an acceptable and established ground for disciplinary measures taken against physicians either by licensing authorities or professional organizations.

Interestingly enough, the court did not foreclose the matter of whether the psychiatrist should be deprived of his license or sanctioned by his professional organization:

> Whether defendant acted in such manner as to seriously affect his performance as a practitioner in the psychiatric field should be left to these more competent fora. The only thing that the record herein supports is that his prescribed treatment was in negligent disregard of the consequences. For that and that alone he must be held liable.

Professional Boards and Associations

As one looks at the capability of licensing boards and professional associations, which were considered "the more competent fora" by that court, according to my research there is an almost total lack of capacity to act. The professional associations have no subpoena power and no expertise in criminal or other evidentiary investigation. They have neither formulated necessary procedures nor employed sufficient legal staff to protect the due process rights of a doctor charged with some such act or themselves if the charged doctor sues them. Indeed, it often happens that, because his or her whole career is at stake, a doctor charged with any ethical complaint hires a lawyer who immediately threatens to sue the society, the association, and its ethics committee, all of whom have no indemnification. That characterization, I must confess, is up to this point an accurate description of APA. However, we are not alone. Lawyers expert in private association law tell me that none of the associations has the proper machinery and that many of them behave as we do, by postponing any and all action until all legal appeals are exhausted in the criminal and/or civil area.

Finally, then, we turn to the licensing boards in hopes that something can be done there. The fact that a number of cases exist in which licensing boards have actually revoked licensure for sexual activity of doctors with patients suggests that some power resides in these boards and is being used.[4] However, the licensing boards in each of the states are organized quite differently. Some have a close relationship to the medical society, others do not, and some are impotent bureaucracies reluctant to do anything. Therefore, one cannot expect real consistency across the different jurisdictions. Each jurisdiction has enabling statutes that limit the scope of authority.

In one western state, for instance, a doctor guilty of the grossest sexual impropriety could not have his license revoked because the only ground was "grossly negligent or ignorant malpractice"; his board found that he was guilty of "grossly negligent or immoral malpractice."

Comment

I have briefly described four possible avenues for punishing, disciplining, or deterring sexual activity between therapist and patient. None of these avenues seems to provide an effective system of control. In the end, in this as in most other things, patients must depend on the decent moral character of those entrusted to treat them.

NOTES

1. W. H. Masters, and V. E. Johnson, "Principles of the New Sex Therapy," *American Journal of Psychiatry*, vol. 133, p. 548, 1976.

2. J. Goldstein, A. Dershowitz, and R. D. Schwartz, *Criminal Law: Theory and Process*, Free Press, New York, 1974.

3. H. S. Shapo, "Note: Recent Statutory Developments in the Definition of Forcible Rape," *Virginia Law Review*, vol. 61, p. 1500, 1975.

4. There have been at least eight reported appeals from license revocation that were grounded on sexual impropriety by a physician. Several were by psychiatrists.

Placebos

86. *The Placebo Dilemma*   Leo Schindel

An observation made in 1971 on a number of Mexican-American women, at a family planning clinic for contraceptives, describes most impressively the problems related to the prescription and use of placebos, in other words, the placebo dilemma confronting the medical profession.

One group of the women had been given contraceptives, and another group had received identical-appearing placebos in order to determine what side effects could be found in each group. None of the women knew what type of pill they had taken. One side effect of the placebo group could definitely be predicted, namely, pregnancy, and in 10 women pregnancy actually occurred.

The fact that a number of the placebo-receiving women became pregnant started a chain reaction of dilemmas. Had the women actually been told what might happen? Did they consent to the trial? Did the physician in charge have the legal right to induce an artificial abortion? How clear was the doctor's conscience, or was he aware of deceitful behavior? But do not such problems always exist when a doctor intends to prescribe a placebo for therapeutic reasons or experimental evaluation of a new drug principle? The same doctor is faced with the potential risk for the patient and for himself and he can never presume what the real benefit may be.

It is certainly true that 40 to 50 years ago, most of the prescribed medicaments or therapeutic procedures primarily had a placebo effect, not specific for the disease, but given in good faith by the medical attendant. And this is a further dilemma. The prescribing physician may be convinced that an antibiotic has a beneficial action in a viral infection or that vitamin supplementation, especially vitamin B_{12} injection, improves the strength and well-being of a patient, even if pernicious anemia is not present. In K. L. Melmon and H. F. Morrelli's *Textbook of Clinical Pharmacology,* mention is made that 35 to 45 percent of all prescriptions are for substances that are incapable of having an effect on the condition for which they are prescribed. The patient's expectation, and that of the doctor, for successful treatment, cause increasing reliance on a therapeutic action which, in reality, is nothing but a placebo effect.

We know from Henry K. Beecher's clinical study[3] that about 35 percent of his patients receiving placebo injections had satisfactory relief of postoperative pain or angina pectoris. Doesn't this observation—repeatedly made by many serious clinicians—suggest that we almost never know what is meaningful in our therapeutic approach, and how doubtful may be the information which we give to patients or to their relatives in answer to their questions about the potential therapeutic effect of the treatment? In principle, placebos may have the same effects and side effects as clinically used therapeutic agents but a positive placebo effect can never be predicted (Anschuetz[2]). Here again, we face a personal dilemma. Should we disclose to our patient the uncertainties of our estimation of the healing process or how problematic our diagnostic or therapeutic prognosis is?

Source: *European Journal of Clinical Pharmacology,* vol. 13, p. 231, 1978.

Does the powerful placebo effect obscure our judgment and keep both the patient and the doctor in the dark?

Would this obscurity be clarified if the patient had given his consent to any treatment, including a placebo? No doubt the value of the placebo would be reduced if the patient's consent were sought, since the "positive therapeutic action" depends on his ignorance. A different question is whether prescription of a placebo requires the patient's consent, since such a harmless, but at the same time highly potent and even beneficial medication is not a drug in the usual sense. This consideration is a further link in the chain of dilemmas about the use of placebos. Would it be sufficient to tell a patient that "this tablet which he will receive may help him?" It is certainly neither lie nor deceit, but if the patient were to agree to the treatment, would it be informed consent?

Looking further reveals an additional dilemma confrontation associated with the use of placebos—the observation of side effects after medication with an inactive placebo material. In his paper "Placebo-Induced Side Effects,"[12] Schindel reviewed placebo-induced symptoms and their frequency. Symptoms ranging from headache to urticaria, diarrhea, sleeplessness, dyspepsia, edema, faintness, anxiety conditions, mental confusion, tremor, tachycardia, and diuresis, and even more have been observed and described with a frequency up to 30 to 40 percent. A recent Japanese publication by Tada Ishioka[14] presented similar results from Japanese people, and also referred to the similarity of the "toxic" effects of active drug principles and those of placebos.

Oliver Wendell Holmes[16] is often cited as having written in 1860 that "if all the materia medica were thrown into the sea, it would help the human race, but it would not help the fish much." This comment was repeated by Douglas J. Whalan,[15] in a symposium on clinical trials and the pharmacists' responsibilities, held in October 1975, in Canberra, Australia, and he continued "of course, these days, the fish are in much greater danger from other sorts of pollution. I understand that in some Australian estuaries the mercury content is so high that when anyone is sick, their temperature is not taken with a thermometer, but with a sardine."

Holmes' statement was a sarcastic exaggeration. However, at the same time he did not know about the highly potent therapeutic drugs which may be both life-saving and life-threatening and herein arises another doctor's dilemma: can we compare a highly potent drug principle—possibly with a narrow therapeutic-toxic margin—with a placebo? It is like a comparison between a 100 percent active compound and a 0 percent material. This problem is especially important in the evaluation of a new compound. If a new antibiotic is to be tested, initially it can only be compared with an antimicrobially effective substance and not with material of no potency.

A particularly unexpected dilemma, which may be regarded as a most undesirable side effect of placebo use, is the development of dependency. Sissela Bok[5] referred to a psychotic patient who was given placebo pills and was told that they were "a new major tranquillizer without any side effects." After having taken this placebo, up to 12 tablets a day for 4 years, she complained of insomnia and anxiety. "When self-medication had reached 25 tablets daily, a crisis occurred, the physician intervened, talked over the addictive problem (but not the deception) with the patient, and succeeded in reducing the dose to two a day, a level which was still being maintained a year later." Many other cases of dependency have been described and they have appeared most frequently in neurotic patients in whom anxiety and sleeplessness have been prominent.

One of my patients represents a good example of how readily dependency can develop: a 40-year-old woman suffered from a duodenal ulcer and kept more or less to a balanced diet. However, she was under the influence of a weight-watcher society, and her diet was "adapted" to the demands of the regulations which this group thought essential for her well-being. The result was quite satisfactory as far as her weight and ulcer condition was concerned, but her sleep was increasingly disturbed. The hypnotic agent which she usually took (nitrazepam, Mogadon) lost its efficacy and her demand for a new hypnotic steadily increased. One day, a placebo tablet, sprinkled with many color spots from crushed colored tablets, was added to the nitrazepam (Mogadon). The result during the weeks that followed was excellent. She slept for 8 hours or more with no disturbing dreams and awoke fresh and without a hangover. After about 12 to 14 nights, the effect of the additional sprinkled tablet material faded away. The addition of second placebo tablets of the same shape, color, and size again brought a good therapeutic result. After a further 3 weeks she was able to sleep with the two placebos alone, since one sprinkled placebo tablet was not sufficient. The medication was maintained for many months until this type of placebo was exhausted and she was transferred to a commercial sedative, again with satisfactory results.

Do placebos alter sleep? Bearing in mind the many patients who have received a placebo instead of a hypnotic, or in addition to one, the answer should be "yes." But reading the paper by K. Adam et al.[1] may raise some doubts.

In 10 volunteers, the deliberate suggestion that an inert capsule was a sleeping pill was found not to influence subjective ratings of sleep quality or anxiety, or electro-physiologically recorded features of sleep. Isn't this fact yet another link in the chain of the placebo dilemma?

In a publication in the British Medical Journal, Kurt Schapira[10] mentioned that the response of patients to differently colored tablets varied remarkably. Thus, "patients with anxiety symptoms showed a more favorable response to green tablets, while the same product as a yellow tablet was more effective in relieving depression." This result is valid at least for the selected group which had been under Schapira's observation and treatment.

The significance of color was also mentioned by Huskisson[7] in his experimental investigation of analgesics in arthritis. Aspirin, Codis, and Distalgesic were the most effective analgesics tested. Concerning placebos, he confirmed earlier observations that placebo given after an active analgesic was more effective than when given before. This phenomenon was still observed when the patient was told that apparently identical tablets were in fact different, or by marking them in a different color. The effectiveness of soluble placebo depended on its color, red being the most effective.

To improve the therapeutic action of an active drug principle by choosing the preferred, individual color for the tablets is a useful hint—already given by Schindel in 1967[11]—but only adds yet another intellectual stress to the existing placebo-dilemma situation.

A dilemma which can probably never be overcome is the situation in which a person "treated" with placebo discovers that he received an "inert nothing." But a similar situation may arise when an antibiotic has been prescribed unintentionally for a virally caused fever and the patient asks again for an antibiotic whenever he or a member of his family, especially children, develop fever.

In the voluminous literature on placebos the distinction is drawn between pure and impure placebos. What pure placebos are can easily be understood, namely the "inert nothing." An impure placebo can be anything administered with the intention to influence a disease condition in man. It is not always easy to differentiate a somewhat active substance from a more active substance. If a known, commercially available drug is given in a dose considered too small to produce a therapeutic effect, i.e., in a subtherapeutic dose, this may be considered a masked "impure placebo." It is not an inert substance, because the patient and doctor believe in its therapeutic action and efficacy. How often are highly active drugs administered in subtherapeutic doses? In recent years we have learned much about faulty digitalization. This impure placebo "treatment" is a serious dilemma for both the sick patient and the doctor. To a certain degree, bioavailability tests are able to help us to overcome this problem. But here, too, it is the therapeutic effect which is decisive and not the time of absorption, the blood level, or the duration of a certain concentration of the active compound in blood.

"The truth and deception in medicine" was the subject of a paper which R. C. Cabot wrote in 1909,[17] where the following statement was made: "The majority of placebos are given because we believe the patient . . . has learned to expect medicine for every symptom, and without it he simply won't get well. True, but who taught him to expect a medicine for every symptom? He was not born with that expectation . . . it is we, the physicians, who are responsible for perpetuating false ideas about disease and its cure . . . With every placebo we give, we do our part in perpetuating error, and harmful error at that" (according to Sissela Bok).

But ever more problems face us when we review critically the famous "double-blind" test procedure. No doubt one can speak of a "double-blind dilemma" (Kligman[9]). Sometimes results of a therapeutic assay remind one of the "blind leading the blind." A fixed dosage regime not adjusted to the needs of the individual, e.g., as for an analgesic, may represent too small or too large a dose. The result is either no effect, because of underdosage, or a toxic adverse effect because of overdosage. What can clinical evaluation or comparison with a placebo achieve in this case? Comparison of morphine with a new analgesic must take into consideration that part of the morphine effect is based on its euphoric component. If a patient has once received a morphine injection he certainly will remember how such side effects as euphoria or nausea affected his personal feelings. Such a patient injected with a placebo (with a different, morphine-like analgesic action) will recognize immediately if he has received morphine or something else when the "side effects" are missing. How can one perform a double-blind study of retinoic acid vs. a placebo in acne, when erythema and peeling will immediately identify the active agent, or a cytostatic agent in psoriasis when clearing is preceded by erosions? How blind must one be not to recognize that after a dose of rifampicin the urine is discolored, or the linen is stained after ingestion of p-aminosalicylic acid? Quite often their color and taste change when placebo preparations are stored for a long time, so that neither the patient nor the doctor needs to be "blind" to identify the original and the comparison agent.

The appropriate selection of patients is a most important decision in separation of biased wishful thinking from realistic results.

What about the "human factor" in evaluation of double-blind controls? L. E. Hill et al.[6] described this dilemma in a recent paper. A panel of observers studied 22 pairs of agents; 5 pairs of substances were an excellent match, which were virtually indistinguishable, but 7 pairs were prepared in such a way that 4 observers easily detected the differences between the natural original and the synthetic-adapted material. One panel member was especially successful and was able to detect 3 times more often than the other observers the differences between the pairs of preparations. However, the panel was inspecting pairs, side by side, and thus were able to state that two preparations were different. This is not the same as saying which was the real drug and which was the placebo. D. S. Blumenthal et al.[4] dealt with the "Validity of Identical Matching Placebos" in an experimental study and found two particular shortcomings. When tasting two different types of medication, some subjects found that one sample (which was actually the active preparation) numbed the tongue, and therefore could be identified as different from the other one (which was the placebo). When capsules containing an antidepressant had to be compared with other capsules (placebo), the fact that they were not identical was demonstrated by putting both types into a water pan. One sample floated on the surface (the placebo) and the other sank to the bottom.

A patient does not usually inform the doctor of the symptoms which appear in a placebo trial, but instead tells the attending nurse. In a study of "placebo and placebo effect in clinic and research," the summary of a report on side effects communicated to doctors or nurses was published, which was based on figures collected by Greenblatt. When patients were asked how they felt and if they had any complaints, the doctors were informed of 72 side effects, and the nurses of 36. When the patients were asked specifically if disturbances of the heart, intestinal organs, etc., were observed after the medicament had been given, the doctors heard such complaints 34 times and the nurses only 4 times. However, when the patients had to write the symptoms on a list after having ingested the individual drug, the doctors found 353 side effects and the nurses only 108. Here again, the human factor—from the patient's side—affected the real value of drug evaluation. In evaluation of a therapeutic effect whether useful or useless, there is a human factor which must be included in the risk of the applied research and realized as an ever-present dilemma.

For the role of the human factor in evaluation of the placebo effect, A. K. Shapiro[13] introduced the term "iatroplacebogenics." It refers to the doctor's personality and attitude, his warmth and his emphasis or hostility toward the patient. Also included is his attitude toward the treatment and the results of his active-enthusiastic or passive-nihilistic intervention. A typical situation was created when a placebo trial was started to evaluate the influence of a placebo on gastric acidity. Two groups of patients received the "inert nothing," one from doctor A, an enthusiastic young researcher. In this group a 12 percent increase in gastric acidity followed placebo administration. The second group, treated and observed by doctor B, a pessimistic, nihilistic, bad-humored bachelor, averaged a 15% decrease in gastric acidity after the same placebo administered in the same quantity and under similar conditions. This is more than a placebo dilemma. It would appear to make evaluation of a drug, the activity of which is to be compared and evaluated, almost impossible.

How problematical a negative therapeutic result can be was demonstrated by E. C. Johnstone et al.[8] in their 6 week double-blind crossover trial of phenelzine (phenethylhydrazine, a well-known MAO inhibitor) versus placebo in 72 patients with neurotic depression. A significant improvement was found in slow acetylators, and in fast acetylators phenalzine was no more effective than placebo.

This study showed that a clinical trial with an "inert nothing" can explain why results are quite often contradictory. It proved furthermore that, in spite of a negative result in a selected group, phenelzine is a useful drug if the genetic phenotype of the patient could be determined before treatment was begun.

Considering the facts, there is no doubt that the existence of the "inert nothing" and the accompanying placebo effect makes evaluation and interpretation of drug testing difficult and complicated.

Only a well-trained and experienced clinical observer should be permitted to use a placebo in establishing the therapeutic value of drugs in order to avoid undesired pitfalls.

NOTES

1. K. Adam, L. Adamson, V. Brezinova, and I. Oswald, "Do Placebos Alter Sleep?" *British Medical Journal*, vol. 195, p. 1, 1976.

2. F. Anschuetz, "Placebo: Wirkung und Indikation," *Diagnostik*, vol. 10, p. 3, 1977.

3. H. K. Beecher, "The Powerful Placebo," *Journal of the American Medical Association*, vol. 159, p. 1602, 1965.

4. D. S. Blumenthal, R. Burke, and A. K. Shapiro, "Validity of Identical Matching Placebos," *Archives of General Psychiatry*, vol. 31, p. 214, 1974.

5. S. Bok, "The Ethics of Giving Placebos," *Scientific American*, vol. 231, p. 17, 1974.

6. L. E. Hill, A. J. Nunn, and W. Fox, "Matching Quality of Agents Employed in Double-Blind Controlled Clinical Trails," *Lancet*, vol. 1, p. 351, 1976.

7. G. C. Huskisson, "Simple Analgesics for Arthritis," *British Medical Journal*, vol. 4, p. 196, 1974.

8. G. C. Johnstone, and W. Marsh, "Acetylator Status and Response to Phenelzine in Depressed Patients," *Lancet*, vol. 1, p. 567, 1973.

9. A. Kligman, "The Double-Blind Dilemma," *Journal of the American Medical Association*, vol. 225, p. 1658, 1973.

10. K. Schapira, "Study on the Effects of Tablet Colour in the Treatment of Anxiety States," *British Medical Journal*, vol. 2, p. 446, 1970.

11. L. Schindel, "Placebo und Placebo Effekte in Klinik u. Forschung," *Arzneimittel-Forschung*, vol. 17, p. 892, 1967.

12. L. Schindel, "Placebo-Induced Side-Effects," in *Drug-Induced Diseases*, vol. 3, p. 232 (ed. L. Meyler and H. M. Peck), Excerpta Medica Foundation, Amsterdam, 1968.

13. A. K. Shapiro, "Iatroplacebogenics," *International Journal of Pharmacopsychiatry*, vol. 2, p. 215, 1969.

14. Tadao Ishioka, "Side Effects of Placebo 1," *Excerpta Medica*, International Congress Series no. 383, Rationality of Drug Development (ISBN 90219 03156), 1976.

15. D. J. Whalan, "Clinical Trials—Ethical and Legal Responsibilities of Pharmacists," *Australian Journal of Hospital Pharmacy*, vol. 5, p. 124, 1975.

16. O. W. Holmes, cited by A. K. Shapiro, "A Contribution to the History of the Placebo Effect," *Behavioral Science*, vol. 5, p. 109, 1960.

17. R. C. Cabot, cited by S. Bok.[5]

87. *Research and Therapeutic Implications* Howard Brody

The Meaning Model

Among several proposed theories of placebo action, the meaning model of Adler and Hammett comes closest to encompassing the essential features. In this model, the subjective sense of *meaning* in the illness experience is factored into (1) *system formation*, or the providing of a coherent explanation of the illness consistent with the patient's world view, and (2) *group formation*, or the gathering of a supportive, caring group around the patient. Together, these factors "are invariably used in all successful interpersonal therapies, and

Source: Howard Brody, *Placebos and the Philosophy of Medicine: Clinical, Conceptual and Ethical Issues*, University of Chicago Press, Chicago, 1977.

are the necessary and sufficient components of the placebo effect." By *system formation* these authors indicate the cultural-symbolic realm; and by *group formation* they point to sociological insights into the workings of the sick role. Thus, the model directs research toward cultural and social aspects of human nature.

The meaning model provides an important corrective for the bulk of placebo research on personality variables, which has focused almost exclusively on the emotional states of subjects without looking at their assumptions or systems of belief. Two cases suggest the central role that belief systems can play in the placebo effect:

Case 1. A woman of Christian Science faith failed to heal despite the relative simplicity of the surgical procedure [to correct retinal detachment] . Afterwards, she indicated to the surgeon that having surgery was in conflict with her Christian Science beliefs. Before reoperating, the surgeon made clear to her that he was only doing a mechanical task akin to realigning a broken bone and that her faith was the major factor in the actual healing. His statement helped her to reconcile her Christian Science beliefs with the necessity of surgery, and she healed quickly after the second operation.

Case 2. A man with far advanced lymph node malignancy, and with readily palpable, large tumor masses in the neck, abdomen, and groins, learned of the appearance of a new "miracle cancer drug," Krebiozen, in the newspapers. At his insistence he was included in a clinical trial of the drug, against protocol regulations, since his physicians felt that he had no more than two weeks to live. Within ten days he had demonstrated marked regression in the size of the tumors; and where he had previously been bedridden and gasping for air, he was well enough to be discharged from the hospital. After two months, however, news reports began to circulate carrying more discouraging news about Krebiozen, and the patient returned to the hospital with return of symptoms and recrudescence of his tumor masses. The physician then announced that it had been discovered that the first batches of Krebiozen had deteriorated with storage, and that a shipment of more potent drug was about to be received. He then proceeded to give the patient injections of plain water. Again, in a short time, the tumors shrank and the patient had nearly total symptom relief.

The patient remained healthy after this for some months until another news report appeared: "Nationwide AMA tests show Krebiozen to be worthless as cancer treatment." Within a few days the patient was readmitted, very depressed, and with far advanced symptoms; he died less than two days later.

Without question the emotional states of the two patients above played a large, if not crucial, role in the clinical outcomes. The point is, however, that descriptions which include reference only to emotional states cannot do full justice to the cases. For example, case 2 could be described as an example of the disappearance and reappearance of cancer symptoms and signs corresponding with cyclic depression. But such a description, making no reference to the changes in cognitive states which precipitated the depressions, is an unsatisfactory explanation. *Meaning* explanations can often give much more specific clues on how to intervene for the patient's benefit.

In medicine, the diagnosis is the primary mechanism for conferring meaning upon an illness event. While medical thinking has tended to distinguish carefully between diagnostic and therapeutic interventions, the meaning model suggests that diagnosis may in part also be treatment. One would hypothesize, then, that from among a group of patients with similar complaints, those given both a placebo and an understandable diagnostic label for their symptoms would have more relief than those given a placebo alone. This is important for group formation also: "We see how important it is that illness be given a legitimate name, that a sufferer have a mantle for his distress that society will accept."

Diagnoses, of course, have been designed by physicians to function within the explanatory system of scientific medicine, but with education of the public, most common diagnoses have become part of the explanatory system of the lay public. Thus, in most cases, the diagnosis will play a role in the patient's system formation, especially if the physician takes the time to explain the diagnosis and answer any questions about it. In most illness episodes, the disease is mild and self-limiting and so knowing the correct diagnosis is likely to exert a positive placebo effect. Even where the prognosis for the disease is very poor, the patient's symptoms might improve once the diagnosis is transmitted to him; a grim certainty is often preferable to paralyzing doubt. In a few cases, such as cancer, where the diagnostic label has been embroidered in the public mind by somewhat unrealistic dread, imparting the diagnosis might exert a negative placebo effect. This explains the traditional reluctance of physicians to report truthfully such diagnoses to the patient although the amount of actual damage that may be done is probably overestimated.

The ways in which diagnostic labeling suggests meaning to the patient need to be studied more fully. It is noteworthy, for example, that people on a waiting list at a psychiatric clinic showed a cure rate significantly above the spontaneous-remission rate for their neuroses before they had actually been seen for treatment. Thus, merely being accepted as a prospective patient by a psychiatric facility may count as sufficient diagnosis to lend enhanced meaning and symbolic coherence to the patient's subjective experience—all the more so because meaninglessness and lack of coherence are key features of the problem. Even though patients typically fear the label of mental illness, the label, once accepted, holds out promise that the condition can be understood and treated. For such patients, the waiting list itself apparently counts as part of the healing context. It would be worthwhile to see if such a phenomenon could be documented among patients on a waiting list to receive treatment for somatic complaints.

Certain behaviors of patients, puzzling at present, become more understandable when the symbolic function of the healing context is taken into account. There is a growing body of medical literature on why patients often fail to comply with the regimen of prescribed treatment. Since most of the literature assumes that the patient comes to the physician to receive the prescription for the regimen, failure to comply constitutes irrational behavior. If, on the contrary, patients come to physicians largely to confer meaning on the illness experience, this function has been completed once the physician pronounces a diagnosis and reinforces it by writing a prescription; the actual taking of the drug may be less important. Research on patient compliance would be more insightful if it took the symbolic functions of the physician-patient encounter into account more explicitly in the experimental design.

Other situations besides the healing context can markedly change one's sense of meaning, and the meaning model suggests that these situations also have the power to influence physical symptoms. A growing body of research has correlated the quantity of "life change," such as changes in residence and jobs, retirement, marriage, and death of a family member, with the likelihood of developing an organic disease in the months following. An important feature of such findings is that the quantity of change is a stronger predictive indicator than whether the change is commonly viewed in positive or negative terms (e.g., marriage and divorce affect health equally).

Another focus for research might be comparisons between the placebo effect and related phenomena. An interesting parallel might be drawn, for example, between the placebo effect and psychotherapy. Jerome Frank, in his very perceptive *Persuasion and Healing,* compares the various contemporary schools of psychotherapy with one another, as well as psychotherapy with the placebo effect, faith healing, shamanistic healing rituals, and religious revivalism. He concludes that there are important shared elements among the psychotherapeutic schools, and that in terms of explaining their general levels of efficacy, their similarities are more important than their differences. Frank lists four features as common to all schools of psychotherapy: (1) the patient's confidence in the therapist's ability and desire to help, (2) a socially sanctioned healing locale, especially one in which the patient can behave in ways that would not be acceptable elsewhere, (3) a "myth" or basic conceptual paradigm to explain the patient's symptoms in broad terms, and (4) a task to perform that involves the patient actively and which, by giving initially successful results, counteracts the demoralization that most patients seeking therapy have experienced in life.

It is immediately apparent that these are precisely the factors that might be expected to enhance system formation and group formation in the meaning model—that is, the factors most responsible for success in psychotherapy might be the same factors responsible for the placebo effect. To say this is certainly not to denigrate psychotherapy in any way. There is ample evidence of the great power of the placebo effect, and anything that can claim for itself even part of this power deserves recognition as an effective therapeutic modality. One might view psychotherapy, in this regard, as a highly organized way of bringing the placebo effect to bear on a special class of patients who otherwise would be resistant to it (except as an immediate and limited response to very specific symptoms).

One additional point of interest in Frank's list of common factors is the fourth factor's emphasis on the importance of having the patient acquire a sense of mastery or control. The meaning model might be said to include mastery and control by implication, since one of the primary reasons for understanding events is to be able to control them. But perhaps mastery and control are important enough concepts to be included explicitly as part of the model. Techniques that increase the patient's sense of control over the illness offer attractive alternatives to deceptive placebo use; one patient has described how being made to feel like a partner in the therapeutic enterprise represented a turning point in his illness.

According to the capacity theory, to have a mind is to confer meaning on the world through the use of symbols, and to use symbols is to have purposes and to engage in responsible behavior. We can see, then, how intimately the concepts of meaning, mastery, and personhood are interconnected. One high priority for the field of philosophy of medicine ought to be the exploration of the impact of illness on the human person in light of these concepts. It has been suggested, for example, that in a very fundamental way, illness restricts one's capacity for rational behavior. To what extent is this true, and to what extent does this influence how we ought to treat the sick? For example, if Cassell's thesis is true to a significant degree, it would not be possible to take seriously any informed consent obtained from a patient who is ill at the time. In this area, empirical issues are closely bound up with philosophical ones; behavioral scientists might engage in a more detailed analysis of how patients move into and out of the sick role and how their subjective sense of meaning and control is altered accordingly.

The discussion of mastery and control suggests a modification of Adler and Hammett's original model which may serve to guide placebo research, as the examples in this section have shown. Although Adler and Hammett stated their two elements were the "necessary and sufficient" conditions for the placebo effect, this is certainly not self-evident. Other important conditions may well be discovered in future study, and so the original language ought to be abandoned. The revised meaning model might read as follows:

> The placebo effect is most likely to occur when the following conditions are optimally met:
> 1. The patient is provided with an explanation for his illness which is consistent with his preexisting view of the world.
> 2. A group of individuals assuming socially sanctioned caring roles is available to provide emotional support for the patient.
> 3. The healing intervention leads to the patient's acquiring a sense of mastery and control over the illness.

While so far we have been focusing primarily on the research implications of this model, there are, as well, obvious implications to be considered in more detail.

Therapeutic Implications of the Meaning Model

While awaiting the results of research, the practicing physician can still draw guidance from the meaning model. The meaning model suggests a number of strategies for eliciting the placebo effect through nondeceptive means.

We have noted periodically that both positive and negative placebo effects may be observed. Even before looking for ways to elicit a positive placebo effect, the physician might be alert for ways to avoid a negative one. In general, a negative effect will result from unconscious neglect or undermining of the conditions of the meaning model. For example, a cold and distant physician may fail to provide suffcient emotional support and hence may interfere with formation of the caring group.

It would appear that a first step toward avoiding negative placebo effects, then, is to promote a greater understanding of the placebo response and to call to the attention of the practitioner the elements that we have included in the meaning model. (As a rule, those physicians who have been recognized by peers and patients for their humane and sympathetic approach have already incorporated into their therapeutic armamentarium all the elements of the meaning model, whether or not they have ever received formal instruction on those points; so the meaning model is often taught implicitly by example even when it has been explicitly unrecognized.) In particular, further education on placebos could overturn several myths still prevalent among practitioners, which data I have shown to be false.

Myth 1. If a patient responds to placebos, his symptom is either feigned or imaginary; hence the placebo can be used in the differential diagnosis of "organic" as opposed to "psychogenic" disorders. (Placebos affect objectively measurable physiological processes, not just subjective reports; see case 2, above, for one example of placebo efficacy in a clearly "organic" condition.

Myth 2. Placebos can relieve only pain or anxiety. (Placebos can influence virtually any condition or symptom upon which they have been tested in controlled trials.)

Myth 3. Placebos, whether they help or not, at least are harmless. (Placebos can produce side effects and addiction like pharmacologically active drugs, and also help reinforce habitual drug taking as a response to illness.)

Myth 4. Only neurotic personality types respond to placebos. (There is no "placebo personality type," and very likely anyone might respond to placebos under the right conditions.)

Once such myths about the placebo effect are exorcised from medical practice, positive guidance can be gained from further attention to the elements of the meaning model. For example, the element of formation of the caring group should alert the physician to the importance of involving the family and other care givers in his team approach to the care of the patient. He ought to reinforce appropriate displays of caring and to be alert for dysfunctional patterns of interpersonal relations that might either deprive the patient of needed support or else continue the sick role beyond its proper limits. Recently, in the field of psychiatry, social work, and family practice, much has been learned about the patterns of family interactions in health and disease, and several new techniques to aid distressed families have emerged.

Group formation, bypassing the family, may sometimes involve instead one of the increasingly popular lay self-help groups. Organizations such as Weight Watchers and Alcoholics Anonymous have achieved impressive records in dealing with chronic health-behavior problems that defy medical management. Where successful, such organizations may be seen to employ all three elements of the meaning model. In addition to the introduction of the individual to a group of people who care about his welfare, the group provides an appealing explanation of the underlying problem which emphasizes its treatable aspects, and the "we licked it, you can too" litany instills a sense of mastery and control. The skillful practitioner will be aware of these self-help groups and will direct his patients to them under the appropriate circumstances.

Regarding mastery, the clinician often has to walk a fine line and be very sensitive to the personal capabilities and psychological resources of each patient. Ideally, in encouraging specific strategies to demonstrate control over symptoms, the physician will begin with modest goals that are well within the patient's capacity. If the physician stresses the concept of control over symptoms and the patient subsequently experiences a worsening of symptoms, the therapeutic course suffers a three-pronged setback: the patient feels guilty for having failed to exercise the control that the physician seemed to expect, the patient fears future rejection by the physician because of this perceived failure, and the failure further cements the idea that control ultimately rests with the disease and not with the patient.

Such setbacks are most likely to occur when the physician goes out on a limb and delivers some sort of evangelical pep talk to the patient. This approach, while appearing to emphasize patient control, actually reinforces physician control, since it is the physician who dictates the proper course of action to the patient. In general, for a placebo effect to occur it is not necessary for the patient to feel himself in control; it is sufficient for him to feel that someone, such as the healer, has mastery over the disease. The physician-control approach is psychologically satisfying to the physician and probably serves the patient well in acute illnesses where faithful adherence to a specified therapeutic regimen offers the best chance for cure. But in chronic illnesses the patient must eventually become his own doctor and must himself manage to integrate continued care of his condition into his overall life plan. Here overdependence upon the physician is most likely to be counterproductive.

The experienced physician is aware of many possible techniques for control of symptoms and can usefully recommend the appropriate techniques to the patient. But instead of recommending or dictating, he may ask the patient what techniques he has discovered for himself that most effectively mitigate symptoms. If the patient has discovered some techniques on his own, the physician may praise him for his resourcefulness and suggest their continued use. If the patient has never thought in terms of his own ability to control symptoms, the physician may suggest that he experiment with some new techniques and report on the results at the next visit. This approach, emphasizing the responsibility of the patient in dealing with chronic symptoms, contrasts markedly with the approach of giving a sugar pill. The latter approach, as Cabot noted, gives the message that the all-powerful physician can offer immediate relief through drugs, and that failure to accomplish this represents a failure of the medical art. The former approach gives the message that symptoms are indeed controllable, but often through a variety of nonpharmacological and commonplace techniques, usually involving a certain amount of trial and error before relief appears.

The final element of the meaning model calls attention to the patient's own explanation for illness. Despite a growing literature on patient education and physician-patient communication, the emphasis in medical thinking has been on transmitting the approved medical-scientific explanation to the patient, instead of eliciting from the patient whatever explanatory model he may already have devised or learned within his own sociocultural environment. In anthropological studies of healing practices in primitive cultures, the disparity between the culturally accepted explanation for the disease and the Western-scientific explanation is striking. It has been realized only recently that the encounter between a physician and a middle-class, educated patient in the United States differs in this regard only in degree, and not in kind, from the encounter between the Western physician and the primitive tribesman. In both cases the patient's own, unstated explanatory model is likely to differ from the physician's model, even if the differences are subtle. Failure to be aware of these differences can, at worst, impede cure, and at best will deprive the physician of a powerful tool for eliciting the placebo effect.

Kleinman, Eisenberg, and Good have suggested that a "clinical social science" should be understood as a study of the means for eliciting from the patient his own explanatory model, so that, if necessary, crucial disparities between the patient's and the physician's models can be dealt with explicitly. They recommend that the following questions be made a part of every therapeutic encounter between doctor and patient: What do you think caused your problem? Why do you think it started when it did? How does your sickness produce its symptoms? How severe is it? How long will it last? What treatment is most appropriate?

The first impulse of the physician after uncovering a divergent explanatory model in the patient is to try to "correct" the explanation to suit scientific views. In some cases, however, especially in cases with hypochondriacal components or wherever the patient has a strong psychological stake in clinging to his existing explanation, the physician may draw out a more powerful placebo effect if he is able to work within the patient's explanatory system.

Case 3. A middle-aged widow was assigned to my practice and came to the office or called with a multitude of nonspecific complaints for which tests revealed no underlying bodily pathology. I attempted to explain to her that emotional stress often results in bodily symptoms, and I tried to help her instead to verbalize these stresses. She responded to this by arguing that she could see no connection between particular stressful situations and her symptoms, and delighted in describing symptoms that had occurred on days when she was feeling happy and at ease emotionally. During this period her visits and phone calls increased in frequency. Finally I dropped all discussion of emotions and began to focus on her symptoms, sympathizing with her plight and complimentating her on her ability to lead a somewhat normal life despite such aggravating illnesses. After several visits her phone calls and unscheduled office calls decreased markedly, and at her regular visits she reported less interference in her daily activities due to symptoms. She also gradually became more willing to discuss her emotional reactions to specific stresses, and her doses of several medications were tapered successfully.

According to my "enlightened" explanatory model, physicians ought to respond to both bodily and emotional distress, but they ought to label precisely the nature of the distress and to apply specific remedies in accordance with the label. According to the patient's explanatory model, physicians are supposed to focus on bodily complaints. My appearing to belittle her symptoms seemed to her to threaten a rejection, as the symptoms, by her model, were her only legitimate ticket of entry into the emotionally satisfying doctor-patient relationship; her only possible response to ward off such rejection was to escalate the severity of her symptoms.

Occasionally a divergent explanatory model may not only inhibit therapy but may indeed cause illness.

Case 4. Workers in an English ceramics factory complained of the recent onset of skin rashes and attributed these to the materials used in the plant. Extensive dermatologic testing failed to reveal sensitivity in any of the workers to substances found in the factory. The first woman to complain of symptoms was found to have an unrelated skin problem, and she had described her symptoms along with her hypothesis as to their origin to her coworkers in vivid terms. When the other workers were told of the negative results of the skin tests and that nervousness over their fellow worker's symptoms was the most likely cause for their complaints, they expressed relief and the epidemic of rashes immediately ceased (Maguire 1978).

Why have scientifically trained physicians been so reluctant to ask about, and then to work with, the explanatory models of their patients? It has been exasperatingly difficult to banish from the medical mentality the false dichotomy between the stereotyped scientific clinician, cold, aloof, and "professional" while superbly skilled in the latest rational therapy, and the stereotyped horse-and-buggy doctor of old—friendly, supportive, and beloved by his patients, yet totally helpless in the realm of scientific diagnosis and therapy. Carefully reasoned assaults on this false dichotomy, emphasizing that medicine requires both scientific and humanistic skills (Pelligrino 1974; Reiser 1978), have not changed the basic reality that the most severe intraprofessional penalties are for lack of scientific skills, rather than lack of humanistic and interpersonal skills. Promulgation of the meaning model might be one small additional contribution to banishing this dichotomy, since the growing body of research on the workings of the importance of the placebo effect demonstrates that the practitioner who holds interpersonal and humanistic skills in disdain is *therefore* an unscientific practitioner.

Abortion

88. *A Defense of Abortion* Judith Jarvis Thomson

Most opposition to abortion relies on the premise that the fetus is a human being, a person from the moment of conception. The premise is argued for, but, as I think, not well. But I shall not discuss any of this. For it seems to be to be of great interest to ask what happens if, for the sake of argument, we allow the premise. How, precisely, are we supposed to get from there to the conclusion that abortion is morally impermissible? Opponents of abortion commonly spend most of their time establishing that the fetus is a person, and hardly any time explaining the step from there to the impermissibility of abortion. Perhaps they think the step too simple and obvious to require much comment. Or perhaps instead they are simply being economical in argument. Many of those who defend abortion rely on the premise that the fetus is not a person, but only a bit of tissue that will become a person at birth; and why pay out more arguments than you have to? Whatever the explanation, I suggest that the step they take is neither easy nor obvious, that it calls for closer examination than it is commonly given, and that when we do give it this closer examination we shall feel inclined to reject it.

I propose, then, that we grant that the fetus is a person from the moment of conception. How does the argument go from here? Something like this, I take it. Every person has a right to life. So the fetus has a right to life. No doubt the mother has a right to decide what shall happen in and to her body; everyone would grant that. But surely a person's right to life is stronger and more stringent than the mother's right to decide what happens in and to her body, and so outweighs it. So the fetus may not be killed; an abortion may not be performed.

It sounds plausible. But now let me ask you to imagine this. You wake up in the morning and find yourself back to back in bed with an unconscious violinist. A famous unconscious violinist. He has been found to have a fatal kidney ailment, and the Society of Music Lovers has canvassed all the available medical records and found that you alone have the right blood type to help. They have therefore kidnapped you, and last night the violinist's circulatory system was plugged into yours, so that your kidneys can be used to extract poisons from his blood as well as your own. The director of the hospital now tells you, "Look, we're sorry the Society of Music Lovers did this to you—we would never have permitted it if we had known. But still, they did it, and the violinist now is plugged into you. To unplug you would be to kill him. But never mind, it's only for nine months. By then he will have recovered from his ailment, and can safely be unplugged from you." Is it morally incumbent on you to accede to this situation? No doubt it would be very nice of you if you did, a great kindness. But do you *have* to accede to it? What if it were not nine months, but nine years? Or longer still? What if the director of the hospital says, "Tough luck, I agree, but

Source: *Philosophy and Public Affairs,* vol. 1, no. 1, p. 47, 1971.

you've now got to stay in bed, with the violinist plugged into you, for the rest of your life. Because remember this. All persons have a right to life, and violinists are persons. Granted you have a right to decide what happens in and to your body, but a person's right to life outweighs your right to decide what happens in and to your body. So you cannot ever be unplugged from him." I imagine you would regard this as outrageous, which suggests that something really is wrong with that plausible-sounding argument I mentioned a moment ago.

In this case, of course, you were kidnapped; you didn't volunteer for the operation that plugged the violinist into your kidneys. Can those who oppose abortion on the ground I mentioned make an exception for a pregnancy due to rape? Certainly. They can say that persons have a right to life only if they didn't come into existence because of rape; or they can say that all persons have a right to life, but that some have less of a right to life than others, in particular, that those who came into existence because of rape have less. But these statements have a rather unpleasant sound. Surely the question of whether you have a right to life at all, or how much of it you have, shouldn't turn on the question of whether or not you are the product of a rape. And in fact the people who oppose abortion on the ground I mentioned do not make this distinction, and hence do not make an exception in case of rape.

Nor do they make an exception for a case in which the mother has to spend the nine months of her pregnancy in bed. They would agree that would be a great pity, and hard on the mother; but all the same, all persons have a right to life, the fetus is a person, and so on. I suspect, in fact, that they would not make an exception for a case in which, miraculously enough, the pregnancy went on for nine years, or even the rest of the mother's life.

Some won't even make an exception for a case in which continuation of the pregnancy is likely to shorten the mother's life; they regard abortion as impermissible even to save the mother's life. Such cases are nowadays very rare, and many opponents of abortion do not accept this extreme view. All the same, it is a good place to begin: a number of points of interest come out in respect to it.

Let us call the view that abortion is impermissible even to save the mother's life "the extreme view." I want to suggest first that it does not issue from the argument I mentioned earlier without the addition of some fairly powerful premises. Suppose a woman has become pregnant, and now learns that she has a cardiac condition such that she will die if she carries the baby to term. What may be done for her? The fetus, being a person, has a right to life, but as the mother is a person too, so has she a right to life. Presumably they have an equal right to life. How is it supposed to come out that an abortion may not be performed? If mother and child have an equal right to life, shouldn't we perhaps flip a coin? Or should we add to the mother's right to life her right to decide what happens in and to her body, which everybody seems to be ready to grant—the sum of her rights now outweighing the fetus' right to life?

The most familiar argument here is the following. We are told that performing the abortion would be directly killing[1] the child, whereas doing nothing would not be killing the mother, but only letting her die. Moreover, in killing the child, one would be killing an innocent person, for the child has committed no crime, and is not aiming at his mother's death. And then there are a variety of ways in which this might be continued: (1) but as directly killing an innocent person is always and absolutely impermissible, an abortion may not be performed. (2) As directly killing an innocent person is murder, and murder is always and absolutely impermissible, an abortion may not be performed.[2] (3) As one's duty to refrain from directly killing an innocent person is more stringent than one's duty to keep a person from dying, an abortion may not be performed. (4) If one's only options are directly killing an innocent person or letting a person die, one must prefer letting the person die, and thus an abortion may not be performed.[3]

Some people seem to have thought that these are not further premises which must be added if the conclusion is to be reached, but that they follow from the very fact that an innocent person has a right to life.[4] But this seems to me to be a mistake, and perhaps the simplest way to show this is to bring out that while we must certainly grant that innocent persons have a right to life, the theses in (1) through (4) are all false. Take (2), for example. If directly killing an innocent person is murder, and thus is impermissible, then the mother's directly killing the innocent person inside her is murder, and thus is impermissible. But it cannot seriously be thought to be murder if the mother performs an abortion on herself to save her life. It cannot seriously be said that she *must* refrain, that she *must* sit passively by and wait for her death. Let us look again at the case of you and the violinist. There you are, in bed with the violinist, and the director of the hospital says to you, "It's all most distressing, and I deeply sympathize, but you see this is putting an additional strain on your kidneys, and you'll be dead within the month. But you *have* to stay where you are all the same. Because unplugging you would be directly killing an innocent violinist, and that is murder, and that's impermissible." If anything in the world is true, it is that you do not commit murder, you do not do what is impermissible, if you reach around to your back and unplug yourself from that violinist to save your life.

The main focus of attention in writings on abortion has been on what a third party may or may not do in answer to a request from a woman for an abortion. This is in a way understandable. Things being as they are, there isn't much a woman can safely do to abort herself. So the question asked is what a third party may do, and what the mother may do, if it is mentioned at all, is deduced, almost as an afterthought, from what it is concluded that third parties may do. But it seems to me that to treat the matter in this way is to refuse to grant to the mother that very status of person which is so firmly insisted on for the fetus. For we cannot simply read off what a person may do from what a third party may do. Suppose you find yourself trapped in a tiny house with a growing child. I mean a very tiny house, and a rapidly growing child—you are already up against the wall of the house and in a few minutes you'll be crushed to death. The child on the other hand won't be crushed to death; if nothing is done to stop him from growing he'll be hurt, but in the end he'll simply burst open the house and walk out a free man. Now I could well understand it if a bystander were to say, "There's nothing we can do for you. We cannot choose between your life and his, we cannot be the ones to decide who is to live, we cannot intervene." But it cannot be concluded that you too can do nothing, that you cannot attack it to save your life. However innocent the child may be, you do not have to wait passively while it crushes you to death. Perhaps a pregnant woman is vaguely felt to have the status of house, to which we don't allow the right of self-defense. But if the woman houses the child, it should be remembered that she is a person who houses it.

I should perhaps stop to say explicitly that I am not claiming that people have a right to do anything whatever to save their lives. I think, rather, that there are drastic limits to the right of self-defense. If someone threatens you with death unless you torture someone else to death, I think you have not the right, even to save your life, to do so. But the case under consideration here is very different. In our case there are only two people involved, one whose life is threatened, and one who threatens it. Both are innocent: the one who is threatened is not threatened because of any fault; the one who threatens does not threaten because of any fault. For this reason we may feel that we bystanders cannot intervene. But the person threatened can.

In sum, a woman surely can defend her life against the threat to it posed by the unborn child, even if doing so involves its death. And this shows not merely that the theses in (1) through (4) are false; it shows also that the extreme view of abortion is false, and so we need not canvass any other possible ways of arriving at it from the argument I mentioned at the outset.

The extreme view could of course be weakened to say that while abortion is permissible to save the mother's life, it may not be performed by a third party, but only by the mother herself. But this cannot be right either. For what we have to keep in mind is that mother and the unborn child are not like two tenants in a small house which has, by an unfortunate mistake, been rented to both: the mother *owns* the house. The fact that she does adds to the offensiveness of deducing that the mother can do nothing from the supposition that third parties can do nothing. But it does more than this: it casts a bright light on the supposition that third parties can do nothing. Certainly it lets us see that a third party who says "I cannot choose between you" is fooling himself if he thinks this is impartiality. If Jones has found and fastened on a certain coat, which he needs to keep him from freezing, but which Smith also needs to keep him from freezing, then it is not impartiality that says, "I cannot choose between you" when Smith owns the coat. Women have said again and again, "This body is *my* body!" and they have reason to feel angry, reason to feel that it has been like shouting into the wind. Smith, after all, is hardly likely to bless us if we say to him, "Of course it's your coat, anybody would grant that it is. But no one may choose between you and Jones who is to have it."

We should really ask what it is that says "no one may choose" in the face of the fact that the body that houses the child is the mother's body. It may be simply a failure to appreciate this fact. But it may be something more interesting, namely, the sense that one has a right to refuse to lay hands on people, even where it would be just and fair to do so, even where justice seems to require that somebody do so. Thus justice might call for somebody to get Smith's coat back from Jones, and yet you have a right to refuse to be the one to lay hands on Jones, a right to refuse to do physical violence to him. This, I think, must be granted. But then what should be said is not "no one may choose, but only "*I* cannot choose," and indeed not even this, but "*I* will not *act*," leaving it open that somebody else can or should, and in particular that anyone in a position of authority, with the job of securing people's rights, both can and should. So this is no difficulty. I have not been arguing that any given third party must accede to the mother's request that he perform an abortion to save her life, but only that he may.

I suppose that in some views of human life the mother's body is only on loan to her, the loan not being one which gives her any prior claim to it. One who held this view might well think it impartiality to say "I cannot choose." But I shall simply ignore this possibility. My own view is that if a human being has any just, prior claim to anything at all, he has a just, prior claim to his own body. And perhaps this needn't be argued for here anyway, since, as I mentioned, the arguments against abortion we are looking at do grant that the woman has a right to decide what happens in and to her body.

But although they do grant it, I have tried to show that they do not take seriously what is done in granting it. I suggest the same thing will reappear even more clearly when we turn away from cases in which the mother's life is at stake, and attend, as I propose we now do, to the vastly more common cases in which a woman wants an abortion for some less weighty reason than preserving her own life.

Where the mother's life is not at stake, the argument I mentioned at the outset seems to have a much stronger pull. "Everyone has a right to life, so the unborn person has a right to life." And isn't the child's right to life weightier than anything other than the mother's own right to life, which she might put forward as ground for an abortion?

This argument treats the right to life as if it were unproblematic. It is not, and this seems to me to be precisely the source of the mistake.

For we should now, at long last, ask what it comes to, to have a right to life. In some views having a right to life includes having a right to be given at least the bare minimum one needs for continued life. But suppose that what in fact *is* the bare minimum a man needs for contined life is something he has no right at all to be given? If I am sick unto death, and the only thing that will save my life is the touch of Henry Fonda's cool hand on my fevered brow, then all the same, I have no right to be given the touch of Henry Fonda's cool hand on my fevered brow. It would be frightfully nice of him to fly in from the West Coast to provide it. It would be less nice, though no doubt well meant, if my friends flew out to the West Coast and carried Henry Fonda back with them. But I have no right at all against anybody that he should do this for me. Or again, to return to the story I told earlier, the fact that for continued life that violinist needs the contined use of your kidneys does not establish that he has a right to be given the continued use of your kidneys. He certainly has no right against you that *you* should give him continued use of your kidneys. For nobody has any right to use your kidneys unless you give him such a right; and nobody has the right against you that you shall give him this right—if you do allow him to go on using your kidneys, this is a kindness on your part, and not something he can claim from you as his due. Nor has he any right against anybody else that *they* should give him continued use of your kidneys. Certainly he had no right against the Society of Music Lovers that they should plug him into you in the first place. And if you now start to unplug yourself, having learned that you will otherwise have to spend nine years in bed with him, there is nobody in the world who must try to prevent you, in order to see to it that he is given something he has a right to be given.

Some people are rather stricter about the right to life. In their view, it does not include the right to be given anything, but amounts to, and only to, the right not to be killed by anybody. But here a related difficulty arises. If everybody is to refrain from killing that violinist, then everybody must refrain from doing a great many different sorts of things. Everybody must refrain from slitting his throat, everybody must refrain from shooting him— and everybody must refrain from unplugging you from him. But does he have a right against everybody that they shall refrain from unplugging you from him? To refrain from doing this is to allow him to continue to use your kidneys. It could be argued that he has a right against us that *we* should allow him to coninue to use your kidneys. That is, while he had no right against us that we should give him the use of your kidneys, it might be argued that he anyway has a right against us that we shall not now intervene and deprive him of the use of your kidneys. I shall come back to third-party interventions later. But certainly the violinist has no right against you that *you* shall allow him to continue to use your kidneys. As I said, if you do allow him to use them, it is a kindness on your part, and not something you owe him.

The difficulty I point to here is not peculiar to the right to life. It reappears in connection with all the other natural rights; and it is something which an adequate account of rights must deal with. For present purposes it is enough just to draw attention to it. But I would stress that I am not arguing that people do not have a right to life—quite to the contrary, it seems to me that the primary control we must place on the acceptability of an account of rights is that it should turn out in that account to be a truth that all persons have a right to life. I am arguing only that having a right to life does not guarantee having either a right to be given the use of or a right to be allowed continued use of another person's body—even if one needs it for life itself. So the right to life will not serve the opponents of abortion in the very simple and clear way in which they seem to have thought it would.

There is another way to bring out the difficulty. In the most ordinary sort of case, to deprive someone of what he has a right to is to treat him unjustly. Suppose a boy and his small brother are jointly given a box of chocolates for Christmas. If the older boy takes the box and refuses to give his brother any of the chocolates, he is unjust to him, for the brother has been given a right to half of them. But suppose that, having learned that otherwise it means nine years in bed with that violinist, you unplug yourself from him. You surely are not being unjust to him, for you gave him no right to use your kidneys, and no one else can have given him any such right. But we have to notice that in unplugging yourself, you are killing him; and violinists, like everybody else, have a right to life, and thus in the view we were considering just now, the right not to be killed. So here you do what he supposedly has a right you shall not do, but you do not act unjustly to him in doing it.

The emendation which may be made at this point is this: the right to life consists not in the right not to be killed, but rather in the right not to be killed unjustly. This runs a risk of circularity, but never mind: it would enable us to square the fact that the violinist has a right to life with the fact that you do not act unjustly toward him in unplugging yourself, thereby killing him. For if you do not kill him unjustly, you do not violate his right to life, and so it is no wonder you do him no injustice.

But if this emendation is accepted, the gap in the argument against abortion stares us plainly in the face: it is by no means enough to show that the fetus is a person, and to remind us that all persons have a right to life—we need to be shown also that killing the fetus violates its right to life, i.e., that abortion is unjust killing. And is it?

I suppose we may take it as a datum that in a case of pregnancy due to rape the mother has not given the unborn person a right to the use of her body for food and shelter. Indeed, in what pregnancy could it be supposed that the mother has given the unborn person such a right? It is not as if there were unborn persons drifting about the world, to whom a woman who wants a child says "I invite you in."

But it might be argued that there are other ways one can have acquired a right to the use of another person's body than by having been invited to use it by that person. Suppose a woman voluntarily indulges in intercourse, knowing of the chance it will issue in pregnancy, and then she does become pregnant; is she not in part responsible for the presence, in fact, the very existence, of the unborn person inside her? No doubt she did not invite it in. But doesn't her partial responsibility for its being there itself give it a right to the use of her body?

If so, then her aborting it would be more like the boy's taking away the chocolates, and less like your unplugging yourself from the violinist—doing so would be depriving it of what it does have a right to, and thus would be doing it an injustice.

And then, too, it might be asked whether or not she can kill it even to save her own life: If she voluntarily called it into existence, how can she now kill it, even in self-defense?

The first thing to be said about this is that it is something new. Opponents of abortion have been so concerned to make out the independence of the fetus, in order to establish that it has a right to life, just as its mother does, that they have tended to overlook the possible support they might gain from making out that the fetus is *dependent* on the mother, in order to establish that she has a special kind of responsibility for it, a responsibility that gives it rights against her which are not possessed by any independent person—such as an ailing violinist who is a stranger to her.

On the other hand, this argument would give the unborn person a right to its mother's body only if her pregnancy resulted from a voluntary act, undertaken in full knowledge of the chance a pregnancy might result from it. It would leave out entirely the unborn person whose existence is due to rape. Pending the availability of some further argument, then, we would be left with the conclusion that unborn persons whose existence is due to rape have no right to the use of their mothers' bodies, and thus that aborting them is not depriving them of anything they have a right to and hence is not unjust killing.

And we should also notice that it is not at all plain that this argument really does go even as far as it purports to. For there are cases and cases, and the details make a difference. If the room is stuffy, and I therefore open a window to air it, and a burglar climbs in, it would be absurd to say, "Ah, now he can stay, she's given him a right to the use of her house— for she is partially responsible for his presence there, having voluntarily done what enabled him to get in, in full knowledge that there are such things as burglars, and that burglars burgle." It would be still more absurd to say this if I had had bars installed outside my windows, precisely to prevent burglars from getting in, and a burglar got in only because of a defect in the bars. It remains equally absurd if we imagine it is not a burglar who climbs in, but an innocent person who blunders or falls in. Again, suppose it were like this: people-seeds drift about in the air like pollen, and if you open your windows, one may drift in and take root in your carpets or upholstery. You don't want children, so you fix up your windows with fine mesh screens, the very best you can buy. As can happen, however, and on very, very rare occasions does happen, one of the screens is defective; and a seed drifts in and takes root. Does the person-plant who now develops have a right to the use of your house? Surely not—despite the fact that you voluntarily opened your windows, you knowingly kept carpets and upholstered furniture, and you knew that screens were sometimes defective. Someone may argue that you are responsible for its rooting, that it does have a right to your house, because after all you *could* have lived out your life with bare floors and furniture, or with sealed windows and doors. But this won't do—for by the same token anyone can avoid a pregnancy due to rape by having a hysterectomy, or anyway by never leaving home without a (reliable!) army.

It seems to me that the argument we are looking at can establish at most that there are *some* cases in which the unborn person has a right to the use of its mother's body, and therefore *some* cases in which abortion is unjust killing. There is room for much discussion and argument as to precisely which, if any. But I think we should sidestep this issue and leave it open, for at any rate the argument certainly does not establish that all abortion is unjust killing.

There is room for yet another argument here, however. We surely must all grant that there may be cases in which it would be morally indecent to detach a person from your body at the cost of his life. Suppose you learn that what the violinist needs is not nine years of your life, but only one hour: all you need to do to save his life is to spend one hour in bed with him. Suppose also that letting him use your kidneys for that one hour would not affect your health in the slightest. Admittedly you were kidnapped. Admittedly you did not give anyone permission to plug him into you. Nevertheless it seems to me plain you *ought* to allow him to use your kidneys for that hour—it would be indecent to refuse.

Again, suppose pregnancy lasted only an hour, and constituted no threat to life or health. And suppose that a woman becomes pregnant as a result of rape. Admittedly she did not voluntarily do anything to bring about the existence of a child. Admittedly she did nothing at all which would give the unborn person a right to the use of her body. All the same it might well be said, as in the newly emended violinist story, that she *ought* to allow it to remain for that hour—that it would be indecent in her to refuse.

Now some people are inclined to use the term "right" in such a way that it follows from the fact that you ought to allow a person to use your body for the hour he needs, that he has a right to use your body for the hour he needs, even though he has not been given that right by any person or act. They may say that it follows also that if you refuse, you act unjustly toward him. This use of the term is perhaps so common that it cannot be called wrong; nevertheless it seems to me to be an unfortunate loosening of what we would do better to keep a tight rein on. Suppose that box of chocolates I mentioned earlier had not been given to both boys jointly, but was given only to the older boy. There he sits, stolidly eating his way through the box, his small brother watching enviously. Here we are likely to say, "You ought not to be so mean. You ought to give your brother some of those chocolates." My own view is that it just does not follow from the truth of this that the brother has any right to any of the chocolates. If the boy refuses to give his brother any, he is greedy, stingy, callous—but not unjust. I suppose that the people I have in mind will say it does follow that the brother has a right to some of the chocolates, and thus that the boy does act unjustly if he refuses to give his brother any. But the effect of saying this is to obscure what we should keep distinct, namely, the difference between the boy's refusal in this case and the boy's refusal in the earlier case, in which the box was given to both boys jointly, and in which the small brother thus had what was from any point of view clear title to half.

A further objection to so using the term "right" that from the fact that A ought to do a thing for B, it follows that B has a right against A that A do it for him, is that it is going to make the question of whether or not a man has a right to a thing turn on how easy it is to provide him with it; and this seems not merely unfortunate, but morally unacceptable. Take the case of Henry Fonda again. I said earlier that I had no right to the touch of his cool hand on my fevered brow, even though I needed it to save my life. I said it would be frightfully nice of him to fly in from the West Coast to provide me with it, but that I had no right against him that he should do so. But suppose he isn't on the West Coast. Suppose he has only to walk across the room, place a hand briefly on my brow—and lo, my life is saved. Then surely he ought to do it, it would be indecent to refuse. Is it to be said, "Ah, well, it follows that in this case she has a right to the touch of his hand on her brow, and so it would be an injustice in him to refuse"? So that I have a right to it when it is easy for him to provide it, though no right when it's hard? It's rather a shocking idea that anyone's rights should fade away and disappear as it gets harder and harder to accord them to him.

So my own view is that even though you ought to let the violinist use your kidneys for the one hour he needs, we should not conclude that he has a right to do so—we should say that if you refuse, you are, like the boy who owns all the chocolates and will give none away, self-centered and callous, indecent in fact, but not unjust. And similarly, that even supposing a case in which a woman pregnant due to rape ought to allow the unborn person to use her body for the hour he needs, we should not conclude that he has a right to do so; we should conclude that she is self-centered, callous, indecent, but not unjust, if she refuses. The complaints are no less grave; they are just different. However, there is no need to insist on this point. If anyone does wish to deduce "he has a right" from "you ought," then all the same he must surely grant that there are cases in which it is not morally required of you that you allow that violinist to use your kidneys, and in which he does not have a right to use them, and in which you do not do him an injustice if you refuse. And so also for mother and unborn child. Except in such cases as the unborn person has a right to demand it—and we were leaving open the possibility that there may be such cases—nobody is morally *required* to make large sacrifices, of health, of all other interests and concerns, of all other duties and commitments, for nine years, or even for nine months, in order to keep another person alive.

We have in fact to distinguish between two kinds of Samaritan: the Good Samaritan and what we might call the Minimally Decent Samaritan. The story of the Good Samaritan, you will remember, goes like this:

> A certain man went down from Jerusalem to Jericho, and fell among thieves, which stripped him of his raiment, and wounded him, and departed, leaving him half dead.
>
> And by chance there came down a certain priest that way; and when he saw him, he passed by on the other side.
>
> And likewise a Levite, when he was at the place, came and looked on him, and passed by on the other side.
>
> But a certain Samaritan, as he journeyed, came where he was; and when he saw him he had compassion on him.
>
> And went to him, and bound up his wounds pouring in oil and wine, and set him on his own beast, and brought him to an inn, and took care of him.
>
> And on the morrow, when he departed, he took out two pence, and gave them to the host, and said unto him, "Take care of him; and whatsoever thou spendest more, when I come again, I will repay thee."   (Luke 10:30~35)

The Good Samaritan went out of his way, at some cost to himself, to help one in need of it. We are not told what the options were, that is, whether or not the priest and the Levite could have helped by doing less than the Good Samaritan did, but assuming they could have, then the fact they did nothing at all shows they were not even Minimally Decent Samaritans, not because they were not Samaritans, but because they were not even minimally decent.

These things are a matter of degree, of course, but there is a difference, and it comes out perhaps most clearly in the story of Kitty Genovese, who, as you will remember, was murdered while thirty-eight people watched or listened, and did nothing at all to help her. A Good Samaritan would have rushed out to give direct assistance against the murderer. Or perhaps we had better allow that it would have been a Splendid Samaritan who did this, on the ground that it would have involved a risk of death for himself. But the thirty-eight not only did not do this, they did not even trouble to pick up a phone to call the police. Minimally Decent Samaritanism would call for doing at least that, and their not having done it was monstrous.

After telling the story of the Good Samaritan, Jesus said, "Go, and do thou likewise." Perhaps he meant that we are morally required to act as the Good Samaritan did. Perhaps he was urging people to do more than is morally required of them. At all events it seems plain that it was not morally required of any of the thirty-eight that he rush out to give direct assistance at the risk of his own life, and that is is not morally required of anyone that he give long stretches of his life—nine years or nine months—to sustaining the life of a person who has no special right (we were leaving open the possibility of this) to demand it.

Indeed, with one rather striking class of exceptions, no one in any country in the world is *legally* required to do anywhere near as much as this for anyone else. The class of exceptions is obvious. My main concern here is not the state of the law in respect to abortion, but it is worth drawing attention to the fact that in no state in this country is any man compelled by law to be even a Minimally Decent Samaritan to any person; there is no law under which charges could be brought against the thirty-eight who stood by while Kitty Genovese died. By contrast, in most states in this country women are compelled by law to be not merely Minimally Decent Samaritans, but Good Samaritans to unborn persons inside them. This doesn't by itself settle anything one way or the other, because it may well be argued that there should be laws in this country—as there are in many European countries—compelling at least Minimally Decent Samaritanism.[5] But it does show that there is a gross injustice in the existing state of the law. And it shows also that the groups currently working against liberalization of abortion laws, in fact working toward having it declared unconstitutional for a state to permit abortion, had better start working for the adoption of Good Samaritan laws generally, or earn the charge that they are acting in bad faith.

I should think, myself, that Minimally Decent Samaritan laws would be one thing, Good Samaritan laws quite another, and in fact highly improper. But we are not here concerned with the law. What we should ask is not whether anybody should be compelled by law to to be a Good Samaritan, but whether we must accede to a situation in which somebody is being compelled—by nature, perhaps—to be a Good Samaritan. We have, in other words, to look now at third-party interventions. I have been arguing that no person is morally required to make large sacrifices to sustain the life of another who has no right to demand them, and this even where the sacrifices do not include life itself; we are not morally required to be Good Samaritans or anyway Very Good Samaritans to one another. But what if a man cannot extricate himself from such a situation? What if he appeals to us to extricate him? It seems to me plain that there are cases in which we can, cases in which a Good Samaritan would extricate him. There you are, you were kidnapped, and nine years in bed with that violinist lie ahead of you. You have your own life to lead. You are sorry, but you simply cannot see giving up so much of your life to the sustaining of his. You cannot extricate yourself, and ask us to do so. I should have thought that—in light of his having no right to the use of your body—it was obvious that we do not have to accede to your being forced to give up so much. We can do what you ask. There is no injustice to the violinist in our doing so.

Following the lead of the opponents of abortion, I have throughout been speaking of the fetus merely as a person, and what I have been asking is whether or not the argument we began with, which proceeds only from the fetus's being a person, really does establish its conclusion. I have argued that it does not.

But of course there are arguments and arguments, and it may be said that I have simply fastened on the wrong one. It may be said that what is important is not merely the fact that the fetus is a person, but that it is a person for whom the woman has a special kind of responsibility issuing from the fact that she is its mother. And it might be argued that all my analogies are therefore irrelevant—for you do not have that special kind of responsibility for that violinist, Henry Fonda does not have that special kind of responsibility for me. And our attention might be drawn to the fact that men and women both *are* compelled by law to provide support for their children.

I have in effect dealt (briefly) with this argument above; but a (still briefer) recapitulation now may be in order. Surely we do not have any such "special responsibility" for a person unless we have assumed it, explicitly or implicitly. If a set of parents do not try to prevent pregnancy, do not obtain an abortion, and then at the time of birth of the child do not put it out for adoption, but rather take it home with them, then they have assumed responsibility for it, they have given it rights, and they cannot *now* withdraw support from it at the cost of its life because they now find it difficult to go on providing for it. But if they have taken all reasonable precautions against having a child, they do not simply by virtue of their biological relationship to the child who comes into existence have a special responsibility for it. They may wish to assume responsibility for it, or they may not wish to. And I am suggesting that if assuming responsibility for it would require large sacrifices, then they may refuse. A Good Samaritan would not refuse—or anyway, a Splendid Samaritan, if the sacrifices that had to be made were enormous. But then so would a Good Samaritan assume responsibility for that violinist; so would Henry Fonda, if he is a Good Samaritan, fly in from the West Coast and assume responsibility for me.

My argument will be found unsatisfactory on two counts by many of those who want to regard abortion as morally permissible. First, while I do argue that abortion is not impermissible, I do not argue that it is always permissible. There may well be cases in which carrying the child to term requires only Minimally Decent Samaritanism of the mother, and this is a standard we must not fall below. I am inclined to think it a merit of my account precisely that it does *not* give a general yes or a general no. It allows for and supports our sense that, for example, a sick and desperately frightened fourteen-year-old schoolgirl, pregnant due to rape, may *of course* choose abortion, and that any law which rules this out is an insane law. And it also allows for and supports our sense that in other cases resort to abortion is even positively indecent. It would be indecent in the woman to request an abortion, and indecent in a doctor to perform it, if she is in her seventh month, and wants the abortion just to avoid the nuisance of postponing a trip abroad. The very fact that the arguments I have been drawing attention to treat all cases of abortion, or even all cases of abortion in which the mother's life is not at stake, as morally on a par ought to have made them suspect at the outset.

Second, while I am arguing for the permissibility of abortion in some cases, I am not arguing for the right to secure the death of the unborn child. It is easy to confuse these two things in that up to a certain point in the life of the fetus it is not able to survive outside the mother's body; hence removing it from her body guarantees its death. But they are importantly different. I have argued that you are not morally required to spend nine months in bed, sustaining the life of that violinist; but to say this is by no means to say that if, when you unplug yourself, there is a miracle and he survives, you then have a right to turn round and slit his throat. You may detach yourself even if this costs him his life; you have no right to be guaranteed his death, by some other means, if unplugging yourself does not kill him. There are some people who will be dissatisfied by this feature of my argument. A woman may be utterly devastated by the thought of a child, a bit of herself, put out for adoption and never seen or heard of again. She may therefore want not merely that the child be detached from her, but more, that it die. Some opponents of abortion are inclined to regard this as beneath contempt—thereby showing insensitivity to what is surely a powerful source of despair. All the same, I agree that the desire for the child's death is not one which anybody may gratify, should it turn out to be possible to detach the child alive.

At this place, however, it should be remembered that we have only been pretending throughout that the fetus is a human being from the moment of conception. A very early abortion is surely not the killing of a person, and so is not dealt with by anything I have said here.

NOTES

1. The term "direct" in the arguments I refer to is a technical one. Roughly, what is meant by "direct killing" is either killing as an end in itself, or killing as a means of some end, for example, the end of saving someone else's life.

2. Cf. *Encyclical Letter of Pope Pius XI on Christian Marriage,* St. Paul Editions, Boston, p. 32: "However much we may pity the mother whose health and even life is gravely imperiled in the performance of the duty allotted to her by nature, nevertheless what could ever be a sufficient reason for excusing in any way the direct murder of the innocent? This is precisely what we are dealing with here." Noonan, in *The Morality of Abortion,* reads this as follows: "What cause can ever avail to excuse in any way the direct killing of the innocent? For it is a question of that."

3. The thesis in (4) is in an interesting way weaker than those in (1), (2), and (3): they rule out abortion even in cases in which both mother

and child will die if the abortion is not performed. By contrast, one who held the view expressed in (4) could consistently say that one needn't prefer letting two persons die to killing one.

4. Cf. the following passage from Pius XII, *Address to the Italian Catholic Socity of Midwives:* "The baby in the maternal breast has the right to life immediately from God. Hence there is no man, no human authority, no science, no medical, eugenic, social, economic or moral 'indication' which can establish or grant a valid juridical ground for a direct deliberate disposition of an innocent human life, that is a disposition which looks to its destruction either as an end or as a means to another end perhaps in itself not illicit. The baby, still not born, is a man in the same degree and for the same reason as the mother" (quoted in Noonan, *The Morality of Abortion,* p. 45).

5. For a discussion of the difficulties involved, and a survey of the European experience with such laws, see *The Good Samaritan and the Law,* ed. James M. Ratcliffe, New York, 1966.

89. *The Supreme Court and Abortion: The Irrelevance of Medical Judgment*   George J. Annas

Bob Woodward and Scott Armstrong persuasively argue that Justice Harry Blackmun saw his task in writing the 1973 Supreme Court abortion decision (*Roe v. Wade*) as eliminating "needless infringement of the discretion of the medical profession" and ratifying "the best possible medical opinion."[1] Blackmun calls his ten years as counsel for the Mayo Clinic "the best . . . of his life," and has a tremendous respect for "what dedicated physicians could accomplish."

Most would agree that Blackmun's opinion accomplished his goal. It permitted a woman

Source: *Hastings Center Report*, vol. 10, October 1980.

and her physician to decide about an abortion without any state interference in the first
trimester; and even in the second and third trimester it forbade the state to place the interests of the fetus higher than the "life and health" of the pregnant woman. The decision not
only upheld the individual rights of women, but also evidenced strong judicial support of
sound medical judgment.

It therefore came as somewhat of a surprise to Justice Blackmun (and three other members of the Court) that when the Court reversed Judge John Dooling's decision in the U.S.
District Court for the Eastern District of New York and decided in June that denial of Medicaid funds for *medically necessary* abortions was constitutional, the majority did not even
discuss the role of either the doctor-patient relationship or medical judgment.

Like all other U.S. Supreme Court decisions concerning abortion, this one is highly controversial. Most commentators are choosing sides based not on the logic of the opinion, but
on their agreement or disagreement with the outcome. This may be perfectly appropriate,
since this 5 to 4 decision is not one mandated by past precedent or constitutional law, but
one made primarily on political grounds. Nevertheless, it is worthwhile to summarize the major arguments presented by the majority and minority, primarily because two new voices in
the abortion debate carry the brunt of the argument: Justices Potter Stewart and John Paul
Stevens.

The Majority

Justice Stewart, writing for the majority, sees the case as a straightforward and logical extension of the Court's previous decision that the U.S. Constitution did not require Medicaid
to fund "elective abortions" even if it funded childbirth because the state could legitimately
favor childbirth over abortion.[2]

At issue in this case is the constitutionality of the Hyde Amendment. The applicable 1980
version provides:

> [N]one of the funds provided by this joint resolution shall be used to perform abortions
> *except where the life of the mother would be endangered* if the fetus were carried to
> term; *or* except for such medical procedures necessary for *the victims of rape or incest*
> when such rape or incest has been reported promptly to a law enforcement agency or pub-
> lic health service. (emphasis supplied)

The pivotal constitutional issue is: does the Hyde Amendment, by denying public funds
for some medically necessary abortions, "*impinge* upon a fundamental right explicitly or implicitly secured by the Constitution?" (emphasis supplied) All the Justices agree that the
right to decide whether or not to terminate a pregnancy is a "fundamental right." Therefore,
the only real issue in the case is that of "impingement." The majority simply, and without
much discussion, adopts the *Maher* analysis as directly applicable. There the Court had held
that "encouraging an alternative" (that is, childbirth) by "unequal subsidization" did not impinge upon a woman's right because it was not "direct state interference." Stated another
way, the government's refusal to fund abortions "places no obstacle" before the woman that
did not already exist, and imposes no independent "penalty" on a woman's exercise of her
constitutional right. Using this analysis, Justice Stewart concludes that the difference between
medically necessary and elective abortions is constitutionally irrelevant—the government

does not have to fund either. But he does suggest some limits. The government cannot penalize a woman who has an abortion by withholding all Medicaid benefits from her because this would amount to a "penalty" for exercising a constitutional right.

Since the majority finds no "impingement," the Hyde Amendment is only required to be "rationally related to a legitimate governmental objective" to be constitutional. This test as traditionally applied has led to the almost universal approval of statutes, since determination of such a relationship is generally considered the province of the legislature, not the courts. The result is therefore predictable. Even though Justice Stewart announces that a majority of the Court believe that the Hyde Amendment is not "wise social policy," they nonetheless uphold it on the basis that such a decision is properly one for the legislature: "By encouraging childbirth except in the most urgent circumstances, [the Hyde Amendment] is rationally related to the legitimate governmental objective of protecting fetal life."

The Dissenters

The dissents by Justices William Brennan, Thurgood Marshall, and Blackmun parallel their dissent in *Maher,* and need not be repeated here. But a new member has been added to the court since *Maher,* and Justice Stevens's dissent merits a careful review. In his view the case is substantially different from *Maher.* In *Maher* the right in question was Medicaid payment for an "elective" or *unnecessary* abortion, one that by definition did not raise the issue of maternal health. But here, as he sees it, the woman's choice is "between two serious harms: serious health damage to [herself] on the one hand and abortion on the other." Since under *Roe* v. *Wade* the state may not protect fetal life when its protection conflicts with the health of the pregnant woman, Stevens argues that the state may "not exclude a woman from medical benefits to which she would otherwise be entitled [that is, coverage for *necessary* medical care as determined by her physician] solely to further an interest in potential life when a physician, 'in appropriate medical judgment,' certifies that an abortion is necessary 'for the preservation of the life or health of the mother.'"

Such a policy is by definition not "neutral" but violates the equal protection clause by penalizing those indigents in need of abortion who cannot afford one. In the words of Justice Stevens, the government may not:

> deny benefits to a financially and medically needy person simply because he is a Republican, a Catholic, or an Oriental—or because he has spoken against a program the government has a legitimate interest in furthering . . . it may not create exceptions for the sole purpose of furthering a governmental interest that is constitutionally subordinate to the individual interest that the entire program was designed to protect.

Justice Marshall argues that, even if one does not see jeopardy of a woman's health as a penalty, the Hyde Amendment bears no rational relationship to a legitimate state interest. He observes that the Hyde Amendment refuses funding even in cases where "normal childbirth" will not result—where the child will die shortly after birth or where the mother's life will be shortened or her health greatly impaired by the birth. Since this is the result, Marshall argues that the only rational basis for the Hyde Amendment is that it was "designed to deprive poor and minority women of the constitutional right to choose abortion." And this is, of course, not a constitutionally permissible reason for legislation.

Inadequacies of the Decision

A number of observations are in order. First, the term "infringement" and its specific application are subject to wide interpretation. The majority of the justices did not view refusal to fund a medically necessary abortion as an infringement on the right of a poor woman to have one, or as a penalty to discourage exercising a constitutional right. The minority differed. I personally find the majority's view insensitive to reality. Justice Blackmun correctly notes, "There is another world out there, the existence of which the Court, I suspect, either chooses to ignore or fears to recognize." By the late spring of 1980, federal and state courts in fourteen jurisdictions (affirmed by four U.S. Courts of Appeals) had ruled that states participating in the Medicaid program were constitutionally required to fund *all* medically necessary abortions as determined by a physician. Two federal courts had found the Hyde Amendment unconstitutional, and no court had ruled otherwise. All these judges must have been surprised at this decision.

> The Hyde Amendment is a transparent attempt by the Legislative Branch to impose the political majority's judgment of the morally acceptable and socially desirable preference on a sensitive and intimate decision that the Constitution entrusts to the individual. Worse yet, the Hyde Amendment does not foist that majoritarian viewpoint with equal measure upon everyone in our Nation, rich and poor alike; rather, it imposes that viewpoint only upon that segment of our society which, because of its position of powerlessness, is least able to defend its privacy rights from the encroachments of state-mandated morality.
> (Justice William Brennan, dissenting in *McRae*)

Second, by permitting the state to place the welfare of the fetus ahead of the health and welfare of the pregnant woman, this case effectively overrules *Roe* v. *Wade* in terms of what interests the state may properly favor over others. And even if one believes that *Roe* should be so overruled on this issue, the Hyde Amendment does not rationally protect fetal life by forbidding funding for even those cases in which the child will die during childbirth or shortly thereafter.

Third, the primary motivation behind the majority's decision seems to have been their reluctance to tell Congress and the states how to spend the taxpayers' money. But Justice Stevens responds that this scheme will cost the government considerably more money (since abortion costs less than childbirth); and that the harm to the woman whose health is injured by childbirth must also be paid for by government funds. He concludes that "there are some especially costly forms of treatment that may reasonably be excluded from the program in order to preserve the assets in the pool and extend its benefits to the maximum number of needy persons." But the Hyde Amendment is not rationally related to such a legitimate governmental policy. Refusing to fund heart transplants or artificial hearts, of course, could be.

Fourth, the majority lack of discussion of the role of the physician is remarkable. It seems to assume either that the physician's judgment of the medical necessity of the abortion is irrelevant or that the physician will (should?) perform the abortion without pay if he or she really believes that it is medically necessary. Neither assumption is tenable.

Finally, the decision again affects only those least able to protect themselves—the poor. While poverty is not a "suspect classification" that requires "strict scrutiny" of the statute in question, Justice Marshall is surely correct in arguing that when a governmental enactment directly affects the very lives and health of poor women who seek to exercise a constitutional right, it is unfair and unjust to judge that statute by the same mechanistic test designed primarily to give judicial deference to legislation about competing business interests.

The funding battle for abortions for poor women has been lost in the courts. It is now up to Congress and the individual states to pass reasonable legislation on this issue, an unlikely outcome given the present political climate. After the Court's previous decision in *Maher*, one supporter wrote, "It's like bringing some of the troops home from Vietnam: we didn't save all fetuses, but we saved some." The analogy, of course, is not quite accurate. It is like bringing some troops home—those who can pay for their own plane tickets.

NOTES

1. *The Brethren*, Simon & Schuster, New York, 1980, p. 175.

2. *Maher v. Roe*. See *Hastings Center Report*, August 1977, p. 8.

Genetic Counseling and Screening

90. The Morality and Ethics of Prenatal Diagnosis
John C. Fletcher

Moral Problems and Ethical Issues

The structure of this chapter will be an examination of the major moral problems in the application of prenatal diagnosis followed by a discussion of the larger ethical issues that flow from the moral problems. In both parts, each side of the arguments will be fully presented. The theses presented are that (1) selective abortion is the major moral problem associated with prenatal diagnosis, and (2) an ethical view attempting to mediate between concern for the life of the fetus and reduction of suffering caused by genetic disease will restrain more bad consequences and maximize more good consequences in the application of prenatal diagnosis than views that stress only fetal rights or maternal-societal rights.

Moral Problems in Prenatal Diagnosis

Table 1 illustrates the process of genetic counseling with prenatal diagnosis and the structure of moral problems embodied in the questions that arise. These problems were identified through an analysis of the literature on prenatal diagnosis as well as a study of 25 couples in genetic counseling accompanied by amniocentesis.[1]

Source: Aubrey Milunsky (ed.), *Genetic Disorders and the Fetus*, Plenum Publishing Corporation, New York, 1979.

RISKS OF AMNIOCENTESIS

Earlier studies of amniocentesis related to indications and accuracy rather than safety.[2] Interestingly, the morality of risk factors was cited more by advocates of selective abortion than by critics. Fuchs[3] and Littlefield[4] argued that parents who were unwilling to accept abortion ought to be denied amniocentesis because of the unknown risk to fetus and mother. The safety of amniocentesis when performed by trained physicians has been established by controlled studies in the United States[5] and Canada.[6]

In both studies, 95 percent of the diagnoses showed negative findings, confirming a previous finding by Milunsky.[2] These results support the position that prenatal diagnosis serves to save life, because more fetuses are saved from abortions done on unfounded genetic risk than are aborted following diagnosis of defects.[7]

Now that a firm baseline for risk assessment has been established, one can separate the abortion issue from the risk question and discuss it separately. Also, those at-risk parents who are opposed to abortion can in good conscience use prenatal diagnosis as a source of information about the health of the expected child.

SELECTIVE ABORTION

Interviews with parents[1] and analysis of the literature show that the use of selective abortion is the prevailing moral problem in prenatal diagnosis. For parents, the structure of the genetic counseling situation prompts a readiness for abortion in case of a positive diagnosis. Since most parents who seek genetic counseling and prenatal diagnosis have already had one or more affected children,[8] they are strongly motivated to have a healthy child. Thus wanting another child (sometimes desperately) and being explicitly committed to abortion pose a tension of severely conflicting loyalties that is perceived as a moral problem.

Opposing Arguments. Physicians and ethicists who object to prenatal diagnosis do not oppose the technique itself but oppose the use of selective abortion on defective fetuses. Two major lines of argument are followed: (1) the basic purpose of medicine to save life is contradicted by the practice of abortion, and (2) while some abortions may be justified, the practice of prenatal diagnosis functions to segregate certain fetuses as deserving of abortion and thus treats fetuses unequally and unjustly.

Kass,[9] a physician-philosopher, bases his objection to selective abortion on the moral quality of all human beings. Singling out defective fetuses on the basis of arbitrary social and personal reasons threatens the fundamental right to life of all other dependent human beings. Lejeune,[10] a geneticist, organizes his argument on the claim of the biological unity of mankind in order to object to the destruction of certain fetuses. He holds that since all human genotypes are derived from an original genetic heritage it is unjustifiable to condemn what is fundamentally human, albeit defective.

Ramsey[11] was the first ethicist to attempt to show that arguments for selective abortion could be used to support active euthanasia of the defective newborn. He argues[12] that the diseased fetus is a patient and deserving of equal protection. He challenges language about "therapeutic" abortion for fetuses,[13] claiming that abortion is never therapeutic for the fetus. Lebacqz,[14] an ethicist, criticizes the moral reasoning of those who favor selective abortion because of the relativity of choosing categories of fetuses to be aborted, the unequal treatment of the innocent and unconsenting fetus, and the relegation of the physician to a role of a technician rather than healer of disease. Dyck[15] claims that physicians who make decisions

TABLE 1. STRUCTURE OF MORAL PROBLEMS OF PARENTS IN GENETIC COUNSELING:

I. DECISION ABOUT AMNIOCENTESIS

Events	Genetic problem arises →	Information from media, physician, friend, etc. How trustworthy? →	Consultation with physician or spouse. Abortion question: conflict with physician and/or family; autonomy: religious conflict →	Genetic counseling: amniocentesis →
Moral problems		Unresolved guilt: questions from previous births or abortions		Impact of counsellor's values: risks vs. benefits; informed consent; indications for amniocentesis

II. DECISION FOLLOWING AMNIOCENTESIS

Events	Postamniocentesis →	Results reported →	*Negative* / *Positive* →	Birth / Abortion/sterilization/birth
Moral problems		Fidelity to family and marriage: anxiety vastly heightened	Decision on abortion and sterilization: reevaluation of childbearing, marriage: "rejection" of living child or sib with same genetic problem while making abortion decision	

III. POSTABORTION/STERILIZATION/BIRTH

Moral problems	Justification of decision: cosmic doubts: self rejection: decision about future birth: fidelity to marriage

From *Theological Studies*, Vol. 33, no. 3, p. 462.

about selective abortion take to themselves unwarranted power as to who shall live or die, when they have no special training to make such decisions.

The strengths of this position are (1) the protection afforded to every life by the concept of equality, (2) the compassion toward the individual fetus regardless of handicap, and (3) the consistency of moral judgments applied to cases varying from severe to minor handicaps. The weaknesses of the position rest on what is excluded from consideration: (1) that the physical or mental problems of the infant will cause great suffering to the mother, the family, and society, and (2) that granting life to the fetus possibly will do it greater injury than denying its life through abortion. The deepest ethical dilemma for those who take this position is how they can justify the increase of suffering to infant, family, and society that their argument allows.

Favoring Arguments. The major arguments for selective abortion grow out of (1) the obligation to reduce or prevent suffering for the affected family, the fetus, and the wider society, and (2) the obligation to prevent genetic diseases and their impact on successive generations in the absence of genetic therapies. Those who advocate or allow selective abortion generally attempt to hold concern for the family's well-being together with concern for the resources of society. Differences in emphasis arise among proponents themselves about the weight one should give to society's interests in any conflict with individual interests and the degree of individual freedom allowed in decisions about selective abortion.

Milunsky[2] states that the basic purpose of prenatal diagnosis is the assurance to parents of unaffected offspring when there is a significant risk of having defective children. He takes pains, however, to prove the economic benefits of selective abortion by showing that the cost to society in maintaining defective individuals is 32 times greater than the cost of prevention. Another physician-geneticist, Motulsky,[16] concentrates on the relief of predictable physical, mental, and economic suffering of the family. In an earlier paper,[17] he had shown that selective abortion would not be a completely effective tool for eliminating genetic diseases unless it were applied to carriers, and he opposed this step because of the prohibitive number of abortions that would be required.

Occasionally, the argument is made that selective abortion must be done on the basis of the obligation to prevent the suffering of the fetus[18-20] and that it is immoral to bring knowingly a seriously defective infant to birth. Camenish[21] challenges this kind of reasoning as illogical since, in his view, we can have obligations only to an existing person and abortion presupposes that the fetus cannot be defined as a person.

Another way of making a strong ethical statement for selective abortion is to insist that the seriously defective fetus has a "right not to be born." Shaw, a geneticist-lawyer,[22] advocated this position along with making the knowing transmission of genetic disease a crime punishable by law. Aikern,[23] a moral philosopher who opposes the argument for equal right to life for fetuses, holds that there is no right to life that is not contingent on the rights of others and the ability of an individual, with the help of others, to make a human life for himself.

Some proponents of selective abortion concentrate more heavily on the protection or improvement of society's genetic health. Neel[24] advocated abortion as the "modern counterpart of infanticide based on congenital defect" to improve the quality of life for all individuals, even though the long-range effect of selective abortion would probably slow the rate of elimination of undesirable genes owing to reproductive compensation. Joseph Fletcher, an ethicist, warned against the trap of sentimentality in some voluntary associations to aid victims of birth defects, since the public may be diverted from its proper task of prevention of such births. Morison,[25] a biologist-philosopher, holds that society has an interest in the quality and quantity of children born and advocated wide use of selective abortion determined by individual choice.

No argument for a program of compulsory abortion has been discussed in medical literature to date. The assumption of all those whose views have been surveyed is that abortion should be voluntary and uncoerced. Crow,[26] a population geneticist, in the context of discussing society's interest in preventing parents from producing uneducable children, refuses to reduce the freedom of the individual by arguing for compulsory abortion or sterilization. Callahan,[27, 28] a philospher, agrees that the vast suffering caused by genetic disease warrants full-scale efforts to prevent, including access to abortion, but he warns that crusading against diseases can create intolerance and antipathy for those who have the disease, thus making them the enemies of the healthy.

The strengths of the argument for selective abortion rest on (1) the increase in human responsibility to control the consequences of reproduction, (2) an increase in the sphere of freedom for affected families, (3) a reduction of human suffering and genetic harm, and (4) the protection of society's resources. One weakness of the argument is related to an assumption about the separability of the biological development of the fetus from the human freedom to act against the fetus. The argument for selective abortion tends to rely so heavily on the freedom to act that it radically separates biology and reasoning, thus bifurcating human existence. A second weakness is that the argument creates precedents in moral reasoning for denying the right to life to other disabled, dying, or defenseless persons.

Mediating positions. Callahan,[29] Gustafson,[30] and the author[20] are ethicists who favor selective abortion in severe cases but attempt to mediate between the opposing positions about selective abortion. A mediating position attempts to include as many contending values, rights, and situational forces as possible. It resists the absolutizing of a particular value (e.g., the life of the fetus or society's interests) to the exclusion of other values. It also recognizes that ideals must be compromised and imperfect solutions attempted if decisions are to be made in the midst of contending forces. Gustafson points out that neither those who argue from a baseline of fetal rights nor those who begin from society's interests proceed to a conclusion without being qualified by the opposing argument. Callahan favors abortion in severe cases while emphasizing that not every deformed or unwanted child is inevitably miserable. The present author advocates practical alternatives to the polarization of fetal rights and the achievement of reduction of suffering. He favors (1) acceptance of selective abortion in medically severe cases for which there is no therapy, along with a policy of financial assistance for families deliberately choosing to accept a defective infant, (2) support for research, including fetal research, required to perfect genetic therapies, and (3) social support for parents who conscientiously object to selective abortion, balanced with application of malpractice to genetic counselors who withhold information about prenatal diagnosis because of their convictions on abortion.

INDICATIONS FOR PRENATAL DIAGNOSIS

Parental anxiety. A moral problem faced by physicians in admitting persons to prenatal diagnosis is posed by parents who threaten abortion unless there is confirmation of "normality" in the fetus, when there is no relevant family history of genetic disease. Is parental anxiety a sufficient cause for prenatal diagnosis? The argument against admission is based on the concept that physicians ought not to use prenatal diganosis to "treat the desires" of parents and become mere technicians for their wishes. [14] Milunsky [2] poses the opposite argument: since the overall risk is 1 in 200 of having a chromosomally defective child, there is an empirical basis for admission, and, further, the probabilities are very high that a life will be saved, since the results of diagnosis are over 95 percent negative. [31] My own views coincide with the latter statement.

SPECIAL PROBLEMS IN SELECTIVE ABORTION

Sex-linked diseases. Some of the most complex moral dilemmas accompany information given by prenatal diagnosis. For example, in muscular dystrophy and hemophilia, the risk of a subsequent male having the disease is 50 percent. When the prenatal test cannot detect affected males, as is currently the case, should all males be aborted? Should all males be brought to term? In muscular dystrophy, affected males will be normal for the first few years of life. What should parents do in this case? Parents and physicians will be guided here by the arguments for or against abortion discussed earlier, but each position is strained by the unknowns and the unintended consequences of these borderline cases. The antiabortionist faces an inevitable addition of suffering through avoiding abortion. The proabortionist will face instances of normal fetuses aborted under the supposition of a birth defect. The strongest argument for abortion here is that a 50 percent risk of disease is very high. The strongest argument against abortion is that a 50 percent chance of normality is too high to justify intervention. In either case, the deeper beliefs of parents and physicians will guide them in what is essentially a decision based on morality. The highest kind of ethical tolerance is required to accept the decisions of parents on either side of the question.

Late abortions. Three kinds of problems attend late abortions. First, there are more frequent and serious physical complications in women who have second trimester abortions. [32] Second, a psychiatric study of 13 couples who underwent abortion for genetic indication [33] showed that 90 percent of the women and 80 percent of the men suffered severe depression, probably revealing the degree of parental loyalty to the developing fetus at that stage. These findings agree with an earlier study of four similar cases [1] done from the viewpoint of the moral suffering of the parents. Caught between the good of wanting a healthy child and the good of wanting to protect themselves and their family from a birth defect, parents suffer intensely following late abortions. Third, abortions done between the 20th and 24th weeks of gestation approach the borderline period for the biological basis of viability, [34] raising the issue of the similarities between the viable fetus and the viable newborn infant.

Ethical Issues of Prenatal Diagnosis

THE ABORTION ISSUE

The major issue caused by prenatal diagnosis is, can abortion be ethically justified as a solution to detection of fetal genetic disease or impairment? Obviously, prenatal diagnosis poses an ethical issue only for those for whom abortion in general is a genuine ethical dilemma. If the fetus is only "tissue" [35] or "matter," [36] then a question of ethics is nonexistent, for the needs of the adults involved would clearly prevail. On the other hand, the equal right to life of the fetus can be argued so exclusively that the needs of adults can be made to appear more egoistic or self-serving than concerned with justice or reduction of suffering.

A case has been made that justifies selective abortion on grounds of reducing the family's suffering and justice due the mother's rights vis à vis the rights of the fetus. [20] In this view, the human being is deserving of protection at every stage of its development, but in conflict situations the degree of protection due the fetus is proportionate to the stage of its development. Thus the claims of the mother and family can more easily override the previable fetus's right to life. When the fetus is viable and a fortiori once it is born, it has an independent status and confronts physicians, parents and legal institutions with claims for care and support. The watershed cases testing this justification occur with fetuses born alive following abortion [37] or with infants born with a genetic disease following a false-negative diagnosis due to human error. [38, 39]

This justification does not satisfy a strict equal right to life argument that makes no ethical relevant distinction between the previable and the viable fetus, or between the fetus and the newborn. The right to life position, while heroic in its defense of the fetus, has two serious negative social effects: in addition to the number of illegal and unsafe abortions that would occur, its observance would add greatly to the predictable suffering of many, especially families genetically at risk. To refrain from preventing suffering when we have opportunities to act is contrary to a major ethical principle that regulates moral conduct. At the same time, framing the justification to abort selectively following prenatal diagnosis as an exception to the valid right to life of a fetus is too strong a defense of the fetus for the argument based solely on maternal or societal rights. This position, sometimes called the "quality of life" argument, has deleterious social effects in that it introduces value judgments that discriminate as to the worth of individual lives and provides grounds for abortion of fetuses that "require any but the most trivial treatment," [17] rather than the most serious cases. There is no evidence that the societies that practice abortion on a wide scale also practice systematic discrimination against the chronically dependent or defenseless. However, insofar as selective abortion creates precedents in reasoning that single out defective fetuses for abortion, there is an obligation to hold this indignity to a minimum and eventually overcome it altogether because these precedents may be used to reduce the dignity of other defenseless persons. A fully developed ethics of selective abortion will provide justification for abortion decisions, but with a sufficiently uneasy conscience to render abortion questionable as an ethically desirable final solution to detection of genetic disease.

Because abortion is never therapeutic for the fetus, [31] even though it can be therapeutic for mother and family, the long-range goal of the use of prenatal diagnosis ought to be the development of therapies for the detected conditions.

THE FUTURE OF PRENATAL DIAGNOSIS AND GENETIC THERAPIES

The second ethical issue raised by prenatal diagnosis is related to the final inadequacy of abortion as an alternative to treatment. Willingness to use abortion in the short term for the relief of particular families creates a need for a more fitting long-term solution in genetic therapies. The issue is, what is the proper goal of prenatal diagnosis and how will priorities be set to ensure the achievement of that goal?

Whether genuine prenatal genetic therapies are achievable can be answered only by the practical results of decades of research, experimentation, and testing. Valenti [40] expresses pessimism about genetic therapies because of the early onset of so many conditions and the probable reluctance of parents to allow experimental therapy for the first time with their fetus because of the risk of failure. Morrow [41] is optimistic about progress in understanding monogenic defects like sickle cell disease, hemophilia, some thalassemias, and the Lesch-

Nyhan syndrome, but he predicts many years of required research and safety tests on a gene therapy scheme.

Because amniocentesis and selective abortion will not significantly reduce genetic diseases, and because compulsory genetic screening before marriage to detect heterozygotes would be unsupportable in terms of the present system of social values,[42] the development of genetic therapies is the long-range goal from which the most tangible medical results can be expected in the field of genetic disease. The planning of policy in the field of human genetics should include increasing resources for basic research and experimentation in gene therapy. Valenti's prediction about the reluctance of parents to participate in gene therapy may be refuted by at-risk parents who are conscientiously opposed to abortion and who would elect experimental gene therapy in preference to donor insemination as a means of having a healthy child.

I hold that medical researchers have an ethical obligation to keep the development of genetic therapies as the major goal of applied human genetics until the goal is achieved or shown to be scientifically impossible.[43] To do less does not keep faith with the imperatives to prevent disease and to do no harm to the patient. The more the unknowns of human development prior to birth are exposed to understanding, the more human status the fetus gains. One of the consequences of fetal research and attempts to do genetic therapy will be treatment of the fetus as human from the earliest stages of development. The planning of the field of applied human genetics must keep faith with both sides of the ethical dilemma that the use of abortion has posed. If gene therapy is truly realized, it will reduce the need for abortion proportionate to its success, as well as bring great benefits from the treatment of the most common disorders. Opponents of abortion and fetal research must be made aware that one of the consequences of their opposition is the potential restriction of discoveries in gene therapy, which would inevitably result in more abortions.

A high degree of ethical tolerance is required of all who work in this field, so that relief can be sought for at-risk individuals, other individuals can be protected from contempt if they oppose abortion, and the goals can be pursued that will complement the skill of diagnosis with the reality of healing.

Addendum

Prenatal diagnosis of the hemoglobinopathies has been increasingly reported by investigators using aspiration or fetoscopy to obtain samples of fetal blood.[44] There are three key moral problems in this developing field: (1) questions of diagnostic accuracy and safety for the mother and fetus, (2) abortion of a fetus diagnosed as homozygous for thalassemia or sickle-cell disease, and (3) access to prenatal diagnosis for parents who need it but cannot afford it.

A February 1978 conference, cosponsored by the Sickle Cell Disease Branch (NHLBI), the Charles Drew Postgraduate School of Medicine, and the Martin Luther King Jr. Hospital in Los Angeles, heard reports from the most active investigators concerning more than 300 procedures. The fetal loss rate in total cases of continuing fetoscopies and aspirations was estimated at 8 percent with strong evidence that the risk level decreases as experience increases. Diagnostic error was less than 5 percent at that date. These figures are too high to designate these techniques as "standard practice," and they are at best "applied research." Further, the author argues that, at this level of risk, parents who desire the test but who state that they do not intend to abort should be discouraged. The risk outweighs the benefit. It is too coercive to require that parents sign a form stating their intention to abort, but the issue should be raised with them.

In thalassemia the burden of disease is clear in its predictable course, relatively early mortality, additional complications of iron overload caused by transfusions, and the chance of a normal life being nil. Abortion can clearly be justified for thalassemia, if one agrees with the criteria for selective abortion expressed above. In sickle-cell disease, the variability of the severity of the disease makes defining the burden more difficult. Powars[45] showed that the peak morbidity occurs between the second and third year and that 10 percent of those children with sickle-cell disease will die in the first decade of life. At the opposite end of the spectrum are patients with slight infections and minor pain. Counselors can give parents scenarios of the worst and best cases. Given the variability, the criterion of family factors takes on more significance. Ethical support could be offered to differing decisions in different families, based on a view of ethics that is contextual. Parental choice about abortion should be respected.

The access issue will become more prominent when the procedures are firmly established as safe and accurate. To date, the use of amniocentesis has been distributed such that it is used mainly by individuals in the middle to upper income levels. The total costs of prenatal diagnosis for the hemoglobinopathies is estimated at $1100, covering hospitalization, additional equipment, and precautions. Since the disease states occur frequently in minority groups, the cost alone will prohibit many families from obtaining a test if they desire it.

The author argues that in 1977 Congress encouraged a serious double standard by passing, on the one hand, a National Genetic Diseases Act emphasizing early screening and individual voluntary action, and omitting, on the other hand, any reference to the fetus diagnosed with serious disease in its language on the grounds for expenditure of public funds for abortion. Many families affected by the hemoglobinopathies have already been cruelly abused by social forces. To continue the double standard is, in the author's view, a further abuse and should be quickly remedied by providing for expenditures under Medicaid for genetic counseling, prenatal diagnosis, and abortion, if parents should choose the abortion alternative in the event of a positive diagnosis.

NOTES

1. J. C. Fletcher, "Parents in Genetic Counseling: The Moral Shape of Decision-Making," in *Ethical Issues in Human Genetics*, B. Hilton, D. Callahan, M. Harris, P. Condliffe, and B. Berkeley (eds.), p. 301, Plenum Press, New York, 1973.

2. A. Milunsky, *The Prenatal Diagnosis of Hereditary Disorders*, Thomas, Springfield, Ill., 1973.

3. F. Fuchs, "Amniocentesis: Techniques and Complications," in *Early Diagnosis of Human Genetic Defects*, M. Harris, (ed.), Government Printing Office, Washington, D.C., 1972.

4. J. W. Littlefield, "The Pregnancy at Risk for Genetic Disorder," *New England Journal of Medicine*, vol. 282, p. 627, 1970.

5. NICHD National Registry for Amniocentesis Study Group, "Midtrimester Amniocentesis for Prenatal Diagnosis: Safety and Accuracy," *Journal of the American Medical Association*, vol. 236, p. 1471, 1976.

6. N. E. Simpson, L. Dallaire, J. R. Miller, et al., "Prenatal Diagnosis of Genetic Disease in Canada: Report of a Collaborative Group," *Canadian Medical Association Journal*, vol. 115, p. 739, 1976.

7. N. M. MacIntyre, "Professional Responsibility in Prenatal Genetic Evaluation," *Birth Defects*, vol. 8, p. 31, 1972.

8. C. O. Leonard, G. A. Chase, and B. Childs, "Genetic Counseling: a Consumer's View," *New England Journal of Medicine*, vol. 287, p. 433, 1972.

9. L. Kass, "Implications of Prenatal Diagnosis for the Human Right to Life," in *Ethical Issues in Human Genetics*, B. Hilton, D. Callahan, M. Harris, P. Condliffe, and B. Berkeley (eds.), Plenum Press, New York, 1973.

10. J. Lejeune, "On the Nature of Man," *American Journal of Human Genetics*, vol. 22, p. 121, 1970.

11. P. Ramsey, "Points in Deciding on Abortion," in *The Morality of Abortion*, J. T. Noonan, (ed.), Harvard University Press, Cambridge, Mass., 1970.

12. P. Ramsey, "The Ethics of a Cottage Industry in an Age of Community and Research Medicine," *New England Journal of Medicine*, vol. 284, p. 700, 1971.

13. P. Ramsey, "Screening: An Ethicist's View," in *Ethical Issues in Human Genetics*, B. Hilton, D. Callahan, M. Harris, P. Condliffe, and B. Berkeley (eds.), Plenum Press, New York, 1973.

14. K. A. Lebacqz, "Prenatal Diagnosis and Selective Abortion," *Linacre Quarterly*, vol. 11, p. 109, 1973.

15. Dyck, A. J., "Ethical Issues in Community and Research Medicine," *New England Journal of Medicine*, vol. 284, p. 725, 1971.

16. A. G. Motulsky, "The Significance of Genetic Disease," in *Ethical Issues in Human Genetics*, B. Hilton, D. Callahan, M. Harris, P. Condliffe, and B. Berkeley (eds.), Plenum Press, New York, 1973.

17. A. G. Motulsky, G. R. Fraser, and J. Felsenstein, "Public Health and Long-Term Genetic Implications of Intrauterine Diagnosis and Selective Abortion," *Birth Defects*, vol. 7, p. 31, 1971.

18. S. Bok, "Ethical Problems of Abortion," *Hastings Center Studies*, vol. 2, p. 33, 1974.

19. J. C. Fletcher, "Abortion, Euthanasia, and Care of Defective Newborns, *New England Journal of Medicine*, vol. 292, p. 75, 1975.

20. J. C. Fletcher, "Moral and Ethical Problems of Prenatal Diagnosis," *Clinical Genetics*, vol. 8, p. 251, 1975.

21. P. F. Camenisch, "Abortion: For the Fetus's Own Sake?" *Hastings Center Report*, vol. 6, p. 40, 1976.

22. B. Hilton, D. Callahan, H. Harris, P. Condliffe, and B. Berkeley (eds.), *Ethical Issues in Human Genetics*, Plenum Press, New York, 1973.

23. H. D. Aiken, "Life and the Right to Life," in *Ethical Issues in Human Genetics*, B. Hilton, D. Callahan, M. Harris, P. Condliffe, and B. Berkeley (eds.), Plenum Press, New York, 1973.

24. J. V. Neel, "Ethical Issues Resulting from Prenatal Diagnosis," in *Early Diagnosis of Human Genetic Defects*, M. Harris (ed.), Government Printing Office, Washington, D.C., 1972.

25. R. S. Morison, "Implications of Prenatal Diagnosis for the Quality of, and Right to, Human Life: Society as a Standard," in *Ethical Issues in Human Genetics*, B. Hilton, D. Callahan, M. Harris, P. Condliffe, and B. Berkeley (eds.), Plenum Press, New York, 1973.

26. Crow, J. F., "Conclusion," *Birth Defects*, vol. 8, p. 115, 1972.

27. D. Callahan, "The Meaning and Significance of Genetic Disease: Philosophical Perspectives," in *Ethical Issues in Human Genetics*, B. Hilton, D. Callahan, M. Harris, P. Condliffe, and B. Berkeley (eds.), Plenum Press, New York, 1973.

28. Callahan, D., "Abortion: Some Ethical Issues," in *Abortion, Society, and the Law*, D. Walbert and J. Butler, (eds.), Press of Case Western Reserve University, Cleveland, Ohio, 1973.

29. D. Callahan, *Abortion: Law, Choice and Morality*, Macmillan, New York, 1970.

30. J. M. Gustafson, "Genetic Counseling and the Uses of Genetic Knowledge: An Ethical Overview," in *Ethical Issues in Human Genetics*, B. Hilton, D. Callahan, M. Harris, P. Condliffe, and B. Berkeley (eds.), Plenum Press, New York, 1973.

31. The term "elective abortion" is now preferred.

32. Institute of Medicine, *Legalized Abortion and the Public Health*, National Academy of Sciences, Washington, D.C., 1975.

33. B. D. Blumberg, M. S. Gulbus, and K. H. Hanson, "The Psychological Sequelae of Abortion Performed for a Genetic Indication," *American Journal of Obstetrics and Gynecology*, vol. 122, p. 802, 1975.

34. R. Behrman, and T. Rosen, *Report on Viability and Non-viability of the Fetus*, The National Commission for the Protection of Human Subjects of Biomedical and Behavioral Research, Washington, D.C., 1975.

35. T. S. Szasz, "The Ethics of Abortion," *Humanist*, Sept.-Oct., 1966, p. 148.

36. H. B. Munson, "Abortion in Modern Times: Thoughts and Comments," *Renewal*, February, 1967, p. 9.

37. S. Bok, B. N. Nathanson, D. C. Nathan, et al., "The Unwanted Child: Caring for the Fetus Born Alive after an Abortion," *Hastings Center Report*, vol. 6, p. 10, 1976.

38. Culliton, B., "Amniocentesis: HEW Backs Test for Prenatal Diagnosis of Disease," *Science*, vol. 190, p. 537, 1975.

39. T. Powledge, "Prenatal Diagnosis—Now the Problems," *New Science*, vol. 69, p. 332, 1976.

40. C. Valenti, "Prenatal Treatment of Heredi-tary Diseases?" *Lancet,* vol. 2, p. 797, 1973.

41. J. F. Morrow, "The Prospects for Gene Therapy in Humans," *Annals of the New York Academy of Science,* vol. 265, p. 13, 1976.

42. I failed in Boston even to establish a *volun-tary* system whereby young couples seeking a marriage license would be offered a *free* oppor-tunity to obtain genetic counseling.

43. Society, too, has obligations to provide op-portunities to ensure the health of its future mem-bers. In Massachusetts, for example, legislation pushed by so-called prolife groups has effectively impeded extremely promising fetal research aimed at both prenatal diagnosis and fetal therapy.

44. B. P. Alter, C. B. Modell, D. Fairweather, et. al., "Prenatal Diagnosis of Hemoglobinopathies. A Review of 15 Cases," *New England Journal of Medicine,* vol. 295, p. 1437, 1976.

45. D. R. Powars, "Natural History of Sickle Cell Disease—The First Years," *Seminars in Hematology,* vol. 12, p. 275, 1975.

91. *Ethics and Amniocentesis for Fetal Sex Identification*
John C. Fletcher

Two types of parents request fetal sex identification by amniocentesis: the first group risk transmitting a sex-linked hereditary disorder and the second want to select the gender of their next child. Physicians generally encourage the first type of parent but discourage the second.

Prenatal diagnosis for sex choice is controversial because of ethical objections to the use of abortion for such a reason and because of the question of whether amniocentesis, a scarce medical resource, can prudently be used for this purpose.[1] The issue is complex and involves many competing ethical claims.

I have reevaluated my position on this issue as a result of participation in a Hastings Cen-ter study group[2] and consultation with staff of the Prenatal Diagnostic Center of the Johns Hopkins Hospital on their policy on amniocentesis for sex choice.

My earlier position was based on four main points. In the first place, I argued that parents with this request ought to be discouraged because sex is not a disease. I saw prenatal diag-nosis as a tool that ethically could be used to diagnose hereditary diseases or congenital defects in the fetus. Second, I stressed that abortion for sex choice could contribute to social inequal-ity between the sexes because of a preference for male offspring. Third, I criticized sex choice as a "frivolous" reason for abortion that could not be successfully defended in the company of serious moral persons. My fourth point was that amniocentesis was a scarce resource in the light of the total number of pregnancies at risk. Requests for fetal sex identification could swamp an already overloaded system or delay laboratory work in cases of serious genetic diseases.

A legal and a public-relations consideration buttressed these reasons and secured my posi-tion. Physicians cannot legally be forced to provide procedures that are not "lifesaving." Furthermore, if parents were accommodated with this request, antiabortion forces might raise a public outcry that would discourage parents genuinely at risk from seeking prenatal test-ing. I supported the prevailing policy of discouragement and defended the practice in some laboratories of refusing to do karyotyping when fetal sex alone was the presenting indication.

Reevaluation

My reevaluation assumes that the basis for the policy of discouragement is the belief of most physicians who perform prenatal diagnosis that abortion for sex choice is morally

Source: *New England Journal of Medicine,* vol. 301, p. 550, 1979.

unjustifiable. Those who reason as I did also use the scarce-resource argument[3] and are wary of the use of prenatal diagnosis for "social engineering" to plan the sex of children. In practice, however, discouragement based on opposition to abortion for sex choice is weightier than the other two reasons. Most of us have an uneasy conscience about the number of abortions performed in the United States and about the lack of moral seriousness with which abortion is sometimes requested and carried out. We have preferred to use prenatal diagnosis in the context of saving fetal lives. I personally believe that sex choice is not a compelling reason for abortion. The first moral response of most who think about the issue is close to queasiness. Yet, the issue does not turn on the validity of opposition to abortion for sex choice. The issue turns on the validity of the legal rules on abortion defined by the Supreme Court, which do not require that a woman state reasons in a public or medical forum for early to mid-trimester abortion. No one is presumed to be a public judge of her reasons except herself. Family, friends, counselors, or physicians may challenge her reasons if she chooses to confide in them. But the rule is that no public test of reasons is required.

Is this the best rule to apply in abortion? Yes, if one holds, as I do, that the woman's right to decide is the overriding consideration in the abortion issue. The rationale for the legal rule omitting a test of reasons is that a woman has the right to control her reproduction and the risks involved in a pregnancy. To employ public or medical tests of reasons provides opportunities to obstruct and defeat society's obligation to grant women the freedom to determine their own reproductive futures. To prevent obstruction of self-determination, it is better to have no public tests of reasons.

The Supreme Court took the position that the state has no interest in refusing an adult woman the right of self-determination in reproduction through the second trimester of pregnancy. Although a Supreme Court decision is not itself an ethical consideration, the legal guideline on abortion points beyond itself to the principles of justice and respect for persons. Justice in the modern state requires that women be freed from restrictions on their freedom and opportunity to compete for the social and economic rewards of citizenship. Respect for persons requires that a woman's autonomy and personal responsibility be the standards that govern the final resolution of conflicts about reproduction and abortion.

The Supreme Court justices probably did not imagine in 1973 that their decision on abortion was related to the right of parents to choose the sex of children through amniocentesis. However, even if the justices were then aware of the potential use of amniocentesis for this purpose, it did not figure in their reasoning. The position that they took made abortion on request a legal practice and the conscience of the individual woman the sole arbiter of the reasons. Abortion for sex choice is legal, and if we are to act in accordance with the principles that should now inform decision making on abortion, all forms of tests should be removed.

Given the ethical and legal posture discussed above, one must be willing to accept the fact that some abortions will be performed for trivial reasons. The existence of some trivial reasons should not deter us from the larger goal of protecting the right of women to make such decisions in the first place. That is what is at stake in the issue under discussion. My major argument is that it is inconsistent to support an abortion law that protects the absolute right of women to decide and, at the same time, to block access to information about the fetus because one thinks that an abortion may be foolishly sought on the basis of the information.

An Example

Another way to measure the degree of ethical inconsistency in the policy of discouragement is to reflect on an example. An obstetrician-gynecologist is asked by a 30-year-old woman in the second month of gestation to perform an abortion. The physician does not inquire about her reasons. As it turns out, she desired the abortion so that she could make a trip to Europe. The same physician is a cooperating member of a prenatal diagnostic center in a university hospital with a policy of discouraging access for prenatal sex identification and a prohibition against laboratory cultures for this purpose. The mother of three children of one gender requests fetal sex identification in the fourth pregnancy. The physician must either refer her to another center at some distance or do the amniotic tap in the office and send the sample to a commercial laboratory where no questions are asked.

If the sometimes trivial reason for abortion must be accepted to protect the rights of many women, how could it be acceptable for the same physician to participate in a system that discriminates because of reasons for abortion? To hold to this inconsistency is morally self-defeating and leads to hypocrisy. Furthermore, amniocentesis and laboratory work should be done under the very best of conditions, if done at all. The physician should not be forced to defend an inconsistent policy and practice less than optimum medicine and science.

Informed Consent

When physicians counsel parents who want to know the sex of the fetus, they should carefully inform them about several areas of risk.

Amniocentesis carries a small but nonetheless real risk of death to the fetus and injury to the mother. The risk of fetal death from amniocentesis has been shown to be less than 1 percent in controlled studies in the United States and Canada.[4,5] A British study that suggested a 1.5 percent fetal loss[6] has been challenged on the ground that selection of controls was biased. Until this controversy is resolved, the previous risk figures and the fact that risk factors are still being studied should be communicated to the parents.

A very small number of technical errors are still made in laboratories. A recent review of 3000 consecutive amniocenteses showed the karyotyping-error rate to be 0.07 percent, or 7 in 10,000.[7]

Mid-trimester abortion is a major procedure, and depression has been reported in both parents after genetically indicated abortions.[8]

Finally, an unknown risk of insult to other members of the family and to the wider society is involved in a decision to abort for sex choice. The physician can, if he or she chooses, state an opposing view in moral terms. What the physician should not do is withhold amniocentesis if informed parents desire to proceed. To do so would be to test the parents' reasons for abortion. The parents may or may not decide on abortion on the basis of the information gained. In any event, that decision remains theirs to make, legally and morally.

Public and Private Opposition

Individuals and groups who want to test the reasoning of those who may seek abortions are free to do so within the limits of the law. Religious groups opposed to abortion can attempt to convince anyone in society that abortion is morally wrong. Any group is free to work toward amending the Constitution so that public tests of reasons on abortion are required. Parents are free to instruct children about human sexuality in a manner that reduces the likelihood that abortion will ever be needed in their families. Spouses and companions are free to challenge the reasoning used in any instance of contemplation of abortion. Social critics and moralists are free to write and speak against the current rules on abortion and the ethical perspective behind the rules. What none of these persons is free to do is to construct a public or medical test of a woman's reasons.

Competing Ethical Claims

Wherever possible, competing ethical claims should be acknowledged in practice. There are three major ethical claims on the other side of the issue: scarcity of amniocentesis, risks and costs of the procedure, and social engineering without full appreciation of the consequences.

When there is a genuine scarcity of amniocentesis in any center, its use for sex choice should be given the lowest priority. Parents who request amniocentesis for sex choice should bear all expenses, since society is not confronted with a disease in the fetus that should be prevented in the interest of the family in society. Because of risks to the mother and fetus, the procedure should be performed only when there is adequate counseling and access to high-quality laboratory work.

Forecasting the long-range consequences of sex preselection is a complex task[9] that deserves more encouragement and support. An earlier study based on data from the 1970 National Fertility Survey showed that the major consequence of sex determination would be planning the order of children (male first, female second) rather than increasing the number of boys.[10] Coombs's excellent study of the preferences for sex of children among American couples showed that wives are much more likely to prefer a son than a daughter and more likely to prefer either one than to have a positive underlying desire for an equal number of boys and girls.[11] The exceptions to this finding were wives of Hispanic heritage, who preferred girls. These findings suggest that if a safe, inexpensive preconception method of sex selection were available, firstborns would increasingly be male. Would these first-born boys receive such a disproportionate share of the emotional and economic resources of the parents that second-born girls would be seriously disadvantaged? More work needs to be done connecting forecasts of technologic advances in sex control with psychologic research in gender roles and birth order. The immediate ethical question is whether a more permissive policy on amniocentesis for sex choice will precipitate a social experiment in sex selection before there is sufficient study of the consequences. The parents who now need amniocentesis for sex choice are presumably motivated to have one child of the opposite gender from their living children. If this is true, these parents and their needs are not accurate predictors of the long-range consequences of sex determination in a planned birth order. Those consequences should be researched in the framework of sex-control methods that are more easily diffused and involve fewer risks than abortion.

Conclusions

In my revised view, it is not ethically required that physicians withhold amniocentesis from fully informed parents who may use the results in deciding to abort for sex choice. Even though the physician may personally disapprove of the request, it is fairer to the parents to grant it within the limits of availability of amniocentesis. Physicians who agree with the social-ethical perspective that informs the legal rules on abortion will finally want to keep faith with the moral intent of the law. Policymakers in this field should now reconsider their obligation to be responsive and consistent in their beliefs. I include myself in the company of those who need to be changed.

NOTES

1. J. C. Fletcher, "Prenatal Diagnosis: Ethical Issues," *Encyclopedia of Bioethics,* Macmillan, New York, p. 1336, 1978.

2. T. M. Powledge and J. Fletcher, "Guidelines for the Ethical, Social and Legal Issues in Prenatal Diagnosis: A Report from the Genetics Research Group of the Hastings Center, Institute of Society, Ethics and the Life Sciences," *New England Journal of Medicine,* vol. 300, p. 168, 1979.

3. A. Milunsky, *Know Your Genes,* Houghton Mifflin Company, Boston, 1977.

4. The NICHD National Registry for Amniocentesis Study Group, "Mid-trimester Amniocentesis for Prenatal Diagnosis: Safety and Accuracy," *Journal of the American Medical Association,* vol. 236, p. 1471, 1976.

5. N. E. Simpson, L. Dallaire, J. R. Miller, et al., "Prenatal Diagnosis of Genetic Disease in Canada: Report of a Collaborative Study," *Canadian Medical Association Journal,* vol. 115, p. 739, 1976.

6. "An Assessment of the Hazards of Amniocentesis: Report to the Medical Research Council by Their Working Party on Amniocentesis," *British Journal of Obstetrics and Gynaecology,* vol. 85, suppl. 2, p. 1, 1978.

7. M. S. Golbus, W. D. Loughman, C. J. Epstein, et al., "Prenatal Genetic Diagnosis in 3000 Amniocenteses," *New England Journal of Medicine,* vol. 300, p. 157, 1979.

8. B. D. Blumberg, M. S. Golbus, and K. H. Hanson, "The Psychological Sequelae of Abortion Performed for a Genetic Indication," *American Journal of Obstetrics and Gynecology,* vol. 122, p. 799, 1975.

9. G. Largey, "Reproductive Technologies: Sex Selection," *Encyclopedia of Bioethics,* Macmillan, New York, 1978.

10. C. F. Westoff and R. R. Rindfuss, "Sex Preselection in the United States: Some Implications, " *Science,* vol. 184, p. 633, 1974.

11. L. C. Coombs, "Preferences for Sex of Children among U.S. Couples," *Family Planning Perspectives,* vol. 9, p. 259, 1977.

92. *The Supreme Court and Sex Choice*
Margaret O'Brien Steinfels

The apparent logic of John Fletcher's argument favoring amniocentesis for sex choice stands only so long as his premise is not compared with what the Supreme Court actually said in 1973. Fletcher's premise: *Roe* v. *Wade* enunciated the absolute right of a woman to obtain an abortion without state interference, including the requirement that she state a reason; His conclusion then follows: a woman also has the right to have amniocentesis to ascertain the sex of a fetus, because to deny the right to amniocentesis for sex choice establishes a test that in effect denies the absolute right to an abortion. By extending the right to abortion, Fletcher uncovers a new absolute right—amniocentesis for sex choice.

It is true that the Court gave little, if any, thought to the matter of amniocentesis —only on the horizon in 1973. But contrary to Fletcher's reading, I see nothing in *Roe* pointing to principles of justice and respect for persons that would allow by extension a right to amniocentesis. *Roe* v. *Wade* speaks only of the right of privacy being "broad enough to encom-

Source: *Hastings Center Report,* vol. 10, February 1980, p. 19.

pass a woman's decision whether or not to terminate her pregnancy"—a decision that the Court saw a woman making in consultation with her physician. Furthermore, while the decision cannot be subject to a state test through the second trimester, the Court does not forbid physicians from inquiring into the reason for abortion; nor presumably would it prohibit a physician from saying "no," if a woman's reason did not meet the test of his or her own standards of practice. Presumably there are physicians who perform abortions only for grave cause, such as saving the life of the mother and who will refuse for less serious reasons. Thus the physician's obligation to perform an abortion is not absolute, nor is the woman's claim absolute. The Court specifically disagreed with the proposition "that the woman's right is absolute and that she is entitled to terminate her pregnancy at whatever time, in whatever way, and for whatever reason she alone chooses."

The Court's decision has been subject to many rhetorical deletions, and Fletcher has accepted the feminist edition—an ironic situation for feminists, who I doubt would be willing to grant Fletcher's new right under the umbrella of the old. If physicians were to accept Fletcher's reading of *Roe* v. *Wade*, they could oppose amniocentesis for sex choice only by opposing abortion and amniocentesis in toto. Conversely physicians who do abortions and amniocentesis would be compelled to do them for sex choice—or for any reason. That can hardly be an obligation imposed on the basis of *Roe* v. *Wade*.

But if Fletcher uncovers a new right on grounds not laid for the old, is there another kind of logic than that of the Court that fuels the argument favoring amniocentesis and abortion for sex choice? Perhaps it is the logic of the technology itself: (1) amniocentesis was developed to identify in utero a fetus with a serious genetic disease and was at first limited to women who previously had given birth to such a child or was at known risk of doing so; (2) after a time the use of the technology was expanded and made routinely available to women at statistical risk because of age; (3) now there is an appeal to another risk and another form of human suffering: bearing a child of the wrong sex. True, the child will not suffer a terrible death or a life filled with stigmatization or agonizing pain, but the mother or father will suffer from having a daughter when a son is needed or a son when a daughter is wanted. The expansive nature of the argument might even give rise to the proposition that the psychological suffering attendant on being an unwanted son or daughter is worse than never having been born at all. So it goes. The technology is there and if new desires supplement the original purposes for its development, what reason is there to oppose its use?

There are many good reasons that physicians use everyday in prenatal clinics; Fletcher enumerates many sound ones, which I will not repeat, and several more could be added including: (1) turning gender into a disease subject to medical "cure"; (2) fostering cultural and social prejudice that values one sex over the other; (3) confirming the prejudice that sex is the governing factor in behavior, status, and vocation. Thus even those not opposed absolutely to abortion or amniocentesis ought to have no difficulty opposing amniocentesis for sex choice. Even if no single principle unites the opposition to such a practice, there are a sufficient number of overlapping reasons to suggest that no physician should feel obliged to perform the procedure in order, as Fletcher would have it, "to keep faith with the moral intent of the law."

93. Selective Birth in Twin Pregnancy with Discordancy for Down's Syndrome   Thomas D. Kerenyi   Usha Chitkara

Amniocentesis for genetic evaluation is now a well-established prenatal diagnostic procedure. The discovery of twins at the time of amniocentesis, however, necessitates additional measures, and in the event of detection of discordancy for an abnormality, it poses a challenging problem. In 1975, Bank et al. reported the first successful amniocentesis and karyotyping in twins. They also forecast the inevitable dilemma: "One unsolved question is the consequence of finding one abnormal and one normal fetus."[1]

At least five recent articles have described cases in the mid-trimester in which one fetus had a major congenital malformation and the other one was normal. Three reports [2-4] involved discordancy for trisomy 21, one for Hurler's disease,[5] and one for spina bifida with hydrocephalus.[6] Interestingly enough, the management and outcome in all five cases was different. In one of the three trisomy 21 cases, the parents chose to abort both twins.[4] In the other two cases the parents elected to continue the pregnancy for the sake of the normal twin. Both pregnancies were carried to term; delivery of a normal infant and a macerated stillborn fetus occurred in one case,[3] and delivery of a normal infant and an infant with trisomy 21, both living, in the other.[2] In the case of discordancy for neural-tube defect,[6] although both twins were born alive, the twin with the spina bifida and hydrocephalus died two days after birth.

The most aggressive management of this problem has been reported from Sweden; in that case there was a prenatal diagnosis of Hurler's disease[5] in one twin. At 24 weeks' gestation, intracardiac puncture resulting in cardiac arrest in the affected fetus was successfully performed without a detectable effect on the normal twin, except for premature labor and delivery at 33 weeks' gestation. We are aware of another, unpublished case from Denmark, in which attempted cardiac punctures were followed by abortion of both twins three weeks later.

In this report we describe a case of twin pregnancy with discordancy for trisomy 21, in which an aggressive approach was undertaken for selective termination of the abnormal fetus by intracardiac puncture and exsanguination at 20 weeks' gestation. The normal fetus was subsequently delivered at term.

The patient, a 40-year-old nullipara with an 18-month history of infertility, underwent genetic amniocentesis at 17 weeks' gestation for the indication of advanced maternal age. Her medical history was unremarkable except for hypothyroidism, for which she had received dessicated thyroid extract, 3 g daily, since 1960. An ultrasound scan before the procedure revealed a twin pregnancy with biparietal diameters of both fetuses compatible with 17.5 weeks' gestation, two clearly defined amniotic sacs, and one placenta on the posterior uterine wall. Amniotic fluid from each sac obtained separately for chromosomal studies revealed two male fetuses. Twin A had a normal male karyotype (46,XY), but chromosomal analysis of Twin B indicated trisomy 21 (47,XY + 21).

Presented with the diagnosis of carrying one normal and one affected fetus, the parents were confronted with the difficult task of making one of two decisions: to induce abortion and lose both fetuses, or to continue the pregnancy. The mother desperately wanted to have the normal child but could not face the burden of caring for an abnormal

Source: *New England Journal of Medicine*, vol. 304, no. 25, June 18, 1981.

child for the rest of her life. Having been made aware of the case report from Sweden in which selective termination of an abnormal twin had been successfully performed even though the unaffected twin was delivered prematurely, she asked if a similar procedure could be offered to her. If it had been refused, she would have chosen to abort both fetuses. At that point, she was referred to us.

Extensive medical and legal counseling and an explanation of the many risks were provided. These risks included abortion of both fetuses, premature delivery of the surviving fetus, performing the procedure on the wrong twin since markers for sac A or B were lacking, and the development of disseminated intravascular coagulation in the mother as a result of fetal death in utero. After careful consideration, the patient decided to undertake the procedure anyway. In view of the fact that the procedure had never been performed in this country, we decided, out of an abundance of caution, to obtain confirmation from a court of law of the parents' right to consent on behalf of the normal fetus.

Results

At 20 weeks' gestation, the procedure was carried out under real-time ultrasound guidance. Meperidine hydrochloride (50 mg) and diazepam (10 mg) were administered intravenously before the procedure. The position and lie of each twin was first assessed; twin A (normal) was in an oblique lie with its head over the pubic symphysis on the right and the breech toward the left side. Twin B (thought to be the affected fetus) was in a transverse lie with its head on the left side and its breech on the right; the face and chest were pointing toward the maternal anterior abdominal wall. Biparietal measurements were 5.0 cm in twin A and 4.9 cm in twin B. Active fetal movements and fetal heartrates of 140 and 150 beats per minute were noted in both twins. Placental implantation was posterior, and the dividing membrane between the two amniotic sacs was clearly identified. The position of the heart of twin B was localized, and its distance from the maternal abdominal wall measured.

Under local anesthesia, 40 ml of amniotic fluid was removed from the sac of twin B with a No. 18 spinal needle. The needle was then advanced into the fetal chest but missed the heart. A second insertion led to cardiac puncture and exsanguination of 25 ml of blood. Immediate analysis for cell size on the Coulter Channelyzer confirmed that the sample was 100 percent fetal blood. Chromosomal analysis of the blood sample three days later confirmed it to be from the twin with trisomy 21. After the procedure movements of the affected fetus and cardiac activity ceased. The heartbeat and movements of the normal twin A were unaffected during and after the procedure. A repeat ultrasound scan on the next day again confirmed that heart rate and motion were normal in twin A and absent in twin B.

The mother's condition remained stable throughout the procedure and afterward. She was given prophylactic antibiotics (ampicillin, 500 mg, and dicloxacillin, 250 mg) every six hours for five days. The rest of the prenatal course was uneventful except for recurring mild uterine irritability, which usually subsided with rest and did not require tocolytic agents. Follow-up biweekly serial sonogram scans indicated appropriate biparietal diameter and fetal growth of twin A and decreasing fetal head and body size of twin B. Blood counts, hematocrit, hemoglobin, red cell indexes, platelets, and fibrinogen were stable throughout the pregnancy. Labor started at 40 weeks' gestation, one day after stripping of membranes. Uneventful delivery of a 2980-g living male infant occurred after nine hours of labor. The birth was soon followed by delivery of the placenta and of twin B in the form of a fetus papyraceus weighing 120 g. The placenta weighed 530 g and was remarkable only in that the area corresponding to twin B was small, fibrosed, and infarcted.

After delivery, the conditions of the mother and baby were stable, and now, seven months later, they continue to do well.

Discussion

The two almost universally accepted medical indications for therapeutic abortion are the diagnosis of a congenital disease incompatible with life and the diagnosis of a disease leading to a life of prolonged suffering for the child and family. The classic examples are Tay-Sachs disease and Down's syndrome (trisomy 21). Although only 30 percent of the patients with Down's syndrome currently in mental institutions were born to women 35 years old or older, 54 to 75 percent of the prenatal genetic amniocenteses performed in 1978 were for advanced maternal age.[7,8] The highest frequency of dizygotic twins occurs between the ages of 37 and 40.[9] Therefore, with the increasing use of genetic amniocentesis, one may expect to be faced with the possibility of detecting Down's syndrome in one twin and not the other. This is well illustrated by recent case reports,[2-4] including our own.

What is the appropriate advice for such a patient? Several recent publications [1-3,5,10,11] have discussed the problems of counseling when twins are involved, and the consensus has been that the final decision should be made by the parents. Although we concurred, we also noted that the specific issues that had to be faced when contemplating selective abortion of one twin while preserving the other were not directly addressed in these articles. Therefore, to ensure that counseling was appropriate, we elected to discuss all the technical difficulties inherent in the procedure with the patient and her husband.

After the parents decided to go ahead with the procedure, we were mainly concerned about performing it without inadvertently bringing harm to the normal fetus. We realized that this was more important than the fate of the affected twin, and that acceptance of this procedure in the future would hinge on the outcome for the normal unaffected twin.

There are several specific technical considerations in this type of procedure. First of all, in the absence of a persisting marker differentiating the two fetuses, it may be difficult to identify the fetus with the abnormality three or four weeks after the initial amniocentesis, when the chromosomal analysis is reported. Therefore, it is conceivable that a destructive procedure could be performed on the wrong fetus. Thus, when twins are encountered at amniocentesis for genetic studies, careful mapping out and identification of the separate sacs— e.g., upper versus lower, right versus left—is imperative. Videotape recording of the real-time scanning of both fetuses may be the best way to facilitate subsequent identification. In our case, even though twin B (with trisomy 21) altered its position, with the head changing from the mother's left side to her right, we were reasonably certain that the relative positions of twin A and B (with twin A lower than twin B) had not changed. The correct selection was not verified on the basis of karyotyping from the fetal blood until three days after the procedure, when fetal demise had already occurred.

The procedure and the subsequent follow-up scans were videotaped. The plotted cephalometry showed a normal growth pattern in the surviving twin and an almost mirror image-like regression in the affected twin. It was a very gratifying experience in such an endangered pregnancy to follow the normal fetus to full term and through vaginal delivery.

NOTES

1. J. Bang, H. Nielsen, and J. Philip, "Prenatal Karyotyping of Twins by Ultrasonically Guided Amniocentesis," *American Journal of Obstetrics and Gynecology*, vol. 123, p. 695, 1975.

2. M. N. Jassani, I. R. Merkatz, J. N. Brennan and M. N. Macintyre, "Twin Pregnancy with Discordancy for Down's Syndrome," *Obstetrics and Gynecology*, vol. 55, suppl. 45S, 1980.

3. R. H. Heller and L. S. Palmer, "Trisomy 21 in One of Twin Fetuses," *Pediatrics*, vol. 62, p. 52, 1978.

4. K. Filkins, T. Kushnick, N. Diamond, B. Searle and F. Desposito, "Prenatal Diagnosis of Down Syndrome in One of Dizygotic Twins," *American Journal of Obstetrics and Gynecology*, vol. 131, p. 584, 1978.

5. A. Aberg, F. Mitelman, M. Cantz, and J. Gehler, "Cardiac Puncture of Fetus with Hurler's Disease Avoiding Abortion of Unaffected Co-twin," *Lancet*, vol. 2, p. 990, 1978.

6. S. Campbell, M. Grundy and J. D. Singer, "Early Antenatal Diagnosis of Spina Bifida in a Twin Fetus by Ultrasonic Examination and Alpha-Fetoprotein Estimation," *British Medical Journal*, vol. 2, p. 676, 1976.

7. M. S. Golbus, "Prenatal Diagnosis of Genetic Defects—Where It Is and Where It Is Going," in J. W. Littlefield and J. de Grouchy (eds.), *Birth Defects: Proceedings of the Fifth International Conference*, Montreal, Canada, August 21–27, 1977, *Excerpta*

Medica, 1978, p. 330, (International Congress Series no. 432).

8. P. Chandra, H. M. Nitowsky, R. Marion, M. Koenigsberg, E. Taben and H. W. Kava, "Experience with Sonography as an Adjunct to Amniocentesis for Prenatal Diagnosis of Fetal Genetic Disorders," *American Journal of Obstetrics and Gynecology*, vol. 135, p. 519, 1979.

9. D. W. Fielding and S. Walker, "Dizygotic Twins with Down's Syndrome," *Archives of Disease in Childhood*, vol. 47, p. 971, 1972.

10. A. G. W. Hunter and D. M. Cox, "Counselling Problems When Twins Are Discovered at Genetic Amniocentesis," *Clinical Genetics*, vol. 16, p. 34, 1979.

11. P. M. Layde, J. D. Erickson, A. Falek and B. J. McCarthy, "Congenital Malformation in Twins," *American Journal of Human Genetics*, vol. 32, p. 69, 1980.

12. T. D. Kerenyi and B. Walker, "The Preventability of "Bloody Taps" in Second Trimester Amniocentesis by Ultrasound Scanning," *Obstetrics and Gynecology*, vol. 50, p. 61, 1977.

13. J. A. Morris, R. F. Hustead, R. G. Robinson and G. L. Haswell, "Measurement of Fetoplacental Blood Volume in the Human Previable Fetus," *American Journal of Obstetrics and Gynecology*, vol. 118, p. 927, 1974.

14. M. Melnick, "Brain Damage in Survivor after In-utero Death of Monozygous Co-twin," *Lancet*, vol. 2, p. 1287, 1977.

94. *Nondirective Genetic Counseling*   Robert Redmon

Recently, as part of a medical residency program for humanists,[1] I listened to a presentation of a case in a postcounseling session in a genetics department of a large medical school. The case is outlined below.

Mrs. Conn is a 38-year-old, 8-week-pregnant woman who was referred to the Genetic Counseling Clinic for information on the possible teratogenic effects of valium (diazepam). She reported that she began taking Valium (20 mg/day) on the day before she became pregnant, continued it for about a month until she suspected she was pregnant, and then discontinued it. She also reported that once during this period she took more (35 mg) than her prescribed dosage. She was told by the genetic counselor that the only reported effects of Valium on pregnancy was a three-to fourfold increase of cleft lip and/or palate. Since the normal risk of such a defect was only 1/1000, this meant that the risk to her child was only 3/1000 to 4/1000. She was also told that this risk is quite small com-

Source: Unpublished manuscript.

pared with other possible birth defects (in particular Down's syndrome due to her age and Tay-Sachs disease due to her and her husband's ethnic background), and that this particular defect is minor in light of modern surgical techniques which can correct it. However, she became quite upset over the small possibility of her child having this particular problem and she indicated she would seek an abortion.

The counselor who was involved in this case, Dr. Brown, who has a Ph.D. in genetics, was quite unhappy over the outcome. She stated to the others in the department that she believed that either Mrs. Conn was acting irrationally, or she was extremely self-centered, and thus overly concerned over the stigma of a cleft lip or palate, or she was using the counselor to justify a decision she had made for other reasons. Dr. Brown's colleagues, however, attempted to reassure her by claiming that the role of counseling is to supply information, to be sure the information is understood, and to be supportive. This seems to have been done, and so she should not be concerned with the outcome. It was pointed out to Dr. Brown that she would not have been overly concerned if Mrs. Conn had chosen an abortion for any other reason, or for no reason at all.

Dr. Brown's unhappiness about the results of counseling is justified. But it is not justified because counseling should be "directive," that is, counseling is successful only if the patient-client acts in a specific way. The justification for this directive outlook is typically given as follows:

> That the parties involved must ultimately decide for themselves is self-evident; that the geneticist can disclaim all responsibility for influencing the decision is, in our opinion, not really justifiable. There is no such thing as being totally objective. The manner alone in which the facts are represented will influence the decision, and the presentation is unavoidably subjective. Apart from this we do not believe that it is either right or desirable to evade a personal commitment when it is desired and might be of help. It is in the nature of the doctor-patient relationship that the doctor assumes at least some responsibility for the patient, influences his decisions and, therefore, must answer for them as well.[2]

Thus, directive counseling is justified as being included in a paternalistically viewed physician-patient relationship. (If the counselor is not a paternalistically minded physician, I suppose he should act like one.)

The other approach to genetic counseling, the nondirective one, is the one that is held by Dr. Brown's colleagues. On this view the task of counseling is to "communicate" with the "clients" (not "patients") so that they "comprehend the medical facts," "understand the options," are able to "choose the course of action which seems appropriate to them in view of their risk and their family goals," and can "make the best possible adjustment to the disorder."[3] In fact, to do otherwise is seen as unethical since it seems to infringe on the moral autonomy of the patient/client. Dr. Brown, if she follows up the counseling session with Mrs. Conn, seems to have fulfilled these requirements. Yet even if Dr. Brown has this nondirective goal, she still is justified in believing she has failed (although she is not necessarily to blame for failing).

The problem is that the directive-nondirective distinction is a confused one. It is based on both a faulty theory of language and a faulty theory of knowledge. The theory of language it assumes is what may be called an "ideational" one. It is the theory that language consists of symbols used to implant "ideas" in another's head, and that our words refer to these mental objects in ourselves. The test for successful communication is that one can recite the facts which are stated, much as a recorder or computer can.

The theory of knowledge assumed is the passive or "empirical" one. One learns when the "information" received by the senses is stored in the memory and compared with other stored data (again, much as a computer operates). This particular theory of knowledge has an ancient history which predates Plato, and I won't rehash it here. But the theory of language which is assumed in the directive/nondirective debate is much more important for our discussion.

A more adequate theory of language for understanding the present problem is one that views language in terms of "acts" of a certain sort ("speech acts").[4] Language (speaking, writing) is seen as consisting of a series of acts used to accomplish certain goals. Some of these acts are accomplished by simply uttering the words with the *intent* to have a certain effect on the hearer ("illocutionary acts"). Stating, promising, asking, ordering, predicting, etc., occur whether or not the hearer responds in the appropriate way. I have promised to pay you five dollars if I simply say, "I promise to pay you five dollars," even if you don't understand English. Other kinds of speech acts ("perlocutionary acts") take place only if there occurs the desired effect ("perlocutionary effect"). I can't warn you, or startle you, or deceive you, or inform you unless you understand and react appropriately.

The problem with the directive-nondirective debate is that in the description of what it means to be nondirective, no distinction is being made between the act of stating facts, and the act of *informing* with its effects. Informing and communicating occur only if certain effects are produced. And the effects produced are actions and dispositions to act in certain ways, not "ideas" in the listener's head. I have *informed* you that it is raining only when you act in certain ways—you go out to roll up the windows on the car you care about, for example. If you simply say after me, "It is raining" and don't act in these ways, I haven't informed you of anything. Thus, simply informing you of something is, in a certain way, a directive act.

To return to Mrs. Conn and Dr. Brown: Dr. Brown seems to have failed to inform Mrs. Conn because Mrs. Conn's actions, including what she says, are not appropriate. The abortion decision is not the problem. The problem is that she has stated the wrong *reason* for the abortion. If she did not want to burden her new marriage with a baby, or if the fear of other defects was cited as a reason, this would have let Dr. Brown know that she had succeeded in giving information. But citing fear of a 3/1000 risk of a minor defect and ignoring an 8/100 risk of serious problems is *irrational* and shows a failure to *comprehend*. She has *not* been informed, regardless of what facts she recites.

The statement by the Ad Hoc Committee, which is quoted in part above, on the goal of counseling must be supplemented by an adequate view as to what communication, information giving, etc., consist of. The counselor's own views as to what is a *rational* response, in terms of probabilities, facts, and values must govern his judgment as to whether information has been given. He must decide which genetic conditions are more serious (a value judgment) as well as the probabilities of their occurrence. And he must determine if the response is *appropriate* to these facts and values, to be sure the client has been informed. If the nondirective approach is the best one, the counselor must allow for a wide range of responses to the information. But a "wide range" does not include *every* response.

Which brings up my final point: The counselor must be quite clear about his own values. In order to tell if someone is responding irrationally, we must have criteria for rationality, and "rational" *is* a value term. Two of the major components of rationality are (1) an appropriate belief structure about reality, including probabilities and reasoning processes and

(2) an appropriate value structure which, for example, places a higher value on a human life than on that of a mouse, or which places a greater dysvalue on Tay-Sach's disease than on a cleft palate. (Mrs. Conn seems to have failed both tests.) We all require such factual and value structures in order to communicate, and the counselor must be especially aware of them in himself and in his clients. The genetic counselor needs study and thought in the area of ethics and moral reasoning as much as the physician. His words and actions do have an effect on his client and he is responsible to and, in some ways, for her.

NOTES

1. Supported by the Virginia Foundation for the Humanities and Public Policy.

2. W. F. F. Vogel, *Genetic Counseling*, Springer-Verlag, New York, p. 97, 1969.

3. Ad Hoc Committee on Genetic Counseling (American Society of Human Genetics), "Genetic Counseling," *American Journal of Human Genetics*, vol. 27, p. 240, 1975.

4. See J. L. Austin, *How to Do Things with Words*, Oxford University Press, London, 1962.

95. *Parents and Genetic Counselors: Moral Issues*
Ruth Macklin

The moral issues that arise in the practice of genetic counseling are primarily those surrounding truth and information in medicine. As noted earlier, there is the overarching issue of whether the genetic counselor's role should be as neutral and objective as possible, or whether it is sometimes permissible or even desirable to offer advice or guide the patient or couple to a decision. This issue appears to be no different, in principle, in the area of genetic counseling from that of a wide range of therapeutic situations in medicine, such as elective surgery or treatment regimens for severely defective newborns. As usual in ethical contexts, it is probably unwise to adhere dogmatically to a rigid principle like "physicians or genetic counselors should never advise, but should always and only inform." While a general presumption in favor of fully autonomous decision making by the patient or client is appropriate, sometimes that presumption may justifiably be overridden. There are cases in which a patient or couple asks directly for advice from the counselor, cases where it is evident to the counselor that the prospective parents fail to comprehend the enormity of caring for and raising a severely defective child, and still other instances where some measure of denial on the part of the parents stands in the way of their facing reality and making a rational decision. As with any other intermediate moral principle, the precept that genetic counselors should remain neutral and objective may justifiably be breached. Although some may argue that the genetic counselor's role includes some eugenic obligations, the purpose of counseling is to help the pregnant woman or prospective parents as much as possible in making an informed choice that is in accord with their own preferred values.[1] It has often been noted that many people suffer guilt, and react unpredictably and often irrationally in the face of information about their role in transmitting defective genes to their offspring. A sensitive and compassionate genetic counselor, observing such situations, would be acting in accordance with a sound and widely held

Source: *Dialogue*, vol. 14, no. 3, p. 375, 1977.

ethical precept in helping such parents come to a decision that is in accordance with their basic value scheme and that they can live with comfortably.

There are special circumstances, in addition to the more common problematic situations in counseling just noted, where the decisions to be made are straightforward medical decisions requiring significant medical expertise. An example is the sex assignment for an intersex child, where the decision depends on knowledge and experience that the parents most likely do not have. As one physician argues:

> Sex assignment is basically a therapeutic problem because it requires surgery to correct the anatomical anomalies of intersex. Once you remove a phallus there's really not much choice any more—you have to raise that child as a female. And the basis for such a decision is medical experience regarding prospective adequacy of sexual performance. There are phalluses that will never be functional no matter how much surgery you do. Therefore, in such a situation it would be advisable to strongly suggest conversion to female gender. . . . We still see many tragedies where the physician makes the wrong decision because of a lack of experience, or because the parents have their minds set on the sex of their child, and the physician allows his decision to be swayed by their attitude. [2]

These observations serve to remind us that although recent work in the field of medical ethics has uncovered a variety of contexts in which decisions formerly considered purely medical ones have been shown not to require special medical expertise, we must nevertheless be careful not to err in the opposite direction by relegating to patients decisions that properly require a knowledgeable medical judgment.

There are still other situations in genetic counseling which pose different sorts of moral dilemmas from those just described. One such problem is whether or not it is ever permissible for a genetic counselor to withhold information from patients. For example, some difficulties might arise if the parents are apprised of the fact that their son's genetic endowment is one that has been found to correlate highly with overly aggressive behavior and even with criminal tendencies. Other sorts of cases usually revolve around potential psychological harm to an individual or damage to a marriage likely to result from disclosure of genetic information. One physician cites the following two instances in which he believes that withholding information is justifiable.

> One example is where the genetic disorder of the child opens the possibility of nonpaternity—where the husband's genotype indicates he may not be the child's father. Disclosure of full information in this case could lead the father to question his acceptance of the child, as well as of his marital relationship.

> Another example would be the case of testicular feminization in which a genotypic 46,XY male develops as a female because of the failure of tissues to respond to testosterone stimulation. One might withhold this information from some parents because they would have difficulty relating to the child or would withhold it from the child herself when she is old enough to be counseled. . . . In cases in which the information can do serious psychological damage, I feel withholding it is justified. [3]

In these sorts of cases, it would seem that a rigid adherence to a moral principle that enjoins persons always to tell the truth, the whole truth, and nothing but the truth is an instance of dogmatism in ethics. Other moral principles sometimes override the precept that mandates truth telling; or, to put it another way, the duty to tell the truth is sometimes superseded by another moral duty, when the two come into conflict. The dilemma here seems to be more of an epistemological one than an ethical one: how can we know in advance when telling the truth or disclosing full information will yield greater harm than good? How can we judge whether it is better, on the whole, for one member of a couple to be told about the infidelity of the other? Do we have an adequate basis for knowing how much and what sorts of psychological harm will be done by informing parents about their child's sexual anomaly, as in the example cited earlier? The ethical principle here seems rather clear: perform that act likely to produce least harm to everyone who stands to be affected. But one can accept this consequentialist moral position and yet still not know how to act because of the epistemological difficulties just noted. This should serve to remind us that not all the problems in moral contexts arise out of uncertainty about which ethical principle to adopt or what to do when two basic moral precepts come into conflict. In the cases just noted, it is likely that general agreement can be secured about the appropriateness of a utilitarian or consequentialist approach. Disagreement is more likely to arise over just which course of action is, in fact, likely to produce more harm, on balance. Aside from other kinds of disputes concerning what properly constitutes harm in such cases, the difficulty does seem to be more of an epistemological one than an ethical one.

The foregoing treatment of moral issues in genetic counseling has rested on the presupposition that the genetic counselor's responsibility is to the patient or client. Based on this presupposition, I have supported the general presumption that favors decision-making autonomy on the part of those being counseled. If, however, the genetic counselor were properly viewed as having an obligation to society at large or to future generations, the presumption about autonomy might have to be overridden in some cases. In answer to the question, "To whom is the genetic counselor responsible?" one geneticist replies:

> Basically, I think that genetic counselors may be misguided if they feel that their ethical obligation is in *any way* to future generations. . . . [A]ll too often, I get the feeling that some genetic counselors are acting on the hidden assumption that they are somehow participating in that particularly Western predilection for attempting to create "ideal situations," in this instance, that of building a better gene pool through "negative eugenics." . . . The genetic counselor's obligation, I will maintain, never should extend beyond the family within his purview. . . . Properly, a genetic counselor's job should not, in any way, be construed as eugenic in practice.[4]

NOTES

1. A view similar to this is argued by Marc Lappé, "The Genetic Counselor: Responsible to Whom?" *The Hastings Center Report*, No. 2, September, 1971.

2. Kurt Hirschhorn, "Symposium: Ethics of Genetics Counseling," *Contemporary OB/GYN*, vol. 2, no. 4, p. 117.

3. Robert F. Murray, Jr., ibid., 120.

4. Marc Lappé, op. cit., 6.

96. Genetic Screening: Whose Responsibility?
Peter T. Rowley

Genetic screening may be defined as the identification of individuals who may profit from genetic information. Criteria for conditions for which genetic screening is appropriate include (1) existence of implications for action for those individuals so identified, (2) ability to determine who is at risk (this may involve performing a laboratory test or simply determining relationship to an affected individual), (3) the likelihood of benefits of notification outweighing its burdens, and (4) availability of adequate means for counseling and follow-up.

Screening for nongenetic conditions (e.g., lead intoxication) is usually intended to discover people with diseases due to extrinsic influences. Genetic screening discovers something within a person's own makeup and may make him feel unworthy or guilty. This raises social, ethical, and legal questions having to do with consent, privacy, confidentiality, and stigmatization. Hence the need for adequate counseling and follow-up. Genetic screening should be followed by genetic counseling of individuals thus identified.

Genetic counseling has been defined by Fraser[1] as a communication process that deals with the human problems associated with the occurrence, or the risk of occurrence, of a genetic disorder in a family. The process involves an attempt to help the individual or family (1) comprehend the medical facts including the diagnosis, the probable course of the disorder, and available management, (2) appreciate the risk of recurrence in specified relatives, (3) understand the options of dealing with the risk of recurrence, (4) choose a course of action which seems appropriate to them in view of their risk and their family goals, and (5) make the best possible psychological adjustment to this risk.

Public Programs

The personal physician's role can be clarified by considering public screening programs and their limitations. The best-known public genetic screening programs are those concerned with phenylketonuria, sickle cell disease, and Tay-Sachs disease.

Screening newborns for phenylketonuria has taught us several lessons. First, evidence of effective intervention shoud precede mandatory screening legislation; at the time mandatory screening of newborns for phenylketonuria was legislated, there was no convincing evidence that treatment would prevent mental retardation. Second, dietary treatment for metabolic errors should be carefully monitored; phenylalanine deprivation, if excessive, can itself cause mental retardation. Third, genetic screening may lead to the discovery of genetic heterogeneity, which complicates diagnosis. Phenylketonuria, for instance, must be distinguished from benign hyperphenylalaninemia. The former, if untreated, nearly always results in mental retardation, but benign hyperphenylalaninemia requires no treatment. Finally, detection must be accompanied by appropriate follow-up. This must be prompt, when prompt treatment is necessary to prevent morbidity, as in metabolic errors in newborns that cause mental retardation. In the case of phenylketonuria, the low phenylalanine diet must be started within a few weeks of birth to prevent brain damage. The state's role in case finding is well-defined, but informing the parents, the prompt institution of treatment, and genetic counseling are the responsibility of the personal physician.

Extensive screening for sickle cell trait in the past five years has taught us several lessons.

Source: *Journal of the American Medical Association*, vol. 236, no. 4, July 26, 1976.

When the individual affected (in this case with sickle cell trait) is not expected to be symptomatic himself, but rather at risk of having a symptomatic child, careful counseling must be provided so that the benefit is not outweighed by the risks. These risks include misunderstanding, impaired self-image, restrictions on employment or insurability, inappropriate restriction of activities of children, and discovery of nonpaternity. When a screening program is targeted for a specific population (in this case blacks), that group should have a role in planning and execution of the screening program. In this way the group can make a judgment about the risks just mentioned before the program is started. If lay individuals are taking major responsibility for screening or counseling, special attention must be paid to assure technical excellence, confidentiality of the data, and referral to conventional medical resources when indicated. For most types of genetic screening, mandatory legislation is not desirable and the initiative is properly left to the individual physician.

Tay-Sachs disease has several favorable characteristics for genetic screening. First, it is mainly confined to a defined population, the Ashkenazi Jews. Second, there is a simple, reliable, automated, and relatively inexpensive test for identification of the carrier state. Finally, there is a reproductive alternative for couples both of whom are carriers, i.e., prenatal diagnosis and the option of aborting an affected fetus.

Many biochemical genetic defects and all chromosomal abnormalities can be diagnosed prenatally by amniocentesis, thus permitting the option of abortion. Recently, the National Institutes of Health has announced results of a study of 1,040 second-trimester amniocenteses.[2] There were no statistically significant differences in rate of fetal loss, prematurity, newborn status, birth defects, or developmental status at 1 year of age. Therefore, midtrimester amniocentesis performed by a properly trained physician does not pose an excessive risk to the pregnancy.

Difficulties that have surfaced in community and government screening programs are not likely to be overcome quickly. For a long time to come, the personal physician will bear the major responsibility for offering genetic screening services for his own patients. In the majority of cases, the role of the personal physician makes him an ideal counselor.

Guidelines

Some guidelines for genetic screening and counseling by the personal physician are as follows:

1. Take a careful family history. This is the single most valuable tool for genetic screening. On your initial workup of a patient, always draw a pedigree. Indicate age, any illness, and, if dead, the cause.

2. If any familial or genetic condition is present, make a specific diagnosis. This may require obtaining records on relatives and investigating them further.

3. Determine the risk to the patient. This involves determining the method of inheritance.

4. Communicate the relevant information to the patient. The physician should be aware of barriers to comprehension in counseling. These include the patient's unfamiliarity with genetics, the concept of probability, and various psychological defense reactions. Before counseling, it is helpful to ask the patient what he already knows about the condition, and what he thinks his degree of risk is, in order to individualize counseling. After counseling, it is helpful to ask him what he understands he has been told to determine his degree of comprehension so that errors in understanding can be corrected.

5. Assist with adjustment. When told of his risk for a serious genetic disease, a patient may react in a way analogous to being informed of a fatal illness: first, with denial; then, anger; next, depression; and finally, resignation.[3] Multiple visits are commonly necessary to assist the patient to adjust. In talking with patients about their genetic makeup, it may be helpful to point out that each of us is an individual in part because our genes are different, that genetic traits that may be harmful in one context may be advantageous in another, that so-called normality is a myth of statisticians, and that genetic uniformity is neither possible nor desirable.

6. Follow-up includes avoidance of precipitating environmental factors, testing for early stages of the disease, and consideration of whether other relatives at risk should be contacted.

The obligation of the personal physician to relatives of his patient is not well defined. It is desirable to at least raise this matter with the patient. At present, one must be guided by his wishes in this regard when the relatives are not also under one's care. Although the patient may feel anxiety in being identified as the source of bad news, he may suffer guilt when individuals later become ill if he had advance knowledge of their risk. A major factor in the decision about informing relatives is whether, once an individual knows he is at risk, any constructive intervention is possible.

Summary

Genetic screening offers the possibility of reducing the suffering due to genetic defects. For the foreseeable future, genetic screening by lay or governmental organizations can do only a small part of the job needed. Hence, the major responsibility falls on the personal physician. A careful family history is the best single genetic screening device. Discussing genetic risks with patients requires careful attention to the patient's difficulties in understanding the concept of probability, his psychological defense reactions, and differences in individual values. For complex cases, help is available in your region.

NOTES

1. F. C. Fraser, "Genetic Counseling," *American Journal of Human Genetics,* vol. 26, p. 636, 1974.

2. *Symposium on the NICHD National Registry for Amniocentesis,* U.S. Department of Health, Education, and Welfare, Oct. 20, 1975.

3. A. Falek, "Application of the Coping Process to Genetic Counseling," read before the Genetic Counseling Meeting, Colorado Springs, Colo., February 26–27, 1975.

Reproductive Technologies

97. *Artificial Insemination: Beyond the Best Interests of the Donor*   George J. Annas

Recent ethical and legal discussion concerning novel ways of reproduction has focused on in vitro fertilization, a process that has never been successfully used in this country, while assuming that most of the issues surrounding another technique that has been successfully used an estimated 250,000 times have been more or less resolved. Artificial insemination by donor (AID) is a cottage industry on the verge of mass marketing. The May 14, 1979, issue of *Advertising Age* noted that two commercial sperm banks each fill over 100 orders a month, and one is preparing to market sperm directly to consumers. In the near future, a "home insemination kit," complete with sperm and instructions on use, is possible. The following ad, now directed to physicians, could appear soon in popular magazines and newspapers: "From our panel of excellent donors, you select one for yourself based on blood type, ethnic origin, race, height, weight, and coloration of skin, hair and eyes."

In *Island,* his vision of the ideal society, Aldous Huxley writes of a time when everyone will use AID voluntarily (at least for a third child) with donors picked from a "central bank of superior stocks" to increase the general IQ of the population. In George Orwell's more sinister society, described in *1984,* artificial insemination is mandatory and all marriages must be approved in advance by the Party. While neither of these futures seems an immediate threat, the perceived legal difficulties, general desire for secrecy, and cottage-industry nature of AID have all conspired to prevent any meaningful standards from developing, and make any future for AID the product of chance rather than policy.

We are faced with a technology that has the potential to make major changes in our reproductive habits, that has been poorly thought out, and if it is "gaining public acceptance," is probably doing so under false pretenses. Until very recently the best one could do was conjecture about the practices in doctors' offices and infertility clinics. However, three researchers from the University of Wisconsin recently published the results of their survey of 379 practitioners of AID who accounted for approximately 3,500 births in 1977 (of an estimated total of 6,000 to 10,000 annually in the United States).[1]

The results are disturbing. Besides pointing to a general lack of standards and the growing use of AID for husbands with genetic defects and for single women, the findings tend to indicate that current practices are based primarily on protecting the best interests of the sperm donor rather than those of the recipient or resulting child. Two areas merit immediate attention: donor selection and record keeping.

Source: *Hastings Center Report,* vol. 9, August 1979.

Donor Selection

The term "donor" is a misnomer. Virtually all respondents in the Curie-Cohen study bought ejaculates, 90 percent paying from $20 to $35 per ejaculate. A more accurate term would be "sperm vendors." While this distinction may seem trivial, it has legal consequences. For example, it makes no sense to designate the form signed by the vendor as a "consent form" since he is not a patient and is not really consenting to anything. It is a contract in which the vendor is agreeing to do certain things for pay. Moreover, continued use of the term "donor" gives the impression that the sperm vendor is doing some service for the good of humanity and deserves some special protection, rather than simply performing a service for pay. The problems with paid "donors" have been amply explored in Richard M. Titmuss's classic study of the blood market, *The Gift Relationship;* similar problems arise in the sperm business.

The actual selection and screening of sperm vendors, however, is more important than the term employed to describe them. The Curie-Cohen study found that 80 percent of all physicians use medical students and hospital residents all or most of the time. In this regard sociobiologists have found that animals will employ that reproductive strategy that maximizes the spread of their genes. In the words of Richard Dawkins in *The Selfish Gene:* "Ideally what an individual would 'like' (I don't mean physically enjoy, although he might) would be to copulate with as many members of the opposite sex as possible, leaving the partner in each case to bring up the children."Artificial insemination, of course, adds an entirely new technology to use in pursuing this strategy.

There can be little debate that physicians in all of these situations are making eugenic decisions—selecting what they consider "superior" genes for AID. In general they have chosen to reproduce themselves (or those in their profession), and this is what sociobiologists would probably have predicted. While this should not be surprising, it should be a cause for concern. Physicians may believe that society needs more individuals with the attributes of physicians, but it is unlikely that society as a whole does. Lawyers would be likely to select law students; geneticists, graduate students in genetics; military personnel, students at the military academies, and so on. The point is not trivial. Courts have found in other contexts that physicians have neither the training nor the social warrant to make "quality of life" decisions. In the *Houle* case, for example, a physician's decision not to treat a defective newborn was overruled on the basis that "the doctor's qualitative evaluation of the value of the life to be preserved is not legally within the scope of his expertise." Selecting donors in this manner, rather than matching for characteristics of the husband, for example, seems to be primarily in the best interests of the physician rather than the child, and probably cannot be justified.

More than this, the Curie-Cohen survey revealed that even on the basis of simple genetics, physicians administering AID "were not trained for the task" and made many erroneous and inconsistent decisions. Specifically 80 to 95 percent of all respondents said they would reject a donor if he had one of the following traits, and more than 50 percent of all respondents would reject that same donor if one of these traits appeared in his immediate family: Tay-Sachs, hemophilia, cystic fibrosis, mental retardation, Huntington's chorea, translocation or trisomy, diabetes, sickle-cell trait, and alkaptonuria. This list includes autosomal recessive diseases in which carriers can be identified, and those in which they cannot, dominant, X-linked, and multigenic diseases.

The troubling findings are that the severity and genetic risk of the condition was not reflected in rejection criteria, and that genetic knowledge appears deficient. For example, 71 percent would reject a donor who had hemophilia in his family, even though this X-linked gene could *not* be transmitted unless the donor himself was affected. Additionally, although 92 percent said they would reject a donor with a translocation or trisomy, only 12.5 percent actually examined the donor's karyotype. Similarly, while 95 percent would reject a carrier of Tay-Sachs, fewer than 1 percent actually tested donors for this carrier state.

Physicians might be giving medical students far more credit than they deserve for a knowledge of their own genetic and family history, honesty, and freedom from venereal disease. Even so, the conclusion must be that while prevention of genetic disease is a goal, it cannot be accomplished by the means currently in use. The findings also raise serious questions about the ability of these physicians to act as genetic counselors, and suggest that other non-medical professionals may be able to do a better job in delivering AID services in a manner best calculated to maximize the interests of the child and not just those of the sperm donor.

Record Keeping

While the Curie-Cohen survey found that 93 percent of physicians kept permanent records on recipients, only 37 percent kept permanent records on children born after AID and only 30 percent kept any permanent records on donors. The fear of record keeping seems to be based primarily on the idea, common in the legal literature, that if identifiable, the donor might be sued for parental obligations (for example, child support, inheritance, and so on) by one of his "biological children" sired by the AID process, and that this suit might be successful. The underlying rationale is that unless anonymity is assured, there would be no donors. There are a number of responses to this argument:

1. It is important to maintain careful records to see how the sperm "works" in terms of outcome of the pregnancy. If a donor is used more than once, a defective child should be grounds for immediately discontinuing use of the sperm for the protection of potential future children. Since the survey disclosed that most physicians have no policy on how many times they use a donor and 6 percent had used one for more than 15—with one using a donor for 50 pregnancies—this issue is more likely to affect the life of a real child than the highly speculative lawsuit is to affect the life of a donor.

2. No meaningful study of the characteristics and success of donors can ever be made if no records are kept concerning them.

3. In those cases where family history is important (and it is important enough to ask every donor about his) the AID child will never be able to respond accurately.

4. Finally, and most important, if no records are kept, the child will never, under any circumstances, be able to determine its genetic father. Since we do not know what the consequences of this will be, it cannot be said that destroying this information is in the best interests of the child. The most that can be said for such a policy is that it is in the best interests of the donor. But this is simply not good enough. The donor has a choice in the matter; the child has none. The donor and physician can take steps to guard their own interests; the child cannot.

Given the recent history of adopted children and their efforts to identify their biological parents, it is likely that if AID children learn they are the products of AID, they will want to be able to identify their genetic father. It is now accepted practice to tell adopted children that they are adopted as soon as possible, and make sure they understand it. It is thought that they will inevitably find out some day, and the blow will be severe if they have been deceived. In AID the consensus seems to be not to tell on the grounds that no one is likely to find out the truth since to all the world the AID pregnancy appears to have occurred normally.

Moralists would probably agree with Joseph Fletcher, who has argued that the physician should not accept the suggestion that a husband's brother be used as a donor without the wife's knowledge (the husband's intent is to keep the "blood line" in his children) because this would be a violation of "marital confidence." It would seem that a similar argument can be made of consistently lying to the child, that is, that it is a violation of "parental confidence." There is some evidence that AID children do learn the truth, and the only thing that the fifteen state legislatures that have laws pertaining to AID agree on is that the resulting child should be considered legitimate—an issue that will *never* arise unless the child's AID status is discovered by someone.

Not keeping records can also lead to bizarre practices. For example, some physicians use multiple donors in a single cycle to obscure the identity of the genetic father. The Curie-Cohen survey found that 32 percent of all physicians utilize this technique, which could be to the physical detriment of the child (and potential future children of a donor with defective sperm) and cannot be justified on any genetic grounds whatsoever.

A number of policies would have to be changed to permit open disclosure of genetic parenthood to children. The first is relatively easy: a statute could be enacted requiring the registration of all AID children in a court in a sealed record that would only be available to the child; the remainder of the statute would provide that the genetic father had no legal or financial rights or responsibilities to the child. Variations would be to keep the record sealed until the death of the donor, or until he waived his right to privacy in this matter, or to only disclose genetic and health information. In the long term, a more practical solution may lie in only using the frozen sperm of deceased donors, in which case full disclosure could be made without any possibility of personal or financial demands on the genetic father by the child.

Conclusions

Current AID practices on donor screening and record keeping are based primarily on protecting the interests of practitioners and donors rather than recipients and children. The most likely reason for this is found in exaggerated fears of legal pitfalls. Policy in this area should be dictated by maximizing the best interests of the resulting children. The evidence is that current practices are dangerous to children and must be modified. Specifically, consideration should be given to:

1. Removing AID from the practice of medicine and placing it in the hands of genetic counselors or other nonmedical personnel (alternatively, a routine genetic consultation could be added to each couple who request AID).

2. Development of uniform standards for donor selection, including national screening criteria.

3. A requirement that practitioners of AID keep permanent records on all donors that they can match with recipients (I would prefer this to become common practice in the profession, but legislation requiring court filing may be necessary).

4. As a corollary, mixing of sperm would be an unacceptable practice and the number of pregnancies per donor would be limited.

5. Establishment of national standards regarding AID by professional organizations, with public consultation.

6. Research on the psychological development of children who have been conceived by AID, and their families.

In the *New England Journal of Medicine,* Dr. S. J. Behrman concludes his editorial on the Curie-Cohen survey by questioning the "uneven and evasive" attitude of the law in regard to AID, and recommending immediate legislative action: "The time has come—in fact, is long overdue—when legislatures must set standards for artificial insemination by donors, declare the legitimacy of the children, and protect the liability of all directly involved with this procedure. A better public policy on this question is clearly needed."

Agreement with the need for "a better public policy" is not synonymous with immediate legislation. The problem with AID is that there are many unresolved problems with it, and few of them are legal. It is time to stop thinking about uniform legislation and start thinking about the development of professional standards. Obsessive concern with self-protection needs to give way to concern for the child.

NOTE

1. M. Curie-Cohen, L. Luttrell, and S. Shapiro, "Current Practice of Artificial Insemination by Donor in the United States," *New England Journal of Medicine,* vol. 300, p. 585, March 15, 1979.

98. Shall We "Reproduce"? The Medical Ethics of In Vitro Fertilization   Paul Ramsey

I must judge that in vitro fertilization constitutes unethical medical experimentation on possible future human beings, and therefore it is subject to absolute moral prohibition. I ask that my exact language be noted: I said, unethical experimentation on *possible future human beings.* By this, I mean the child-to-be, the "successful" experiments when they come.

I mean to exclude three things that could be said additionally to make a showing of medical immorality and a notation of illicitness upon the trials that are currently being performed. Excluded are (1) the charge that before going to human experimentation physicians should not have omitted first proving their technique in species more closely related to man, on the primates, e.g., monkeys. This is a question of the background needed in the experimental design which an amateur cannot judge. Still I do know enough about discussions among ethical physicians concerning the need to complete the "animal work" before going to "human work" to know that this is a serious charge that requires some answer from the physicians attempting in vitro fertilization and implantation in human females—an answer which I have not seen. Excluded from my chief concern is also (2) the charge that the women "volunteers"—urged on as they are by a desperate desire to overcome their oviduct obstruction and to have a child of their own—have not given a fully understanding consent to what is being

Source: *Journal of the American Medical Association,* vol. 220, no. 10, June 5, 1972.

done upon them and by means of them. Clearly, the women already submitted to laparoscopy are experimental subjects, not patients who are likely to get children by this unproven technique. It is not enough to say to them, as Dr. Edwards is reported to have said, that "your only hope is to help us."[1] Now, I know that there is a spectrum and no clear lines to be drawn between pure experiment, therapeutic investigation, and proven therapy. Still, one way to make a significant distinction along this spectrum is to suppose one of these women to ask, "Doctor, are you doing this for *me* or am I doing it for you and your research?" The answer to that question to date is that the women are undergoing surgery and other procedures for the sake of medical research; and it is a cardinal principle of medical ethics that they should have knowingly consented to that, and not primarily to a therapy they hoped would relieve their own childlessness.

Excluded also from my present concern is (3) the charge that it is immoral to discard or terminate the lives of the zygotes, the developing cluster of cells, the blastocysts, the embryos, or the fetuses it will be necessary to kill in the course of developing this procedure. Persons who believe that an individual human life begins with conception, or after the time of segmentation, or at implantation, or with the morphologically human fetus, or with heartbeat or ECG readings, or self-movement (or any time before birth) must regard experiments in in vitro fertilization and artificial implantation as ab initio inherently immoral, because the physician must be willing to discard mishaps at any point in that span of time which do not come up to the standards of an acceptable human being. Make no mistake about it, this will extend, through screening by amniocentesis and fetoscopy, well into the period in which hysterotomy would have to be done if a defective result is detected, in order to abort the wrong life begun in the laboratory. I have a great deal of sympathy for the conclusion that this is, therefore, a wrong way to begin a human life. Still, when I say that in vitro fertilization followed by implantation is an immoral experiment on possible future human beings I do not assume any of these notions (for some of which there are better reasons than the socially prevailing notion) of when the possible future human being is an actual human being.

Instead, I assume the going perception of when there is a human life: when we see it before our eyes in the incubator, in a hospital nursery, in a bassinet or a playpen, playing hopscotch on the sidewalk, or going to kindergarten, and I assert that it clearly seems to me that in vitro fertilization followed by implantation is an immoral experiment on such a possible future human life.

Dr. Patrick Steptoe, Dr. Edwards' colleague, is reported[2] to have said that the decision to implant a given embryo, based on statistical evidence and hope—an embryo which cannot be karyotyped for genetic or other damage as a final procedure before implantation without too grave risk of further, more serious damage—will "call for a 'brave decision.'" Bravery, courage, used to be the word for a man's moral virtue in the face of danger or adversity. If (as I believe) we should watch our language as we watch our morals, Dr. Steptoe seriously misused language. What he meant was "rashness" in action regardless of the consequences to another human life, and not "courage," facing one's own perils or adversities. That, in former, more moral ages of mankind, was viewed as a vice.

Dr. Daniele Petrucci of the University of Bologna is a rather discredited pioneer among these adventurers. He is discredited, however, for not having published a scientific article; his experiment was "insufficiently documented"; other scientists could not repeat his procedures or check his results, or even know his claims were not fraudulent. He was not discredited, however, for doing what he said he did to a human fetus; for what he might well have done to a possible future human life if his experiment had been continued or had that in view. In 1961, Petrucci reported that after more than 40 failures he had successfully fertilized a human egg in vitro, cultured the embryo for 29 days ("a heartbeat was discernible"), and then destroyed it because "it became deformed and enlarged—a monstrosity." Nor, so far as I know, has Petrucci's end-in-view been generally excluded from among the possible purposes of manipulating embryos; indeed, one finds frequent mention of related designs in experimental biology: Petrucci told Italian newspapermen that he only meant to find a way to culture organs that would resist the rejection phenomenon when transplanted. With that, Petrucci yielded to his church's condemnation of producing a human being without "the most supreme assistances of love, nature and conscience" (editorial, *L'Osservatore Romano*) and became a forgettable episode in the history of in vitro fertilization research—unless, while in Russia to receive a medal, he passed on his arts to experimental biologists there.[3]

My reason for bringing up the Petrucci episode is not, rhetorically and emotionally, to tar more responsible scientists with the damage he was willing to accept. It is rather to say simply that unless the *possibility* of such damage can be definitively excluded, in vitro fertilization is an immoral experiment on possible future human beings. And it is to say that this condition cannot be met, at least not by the first "successful" cases; and therefore that any man's or any woman's venture to begin human life in this way is morally forbidden. We cannot morally *get to know* how to perfect this technique to relieve human infertility (even if, once perfected, it would not be a disastrous further step toward the evil design of manufacturing of our posterity).

We all know from the popular and the scientific accounts that in order to accomplish in vitro fertilization, scientists must mimic nature perfectly.

> The mammalian egg has been carefully adapted over many centuries of evolution and natural selection to a very delicate balanced environment in the ovarian follicle, the fallopian tube, and the womb. Likewise, the mammalian and human sperm has been adapted through millennia by natural selection to survive in the environment of the vaginal canal and the uterus and achieve fertilization in the fallopian tubes. . . . The scientist must duplicate almost exactly this delicately balanced internal environment of the female reproductive tract, or fail in his attempt to achieve in vitro fertilization.[4]

This artificial mimicry of nature has been accomplished in the matter of fertilization and the culture of human life until well beyond the time implantation would take place naturally. Along the way, the scientists have learned a great deal about duplicating the environment in which the sperm can be "capacitated"; they have learned that fertilization is not a "moment" but a process, that cells that seem to be fertilized may only be dying. (Claims to scientific fame depend on this latter point!)

The same can be said about those scientists who are at work assaulting and attempting to duplicate human gestation in the middle and later stages. They too must be able to mimic natural human gestation entirely; the slightest lapse or mistake would be disastrous to a possible future human being.

My point as an ethicist is that none of these researchers can *exclude* the possibility that they will do irreparable damage to the child-to-be. And my conclusion is that they cannot morally proceed to their first ostensibly successful achievement of the results they seek, since they cannot assuredly preclude all damage.

However much these experimental embryologists may have mimicked nature perfectly, they cannot guarantee that the last artificial procedure they carry out before implantation (or know they cannot carry through, such as karyotyping, which Dr. Steptoe cited when he erroneously spoke of "bravery") may be the important one. The last procedure may induce damage (or the last procedure known to be possibly damaging may not be able to be used although it might detect damage induced by previous procedures). Damage could be introduced during the transfer procedure, even after the last inspection is made. The last inspection may induce damage, or it may not be done because it could be fatal or damaging. For all we know, the manipulation may implant embryos that, if abnormal, will not be spontaneously aborted with the same frequency as under natural conditions. Finally, detectable natural abnormalities and detectable induced abnormalities may prove inseparable to such a degree that it will be difficult to establish exactly what are the additional risks due to this procedure. If true, that would be a limit upon experimental designs, even if one had gotten over the earlier objections that it is immoral to use the child-to-be to find out.

These are some of the reasons in vitro fertilization followed by implantation must necessarily require (by an amazing degradation of moral language) "courage" on the part of the physician-experimenter. He can never know what he is doing to a possible future human being. Even if he had not omitted experiments on monkeys first, no trial on monkeys would have told him whether he was or was not in the human case inducing mental retardation. It will not be enough to be able to discard grossly damaged embryos; there may well be damage that cannot be grossly scanned (as later on a club foot can be) and which are of crucial importance for the normal human capacity of the child-to-be. This is why experimentation on the primates could never settle the issue I am raising.

Anyone familiar with discussions of the ethics of medical experimentation knows that physicians acknowledge that the passage from "animal work" to work in the human always involves unknown risks that cannot have been tested before. Because of this fact, the move to human experimentation is made only when physicians secure the partnership of an informed, consenting volunteer for nonbeneficial investigation or when they already have a patient suffering from an illness, to cure which they need and he equally needs investigational therapy to be performed. They do not (or should not) first manipulate a patient's consent. Nor do they first manipulate a patient so that he is in some need of possibly harmful treatment. Neither of these two conditions for moving to "human work" can be met in the case of in vitro fertilization and embryo transfer. The child-to-be is not a volunteer; and before his beginning he is in no need of physicians to learn how not to harm him.

There are more cautious physicians and others who seem to believe that these obstacles and objections in the way of justifying in vitro fertilization will fall without the need for immoral experimentation on possible future human beings in the process. They have not, in my opinion, paid attention to the logic of the matter, to the unforecloseable risks involved in moving to the human work or to the necessity of bringing the first cases to term (and beyond) in order ever to learn whether the trial did harm or not. Thus, Dr. Kenneth Greet, a British Methodist, referring to criteria laid down some years ago by the British Council of Churches, stated:

> Provided the fertilization of the ovum is undertaken in order that it should be transplanted into the lining of the uterus, and provided also no harm is done at that stage which would result in malformation, then I think it is something to be welcomed.[5]

And Dr. Luigi Mastroianni, chairman of obstetrics and gynecology at the University of Pennsylvania, is reported[6] to have said,

It is my feeling that we must be very sure we are able to produce normal young by this method in monkeys before we have the temerity to move ahead in the human. . . . In our laboratory, our position is, "Let's explore the thing thoroughly in monkeys and establish the risk." Then we can describe the risk to a patient and obtain truly informed consent before going ahead. We must be very careful to use patients well and not be presumptuous with human lives. We must not be just biologic technicians. [7]

Surely Dr. Mastrioianni's very fine statement falls of its own weight. Because his is a splendidly articulated statement, it is clear that the conditions he lays down for not being "presumptuous with human lives" cannot be fulfilled (or that in the case of the woman's consent, they are not sufficient.) One is apt to miss this when reading Dr. Greet's statement of the basic principle of medical ethics ("do no harm") which is not articulated for the case under consideration; he leaves wide open the possibility that the criteria can be met. While Dr. Mastroianni also seems to believe that this test can be met, his statement makes it evident that it cannot. Work in monkeys would enable scientists to describe the risks accurately for monkeys, but not for possible deep injuries in the human case—for example, hemophilia or mental retardation or multifactoral personality and behavioral defects. These can be known only by work in humans, which because the risks are not known, would be immoral to research by means of a possible case of embryo transplant brought to birth. Moreover, to be able to "describe the risk to a patient" (the woman, only) and to "obtain truly informed consent before going ahead" would relieve the physician of presumptuous manipulation of her consent. But that would in no way relieve the physician of complicity in such a woman's willingness to be "presumptuous" with a human life—her child-to-be—or from guilt for allowing or enticing her to consent to any such thing, even if the risk could be exactly described from work in monkeys.

Is there any answer to this argument against in vitro fertilization—an argument which, I believe, must hold unless we are cloyed by the sentiment that a woman should be enabled to have a child by any means and if we are not simply fascinated by "advancements" in the scientific possibilities of unusual modes of human fecundity?

One answer is that after implantation, intrauterine monitoring by means of amniocentesis, or fetoscopy when it is developed, will enable physician-scientists to scan and screen their results, and by abortion discard their mishaps, i.e., any lives later discovered to have been damaged by the procedures of in vitro fertilization and implantation itself.

The proper reply to this retort is that invading the uterus to make these check-ups may itself induce additional damage to the fetus, not only to the woman. Physicians engaged in amniocentesis usually concentrate on the statistical incidence of this possibility, which is low. One or two percent, they say, which in their practice is to be compared with a like statistical risk that the fetus already conceived may be defective in one way or another. That, I would say, is a different moral problem than if human ingenuity first creates at risk the human life which must thereafter be monitored, at those additional risks, by amniocentesis with abortion as the refuge in case it is discovered that one had seriously impaired the life he meant to produce. To monitor by amniocentesis a fetus already conceived and determined to be at special risk of being genetically damaged *may* be justified by balancing that unborn child's already existent 1 or 2 percent risk of genetic disease against the 1 or 2 percent of risk that the procedure to find out may itself do damage. But even if that is an ethical practice in medicine, the cases we are discussing—in vitro fertilization and artificial implantation—do not already have a patient at risk. The possible future human being is at risk only of being created in this way, of having someone wrongly accept for him an incidence of additional risk of induced damage from the procedure chosen to be used in his creation.

Then there are those physicians who go behind the equilibration of incidence of risk and speak frankly of the depth of what is at risk in every case in which amniocentesis is used. So we must add to the original "daring" venture to create a human life the additional risks, however small, of serious damage which monitoring what we had done itself imposes on a possible future human being. Henry Nadler, M.D., of Children's Memorial Hospital, Chicago, refreshingly says that only defects established before amniocentesis is performed (12 weeks) can be excluded from its possible adverse effects.

> There is no way with present studies . . . of establishing ten or fifteen years from now if these children lose 5 or 10 IQ points. We might be able to get an approximation during the first year of life if their rate of growth is significantly different. However, more subtle damage will be difficult to evaluate.[8]

In short, if in vitro fertilization scientists appeal to intrauterine monitoring as an "out" after what they may have done by their last procedure (which by definition could not at that point be monitored), they may only be adding possible damage to possible damage that cannot be excluded and which may be brought upon a possible future human being whom they thus dare to initiate.

I see no line of moral reasoning that can justify this as an ethical practice of medicine. Nor do I see how any woman could *knowingly* consent to it. But, then, there may be depths I do not fathom in "Women's Lib"!

A negative moral verdict upon in vitro fertilization follows from right-ordered concern for the child that will be produced by the "successful" cases of these experiments. It is not a proper goal of medicine to enable women to have children and marriages to be fertile *by any means*— means which *may* bring hazard form the procedure, *any* additional hazard, upon the child not yet conceived. To suppose otherwise is to believe couples have such an absolute right to have children that this right cannot be overridden by the requirement that we should first have to exclude any incidence of *induced* risk to the child itself. This would be to adopt an extreme pronatalist assumption that an unconceived child somehow already has a title to be conceived. In such pronatalism, extremes meet: artificial modes of conception and gestation find themselves strange bedfellows with the insistence of a few uninstructed Roman Catholics that the life-giving potentiality of sperm and ovum are not artificially to be denied. (An illiterate spokesman for this point of view once told me that this was what Jesus meant when he said "Suffer the little ones to come unto me . . . !) Thus, the justification of in vitro fertilization and the prohibition of contraception both alike exalt—though in different ways—the absolute rights of "nature." The good of the possible future human being is not allowed, in the first case, to "interfere" with getting pregnant artificially, nor in the second case to interfere with natural fecundity.

The conclusion that a child should be conceived at risk of induced damage requires not only the assumption that while yet nothing, he somehow had title to be born (which, if true, might warrant our taking *his* risks in his behalf). In medical circles, this requires also the mind-boggling assumption that an unconceived child is somehow the equivalent of an existing child as already the subject of medical care and, therefore, a proper subject of investigational therapy without his consent. So only can we bring him under the ordinary categories and balancing judgments of medical treatment at risk. By first imagining the qualitative gulf separating being from nonbeing to have been traversed—and only so—can we imagine that proper treatment (of his being) means simply taking every precaution to avoid damaging him, making all possible tests, scanning and screening him to see whether anything has gone awry. By viewing the possible future child, while he is still a hypothetical nothing, as if he were already a patient needing all these precautions—and only so—can we bring ourselves to believe that minimizing the risks is enough. That *is* enough for an ordinary patient in the bush but not enough for a patient in the hand, i.e., literally, "manipulated," in vitro, before he ever was. But to manipulate a patient into being requires at least the far more stringent requirement that to do this we must know that every possibility of damage from the procedure itself has surely been foreclosed. That stipulation the manipulation of embryos is not likely to meet. Anyone familiar with discussions of the moral limits upon human experimentation would say, I think, that the stipulation cannot be met. Medicine must certainly violate it before learning how to meet it, even if the first implanted baby turns out to be a Mahalia Jackson and not a monstrosity or mentally retarded. An experiment must be moral in its inception, as Dr. Henry K. Beecher said so often—it does not become moral because it happens to produce good results.

Since medicine manipulates human beings—sometimes at great risk, always at some risk—in order to persuade ourselves that we are permitted to manipulate a baby into being, at some risk, the unmade baby must be vaguely thought of as somehow already in being. So Dr. Edwards, in a scientific (not a popular) presentation of the state of the art, revealingly referred to one of his patients as "the mother."[9]

Whether physicians engaged in this practice in fact vaguely think in this way or not, they must act as if the baby already has being in order to grant themselves the permission to think it sufficient simply to do everything thereafter to minimize the risks. By the ordinary canons of medical ethics, the unmade child has not "volunteered" to help the scientist—or even his "mother." If the possible future human being can be construed to have "volunteered," we would have first to construe him to be there, in being, or at least with a powerful title to be born, willing to suffer some induced risk in order to be manipulated to "come unto us." To construe his consent requires not only these manifest absurdities; to do so, to consent in his behalf, would also require that he be already exposed to some risk which these procedures are designed to relieve. For, again by the ordinary canons of medical ethics, we are not permitted to give proxy consent except medically in behalf of someone who may not be in a position to give expressed consent, or to impute to him a will to relieve someone else's condition—in his case "his" "mother's" infertility. We ought not to choose for another the hazards he must bear, while choosing at the same time to give him life in which to bear them and to suffer our chosen experimentations. The putative volition of such an unmade child must, anyway, be said to be negative, since researchers who work in human experimentation do not claim that they are allowed to ask volunteers to face possibly suicidal risks or to place themselves at risk of serious deformity.

Before concluding, it is worth calling attention to the fact that a negative moral verdict against in vitro fertilization need invoke no other standards of judgment than *the received principles of medical ethics.* I have appealed to no religious and to no other ethical criteria. Either the accepted principles of medical ethics must give way, or fabricated babies should not be ventured.

NOTES

1. E. Grossman, "The Obsolescent Mother: A Scenario," *Atlantic*, vol. 227, p. 39, May 1971. *Medical World News* (April 4, 1969, p. 27) quotes Dr. Edwards' statement in full: "We tell the women with blocked oviducts, 'Your only hope of having a child is to help us. Then maybe we can help you.' " The question is whether the single word "maybe" communicates the fact that the physicians likely did not *mean* actually to attempt to overcome childlessness in most, if any, of the cases so far. The statement that artificial fertilization is the woman's "only hope" was simply false—unless there were *medical* reasons why none of these women were patients on whom oviduct reconstruction (see below) or superovulation might have been tried. (In one series of 46 women, three promptly became pregnant as a result of the superovulatory drug administered as a part of the procedure to collect oocytes.) And, of course, if "hope" is a proper subject for medical treatment, adoption was also an alternative.

The question of defective consent arises in another form in the case of experiments in the 1950s performed by Dr. Landrum Shettles of Columbia University's College of Physicians and Surgeons. He was *not* trying to overcome the barrier of oviduct trouble to enable his "patients" to have a baby. Instead, as one recent account puts it: "In the course of performing various operations requiring abdominal incision into the peritoneal cavity of the female, Dr. Shettles pierced the ovaries of his patients with a syringe and aspirated . . . some of the eggs from their follicles . . . without harming the patient in any way. . . . (D.M. Rorvik, "The Test-Tube Baby is Coming," *Look*, May 18, 1971, p. 83). The question is not whether Dr. Shettles *harmed* these patients in any way, but whether they *consented* in any way to have a procedure done to them that was wholly unrelated to the condition that called for the abdominal incision to be made.

2. E. Grossman, op. cit., also D. M. Rorvik, op. cit., p. 85. Rorvik also describes Dr. Shettles as one among many "daring" experimenters who have "propelled mankind forward," and as *pressing on* in the face of criticism. This may be courage in the face of a scientist's "adversities." The question is whether this personal and professional "daring" has excluded or can exclude any possible damage to that possible future human being, before the scientist "dares" go ahead. If not, use of words like

"bravery" or "courage" represents a serious degradation of our moral language.

In a scientific article published as late in the course of these advances in experimental embryology as 1970, Dr. Edwards and colleagues stated flatly that "the normality of embryonic development and the efficiency of embryo transfer *cannot* be assessed" [italics added]. (R. G. Edwards, P. C. Steptoe, and J. M. Purdy, "Fertilization and Cleavage in Vitro of Preovulator Human Oocytes," *Nature*, vol. 227, p. 1307, 1970.) That cautionary statement from the scientists is related not only to the quality of courage discussed above; on this, the question will be whether these limits can ever be overcome without actions that are irremediably rash in dealing with viable progeny. The 1970 statement is also decisive in answering the question whether all the women who to date have been experimental subjects were deceived. They were, if no more was told them than "maybe we can help you."

3. Before desisting, Petrucci said he had maintained another fetus, a female, alive for a full 49 days before it died owing to a "technical mistake." In 1966, the Russian scientists announced they had kept 250 fetuses alive beyond the record Petrucci claimed; one lived, they said, for 6 months and weighed 510 g (1 lb 2 oz) before dying. (R. T. Francoeur, Doubleday & Co., Inc. Garden City, N.Y., 1970, p. 58.)

4. Ibid., p. 59.

5. K. Greet, quoted in Francoeur, ibid., p. 74.

6. V. Cohn, "Lab Growth of Human Embryo Raises Doubt of Normality," *Washington Post*, March 21, 1971.

7. Six years ago Dr. Edwards was also more cautious; indeed, he seemed to believe culturing eggs for the treatment of human infertility faced insurmountable practical and moral objections. "If rabbit and pig eggs grown in culture can be fertilized after maturation in culture, presumably human eggs grown in culture could also be fertilized, *although obviously it would not be permissible to implant them in a human recipient*. We have therefore attempted to fertilize human eggs in vitro [italics added]." That is, in order to study the process of human fertilization and early growth, precisely *not* in order to produce a child-to-be. (R. G. Edwards, "Mammalian Eggs in the Laboratory," *Scientific American*, vol. 215, p. 73, August 1966.)

8. M. Harris (ed.), *Early Diagnosis of Human Genetic Defects: Scientific and Ethical Considerations*, Symposium jointly sponsored by the John

E. Fogarty International Center for Advanced Study in the Health Sciences, National Institutes of Health, Bethesda, Md., May 18–19, 1970, U.S. Government Printing Office, 1972, p. 182.

    9. R. G. Edwards, P. C. Steptoe, and J. M. Purdy,

op. cit. p. 1307. If these women were patients for infertility, Leon Kass remarks [M. Hamilton (ed.), *Three Medical Futures,* Wm. B. Eerdmans Publishing Co., Grand Rapids, 1972], then "mothers" is surely the one thing they are not.

99. *Contracts to Bear a Child: Compassion or Commercialism?*
George J. Annas

Many medical students (and others) supplement their income by selling their blood and sperm. But while this practice seems to have been reasonably well accepted, society does not permit individuals to sell their vital organs or their children. These policies are unlikely to change. Where on this spectrum do contracts to bear a child fall? Are they fundamentally the sale of an ovum with a nine-month womb rental thrown in, or are they really agreements to sell a baby? While this formulation may seem a strange way to phrase the issue, it is the way courts are likely to frame it when such contracts are challenged on the grounds that they violate public policy.

In a typical surrogate-mother arrangement, a woman agrees to be artificially inseminated with the sperm of the husband of an infertile woman. She also agrees that after the child is born she will either give it up for adoption to the couple or relinquish her parental rights, leaving the biological father as the sole legal parent. The current controversy centers on whether or not the surrogate can be paid for these services. Is she being compensated for inconvenience and out-of-pocket expenses, or is she being paid for her baby?

Two personal stories have received much media attention. The first involves Patricia Dickey, an unmarried twenty-year-old woman from Maryland who had never borne a child, and who agreed to be artificially inseminated and give up the child to a Delaware couple without any compensation. She was recruited by attorney Noel Keane of Michigan, known for his television appearances in which he has said that for a $5,000 fee he will put "host mothers" in touch with childless couples. Ms. Dickey explained her motivation in an interview with the *Washington Post:* "I had a close friend who couldn't have a baby, and I know how badly she wanted one. . . . It's just something I wanted to do" (Feb. 11, 1980, p. 1). The outcome of Dickey's pregnancy—if one occurred—has not been reported.

More famous is a woman who has borne a child and relinquished her parental rights. Elizabeth Kane (a pseudonym), married and the mother of three children, reportedly agreed to bear a child for $10,000. The arrangement was negotiated by Dr. Richard Levin of Kentucky, who is believed to have about 100 surrogates willing to perform the same services for compensation. Levin says, "I clearly do not have any moral or ethical problems with what we are doing" (*American Medical News,* June 20, 1980, p. 13). Mrs. Kane describes her relationship to the baby by saying, "It's the father's child. I'm simply growing it for him" (*People,* Dec. 8, 1980, p. 53).

Even this brief sketch raises fundamental questions about the two approaches. Should the

Source: *The Hastings Center Report,* vol. 11, April 1981.

surrogate be married or single; have other children or have no children? Should the couple meet the surrogate (they were in the delivery room when Mrs. Kane gave birth to a boy)? Should the child know about the arrangement when he grows up (the couple plans to tell the child when he is eighteen)? Is monetary compensation the real issue (the sperm donor has agreed to give Ms. Dickey more sperm if she wants to have another child for her own—could this cause more problems for both him and her)? What kind of counseling should be done with all parties, and what records should be kept? And isn't this a strange thing to be doing in a country that records more than a million and a half abortions a year? Why not attempt to get women who are already pregnant to give birth instead of inducing those who are not to go through the "experience"?

These questions, and many others, merit serious consideration. So far legal debate has focused primarily on just one: can surrogate parenting properly be labeled "baby selling"? Some have argued that it can be distinguished from baby selling because one of the parents (the father) is biologically related to the child, and the mother is not pregnant at the time the deal is struck and so is not under any compulsion to provide for her child. But the only two legal opinions rendered to date disagree. Both a lower court judge in Michigan and the attorney general of Kentucky view contracts to bear a child as baby selling.

Court Challenge in Michigan

In the mid-1970s most states passed statutes making it criminal to offer, give, or receive anything of value for placing a child for adoption. These statutes were aimed at curtailing a major black market in babies that had grown up in the United States, with children selling for as much as $20,000. Anticipating that Michigan's version of this statute might prohibit him from paying a surrogate for carrying a child and giving it up for adoption, attorney Keane sought a declaratory judgment. He argued that the statute was unconstitutional since it infringed upon the right to reproductive privacy of the parties involved. The court was not impressed, concluding that "the right to adopt a child based upon the payment of $5,000 is not a fundamental personal right and reasonable regulations controlling adoption proceedings that prohibit the exchange of money (other than charges and fees approved by the court) are not constitutionally infirm." The court characterized the state's interest as one "to prevent commercialism from affecting a mother's decision to execute a consent to the adoption of her child," and went on to argue that: "Mercenary considerations used to create a parent-child relationship and its impact upon the family unit strike at the very foundation of human society and are patently and necessarily injurious to the community."

The case is on appeal, but is unlikely to be reversed. The judge's decision meant that Ms. Dickey, and others like her, could not charge a fee for carrying a child. It did not, however, forbid her from carrying it as a personal favor or for her own psychological reasons.

The Kentucky Statutes

One of the prime elements of surrogate mother folklore held that contracts to bear a child were "legal" in Kentucky. On January 26, 1981, Steven Beshear, the attorney general of the Commonwealth of Kentucky, announced at a Louisville news conference that contracts to bear a child were in fact illegal and unenforceable in the state. He based his advisory opinion on Kentucky statutes and "a strong public policy against 'baby buying.'"

Specifically, Kentucky law invalidates consent for adoption or the filing of a voluntary petition for termination of parental rights prior to the fifth day after the birth of a child. The purpose of these statutes, according to the attorney general, is to give the mother time to "think it over." Thus, any agreement or contract she entered into before the fifth day after the birth would be unenforceable. Moreover, Kentucky, like Michigan, prohibits the charging of a "fee" or "remuneration for the procurement of any child for adoption purposes." The attorney general argued that even though there is no similar statute prohibiting the payment of money for the termination of parental rights, "there is the same public policy issue" regarding monetary consideration for the procurement of a child: "The Commonwealth of Kentucky does not condone the purchase and sale of children" (Op. Atty. Gen., 81–18). The attorney general has since brought an action to enjoin Dr. Levin and his corporation from making any further surrogate-mother arrangements in the state.

Who Cares?

Surrogate parenting, open or behind a wall of secrecy, is unlikely ever to involve large numbers of people. Should we care about it; or should we simply declare our disapproval and let it go at that? I don't know, but it does seem to me that the answer to that question must be found in the answer to another: what is in the best interests of the children? Certainly they are more prone to psychological problems when they learn that their biological mother not only gave them up for adoption, but never had any intention of mothering them herself. On the other hand, one might argue that the child would never have existed had it not been for the surrogate arrangement, and so whatever existence the child has is better than nothing.

A Surrogate Mother's View

"Elizabeth Kane" says she felt regret only once—during labor. "I thought to myself, 'Elizabeth, you're out of your mind. Why are you putting yourself through this?' But it was only for a moment." She also says she "felt so many emotions during the pregnancy that I wrote a book," now in the hands of an agent. (*Washington Post*, Dec. 4, 1980.)

One of the major problems with speculating on the potential benefits of such an arrangement to the parties involved is that we have very little data. Only anecdotal information is available on artificial insemination by donor, for example. It does not seem to harm family life. But the role of the mother is far greater biologically than that of the father, and family disruption might be proportionally higher if the mother is the one who gives up the child. The sperm donor in the Patricia Dickey case is quoted as having said:

It may sound selfish, but I want to father a child on my own behalf, leave my own legacy. And I want a healthy baby. And there just aren't any available. They're either retarded or they're minorities, black, Hispanic. . . . That may be fine for some people, but we just don't think we could handle it.

Is this man really ready for parenthood? What if the child is born with a physical or mental defect—could he handle that? Or would the child be left abandoned, wanted neither by the surrogate nor by the adoption couple? The sperm donor has made no biological commitment to the child, and cannot be expected to support it financially or psychologically if it is not what he expected and contracted for.

Perhaps the only major question in the entire surrogate mother debate that does have a clear legal answer is: Whose baby is it? On the maternal side, it is the biological mother's baby. And if she wants to keep it, she almost certainly can. Indeed, under the proper circumstances, she may even be able to keep the child and sue the sperm donor for child support. On the paternal side, it is also the biological child of the sperm donor. But in all states, children born in wedlock are presumed to be the legitimate children of the married couple. So if the surrogate is married, the child will be presumed (usually rebuttable only by proof beyond a reasonable doubt) to be the offspring of the couple and not of the sperm donor. The donor could bring a custody suit—if he could prove beyond a reasonable doubt that he was the real father—and then the court would have to decide which parent would serve the child's "best interests."

It is an interesting legal twist that in many states with laws relating to artificial insemination, the sperm donor would have no rights even to bring such a suit. For example, to protect donors the Uniform Parentage Act provides that "The donor of semen provided . . . for use in artificial insemination of a woman other than the donor's wife is treated in law as if he were not the natural father of a child thereby conceived." The old adage, "Mama's baby, papa's maybe" aptly describes the current legal reaction to a surrogate who changes her mind and decides to keep the child.

Should There be a Law?

The Science and the Family Committee (which I chair) of the Family Law Section of the American Bar Association is currently studying the surrogate mother situation (and the broader issue of in vitro fertilization) in an attempt to determine what, if any, legislation is appropriate in this area. DHEW's Ethics Advisory Board's final recommendation on in vitro fertilization and embryo transfer was that a "uniform or model law" be developed to "clarify the legal status of children born as a result of *in vitro* fertilization and embryo transfer." This seems to make some sense—although it does seem to be premature. We need a set of agreed-on principles regarding artificial insemination by donor and surrogate mothers—both technologies currently in use—if legislation on in vitro fertilization and embryo transplant is to have a reasonable chance of doing more good than harm.

Experimentation

The articles in this section can be seen as addressing two different questions with regard to research on human subjects. The first set of articles focuses on the general ethical and legal questions in experimentation, and the second set explores the ethical problems of doing research on specific populations or in specific contexts.

The major issues posed by the first set of articles are the problems in doing randomized clinical trials. Three dilemmas arise: (1) when is it permissible to start such trials, on the assumption that they are only ethically legitimate if the researcher believes that the alternative treatments are of equal worth; (2) when is it permissible to stop such trials, given the need for statistical accuracy versus protecting one's patients; and (3) how much information should be told to the subjects; in particular, should they be informed of the fact of randomization and the status of the preliminary data. Fried's article is a general review of some basic legal concepts, such as battery and negligence, applied to research, with specific attention to randomized clinical trials (what Fried terms "mixed therapeutic and nontherapeutic research"). With reference to the above issues, Fried argues for a greater duty of disclosure in the research context and the inappropriateness of the so-called "therapeutic privilege."

In addition to these issues, six ethical norms for clinical trials are identified and discussed, especially by Levine and Lebacqz. These include: good research design; balance of harm and benefit; competence of the investigator; informed consent; equitable selection of subjects; and compensation for research related injuries. Kolata's piece highlights some of the general questions in the context of a particular problem—the use of chemotherapies in osteogenic sarcoma.

The second set of articles in this section includes pieces on research with the elderly, children, fetuses, prisoners, and on Huntington's disease. The underlying question posed by these pieces is whether the general ethical norms or guidelines to protect human subjects are sufficient to protect those whose autonomy, capacity for rationality, or vulnerability is less than that of the normal subject. Research on these subjects is necessary since it is not possible to extrapolate medical data from one population to another. The difficult problem is how such research can be conducted and benefits gained while protecting the subjects' rights and interests.

With regard to the elderly, the main questions are competency to consent, autonomy (especially for institutionalized patients), the ability to comprehend information, and the altered nature of the risk-benefit ratio for elderly individuals. With regard to children, the main questions are whether children should be used as subjects in nontherapeutic research, who should be their surrogate decision makers, whether and at what age children should be allowed to refuse to participate in either therapeutic or non-therapeutic research, how the risk-benefit ratio should be understood, and whether institutionalized children should be subjects in research. The permissibility of research on the fetus is partially dependent on one's conception of the nature of the fetus. Feinberg's piece on the concept of a person (under Conceptual Foundations) is therefore relevant to this section as well. Other issues presented by fetal research are its relation to the abortion controversy itself; i.e., if abortion is legitimate does it necessarily follow that fetal research is acceptable, the basis for surrogate decision making for fetal research, and the concept of harm or risk for the fetus. McCormick's piece systematically considers these issues for the different classes of fetuses considered for research—when abortion is planned, when it is not, and for the fetus both ex utero and in utero.

Prisoners are often thought to be good populations for research since it is relatively easy to regulate and monitor various factors of their lives and to follow them carefully over a long period. In the case of prisoners, the difficult ethical issue is usually whether the prison situation itself and/or any possible threats or rewards would be coercive and thus limit the prisoner's freedom to consent to participation. The dispute in the prisoner situation generally revolves around two points: first, whether offers are coercive, and second, what the criteria are for the distinction between threats and offers. Evidence has been offered to suggest that prisoners themselves frequently welcome the opportunity to participate in research. Reasons such as relief of boredom, being treated as a person, having family and friends visit them in the hospital rather than in prison, and developing a relationship with a person outside the penal structure, i.e., the researcher, are all cited as benefits which some prisoners would like the opportunity to obtain. Branson's piece discusses these issues with particular reference to the National Commission's report.

Huntington's disease poses specific difficulties. The primary question is whether to attempt to screen individuals for the future onset of Huntington's disease since at present there is no cure or therapy to offer. With regard to the research itself in developing a presymptomatic test, there are also complicating factors. One problem is the need for great accuracy because the information is to be used to make major life plans for the future and not to begin therapy. Obtaining accuracy is made especially difficult due to a wide variability in age of onset, the problem in defining the subject and control groups, and the length of time needed to validate any hypotheses. Other issues relate to the questionable voluntariness of those to be screened and the problems of what to do with preliminary findings. The piece on Huntington's disease is used as a case example of the special types of issues which can arise in devising particular research protocols. (See Cases *4, 22, 34, 49, 57, 66.*)

100.
Ethical Considerations in Clinical Trials
Robert J. Levine   Karen Lebacqz

The ethical norms established in various codes and regulations are inadequate to resolve some of the ethical problems presented by clinical trials. They are stated too vaguely to provide unequivocal answers to many specific questions. In order to remedy this situation, many commentators have proposed the development of more specific and complex regulations. We propose that a more fruitful approach would be to examine the ethical principles underlying the norms and to apply these principles to the specific problems. We apply this approach to two questions: (1) Is it ethical to select subjects for a randomized clinical trial (RCT) exclusively from Veterans Administration (VA) hospitals? (2) In the conduct of an RCT is it necessary to disclose the fact that therapy will be determined by chance? We conclude that problems of justice arise not only because of the vulnerability of patients in VA hospitals but also because of the loss of the physician-patient relationship in an RCT. However, the use of patients in a VA hospital is not always unjust; in most cases such use can be made more just through various modifications in design. We also conclude that the fact of randomization should be disclosed in any situation in which it might materially affect the prospective subject's decision, and that the values and preferences of the subjects should be taken into account in determining what information might be material. This work is only a preliminary step toward analyzing ethical issues in clinical trials. While some would challenge our conclusions, we hope that our methods will facilitate clarity about the locus of disagreement in current controversies and about the value questions that must be answered in order to set an ethical context for the conduct of clinical trials.

Most discussions of the "ethics" of research tend to concentrate on issues related to "informed consent."[15] Important though such issues are, they are neither the only nor the most important ethical considerations in the design and conduct of clinical trials.[*] As a simple rule of thumb, any time the words "should" or "ought" appear, an ethical question has been raised. For example, the question, "When should a clinical trial be stopped?" is an ethical question in that one cannot answer by looking only to scientific considerations. Along with scientific judgments about how many data are required in order to draw meaningful conclusions will be considerations of possible injury to subjects in the trial or injury to patients waiting for the development of new therapies. The range of ethical problems one encounters in the course of planning and conducting clinical trials is vast; it encompasses nearly all of those presented by all research involving human subjects.

Consequently, in this paper we shall not attempt either a thorough analysis of the issues or a comprehensive survey of the relevant literature. Rather we shall begin by taking seriously several problems: When and how to stop a clinical trial, Who will be effective as a clinical trials investigator, and Patient recruitment: Problems and solutions. From these and one additional question that

Source: *Clinical Pharmacology and Therapeutics*, vol. 25, no. 5, part 2, p. 728, May 1979.

[*]We use the term "research," "practice," and "innovative therapy" as defined by the National Commission for the Protection of Human Subjects of Biomedical and Behavioral Research (Commission).[20, 31] For reasons elaborated elsewhere,[20] we prefer the term "nonvalidated practice" to "innovative therapy." The term "clinical trial," as used here, refers to a class of research activities designed to develop generalizable knowledge about the safety and /or efficacy of either validated or nonvalidated practices.

we propose (should subjects be compensated for injury), we suggest the dimensions of ethical dilemmas in clinical trials, namely, problems in the interpretation or application of underlying norms and principles of ethical conduct. We shall then take issues related to patient recruitment for more careful examination, in order to show how differences in interpretation of basic norms and principles affect decisions about the conduct of trials and in order to suggest possible solutions to some central ethical dilemmas.

Ethical Issues and Basic Norms

Each of the questions or areas of concern mentioned above points to a range of related questions and to one or more basic norms which are commonly understood to apply to the conduct of research on human subjects.

When and how to stop a clinical trial. We begin by posing this area of concern in the form of two questions: When should clinical trials be stopped? How should clinical trials be stopped? These two ethical questions suggest a range of related questions: When should clinical trials be started? If controlled, what should be used as the control intervention? Should interventions be assigned according to a process of randomization? How should information gathered during the course of the trial affect its conduct?

This set of questions points to two basic norms identified in codes of ethics for the conduct of research on human subjects.* The

first of these is the norm of *good research design.*[†] This norm appears in almost all codes and regulations for the conduct of research:

> The experiment should be so designed and based on the results of animal experimentation and a knowledge of the natural history of the disease or other problem under study that the anticipated results will justify the performance of the experiment (Nuremberg 3).

> Biomedical research involving human subjects must conform to generally accepted scientific principles and should be based on adequately performed laboratory and animal experimentation and on a thorough knowledge of the scientific literature. (Helsinki I. 1).

While there are slight variations in the expression of the norm, the basic idea is constant: Research must be sufficiently well designed to achieve its purposes and must be scientifically sound; otherwise, it is not justified. What constitutes good design is, of course, a matter of some debate which is not resolved by the norm itself. But the question of when to stop a clinical trial is at least in part a question of adequate design and is thus covered in part by this norm.

But implicit in the question is also the suggestion that a trial might be stopped *before* its designated time. To the requirement for good design is added concern for the well-being of the subjects. Thus, another basic

---

*The normative statements cited in this paper are taken from the Nuremberg Code, the 1975 revision of the Declaration of Helsinki (both of which are reproduced in a recent book[25]), and from the Regulations of the Department of Health, Education, and Welfare (DHEW).[5] Often, normative statements contained in the Code and in the Declaration will have no parallel in Regulations. There are various reasons for this. Most importantly, the Regulations are not intended to be an ethical code. Rather, they require that an institution submit "a statement of principles which will govern the institution in the discharge of its responsibilities for protecting the rights and welfare of subjects. This may include appropriate existing codes or declarations or statements formulated by the institution itself" (DHEW, 46.106a). However, in some cases there are parallel norms stated in the Regulations. In the event of conflicts the Regulations go on to state: "It is to be understood that no such principles supersede DHEW policy or applicable law" (DHEW, 46.106a).

[†]As a matter of convenience, we shall use brief expressions of the ethical norms in this paper. In general, they may be translated into proper normative statements by incorporating them in suitable declarative sentences—e.g.: There should be good research design. There should be a favorable balance of harms and benefits.

norm is brought into play, the norm that requires an identification of the consequences of action and a *balance of harm and benefit.* * The norm is expressed in codes of ethics in two common forms: First it requires that possible harms to subjects be outweighed by the benefits one expects to accrue from the research:

> The degree of risk to be taken should never exceed that determined by the humanitarian importance of the problem solved by the experiment (Nuremberg 6).

> Biomedical research involving human subjects cannot legitimately be carried out unless the importance of the objective is in proportion to the inherent risk to the subject (Helsinki I.4).

> The risks to the subject [must be] so outweighed by the sum of the benefit to subject and the importance of the knowledge to be gained as to warrant a decision to allow the subject to accept these risks . . . (DHEW, 46.102 b, 1).

Second, it requires that some harms be considered sufficient to outweigh anticipated benefits and, hence, to require stopping a trial in process:

> During the course of the experiment the scientist in charge must be prepared to terminate the experiment at any stage, if he has probable cause to believe . . . that a continuation . . . is likely to result in injury, disability, or death to the experimental subject (Nuremberg 10).

> The investigator or the investigating team should discontinue the research if in his/ her or their judgment it may, if continued, be harmful to the individual (Helsinki III. 3).

Thus, research may not be initiated unless the consequences of conducting it are judged likely to produce more good than harm, and it must be terminated if certain harms appear likely, no matter what good consequences might result.

The question, When and how should clinical trials be stopped? has thus opened up a range of issues related to two basic norms: *good research design and balance of harm and benefit.*

Who will be effective as a clinical trials investigator? As posed, this does not appear to be an ethical question; rather, it seems to be concerned with various matters of fact: What sort of person will be effective in a certain role? However, to judge someone's performance "effective" is to make a value judgment. In order to reveal the underlying ethical content of this question, it may be reformulated: Who should be permitted or encouraged to do clinical research?

The question gives rise to a series of concerns: What training should be required of clinical trials investigators? Should they be licensed especially to do this sort of research? Should students, interns, or others in training be permitted to conduct clinical trials? What disciplines should be represented in the research team? Is it permissible for physicians to conduct clinical trials on their own patients, or must another physician always be involved?

These questions point to the basic norm that requires *competence of the investigator(s):*

> The experiment should be conducted only by scientifically qualified persons. The highest degree of skill and care should be required through all stages of the experiment of those who conduct or engage in the experiment (Nuremberg 8).

---

*This norm is often referred to as a "risk-benefit calculus." However, we prefer to state the norm in terms of balancing harms and benefits for two reasons: (1) Since "risk" means "probability of harm," it is more accurate to balance it against "probability of benefit" rather than against "benefit" per se. (2) Harms and benefits are not merely to be *calculated;* rather, they are required to be in a certain ratio or relationship to each other customarily alluded to as "favorable." A more complete discussion of the factors that should be considered in balancing harms and benefits is published elsewhere.[21]

Biomedical research involving human subjects should be conducted only by scientifically qualified persons and under the supervision of a clinically competent medical person. The responsibility for the human subject must always rest with a medically qualified person . . . (Helsinki I.3).

The norm requires: (1) adequate scientific training and "skill" to accomplish the purposes of the research, and (2) a high degree of professionalism necessary to "care" for the subject.

The 1975 revision of the Declaration of Helsinki and the recently developed DHEW Regulations governing research on the fetus reflect another concern for competence of the investigator:

When obtaining informed consent for the research project the doctor should be particularly cautious if the subject is in a dependent relationship to him or her or may consent under duress. In that case the informed consent should be obtained by a doctor who is not engaged in the investigation and who is completely independent of this official relationship (Helsinki I. 10).

Individuals engaged in the (research) activity will have no part in: (i) any decisions as to the timing, method, and procedures used to terminate the pregnancy, and (ii) determining the viability of the fetus at the termination of the pregnancy . . . (DHEW), 46.206a, 3).

These statements recognize the possibility that a physician-investigator performing in a dual role may have difficulty dealing with the conflicts of interest arising from this double function. They create a requirement to avoid certain situations in which the interests of research might be permitted to override the interests of the patient-subject.

Patient recruitment: Problems and solutions. At first glance, this topic—like its predecessors—seems to reflect concerns about matters of fact: What techniques are effective in attracting subjects to proposed trials?

How can suitable prospective subjects be located? And so on. Once again, however, further examination reveals two basic ethical questions:

1. Whom should we select for possible involvement as subjects in a clinical trial?
2. Once they have been selected, how should we invite them to participate or be involved in the trial? These are, respectively, questions about the ethics of subject selection and of informed consent.

A norm requiring *informed consent* is well established in codes and regulations for the conduct of research:

The voluntary consent of the human subject is absolutely essential (Nuremberg 1).

[E]ach potential subject must be adequately informed of the aims, methods, anticipated benefits and potential hazards of the study and the discomfort it may entail (Helsinki I.9).

Legally effective informed consent will be obtained by adequate and appropriate methods . . . (DHEW, 46.102b,3).

These expressions of the norm would suggest that patients may not be involved in a trial unless they have given informed and voluntary consent.

However, the Declaration of Helsinki makes an apparent exception to this norm (or gives it an alternative interpretation) in which the subjects-to-be are patients and the research involves a new therapeutic intervention intended to benefit them. Here, the Declaration does not make consent mandatory:

If the doctor considers it essential not to obtain informed consent, the specific reasons for this proposal should be stated in the experimental protocol . . . (Helsinki II. 5).

The Declaration of Helsinki may be interpreted to mean that under some circumstances it would be permissible to involve nonconsenting subjects. While DHEW regulations permit no such exceptions, the regulations of the Food and Drug Administration (FDA)[4] permit the following exceptions:

> In "those relatively rare cases in which it is not feasible . . . or in which as a matter of professional judgment exercised in the best interest of a particular patient. . it would be contrary to that patient's welfare to obtain his consent" (Section 310.102d).

The norm of *informed consent* includes not only the right to refuse participation at the outset, but is also usually interpreted to include the right to withdraw at any time:

> During the course of the experiment the human subject should be at liberty to bring the experiment to an end . . . (Nuremberg 9).

> [The subject] should be informed that he or she is at liberty to abstain from participation in the study and that he or she is free to withdraw his or her consent to participate at any time (Helsinki I.9). The basic elements of . . . consent include: . . . (6) an instruction that the person is free to withdraw his consent and to discontinue participation in the project or activity at any time without prejudice to the subject (DHEW 46.103c, 6).

In general, therefore, we may say that the norm of *informed consent* requires the investigator to secure the consent of patients prior to their involvement and to permit them to withdraw at any time without prejudice.*

While the norm related to the involvement of particular subjects is well established—and much debated[15]—less has been said explicitly about requirements for selection of groups or individuals to invite to participate in research. Most codes appear to subsume this question under the norms of scientific design and of consent: Physician-investigators would select patients on the basis of appropriate scientific considerations, and, then, provided the subject (or his or her legal guardian) gives valid consent, the selection of that subject is deemed appropriate.†

In 1970, Hans Jonas[10] published an influential essay in which he argued for a

---

*Surprisingly, there has been little debate as to whether subjects should indeed always be free to withdraw at any time; most of the debate in this area has been over interpretations of what constitutes an adequately "informed" or "voluntary" consent. The requirement that subjects should always be at liberty to withdraw without prejudice seems to be based on the assumption that the subject is always doing something for the good of others; such supererogatory acts are generally not considered mandatory. There are several alternative ways to view the role of research subject: (1) McCormick[22] has argued that participation in some sorts of research is a duty. One might extrapolate from this argument to contend that—under some circumstances—the subject might not have the freedom to withdraw. Parenthetically, McCormick would probably argue that the individual should be free to choose *when* to exercise this duty. (2) Ramsey[23] and Jonas[10] characterize research as a "joint venture" between the subject and the investigator; ideally, they may be considered "coadventurers." If one accepts this argument, the agreement to participate in research may be viewed as a form of *promise*. Ethically, promises may be broken only for certain justifying reasons, not simply at the whim of the promisor. (3) Levine[16] has argued that the subject ordinarily chooses to receive an "innovative therapy" because of the good (benefit) he or she expects to derive from this choice. In some circumstances the subject may be viewed as having assumed a reciprocal obligation" of bearing the *inconvenience* of tests necessary to prove its safety and/or efficacy. The argument that an individual who chooses to receive a benefit from society thereby incurs a reciprocal obligation to serve society by participating in research designed to validate the therapy he or she receives seems highly germane to considerations of clinical trials. It must be emphasized that this obligation is to assume a burden characterized as "mere inconvenience";[16] it is not extended to create an obligation to assume risk of physical or psychological harm.

†As noted above, however, the Declaration of Helsinki makes an exception to the rule of consent for certain patients. As might be expected, then, the criteria for selection of subjects within that group also differ from the normal consent criteria. Selection of patients to receive nonvalidated therapies is left to the discretion of the physician: "In the treatment of the sick person, the doctor must be free to use a

"descending order of permissibility" for the recruitment ("conscription") of subjects for research. His critieria for selection related directly to the person's capacity to understand the goals of the research and to participate in it as a partner with the investigator. Accordingly, he proposed that the most suitable subjects would be researchers themselves because they had the greatest capacity to give a truly "informed" consent. He also argued that very ill or dying subjects should not be used in research even when they give consent unless the research relates directly to their own illnesses. Underlying this argument is a perception of very ill or dying subjects as peculiarly vulnerable to pressures which make their consent insufficiently free or informed. In this way, the strict concern for consent was supplemented by Jonas with a concern for the situation of the subject and the ways in which the situation might render the subject vulnerable; vulnerable subjects were afforded extra protection against selection even if they wished to be selected or to participate.

Recognition that extra protection is required for those who are vulnerable by virtue of their capacities or situations is expressed in the 1975 revision of the Declaration of Helsinki. However, the requirement established in the Declaration is precisely the opposite of what Jonas proposed: Sick persons are to be recruited as subjects of "nontherapeutic research" only when it is unrelated to their illnesses.

Nontherapeutic Biomedical Research: The subjects should be volunteers—either healthy persons or patients for whom the experimental design is not related to the patient's illness (Helsinki III. 2).*

In several of its recent reports, the Commission has made recommendations that regulations be developed to protect the vulnerable. In general, what is being developed is a requirement not to use institutionalized subjects—e.g., prisoners[30]—or persons with limited capacities to consent—e.g., children[29]—if less vulnerable persons are available and would be suitable subjects. For example, in its report on research involving children,[29] recommendation 2 reads, in part:

Research involving children may be conducted or supported provided an Institutional Review Board has determined that . . . (B) where appropriate, studies have been conducted first on animals and adult humans, then on older children, prior to involving infants . . . (E) subjects will be selected in an equitable manner . . .

To lend substance to this recommendation, the following comment is provided:

Subjects should be selected in an equitable manner, avoiding overutilization of any group of children based solely upon administrative convenience or availability of a population. The burdens of participation in research should be equitably distributed among the segments of our society, no matter how large or small those burdens may be.

Thus, a norm of *equitable selection of subjects* is developing which supplements pre-

---

new diagnostic or therapeutic measure . . . (Helsinki II. 1). The assumption is clearly that selection will be based on patient need and expected benefit to the patient: "If in his judgment it offers hope of saving life, re-establishing health, or alleviating suffering" (II. 1).

*A strict interpretation of this principle—in the context of a document that distinguishes between therapeutic and nontherapeutic research—has the following unfortunate (and unintended) consequences: (1) All rational research designed to explore the pathogenesis of diseases would be forbidden. The Declaration would require that it be conducted only on healthy persons or patients not having the disease one wishes to investigate. (2) In a placebo-controlled drug trial, those who receive the placebo must be either healthy persons or patients for whom the experimental design is not related to the patient's illness. Problems created by the spurious distinction between therapeutic and nontherapeutic research are discussed in more detail elsewhere.[13, 19, 20] vious concerns for *informed consent*. It reflects the growing recognition that the voluntary choices of persons are, at times, not sufficient to ensure fair distribution among individuals and groups of the burdens and benefits of research.

"Should subjects of research be conpensated?" To the questions we started with we add a fourth, namely, whether the subjects of clinical trials should be compensated for research-related injury. To date, no code or regulation specifically mentions or requires such compensation, but as attention to questions of fairness in the distribution of burdens and benefits develops, some commentators have suggested that subjects of research be compensated for injuries sustained in their participation.

For example, the recent DHEW Secretary's Task Force on the Compensation of Injured Research Subjects recommends[7] that:

> Human subjects who suffer physical, psychological, or social injury in the course of research conducted or supported by the PHS should be compensated if (1) the injury is proximately caused by such research, and (2) the injury on balance exceeds that reasonably associated with such illness from which the subject may be suffering, as well as with treatment usually associated with such illness at the time the subject began participation in the research.

In justifying this recommendation, the Task Force argues that where society is both the sponsor and the beneficiary of research, it incurs an obligation to compensate those who are injured by research. While the Task Force notes that patients often participate at least in part for personal gain (in the hope of receiving a new and effective therapy), the Task Force concludes that neither this fact nor the fact that such patients also give their consent to participate reduces the obligation of society for those injuries that are specifically related to the *research* aspects of activities in which patients engage.

There thus seems to be emerging another norm for the conduct of research on human subjects: *Compensation for research-related injury.*

Underlying Principles

We have identified six ethical norms for research involving human subjects: (1) good research design, (2) balance of harm and benefit, (3) competence of the investigator(s), (4) informed consent, (5) equitable selection of subjects, and (6) compensation for research-related injury. While not all these norms have been recognized as either compelling or applicable at all times, there is a growing consensus that adherence to each norm is a necessary condition for the ethical conduct of clinical trials.[28]

Yet these norms are variously expressed and interpreted. For example, in considering the requirement for *informed consent,* FDA Regulations and the Declaration of Helsinki permit exceptions to this requirement while DHEW Regulations do not (see above). Moreover, most norms are expressed in such vague language that it is difficult to know exactly how to apply them to particular cases. "There should be a favorable balance of harms and benefits" is a clear statement of a widely recognized norm, but it does not tell the investigator or the Institutional Review Board (IRB) how much benefit to society might justify the imposition of a substantial risk of physical harm on an individual subject:[19] Is it permissible to do kidney biopsies on normal volunteers in order to develop control data for a study of patients with glomerulonephritis? Similarly, "subjects should be selected equitably" is a clear statement of an emerging norm, but it does not say what constitutes "equitable" selections. Is it permissible to involve only veterans in a clinical trial?

Some commentators have tried to resolve such uncertainties by defining the exact content of each norm, for example, by listing all the bits of information that must be given to the subject in order for consent to be adequately "informed." Others, of course, promptly point out that giving information does not ensure that the subject made an informed choice.[15]

We propose here a different approach to the problem of applying norms to specific cases or types of cases. Rather than trying to pin down each norm and to specify its exact content, we propose instead to look behind the norm, as it were, to the underlying principle(s) which it is intended to uphold and embody. It is then the interpretation and interplay of these principles that become important in determining what to do in each instance.

For example, the norms requiring *competence of the investigator(s)* and *good research design* seem to derive from and uphold three basic values or principles:

1. Without a competent investigator (or investigative team) and good research design, there will be no benefits forthcoming from the study. Thus, these norms point to the underlying principle that requires us to do good, which we call *beneficence*.

2. Competent investigators and good research design also protect subjects from harm. Thus, these norms also uphold the principle of *not harming* or *nonmaleficence* (primum non nocere).

3. Finally, even where research presents no risk of harm to subjects, the requirements that the investigator(s) be competent and the research well designed serve to ensure that people's time is not wasted and that their desire to participate in a meaningful activity is not frustrated. These norms thus also serve to uphold the principle of *respect for persons*.

The principle of *respect for persons* requires that persons not be used merely as a means to another's end.[15] The norm of *informed consent* upholds this principle by ensuring that they are not "used" by another without their knowledge and consent. Since the opportunity to give or refuse consent,

and to withdraw from participation, also serves to permit individuals to protect themselves from unpleasant or harmful activities, this norm is secondarily linked to the principles of *beneficence* and *not harming*.

Finally, the norms of *equitable selection of subjects* and *compensation for research-related injury* express different aspects of the basic principle of *justice,* or fairness, which requires that burdens and benefits be distributed fairly.[14]

Thus we find that the six norms taken together rest on four basic principles for human conduct: *doing good (beneficence), not harming (nonmaleficence), respecting persons,* and *distributing goods and evils fairly (justice).*

We propose that clarity about the application of norms to situations is best achieved by examining these underlying principles to see what they require. Most disagreements, e.g., about whether subjects may be involved without their knowledge or consent, arise from differences in the interpretation or balancing of these principles. For example, those who take *respect for persons* to mean primarily or exclusively respect for the individual's autonomous choice and who also give this principle highest weight will usually argue that it is never permissible to involve a subject without that person's consent; but those who interpret the principle to include justifiable instances of paternalism or who give more weight to other principles (such as *beneficence*) may argue that consent is not necessary so long as subjects are benefited and and not harmed.[15] Not until decisions are made about the meaning and balancing of the principles will these two antagonists see eye-to-eye; simply pointing to norms of *informed consent* and *good research design* is not enough.

Of course, there is by no means universal agreement as to the interpretation or weighting of principles. In what follows, we take two current ethical dilemmas in clinical trials and expose the questions that must be raised about underlying principles in order to find their solutions. While we do not propose any final solutions, we hope to further the dialogue on these and other ethical dilemmas in clinical trials.

Application of Principles to Problems

We shall examine some of the issues grouped under the general topic of "patient recruitment" in order to illustrate the application of norms and principles to particular problems in the ethics of clinical trials.

Whom shall we recruit? Numerous complex questions can be raised about the selection of potential subjects or subject populations for research.[16] We shall focus on one that is peculiarly relevant to the conduct of randomized clinical trials (RCTs): Is it ethical to select subjects exclusively from Veterans Administration (VA) hospitals?

Several reasons have been advanced for doing RCTs in VA hospitals: Such hospitals are excellent places for the conduct of trials because of the comprehensive nature of their records, the fact that patients can be located and retained within a protocol even if they move to other geographic locations, and the well-developed administrative coordination between the hospitals in the system. In short, the VA hospital system provides a highly efficient locale for the conduct of an RCT: Statistically significant results can be generated in a relatively short time and at a relatively low cost.

It would seem, then, that the ethical principle of *beneficence* would support the use of patients in VA hospitals as subjects for RCTs. Great good can be done at little cost. The balance of benefits over harms seems to be maximized.

Yet the exclusive use of patients in VA hospitals has been strongly condemned as unfair:

[T]he main participants . . . are now primarily recruited from the temporary or permanent inmates of public institutions, our Veterans Administration Hospitals, our mental institutions, and, often, our prisons. This means that it is mainly the underprivileged of our society who perform these services. . . .[33]

There are certain injustices that are so gross that few would try to defend them. That RCTs should be performed on, say, the poor . . . or those who happened to come for treatment to a Veterans Administration Hospital, while others received the benefit of a fully individualized treatment, would be grossly unfair.[9]

In short, these critics charge that while the use of patients in VA hospitals may serve the cause of efficiency and do good in some ways, it also violates the requirements of the principle of *justice*.

There appears to be, then, a conflict between the requirements of *beneficence* and those of *justice*. Our task is to see whether the two principles can be harmonized, and what their application to the problem of selection of subjects means for the exclusive use of patients in VA hospitals.

First, we acknowledge that there are different interpretations of the requirements of *justice*. While it is generally agreed that *justice* demands a fair sharing of burdens and benefits, just what is an unfair share is the subject of considerable controversy. Is it fair for persons to be treated differently on the basis of their needs—their accomplishments—their past records or future potentials? On what basis should goods and burdens be distributed in order to ensure that the distribution is fair?[12]

While it is sometimes argued that the most "fair" distribution is precisely that which creates the most benefits for society at large,* this interpretation does not accord with either Western concepts of the fundamental

---

*This is the classical utilitarian argument which harmonizes *justice* and *beneficence* by stipulating that there is no conflict: to create good *is* to do justice; just institutions act so as to produce "the greatest good for the greatest number."

equality of persons (e.g., before the law) or the very strong tradition that interprets "fairness" to require extra protection for those who are weaker, more vulnerable, or less advantaged than others. This latter interpretation is reflected in such disparate sources as the injunction in the Judeo-Christian tradition to protect widows and orphans, the Marxist dictum "from each according to ability; to each according to need," and, most recently, John Rawls's contractual derivation of principles of justice. [12, 24]

On this interpretation, which we favor, whether it would be fair to select subjects exclusively from VA hospitals would depend on: (1) whether patients in such hospitals are in some way vulnerable or disadvantaged such that they should receive extra protection from bearing burdens, and (2) whether the clinical trials present burdens from which vulnerable subjects should be protected. Let us examine the case regarding each of these determinations.

Are patients in VA hospitals more vulnerable or less advantaged than patients with similar conditions in private hospitals? We propose that there is at least one condition of being a patient in a VA hospital which tends to render one more vulnerable and less advantaged than other patients, namely, the condition of having limited options. Private patients may choose another physician—or—in most cases—another hospital setting if they prefer not to participate in an RCT. Veterans wishing to exercise such an option, however, will often be obliged to assume a large financial burden. In order to receive the benefits due to them as veterans, they must use certain specified facilities; their options for receiving medical care thus are usually more limited. To this extent, they may be considered more vulnerable and less advantaged than other patients with similar conditions receiving private care. Thus, one could argue that in general they should receive more benefits and bear fewer burdens of research.

But do RCTs present burdens from which vulnerable persons should be protected? One recent study suggests that it may be *less* risky for patients to be involved in clinical trials than to receive treatment in a nonresearch setting. [2] Thus, participation in a clinical trial might be considered a benefit and not a burden. However, the risks measured in this study are primarily those of death or disabling injury. While each RCT will present to the subjects its own peculiar complement of such risks—as well as its own complement of benefits—these risks are not the only burdens to be considered. In the context of medical treatment, the physician-patient relationship itself is generally considered a "good"—as Fried [9] puts it, the "good of personal care." Virtually all physician-investigators who have argued that the standards for informed consent should be less stringent for an RCT than for other forms of research recognize, at least implicitly, the loss of the good of personal care as a burden of the RCT (see below).

There is at least one sense, then, in which the RCT may be said to present burdens from which vulnerable or less advantaged subjects should be protected and at least one sense in which patients in VA hospitals should be considered to be vulnerable or less advantaged. One interpretation of *justice*, therefore, would seem to suggest that patients in VA hospitals should not be used as subjects in RCTs, despite the benefits that might result from their participation.

However, this is not a final conclusion. There are ways to reduce the apparent tension between the requirements of the principles of *beneficence* and *justice*. First, one could take steps to minimize the burdens imposed by the RCT—the loss of the personal physician-patient relationship. For example, patients who participate in RCTs might be afforded the opportunity to maintain a physician-patient relationship with a physician not involved in the RCT but sufficiently familiar with it to facilitate the integration of its components and objectives with those of personal care. [16]

Second, steps might be taken to minimize the "disadvantaged" position of the patient in the VA hospital. For example, patients in the hospital might be given the option of personal care *or* participation in the RCT, thus increasing their options to be more similar to those enjoyed by private patients. Alternatively, veterans refusing participation might be referred for "personal care" to a private hospital at the expense of the VA.

Another mechanism which both decreases vulnerability and helps in the assessment of the true magnitude of the burden involves consultation with the community.[16] We have argued here that the deprivation of the good of "personal care" is a burden. But judging something to be a burden is a value judgment, and it is possible that patients' value judgments might differ from ours. Ordinarily, we learn about the patient's value system through negotiating for consent; if the subject chooses to participate, we assume that, in the judgment of the subject, the burdens are bearable or worth assuming. The concern that is raised here is that prospective subjects are highly dependent upon those who would be seeking consent, and thus they may be intimidated and their freedom to assert their own value systems might be compromised.[18] This is particularly true when there are few or no alternatives available to the prospective subject.[16]

One way to address this problem of intimidation and to provide more opportunity for subjects to assert their own value judgments might be to equalize the balance of power by assembling a group of prospective subjects to discuss the proposed RCT with the investigator(s) at an open meeting.[16] After presenting the research plans, the investigators might ascertain whether subjects would consider participation a burden and whether they would consider it unfair for them to bear those burdens. One might be surprised to learn that the community of prospective subjects does not consider the burdens too great or the selection process unfair. We note, for example, the recent successful performance of a placebo-controlled randomized trial of the efficacy of vitamin C in the prevention of acute illnesses in Navajo schoolchildren performed after consultation with the community.

Finally, of course, one might address the issue of inequitable distribution by including private patients and/or private hospitals in the RCT; in this way, any burdens imposed by the fact of randomization will not be borne solely by those who are less advantaged.

Thus, while there is no clear answer to dilemmas of *justice* applicable to all contingencies, there are ways to modify the design or implementation of the RCT so that the use—and even the exclusive use—of patients in VA hospitals need not be unjust.

How shall we recruit patient-subjects for participation? Involvement of individual subjects requires their informed consent. One aspect of the general issue of informed consent is highly controversial and peculiarly relevant to the conduct of RCTs: Is it necessary to disclose to the prospective patient-subject the fact that his or her therapy will be determined by chance?

Some existing regulations would seem to require disclosure of this fact. In DHEW Regulations (46.103c), the investigator is required to provide: "(1) A fair explanation of the procedures to be followed . . . , including identification of any procedures which are experimental . . . (and) . . . (4) a disclosure of any alternative procedures that might be advantageous for the subject. . . ." Taken together, these requirements suggest minimally that if prospective subjects ask about alternatives or ask why particular alternatives are not to be employed in their cases, an honest response would reveal the plan to randomize. However, the regulations do not *specifically* require disclosure of randomization, and so we turn once again to the basic ethical principles to see whether this fact should indeed be disclosed.

As noted above, the requirement for informed consent is derived from the ethical principle of *respect for persons,* which requires that we respect another's right to self-determination, i.e., to be left alone or to make free choices.[15] In general, respect for the other is shown by negotiating for informed consent.

Such negotiation is truly respecting of the

other only if we provide a complete and honest account of all information relevant to the person's decision. Based on the presumption that we might not anticipate all information relevant to that decision, we "offer to answer any inquiries concerning the procedures . . ." as required by DHEW regulation. Consent is not valid if information relevant to the decision is deliberately withheld or distorted. Thus, we conclude tentatively that if the fact that therapy will be determined by chance is relevant or "material" to the prospective subject's decision, there is a duty to disclose this fact. If we do not disclose a "material" bit of information, we have—in ethical terms—shown disrespect for a person by illegitimately using that person as a means to our own ends.*

It seems, therefore, that the principle of *respect for persons* requires disclosure of the fact of randomization, at least in those instances in which it might reasonably be expected to affect the prospective subject's decision. However, a number of commentators have argued against the disclosure of this fact. Some of these arguments suggest that other ethical principles are also at stake, and other arguments appear to rest on differing interpretations of the principle of *respect for persons*.

One commonly used argument is that if randomization were disclosed, patients would refuse to participate and it would be impossible to conduct a successful RCT.[3,11] As Chalmers[3] puts it: "If they were in their right senses, they would find a doctor who thought he knew which was the better treatment, or they would conclude that if the differences

were so slight . . . they would prefer to take their chances on no operation."

This argument assumes a particular interpretation of patient behavior that can be challenged. More important for our purposes, however, it also appears to be based on a primary concern for *beneficence*: Assuming that RCTs are necessary in order to do good (e.g., to get accurate data) and that the failure of patients to participate will prevent great good from being done, it rests on a balancing of values that puts the good to be done over and above the right of patients to be fully informed. It thus puts *beneficence* over *respect for persons*. Demonstrating that patients do not in fact withdraw or refuse to participate when the fact of randomization is disclosed would help to reconcile this apparent conflict, since it would show that respecting the right of persons to choose will not prevent good from being done. Our experience suggests that this is the case.†

A second argument against disclosure holds that the RCT is so similar to the routine and accepted practice of medicine that the fact of randomization may be considered one of the "details" of treatment that is not normally disclosed in medical practice.[3,8] As Chalmers[3] argues, "It is not customary in the ordinary practice of medicine to inform patients of all the details with regard to how decisions are made in their treatment."

This argument has its ethical basis in the principle of *beneficence*. It also assumes that it is the physician who judges what the "good" is that is to be done. The Oath of Hippocrates[25] puts it this way: "I will use treatment to help the sick according to

---

*In law, the battery theory of informed consent reflects the same line of reasoning: it is wrong a priori to touch, treat, or do research upon a person without that person's consent. As stated by Justice Cardozo in a landmark case, the reason it is wrong is quite simply that "[E]very human being of adult years and sound mind has a right to determine what shall be done with his own body. . . ."[15] Whether or not harm befalls the person is irrelevant; it is the "unconsented touching" that is wrong. The modern trend in malpractice litigation is to treat cases based upon failure to obtain proper consent as *negligence* rather than as battery actions. However, under both battery and negligence doctrines, consent is invalid if any information is withheld that might be considered material to the decision to consent.[15]

†At Yale University School of Medicine, it has been the policy to require disclosure of the fact of randomization on written consent forms for over 5 years.[17] There has been no report that the conduct of RCTs has been hindered because an insufficient number of patients have agreed to participate.

my ability and judgment, but never with a view to injury and wrongdoing." There is no requirement that one consult the patient about what would be a "benefit" or which of several "benefits" the patient might prefer; it is only necessary for the physician to act for the patient's benefit. In this view many aspects of practice may be considered "details" which need not be disclosed. Here, the argument is extended to include the fact of randomization as one such "detail."

This argument may be correct in its assumption that in the routine practice of medicine considerations of patient benefit often do override considerations of respect for autonomy, and that patients are not informed as meticulously in practice as they are in research. Whether this should be the case is, however, a matter of some debate. That is, it is not clear that standards for informed consent should be any less stringent in medical practice than they are in research. In reviewing the debate on this issue, Levine[18] concluded that:

> [P]atients are entitled to the same degree of thoroughness of negotiations for informed consent as are subjects. However . . . the patient should, in general, be allowed more freedom than the subject to relinquish this entitlement . . . (and) to delegate decision-making authority to a physician. . . . The most important distinction . . . is that the prospective subject must be informed that if the proposed activity is research or innovative practice, the subject will be at least in part a means and perhaps only a means to another's end.

Thus, unless patients specifically relinquish the right to be informed, they should be informed and have the opportunity to give consent just as research subjects do.* It is not sufficient, therefore, to argue that the fact of randomization is a "detail" that need not be disclosed because it is likened to the "details" of medical practice.

Of perhaps even more importance is the question of whether this fact, or any other presumed "detail" related to the clinical trial, would be "material" to the patient's decisions to consent, since disclosure of "material" facts is generally required by the principle of *respect for persons*. The third argument against disclosure, therefore, is that the fact of randomization is not "material" to the patient's decision.[3]

The construction of this argument is: It is generally agreed that one should not initiate an RCT if one knows at the outset which of the two therapies is superior—more advantageous for the patients.[3, 11, 16, 26, 27] As one commentator explains, if the physician knows that one therapy is superior, ethically he or she is obligated to give that therapy to each patient needing treatment.[3] Since the clinician's primary duty is to do good for the patient, it would not be ethical to use an intervention known to be inferior.

Given this assumption, then, the physician knows that the choice between the two therapies is arbitrary, in the sense that they are "medically equivalent," and there is no rational basis for choosing between them. The physician will probably find no method for choice superior to that of flipping a coin. Since there are no rational grounds for choice between the two therapies, there is no information to be provided to the patient that could possibly be "material" to the patient's decision. What is material to the patient is to seek treatment or not to seek treatment; the choice between two medically equivalent treatments is not material from the patient's perspective. To disclose how the particular therapy is to be chosen for that patient will not enhance the patient's capacity for rational decision making about accepting therapy and thus will not respect the patient as a rational decision maker. Moreover, it may have the detrimental effect of undermining the patient's confidence in the physician and thus adversely affect any treatment given.

---

*Indeed, the legal grounding for the requirement for consent to participate in research is based on the outcome of litigation of disputes arising almost exclusively in the context of the practice of medicine.[15, 18]

While this is at first glance an attractive argument, there is often cause to question the equality of the two treatments and thus the conclusion that the patient will have no grounds for choosing between them.

When treatments are judged "medically equivalent," what is usually meant is that certain gross measures of outcome are the same, e.g., that two years after the initiation of either course of treatment, the probability that the patient will still be living is equivalent. There are two problems with such gross measures of equivalence.

First, as Fried[9] points out, the apparent medical equipoise would not always exist in respect to a particular patient:

> Consider, for instance, the choice between medical and surgical intervention for acute unstable angina pectoris. I would suppose that a group of patients could be so defined that the risks and benefits of the two available courses of action were quite evenly balanced. But, when a particular patient is involved, with a particular set of symptoms, a particular diagnostic picture, and a particular set of values and preferences, then one may doubt how often a physician carefully going into all of these particularities would conclude that the risks and benefits are truly equal.

In part, what is at stake here is the medical judgment of the physician regarding the treatment for *this* patient with *this* set of *signs* and *symptoms*. Physicians often claim that decisions about treatment have to be based at least in part on their intuitive grasp of what is needed, based on years of experience in responding to slight variations in the "clinical picture"; if this is true, then the physician may have grounds for thinking that even though two therapies are "medically equivalent" in terms of the long-range outcome for a *group* of patients, one may be superior for *this* patient. In that case, the two treatments cannot be judged to be equivalent.

But Fried[9] also points to the second reason for invalidating the claim of "equivalency"

between the treatments: namely, patients differ in their values and preferences and may find the *quality* of life offered by one or the other of the two treatments to be as important for them as the eventual *outcome* of treatment. Thus, even though two treatments may be "medically equivalent" in terms of eventual outcome of life expectancy, they may be radically different in terms of their *meaning* for the patients.

For example, an RCT was performed to compare the results of radical mastectomy with wide excision in the treatment of early breast cancer.[1] The trial was considered justified because evidence had accumulated that the unorthodox method (the restricted surgery) had sufficient evidence in its favor so that "all those engaged in the trial would be willing to allow their own relatives to enter it." Thus, presumably, the two treatments were judged to be potentially medically equivalent. Now we raise the question: Should the women participating in this trial have been told that two different treatments were being tested and that the selection of their treatment would be at random?

Since one of the alternative treatments under consideration was of a "mutilating character" (to quote the investigators), it seems likely that, although the treatments might have been equivalent from the perspectives of long-term morbidity or mortality rate, the women involved might find one of them more acceptable from a personal perspective; thus, many of these women might have preferred to be given the option of receiving treatment without random assignment.

In another well-known example, an RCT was performed to determine the effect of treatment on morbidity and mortality rate in men with mild hypertension.[32] In order to justify the establishment of this RCT, it was necessary to maintain that one could not predict whether such patients would sustain more complications of hypertension (morbidity and mortality rate) during therapy with three standard antihypertensive medications than they would during administration of a placebo. Assuming that this stated null hypothesis is correct, is nondisclosure justified?

Once again, we contend that it is not. The antihypertensive drugs employed had such side effects as depression, exercise intolerance, impotence, and the like. It is reasonable to expect that many of these men, if fully informed, would have preferred to take the placebo rather than to risk the side effects of these drugs, if indeed the chances for reduced morbidity or mortality rate from hypertension were identical. Thus, the possible side effects of the drugs would not be immaterial to the decision to participate, and the fact of randomization would become material to the patient's choice.

Of course, to some patients, only the gross outcome (the morbidity or mortality rate after X years) would matter. As noted above, patients often do choose to participate in RCTs, even when they are fully informed. But we conclude that one cannot *assume* the fact of randomization is immaterial to the patient's decision; only the patient can make that determination. Thus, in order to respect the free choice of persons, patients should generally be told of the plan to randomize and should be given the choice to accept participation in the trial or to accept one of the available standard treatments. In practice, the burden of proof should rest with those who would argue that it is not necessary to inform prospective subjects that their therapy will be determined by chance; unless they can convince reasonable persons (i.e., the IRB members) that this is so, the patients should be informed of their therapy.

In sum, we do not believe that concerns for *beneficence* should outweigh those of *respect for persons,* nor do we accept the interpretation that "material" facts relevant to showing such respect are limited to gross medical equivalency. We therefore hold that patients should be informed that their therapy will be selected randomly. While we have chosen some rather dramatic cases to illustrate the relevance of personal values and preferences, we consider it likely that such values and preferences will affect the relevance of many characteristics of RCTs.

NOTES

1. H. Atkins, J. L. Hayward, D. J. Klugman, and A. B. Wayte, "Treatment of Early Breast Cancer: a Report after Ten Years of a Clinical Trial," *British Medical Journal,* vol. 2, p. 423, 1972.

2. P. V. Cardon, F. W. Dommel, Jr., and R. R. Trumble, "Injuries to Research Subjects," *New England Journal of Medicine,* vol. 295, p. 650, 1976.

3. T. C. Chalmers, "The Ethics of Randomization as a Decision Making Technique and the Problem of Informed Consent," in USDHEW Report of the 14th Annual Conference of Cardiovascular Training Grant Program Directors. Bethesda, Md., 1967. National Heart Institute. (As cited by Fried, below, note 9.)

4. Code of Federal Regulations, 21 CFR 310, revised as of March 29, 1974.

5. Code of Federal Regulations, 45 CFR 46, revised as of April 1, 1977.

6. J. L. Coulehan, S. Eberhard, L. Kapner, F. Taylor, K. Rogers, and P. Garry, "Vitamin C and Acute Illness in Navajo School Children," *New England Journal of Medicine,* vol. 295, p. 973, 1976.

7. DHEW Secretary's Task Force on the Compensation of Injured Research Subjects, DHEW Publication OS-77-003, Washington, D.C., 1977.

8. A. R. Feinstein, "Clinical Biostatistics. XXVI. Medical Ethics and the Architecture of Clinical Research," *Clinical Pharmacology and Therapeutics,* vol. 15, p. 316, 1974.

9. C. Fried, *Medical Experimentation: Personal Integrity and Social Policy,* North-Holland Publishing Co., Amsterdam, 1974.

10. H. Jonas, "Philosophical Reflections on Experimenting with Human Subjects," in P. A. Freund, (ed.), *Experimentation with Human Subjects,* p. 1, Braziller, New York, 1970.

11. L. Lasagna, "Drug Evaluation Problems in Academic and Other Contexts," *Annals of the New York Academy of Science,* vol. 169, p. 503, 1970.

12. K. Lebacqz, "Ethical Issues in Psychopharmacological Research," in D. M. Gallant, and R. Force (eds.), *Ethical and Legal Issues in Psychopharmacologic Research and Treatment,* p. 113,

Raven Press, New York, 1978.

13. K. Lebacqz, "Reflections on the Report and Recommendations of the National Commission: Research on the Fetus," *Villanova Law Review*, vol. 22, p. 357, 1977.

14. K. Lebacqz, "The National Commission and Research in Pharmacology: An Overview," *Federation Proceedings*, vol. 36, p. 2344, 1977.

15. K. Lebacqz, and R. J. Levine, "Respect for Persons and Informed Consent to Participate in Research," *Clinical Research*, vol. 25, p. 101, 1977.

16. R. J. Levine, "Appropriate Guidelines for the Selection of Human Subjects for Participation in Biomedical and Behavioral Research," prepared for the National Commission for the Protection of Human Subjects of Biomedical and Behavioral Research, 1976.

17. R. J. Levine, "Guidelines for Negotiating Informed Consent with Prospective Human Subjects of Experimentation," *Clinical Research*, vol. 22, p. 42, 1974.

18. R. J. Levine, "Informed Consent to Participate in Research" (in 2 parts), *Bioethics Digest*, vol. 1, no. 11. p. 1; no. 12, p. 1, 1977.

19. R. J. Levine, "Nondevelopmental Research on Human Subjects: The Impact of the Recommendations of the National Commission," *Federation Proceedings*, vol. 36, p. 2359, 1977.

20. R. J. Levine, "The Impact of Fetal Research of the Report of the National Commission for the Protection of Human Subjects of Biomedical and Behavioral Research, *Villanova Law Review*, vol. 22, p. 367, 1977.

21. R. J. Levine, "The Role of Assessment of Risk-Benefit Criteria in the Determination of the Appropriateness of Research Involving Human Subjects," *Bioethics Digest*, vol. 1, p. 1, 1976.

22. R. A. McCormick, "Proxy Consent in the Experimentation Situation," *Perspectives in Biology and Medicine*, vol. 18, p. 2, 1974.

23. P. Ramsey, *The Patient as Person*, Yale University Press, New Haven, 1970.

24. J. Rawls, *A Theory of Justice*, Harvard University Press, Cambridge, Mass., 1971.

25. S. J. Reiser, A. J. Dyck, and W. J. Curran, *Ethics in Medicine: Historical Perspectives and Contemporary Concerns*, MIT Press, Cambridge, Mass., 1977.

26. D. D. Rutstein, "The Ethical Design of Human Experiments," in P. A. Freund (ed.), *Experimentation with Human Subjects*, Braziller, New York, 1970.

27. L. W. Shaw, and T. C. Chalmers, "Ethics in Cooperative Clinical Trials," *Annals of the New York Academy of Science*, vol. 169, p. 487, 1970.

28. The National Commission for the Protection of Human Subjects of Biomedical and Behavioral Research, "Identification of Basic Ethical Principles," Draft of June 3, 1976.

29. The National Commission for the Protection of Human Subjects of Biomedical and Behavioral Research, "Research Involving Children," Washington, D.C., 1977, DHEW Publication No. (OS) 77–0004.

30. The National Commission for the Protection of Human Subjects of Biomedical and Behavioral Research, "Research Involving Prisoners," Washington, D.C., 1976, DHEW Publication No. (OS) 76–131.

31. The National Commission for the Protection of Human Subjects of Biomedical and Behavioral Research, "The Boundaries between Biomedical and Behavioral Research and Accepted and Routine Practice," Draft of February 24, 1976.

32. Veterans Administration Cooperative Study Group on Antihypertensive Agents," Effects of Treatment on Morbidity in Hypertension," *Journal of the American Medical Association*, vol. 213, p. 1143, 1970.

33. H. Zeisel, "Reducing the Hazards of Human Experiments through Modifications in Research Design," *Annals of the New York Academy of Science*, vol. 169, p. 475, 1970.

101.

Are Uncontrolled Clinical Studies Ever Justified?

Henry Sacks   Sherman Kupfer   Thomas C. Chalmers and Others

Henry Sacks, Sherman Kupfer, Thomas C. Chalmers

To the Editor: The publication in the June 5 and 19 issues of two therapeutic studies, by Antman and Dzau and their colleagues, that lack control groups raises serious questions about the conduct of such trials. Both articles are written as though they provided strong evidence for the effectiveness of a new drug for a life-threatening condition but in fact both are collections of anecdotal experience, uncontrolled and unblinded. Both papers acknowledge this important defect with a line or two in the Discussion, but obviously neither the investigators nor the reviewers thought that the conclusions were compromised. The use of controls is a basic principle of scientific inquiry; in fact, just one year earlier, the *Journal* published a history of the placebo effect in one of the conditions (angina), which clearly documented the danger in relying on uncontrolled observations.[1]

Publication of such studies may create problems for other investigators and their patients. If they are convinced by these articles of the effectiveness of the drugs, can they ethically do blinded and randomized trials, as was called for in an accompanying editorial,[2] when to do so would mean withholding a "proved" drug from a patient with a life-threatening disease?

Why were these studies approved by human-experimentation committees at major centers? Good experimental design is the sine qua non of ethical research in human beings. The Food and Drug Administration recognizes this necessity when it includes in the proposed rules for human research the requirement that "the research methods are appropriate to the objectives of the research and the field of study."[3] To us, such a statement implies that human-research review committees should ensure that adequate controls are included when sick patients are placed at risk in the investigation of new drugs.

NOTES

1. H. Benson, and D. P. McCallie, Jr., "Angina Pectoris and the Placebo Effect," *New England Journal of Medicine*, vol. 300, p. 1424, 1979.
2. J. N. Cohn, "Progress in Vasodilator Therapy for Heart Failure," *New England Journal of Medicine*, vol. 302, p. 1414, 1980.
3. "Proposed Regulations Amending Basic HEW Policy for Protection of Human Research Subjects," *Federal Register*, vol. 44, p. 47688, 1979.

The above letter was referred to the authors of the articles in question, three of whom offer the following reply (Antman et al. replied to a similar letter in the issue of October 16):

Norman K. Hollenberg, Victor J. Dzau, Gordon H. Williams

To the Editor: The letter from Sacks et al. raises not one issue but two. Should open, uncontrolled clinical trials be performed? If so, should the results be published?

When the possibility of a new therapy is raised, it is necessary to perform a preliminary study. Because of the enormous cost and demands of large, controlled clinical trials, some preliminary evidence of efficacy is mandatory. In the absence of such information, the necessary referral of patients for the study is unlikely. How can one encourage a patient to enter a controlled study unless at least some preliminary indication of efficacy is available? Without the encouragement provided by such preliminary evidence, the resources required for a large, controlled clinical trial simply cannot be mobilized.

The second question is, When should the results of such trials be published? The answer is not straightforward. Perhaps the stance adopted by Sacks et al.—Never publish such observations because they cannot prove efficacy—is reasonable. On the other hand, on occasion one sees such dramatic evidence of therapeutic benefit that it seems reasonable to provide this preliminary information to the medical community. Indeed, one may feel an obligation to present the information, not as final evidence—which clearly requires a controlled clinical trial—but rather as an indication that patients who fall into the category under study may benefit.

The promising results in our initial trial have made it possible for us to undertake a controlled clinical trial, which is now under way. We expect the trial will require two years. Should we have waited the two years before providing the medical community with some notion of the efficacy of the drug? We think not. How dramatic and compelling should the results be to merit publication? To that, we find no easy answer.

102.
Dilemma in Cancer Treatment   Gina Bari Kolata

Nearly every current list of curable cancers includes osteogenic sarcoma. This cancer of the long bones of the arm and leg primarily strikes teenagers, and, until recently, its prognosis was dismal. In the 1960s, virtually everyone who got the disease died within 2 years. Now as many as 50 percent of those whose cancer has not spread at the time of diagnosis are cured, and as many as 70 percent of all patients live 2 years.

Whenever such a dramatic change in cancer survival rates occurs, the question is, why? Most pediatric oncologists used to think they knew the answer, but now many are not so sure. As a result, they are confessing that they no longer know how to treat their osteogenic sarcoma patients.

The conventional wisdom has been that adjuvant chemotherapy, which is chemotherapy given to patients with no evidence of metastasis at the time of diagnosis, helps cure osteogenic sarcoma patients. The idea is that the treatment destroys micrometasta-ses—tiny foci of cancer that cannot be visually detected. Adjuvant chemotherapy is thought to make metastases less likely to develop and, if they do, less numerous and easier to treat. The chemotherapy is always preceded by removal of the cancerous bone.

Prior to the 1970s osteogenic sarcoma patients were treated with surgery alone. Adjuvant chemotherapy was not given because there was no reason to believe that it would help. Those who already had metastases at the time of diagnosis often were not treated at all—their situation was considered hopeless. The prognosis for these patients is still not particularly good, although now they are given chemotherapy and their metastases (which nearly always occur in the lungs) are surgically removed. But these patients often are not cured. The crucial step in curing osteogenic sarcoma, members of the medical community believe, is in preventing it from spreading through the body—which adjuvant chemotherapy was said to do. This chemo-

Source: *Science*, vol. 209, August 15, 1980.

therapy was thought to have been a key factor in the difference between the survival rates for the 1960s and those for the 1970s.

Yet all along there were those who doubted that the case for adjuvant chemotherapy was established. A few investigators, primarily at the Mayo Clinic and the National Cancer Institute (NCI), were suspicious that, because of changes in diagnostic techniques, the pre-1970 patients could not fairly be compared with patients today. Thus, it was felt, the comparisons in survival rates that established the usefulness of adjuvant chemotherapy might be misleading. Perhaps, they said, adjuvant chemotherapy really is not helpful in treating osteogenic sarcoma. The method is toxic and very expensive; it would be of grave concern if it were given needlessly. Until recently, however, the skeptics were given short shrift. "The desire to believe in progress in cancer treatments is so profound that people don't want to hear the disbelievers," says Arthur Levine, who heads the pediatric oncology branch at the NCI.

The story of how adjuvant chemotherapy became an accepted treatment for osteogenic sarcoma and why it is now being questioned illustrates statisticians' worst fears about the use of historical control groups in clinical medicine. It also illustrates the agonizing dilemmas that can occur when doubts are raised about an apparently successful treatment. These dilemmas are commonplace, says Vincent DeVita, acting director of the NCI, and they arise nearly every time there appears to be progress in cancer treatment. Frequently, it is not clear which of several factors is responsible for the encouraging results.

Because osteogenic sarcoma had such a grim prognosis in the 1960s, medical researchers began trying one chemotherapeutic agent after another in an attempt to destroy lung metastases. Nothing worked. Then, in the early 1970s, two new chemotherapeutic agents were tried—adriamycin and high doses of methotrexate. Initial reports were that as many as 80 percent of the patients with metastatic disease responded.

Oncologists were ecstatic over these results. "Everyone went bananas," says Herbert Ableson of Harvard's Sidney Farber Cancer Center. But, as more patients were given this chemotherapy, it became clear that really only a small percentage respond, and then only temporarily.

Caught up on the initial wave of excitement over adriamycin and high-dose methotrexate, James Holland at Mount Sinai Medical Center and, independently, Norman Jaffee, now at the M. D. Anderson Cancer Center in Houston, together with Emil Frei of the Sidney Farber Cancer Center tried using these same chemotherapeutic agents *before* the disease had obviously spread. In 1974, the two groups reported that about 50 percent of patients who had no evidence of metastases and who were treated with adriamycin or high-dose methotrexate lived disease-free for 2 years after their disease was diagnosed. In contrast, only 20 percent of the 1960 patients with no evidence of metastases at the time of diagnosis lived 2 years.

Since 1974, adjuvant chemotherapy has been given in increasingly higher doses. A variety of chemotherapeutic agents has been tried, alone and in combination, but still the most commonly used ones are adriamycin and high-dose methotrexate. Since methotrexate, a folic acid antagonist that prevents DNA synthesis, is extremely toxic when given in high doses, it must be followed by calcium leucovorin, a folic acid analog that allows normal cells to survive. Both methotrexate and adriamycin cause vomiting and hair loss and both can also have more serious side effects. For example, adriamycin can damage the heart, leading to a form of congestive heart failure. There is a maximum cumulative dose of the drug that patients can tolerate in their lifetime.

At the same time as adjuvant chemotherapy was becoming popular, diagnostic techniques were changing. In the 1960s, physicians used chest x-rays to look for metastases. In the 1970s, they switched to the more sensitive technique of chest tomograms, which are x-ray slices of the chest. More recently, a number of medical centers have begun using the even more sensitive technique of computer-assisted tomography.

These changes in diagnostic technique put a question mark over the use of historical control groups. There is a real danger that many of the 1960 patients who were supposed to have been free of metastases might actually have had metastatic disease by 1970 criteria.

Among those who raised these questions about the patient comparisons were investigators at the Mayo Clinic. In 1976 they asked for and received funds from the NCI to conduct a randomized controlled trial comparing adjuvant chemotherapy plus amputation to amputation alone for patients with no visible metastases at the time of diagnosis. The investigators felt that such a trial was warranted for theoretical reasons and because they had just reviewed their data on the survival rates of patients with osteogenic sarcoma. The results were illuminating.

Between 1963 and 1972, they found, the survival of patients at the clinic who had no metastases at the time of diagnosis and who were treated with amputation alone was typical of that at other institutions—about 25 percent lived 2 years after the disease was diagnosed. But from 1972 to mid-1974, the 2-year disease-free survival rate had increased to 50 percent, typical of the rate claimed for patients given adjuvant chemotherapy, even though most of the Mayo Clinic patients had not been given this chemotherapy. "The survival of patients treated with surgery alone is excellent and is getting better all the time," says William Taylor, a Mayo Clinic statistician.

There is no obvious explanation for the Mayo Clinic's experience. "When I look at the data, the dominant variable is still time," Taylor remarks. Other institutions cannot do a similar analysis of survival rates, since they have given patients adjuvant chemotherapy for nearly a decade.

Although the more sensitive diagnostic techniques for detecting lung metastases could have contributed to the improved survival rates of Mayo Clinic patients, it is not yet clear just how many patients with metastatic disease who are now being screened out of study groups would previously have been included. Steven Rosenberg, chief of surgery at the NCI, says that 4 of 11 osteogenic sarcoma patients who had normal chest x-rays were found to have metastatic disease upon referral to the NCI. John Muhm and Douglas Pritchard of the Mayo Clinic report that 20 percent of their patients who have no metastases detectable with chest x-rays have metastases detectable with CAT scans and that 15 percent of patients with no metastases detectable with tomograms have visible metastases when given CAT scans. On the other hand, Jaffee finds that tomograms detect only an additional 3 percent of patients with metastases. "I don't think screening methods make a difference," he says.

Even the Mayo Clinic patients who relapsed, however, seemed to live longer in the 1970s than in the 1960s. The improved survival times obviously were not due to adjuvant chemotherapy, but may have occurred because surgeons in the 1970s began removing lung metastases. They discovered that this process seemed to prevent further relapses. Devita recalls that in the days before this surgery was tried, "I used to go on the wards and see the osteogenic sarcoma patients. Anyone with metastatic disease was considered gone." Surgeons began removing lung metastases, DeVita says, because the patients were young, their situation seemed hopeless, and the surgeons were anxious to do something to help them. No one expected the surgery to do much good. "It was contrary to the theory of metastatic disease," DeVita explains. Physicians generally believe that once a cancer has spread, the visible metastases are only part of the cancer. Microscopic metastases are also thought to be present and these cannot be removed.

Another possible reason for the improved survival rates is that the patient referral patterns changed in the 1970s. The 1960 patients, DeVita explains, "probably reflected a smaller proportion of patients. The minute there was excitement about adjuvant chemotherapy, more patients were referred [to major medical centers]. This always happens when you make some progress." It is conceivable that before the excitement over adjuvant chemotherapy, most of the patients referred to major medical centers were those with the worst prognoses.

These possible explanations of the Mayo Clinic's finding that the clinic patients treated without adjuvant chemotherapy seemed to do well were reasons to conduct a randomized controlled trial, in the opinion of a number of medical investigators. But the Mayo Clinic's trial was not well accepted by many physicians who believed in adjuvant chemotherapy and thought the trial unethical. The Mayo Clinic physicians had great difficulty recruiting patients for their randomized controlled trial. They ended up with only 37 patients, which is less than half the number referred to the clinic and asked to participate.

Some patients, explains John Edmonson, who conducted the Mayo Clinic trial, declined to participate because they decided they definitely wanted chemotherapy. Often these patients were swayed by their personal physicians, who told them that all major medical centers except the Mayo Clinic believe in adjuvant chemotherapy for osteogenic sarcoma. Other patients did not participate because, after being told by the Mayo Clinic investigators that there was some question about whether adjuvant chemotherapy works, that the therapy is toxic, and that they would have to come to the clinic every 3 weeks for 1 year and spend 3 to 5 days there each time, the patients decided that they would rather take their chances without chemotherapy.

The trial went ahead anyway, and Edmonson presented preliminary results at the end of May at a meeting of the American Society of Clinical Oncology. More than half the trial's patients, he reported, were continuously disease-free 2 years after surgery, and 75 percent survived 2 years. There was no difference between the treatment groups in time to first metastasis, and there was no difference between the groups in number of metastatic nodules appearing at relapse. Still, 37 patients is a very small number. "These results cry out for corroboration," Taylor says.

The Mayo Clinic results, however, have not been enthusiastically embraced by all oncologists. "We hurt a lot of people's feelings. This is not something people take lightly," said Edmonson. Others, however, say it is not that their feelings are hurt. Rather, they remain unconvinced by this trial. First, they say that only the Mayo Clinic reports such good survival data for patients not given adjuvant chemotherapy. "What is different about the Mayo Clinic population?" asks Charles Pratt of St. Jude's Hospital in Memphis. He points out that the patients are mostly white, middle- or upper-middle-class, and may receive treatment earlier in the course of the disease than poorer patients from urban areas or the rural South.

Abelson points out that it is hard to draw conclusions about a trial consisting of only 37 patients. This is not to fault the Mayo Clinic—only about 1000 people in this country develop osteogenic sarcoma each year. But in order to detect a 20 percent difference in survival between two groups, a trial would have to include at least 180 patients, according to Abelson. Even then, he says, there would still be a 5 percent chance of a false negative. "It is patently impossible for a single institution to do [an appropriately sized] study. It's almost mandatory to do a multi-institutional trial."

The NCI has been trying for several years to interest other institutions in joining it in a controlled trial of adjuvant chemotherapy in osteogenic sarcoma. Until very recently, it has had no success. Following the announcement of the Mayo Clinic results, however, six institutions are willing to consider joining the NCI in such a trial, Levine says. Abelson, who is among those now interested in a controlled trial, explains that he believes a trial is warranted because "the historical control problem is so substantial and the issues raised are so provocative." Others, as would be expected, believe so strongly in adjuvant chemotherapy that they feel ethically constrained from participating in such a trial. "I would not like my patients entered in such a trial," says Jaffee.

General Legal Principles Applied to Medical Experimentation
Charles Fried

At the outset we must distinguish between therapeutic and nontherapeutic experimentation. Experimentation is clearly nontherapeutic when it is carried out on a person solely to obtain information of use to others, and in no way to treat some illness that the experimental subject might have. Experimentation is therapeutic when a therapy is tried with the sole view of determining the best way of treating that patient. There is a sense, as a number of commentators have observed, in which so far as there is more or less uncertainty about the best way to proceed in the patient's case, treatment is often experimental. Also what is learned in treating one patient will be of use in treating others. This may be so, but it in no way obscures the distinction between therapeutic and nontherapeutic research, since therapeutic research is carried out only and only so far as that subject's interests require. Any benefits to others are incidental to this dominant goal. These are the clear cases at the extreme.

There are in practice large numbers of gradations in between. Much research is mainly therapeutic, in the sense that the patients' interests are foremost, but nevertheless things may be done which are not dictated solely by the need to treat that patient: tests may be continued even after all the information needed to determine the best treatment of the particular patient has already been gathered; or substances may be injected for a period or in doses not strictly necessary for the cure of that patient, but with the motive of developing information of use to others. Moving in from the clear case at the other extreme, that of nontherapeutic research, it must be recognized that persons who become research subjects in nontherapeutic experimentation may often be the beneficiaries of a degree of medical attention which they might not otherwise enjoy, and which thus redounds to their benefit. And there are all possible degrees and gradations in between.

Nontherapeutic Experimentation

No special doctrines apply to nontherapeutic experimentation. Indeed, to the extent that the experimentation is nontherapeutic, the fact that it is being carried out by doctors should be entirely irrelevant. The usual privileges under which doctors work, and the usual special doctrines according to which the liabilities of doctors are judged, should not be applicable, since they proceed from the premise that the doctor must be given considerable latitude as he works in the presumed interests of his patient. But that is not the case in nontherapeutic research. The doctor confronts his subject simply as a scientist.

In general, the law imposes a strict duty of disclosure, wherever an individual with a great deal to lose is exposed to a risk or is asked to relinquish rights by someone with considerably greater knowledge. And this is true, whether the relation is one of buyer and seller or involves some public interest. Persons selling cosmetics, automobiles, or pharmaceuticals are required to make full disclosures of all the hazards involved in the products they sell. But policemen seeking damaging admissions from suspects are also required to issue a warning of constitutional rights and to offer legal assistance before those rights are waived. There is no reason why the case should be any different where a researcher asks an experimental subject to risk his health.

Indeed the case might be made that the

Source: Charles Fried, *Medical Experimentation: Personal Integrity and Social Policy,* American Elsevier Publishing Co., New York, 1974.

developing doctrines of strict liability would argue for the imposition of liability without fault, and regardless of disclosures for harm occasioned in the course of nontherapeutic experimentation. In general, it is coming to be believed that those who are in a better position to appreciate the risks of a course of conduct, who are in a better position to ensure against those risks or otherwise spread their cost to the broadest group of beneficiaries, and finally whose responsible decisions in evaluating the propriety of the risks we can influence by imposing upon them the costs of those decisions, should be strictly liable (that is liable without fault) for the risks that their conduct imposes. These conditions are amply met in the case of nontherapeutic experimentation. Finally, if the financial pressures of caring for and compensating subjects injured in nontherapeutic experiments meant that experimenters exercised greater caution and carefully evaluated the benefits to be expected from the research, this would be a highly desirable consequence. It is for this reason that a number of commentators have suggested either strict liability for nontherapeutic experimentation or some form of compulsory medical experimentation insurance. In either case the experimental subject would be assured of proper medical care as well as compensatory payments for any injuries he suffers in the experiment. Since most subjects of nontherapeutic experimentation are either idealistic persons for whom the small amounts of compensation are not a significant inducement, or disadvantaged persons for whom the small compensation acts as an all too significant inducement, this added responsibility would seem fair and appropriate.

Therapeutic Experimentation

Legal decisions and commentators have always stated that a practitioner is only justified in using "accepted remedies," unless his patient specifically consents to the use of an "experimental" remedy. This statement has seemed reactionary and unreasonable to doctors, but if one puts it in the context of

general doctrine one might say that its teeth are quite effectively drawn. General principles require the consent of the patient to any therapy, usual or unusual. It is just that as the therapy moves away from the standard and accepted, the need for explicit consent, full disclosure of risks and alternatives, becomes more acute, and more likely to pose an issue. The doctor who prescribes an accepted remedy, under the principles set forth so far, might have a good defense to the claim that he should have told his client about alternative, untried, or experimental remedies.

The obligation to advise the patient of alternative therapies does not extend to all the hypothetical, untried, or experimental remedies that various researchers are in the process of developing. Where, however, the therapy used is in itself experimental, this fact and the existence of either alternatives or professional doubts become material facts, which like all material facts should be disclosed. Beyond this, where the experimentation is truly and exclusively therapeutic, there are no particular legal constraints that do not apply to the practice of medicine generally.[1] It is simply that the implication of those general doctrines may take on a special coloring in this context.

Mixed Therapeutic and Nontherapeutic Research: the Problem of the Randomized Clinical Trial

The kind of medical experimentation which causes the greatest legal and ethical perplexities is what might be called mixed therapeutic and nontherapeutic experimentation: The patient is indeed being treated for a particular illness, and a serious effort is being made to cure him. The systems of treatment, however, are not chosen solely with the view to curing the particular patient of his particular ills. Rather, the treatment takes place in the context of an experiment or a research program to test new procedures or to compare the efficacy of various established procedures. Nor is it the case that this research purpose is limited to carefully reporting the results of treatments in particular cases. Rather, therapies are tried, continued, or varied, and patients are assigned to treatment categories partially in response to the needs of the research design, i.e., not exclusively by considering the particular patient's needs at the particular time. Usually it will be the case that there is genuine doubt about which is the best treatment, or the best treatment modality, so that the doctors participating in the experiment do not believe they are compromising the interests of their patients. Or where this is not completely true, it is often the case that no serious or irreversible harms or risk are imposed in pursuing the research design rather than pursuing single-mindedly the interests of the particular patient. The clearest case, and the one which is the focus of our concern in this essay, is the randomized clinical trial (RCT), in which patients are assigned to treatment categories by some randomizing device, with the thought that in this way any bias of the experimenter and any unsuspected interfering factor can be eliminated by the statistical method used. And generally it is said that the alternative therapies between which patients are randomized both have a great deal to recommend them, so that there is no real sense in which one or the other group is being deliberately disadvantaged—at least until the results of the experiments are in. [2]

What is the legal status of experimentation having both therapeutic and nontherapeutic aspects? Since there is a general obligation to obtain consent to a therapy, and since that obligation becomes more exigent as the treatment to be used departs from the ordinary and the accepted, there is at least the legal obligation to obtain consent for the use of the treatment contemplated, with full disclosure of the expected benefits and hazards. This much is straightforward, and not peculiar to the area of mixed therapeutic and nontherapeutic experimentation and RCTs. Moreover, as we have seen, a number of courts have insisted that the disclosure made in obtaining consent include a disclosure of the existence and characteristics of alternative therapies. Certainly if the therapy proposed is experimental in the sense of innovative, this fact along with some description of more traditional alternatives should be part of the disclosure.

The crucial question, and one as to which there is no decided case, asks whether it is also necessary to disclose first that an experiment is being conducted, and second and more delicately the nature of the experiment and the experimental design.

Specifically, in the case of the RCT must the doctor disclose the fact that the patient's therapy will be determined by a randomizing procedure rather than by an individualized judgment on the part of the physician? Some physicians active in mixed therapeutic and nontherapeutic experimentation have argued that it is both unnecessary and undesirable to make this last disclosure: It is undesirable because some patients might be scared off, withdraw from the experiment, and seek help elsewhere. It is also undesirable because of those patients who, while remaining in the experiment, might be caused such a degree of distress and anxiety that it would interfere with their cure. The disclosure of randomization is argued to be unnecessary since the medical evidence regarding the alternative treatments will often be evenly balanced (that is why the experiment is being conducted—to help resolve the doubts) so that it is in no way inaccurate to tell the patient that medical opinion is divided on the best therapy, and that the patient will receive the best available therapy according to current medical judgments. To tell the patient that he is being randomized, on this view, would add nothing of relevance regarding the expected outcome of his treatment, and thus nothing of relevance to his choice whether or not to consent to the treatment.

There are no authoritative decisions holding that consent in the absence of a disclosure that the patient is being randomized or that his treatment is being determined by reference to factors other than his individual concerns is invalid consent because of incomplete disclosure. The general principle holds that a person must be given all material information relating to the proposed therapy. But is the fact of randomization, or of the existence of an experiment such material information? The information would seem to deal rather with the way in which the therapy is chosen than with the characteristics of the therapy itself. Nevertheless, it would seem that most patients would consider the information regarding the choice of mechanism as highly relevant, and would feel that they had been "had" upon discovering that they had received or not received surgery because of a number in a random number table. But does this sentiment create a duty; does it mean, for instance, that consent to the treatment was ineffective and the participating doctors are guilty of a battery?

Though there is no authoritative decision to point to, there are analogies from other areas of law which would suggest that full candid disclosure should include disclosure of randomization. The very fact that the doctor acts in the dual capacity of therapist and researcher, and that his role as researcher to some degree does or may influence his decisions as a therapist, would argue that the fullest disclosure of all circumstances relating to that dual role, and to the basis on which functions are exercised and decisions made, would be required. If the relation were not that of doctor and patient, but of lawyer and client, or of trustee and beneficiary of a trust fund, or of a director or officer of a corporation and the corporation, there would be a strict duty to disclose the existence of any interest which the fiduciary has that may conflict with or influence the exercise of his functions in his fiduciary capacity. The fiduciary owes a duty of strict and unreserved loyalty to his client.

Imagine the case of a lawyer for a public defender organization who has agreed to participate in a foundation-sponsored research project on sentencing. As part of the research protocol his decision as to whether to plead certain categories of offenders guilty or to go to trial is determined at random. This is intended to discover how that decision affects the eventual outcome of the case at the time of sentencing and parole. His clients are not told that this is how the lawyer's "advice" as to plea is determined.[3]

The law of conflict of interests and of fiduciary relations clearly provides that the fiduciary may not pursue activities that either do in fact conflict with the exercise of his judgment as a fiduciary, or might conflict with or influence the exercise of his judgment, or might appear to do so, without the explicit consent of his client. And if the consent is obtained other than on the basis of the fullest disclosure of all facts not only which the fiduciary deems relevant but which he knows his client might consider relevant, the disclosure is incomplete, the consent is fraudulently obtained, and the fiduciary is in breach of his fiduciary relationship. There is no reason why the doctor should not be held to be in a fiduciary relationship to his patient, and therefore why the same fiduciary obligations that obtain for a lawyer, a money manager, a corporation executive or director should not obtain for a doctor.

However the issue of informing patients of the fact of randomization might be resolved, it would seem that there is a continuing duty on the part of the patient's physician to inform himself about the progress of the experiment and to inform his patient about any significant new information coming out of the experiment that might bear on the patient's choice to remain in the study or to seek other types of therapy. This is an important issue in RCTs involving long-term courses of treatment. If patients abandon one alternative on the basis of early, inconclusive results, no definitive conclusion can be drawn from the trial. Failure to make continuing disclosures and to offer continuing options to the patient in the light of developing information may not constitute the tort of battery, however, since there may be no physical contact requiring a new consent. The wrong which is done to the patient would be in the nature of negligent practice, and as to that the determinative standard is the standard of practice of a respected segment of the profession. The physician who does not keep his patient continuously informed may argue that to do so would interfere with the experiment, and he might find experts to testify that such continuing disclosure in the course of an experiment is not thought to be good practice. The argument should not be accepted uncritically, since the practice which the doctor in the case of an RCT would refer to would not be traditional therapeutic practice, but rather the practice of experimentation itself. Indeed it would seem that the doctrine of the case, holding that a physician had a duty to inform his patient that his broken leg was not healing properly and that there was another method of treatment available in a nearby city which was more likely to result in cure, is equally applicable to the case of a participant in an RCT who has been assigned to a treatment category which, as the experiment progresses and the data come in, appears to be the less successful treatment. Nor would the device by which only a supervising committee and not the patient's physician has access to the results of the experiment for a determined period of time insulate the physician from the consequences of this doctrine.

NOTES

1. There may come a point, of course,where the procedure is so risky, the benefits so uncertain, and the basis of the treatment so speculative that to use it even with consent is tantamount to unprofessional conduct and quackery. The vagueness of the boundary is, of course, a cause for disquiet for practitioners working with new therapies.

2. Thus, for instance, in a major RCT of the efficacy of simple as compared with radical mastectomy for cancer of the breast, Sir John Bruce writes: "One of the important ethical necessities before a random clinical is undertaken is a near certainty that none of the treatment options is likely to be so much inferior that harm could accrue to those allocated to it. In the present instance . . . it looked as if the mode of primary treatment made no significant difference, at least in terms of survival." "Operable Cancer of the Breast—A Controlled Clinical Trial," *Cancer*, vol. 28, p. 1443, 1971.

3. Professor Paul Freund has suggested that it would be improper for a judge to randomize in sentencing (*New England Journal of Medicine*, vol. 273, p. 657, 1965). Whatever the objection to this may be, it is quite different from the objectionts I raise in my hypothetical cases or in medical practice. The convicted criminal is not the client of the judge and the judge does not owe him an undivided duty of loyalty. Indeed it is his job to consider social interests in sentencing the individual, and the randomized experiment may be a way of doing this.

104.

The Ethics of Randomization as a Decision-Making Technique, and the Problem of Informed Consent
Thomas C. Chalmers

"Do no harm while nature heals" was the motto of my father, who practiced medicine at the end of the nineteenth and early part of the twentieth century. This was a relatively easy course for him to follow in those days when the only effective medicines were digitalis and morphine, and life-threatening treatments such as major surgery were just beginning to be used. Nowadays the busy physician makes several decisions a week which are critical to the life and health of his

patient. Whether alone or with consultations, he makes these decisions by means of so-called clinical judgment, a subtle distillation of his personal experience and the knowledge that he has been able to glean from the medical literature.

The major danger in basing action on personal experience is the unavoidable excess influence of the most recent experience. The last case or two, especially if dramatically successful or unsuccessful, cannot help but

Source: *Report of the Fourteenth Conference of Cardiovascular Training Grant Program Directors, National Heart Institute*, U.S. Department of Health, Education, and Welfare, Washington, D.C., 1967.

have more influence on the next decision than those cases encountered in the more distant past. As an aside I should like to suggest that the older clinician is the more able decision maker not only because he has had more experience, but also because a growing defect in memory for recent events allows him to give a more equal weight to his experiences, no matter when they occurred.

The second important component of clinical judgment is a knowledge of the medical literature, both basic and clinical. Unfortunately basic research has, almost by definition, little immediate application to the treatment of patients. The practicing physician must be able to evaluate and rely on the clinical medicine literature when he treats patients, and he must be ready to defend his decisions by referring to the articles written by his peers or to his own research experience. When the treatment is symptomatic, it probably makes little difference what the physician does. The potent factor is his interest in his patient. However, when the treatment is life-threatening, as with major surgery or other drastic regimens, then the physician and his patient are in trouble because the clinical literature is so notoriously unscientific. By this I mean that the conclusions of the authors are seldom borne out by the data. Less than 20 percent of the clinical trials reported in the medical literature are controlled, and unfortunately the more drastic and dangerous the therapy the less are controls employed. The major defect in most reports of new therapies is the complete inability of the author or the reader to separate out the effects of the treatment under study from the effects of selection of patients for that treatment. In addition, the physician attempting to decide about life-threatening therapies rarely considers another important selection factor, the multiple variables that determine whether a series of patients is written up or not, and whether a paper is accepted for publication or not. So the final reported series may represent a very small and unidentifiable subgroup of the total number of patients presenting with the disorder un-

der study, and it is next to impossible to apply that information correctly in making decisions about individual members of the total population with that disease.

It is clear by now that I am trying to develop a case for the controlled clinical trial in the initial investigation of a life-threatening therapy. A carefully constructed protocol will contain a randomization procedure by which clearly defined patients are assigned to the new or conventional therapy. In that case the relative efficacy of the new treatment and the population to which it can be applied can be clearly determined. If the new treatment turns out to be best, the patients assigned to that will have been the lucky ones. If the new treatment is comparatively bad, the controls will be the lucky ones. In either case, the patients will be carefully treated and may thus do better than those who are not studied at all.

From the scientific standpoint, there is no doubt about the need for controlled trials of all new procedures which may on the average be more harmful than helpful. Yet in the last 30 years any number of new procedures have been introduced, only to be discarded or modified many years later when the slow process of individual clinical experience suggested that they were actually dangerous, or at least not as effective as the original proponents had thought. It is unlikely that total ignorance of scientific methodology is the reason for the great scarcity of well-controlled trials of new therapies in clinical medicine. It is more likely that those who introduced and publicized the new methods felt that it was unethical to withhold the possibility of benefit from any available patients, and that they certainly had to decide who was suitable for the operation according to their best clinical judgment rather than according to some very undoctorlike randomization procedure. To me it seems clear that to randomize patients into a group receiving the new therapy being evaluated, and a group receiving the standard therapy, whether it be a similar treatment or no treatment, depending on what is currently accepted for the disease, is much more ethical and is much more in the interest of the individual patients than is treatment of consecutive selected patients as if the new therapy had already been established; or conversely, the withholding of a new therapy from a group of patients as if it had already been proved to be ineffective.

Three problems remain to be discussed with regard to this discussion of randomization: when to start, what to tell the patients, and when to stop.

One often hears experienced clinical investigators insist that a randomized controlled trial should never be started until the techniques of the new therapy have been worked out in a preliminary group of patients. I am convinced that from the ethical standpoint this is very dangerous reasoning. New therapeutic procedures are always changed and are usually improved by experience with the first few patients. However, it is extremely difficult for the investigators not to acquire enthusiasm, or the opposite emotional response, when they have tried out the new therapy in a consecutive series of patients. If they have worked out a good dosage regimen or what they consider an effective operative procedure, they are almost by definition convinced that the new treatment has enough merit so that they cannot ethically deprive a control group from receiving it. Or they might prematurely discard a new treatment because of poor results, when in fact a randomized control group might have done much worse. So I believe that it is important to randomize from the very first patient not only to protect future patients but also to protect the first patients, who should have a chance to fall into the control group when the new treatment may well be ineffective because of the inexperience of the person who is applying it. The control patient can always be removed from that group and placed in the experimental group if and when the new treatment seems to be superior to the old.

The second problem has to do with the obtaining of informed consent in therapeutic trials in life-threatening procedures. There can be no argument against the requirement that the investigating phsyician must obtain completely informed consent from patients taking part in trials which are done for the sake of research and from which they do not necessarily have more to gain than to lose. But I believe that the situation is somewhat different when randomization is carried out because the physician does not know which therapy is better for the individual patients. There are two potent arguments against informing patients with a life-threatening disease that the decision about whether or not he should have a life-threatening operation will be made by chance rather than by clinical judgment. First, it is not in the best interest of the patients because it seems likely that 9 out of 10 would refuse these studies, and therefore the operation, if so informed. If they were in their right senses, they would find a doctor who thought he knew which was the better treatment, or they would conclude that if the differences were so slight that such a trial had to be carried out, they would prefer to take their chances on no operation. Assuming that there is a 50 percent chance that the operation will prove to be effective, then half the patients who were scared out of the operation by having asked for their informed consent would have been mistreated. Furthermore, it is probable that a very sick patient needs to have complete confidence in the fact that his doctor has the knowledge to make the right decisions with regard to his care. In the course of a traumatic illness the loss of that confidence may do great harm to the patient. It is a rare patient who could be expected to be objective enough about his own serious illness to welcome the fact that his physician has enough knowledge to avoid decisions based on ignorance.

The second argument against informing patients that the decision to operate or not will be based on randomization lies in the fact that it is not customary in the ordinary practice of medicine to inform patients of all the details with regard to how decisions are made in their treatment. Few patients would be saved by established surgical procedures if the physician and surgeon had to recount in every detail the complications of the operation. The most vigorous advocates of portacaval shunt surgery would be able to do no more operations if they were required to explain to each patient that of the 50 reports in the literature the only controlled studies showed no effects, and all the enthusiastic reports were totally uncontrolled. The physician must assume some responsibility for making decisions in the best interest of his patients.

Although in my opinion the physician may withhold information from the patient about the exact details of how decisions are made in a randomized study, he must inform the patient of the pros and cons of each therapeutic maneuver under consideration, and he must assure the patient that he will not carry out any therapy that he knows to be wrong. He must inform the patient that he is taking part in a study of a procedure that has not yet been established as efficacious. In other words, the patient should know that he is taking part in a research project and should be free to refuse to take part. And it should go without saying that all physicians concerned in a randomized study must be convinced that the knowledge necessary to make a decision [about] that patient is not available.

This brings me to the third problem, and to me the most serious one, that must be faced by the physician concerned with the ethics of controlled trials, namely, how one makes the decision about when to stop the trial, when a decision should be made to treat all patients according to the apparent results of the trial. The biostatistician tells us that we must determine from the variability before we start the trial what a reasonable number of experiences would be, and that usually we should not stop unless there is less than a 10 or 15 percent chance that we are missing a real difference, or less than a 5 percent chance that the difference we might have demonstrated is a true one and not one due to chance. This is entirely reasonable from the standpoint of the application of the conclusion to future patients. The conclusion can be reached either by the fixed sample technique with occasional peeking by a disinterested person, or by the sequential analysis technique. Either way one should be reasonably sure before stopping a study that the conclusion would be valid and not reversed by further experience. One owes this to the patients who were randomized into the less favorable treatment, if there is a difference.

But what about the rights of the patient who enters a study at a time when one treatment is leading the other, but when the study is being continued because the difference is not significant? One can easily argue that since the difference is not significant, the result can be reversed by further experience. But one can also argue that the welfare of that one patient is more assured if he receives the treatment that is ahead rather than the one that is currently behind in the evaluation. In other words, randomization could be unfair to him because he might be assigned to a treatment that has a less than 50 percent chance of being shown to be the correct one. This argument can then be reduced to the ridiculous by pointing out that the first patient in a study makes it more or less likely that one treatment will come out ahead. The situation is not analogous to the oft-quoted coin flipping rule that the results of previous flips do not influence the next one. In the case of the controlled trial the result of each comparison adds to the evidence for or against the superiority of one or the other treatment. To this problem I can see no solution.

The fact that the investigator is also the patient's physician requires that he tell the subject of the investigation which treatment is ahead. In situations in which both the disease and the treatment are life-threatening, it is unlikely that the patient would consent to be assigned to the treatment that is less likely to prove effective.

In summary, I should like to present three conclusions: (1) in the gradual evolution of our knowledge with regard to the prevention and treatment of disease the controlled clinical trial is by far the most effective way of saving people form the misapplication of dangerous and ineffective treatments. (2) We now know how to design scientifically precise and reliable trials of all preventive and therapeutic maneuvers. (3) Currently there are serious ethical and legal barriers to the conduct of any but the most insignificant trials.

Addenda

Soon after the above discussion of ethical issues involved in clinical trials was presented in 1967, my ideas changed with regard to two items discussed. First, experience developed in talking with patients about the importance of randomization as a decision-making process revealed that they were completely receptive when the alternatives were explained. In fact, they understood the need for randomization much better than practicing doctors usually do. On the basis of this experience, I changed my opinion about withholding exact details of the process and now believe in full disclosure of the decision-making process in clinical medicine, whether it be part of a clinical trial or the application of methods variously established in the literature.

A second modification in my thinking has developed with regard to how to handle the problem of an impending statistically significant difference between two treatments before the planned conclusion of a study. The dilemma is well outlined above. The only practical solution, not included in the document, is the setting up of a data monitoring committee of clinicians, statisticians, and consumer representatives who will look at the trends in studies and consider cessation as soon as the results in that study, or other studies reported since inception of the one in question, indicate that this should be done, and stop the trial whenever it is in the best interests of the participants to do so, recognizing that the patients have agreed in response to the informed-consent document that the study will be continued until a useful answer is obtained.

The application of ethics to the practice of medicine requires an evaluation of all alternatives, and the inclusion of patients in clinical trials must be considered in the light of therapeutics in general. When that is done, it is apparent that on the average the practice of medicine within the well-constructed trial is more ethical than the care of the average patient, which depends so much on ignorance of the true and relative efficacy of therapeutic measures employed.

105.
Being Old Makes You Different: The Ethics of Research with Elderly Subjects
Richard M. Ratzan

In 1963, two researchers and the director of the Department of Medicine at the Jewish Chronic Disease Hospital (JCDH) in Brooklyn injected patients with cells that contained cancerous material.[1] The object of the study was "to test immunological resistance of these patients to cancer"; the result, however, was a well-publicized ethical furor that was influential in establishing the need for more stringent regulation of research involving human subjects.

Many of the issues raised by this case have been broadly debated—problems of informed consent (there was a significant doubt that

Source: *Hastings Center Report*, vol. 10, October 1980, pp. 32–42.

these patients had ever been told that the cells were cancerous) and beneficence (the research was in no way related to the patient's care). However, one important aspect of the case has received less attention: these patients were institutionalized and most were elderly. The general question raised by the case is: do the elderly, simply by virtue of their age, constitute a specially vulnerable group of potential research subjects that requires special protection?

The National Commission for the Protection of Human Subjects of Biomedical and Behavioral Research included the elderly in its *Report and Recommendations in Research Involving Those Institutionalized as Mentally Infirm* [2] (subsequently modified and issued as proposed regulations by the Department of Health, Education and Welfare, now the Department of Health and Human Services),[3] but did not take up the specific problems of elderly research subjects. Yet even a brief look at the changing demography of the elderly in the United States suggests the increasing importance of clinical research in geriatrics, and the seriousness of the inattention to its special ethical questions.

In 1977, there were approximately 20 to 22 million Americans over the age of sixty-five (roughly 10 to 11 percent of the total population), a figure that will probably double in the next fifty years.[4] It is equally important to appreciate the statistics of senile dementia and institutionalization, two closely interrelated conditions that influence clinical geriatric research. Approximately 5 to 10 percent of those over sixty-five, roughly 1.5 million individuals, now suffer from senile dementia; that is, they show symptoms of mental deterioration, such as loss of memory, particularly of recent events; loss of ability to do simple arithmetic problems; and disorientation of time and place.[5] (The terms "senile" and "demented" are often used interchangeably to refer to those affected.) The same percentage of our elderly, including many of these senile persons, are institutionalized for a variety of reasons, not all of them med-

ical and not all of them requiring institutionization if better community-based supports existed.[6] Since the incidence of senile dementia is much higher (15 to 20 percent) in persons over the age of eighty, the absolute number of senile Americans will obviously increase with the projected increase in this category of the elderly population. Thus, if Census Bureau predictions are correct, in 2025 there will be 55 million Americans over the age of sixty-five; more than 2.5 million will be senile unless an effective therapy or cure is discovered in the interim.[7]

Types of Research

When considering types of clinical geriatric research, three areas are especially problematic: the specificity of the research, the degree of risk with relation to intrusiveness, and dementia research in particular.

Specific research. Of relevance to geriatric research intended primarily for knowledge rather than therapy is the issue of "specific" research, that is, whether the research is being performed primarily for knowledge about a disease or condition of that specific subject and whether it is necessary to use that subject instead of another noninstitutionalized, or younger, or nonsenile one. For example, is it ethical to ask institutionalized subjects, whether mentally disabled or not, to volunteer for a study of older persons' post-influenza vaccine serologies when a noninstitutionalized sample would answer the question? Was it ethical for my institution to ask for volunteers for a study designed to establish the correlation (or lack of it) between blood and sweat digoxin levels in adults (not just old adults), when a younger, noninstitutionalized population would have sufficed? Or were we, like the Jewish Chronic Disease Hospital, using a "wealth of patient material,"[1] conveniently captive due to an "accident of propinquity"?[8]

This question is of paramount importance for senile dementia research. For if research primarily intended for knowledge is not permitted to use institutionalized subjects, it may make such research difficult, leaving unanswered many problems of senile dementia, for example, the correlation between psychological testing and cerebrospinal fluid levels of neurotransmitters, and longitudinal studies of the relationship between arteriosclerosis, hypertension, and senile dementia, to name just a few studies that could not now be interpreted as research intended primarily for therapy for a particular subject.

In its *Report and Recommendations on Those Institutionalized as Mentally Infirm,* the National Commission took a definite stand in favor of patient-specific research. However, its Recommendation[2] permits more-than-minimal-risk research authorized by the proxy of an incompetent, institutionalized patient in the interest of future patients. Hans Jonas, a philosopher, has reminded us that "progress is an optional goal," not worth having if it is at the expense of the loss of society's moral values concerning individual worth.[9] Accordingly, Jonas feels that it is "indefensible" to conduct nonspecific research. However, it is as much an abrogation of competent subjects' autonomy to decide their refusal as it is their acceptance and it might be construed by some as paternalism, with all its attendant negative effects.

If we do allow institutionalized elderly subjects to participate in research, specific or otherwise, should there be any limitations? Some have proposed that since institutionalization and/or being mentally disabled is already a burden, such subjects should either not be asked to participate, or if so, only on a proportionate basis. Joseph Goldstein, a legal advocate for the rights of the mentally disabled, says: "The institutionalized mentally infirm should not constitute a greater percentage of subjects than they represent in the total community."[10] The National Commission suggested that the equitable way to select subjects institutionalized as mentally disabled would be in such a fashion that "the burdens of research do not fall disproportionately on those who are least able to consent or assent, nor should one group of patients be offered opportunities to participate in research from which they

may derive benefits to the unfair exclusion of other equally suitable groups of patients."

Warren Reich, a philosopher, argues, however, that "proportionate or disproportionate use of the elderly in research is not simply calculated arithmetically (e.g., in proportion to the percentage of the aged in the population at large), but rather by an assessment of relevant factors,"[11] which he enumerates in part. However, when we analyze his relevant factors (such as "whether the elderly have the same basic obligation as others to promote health through involvement in research" and "whether other less coerced or less vulnerable categories of potential research subjects are available"), most of them reflect paternalistic thinking. For if we recognize the autonomy of the mentally competent, elderly research subject, these questions become no more relevant, and no more difficult to answer (though no less so either), than they are for any other class of competent research subjects. Once the mentally competent, elderly research subject is treated as an autonomous agent, it becomes reasonable and equitable to apply percentages to recruitment for participation.

The mentally incompetent elderly research subject is a different matter. With respect to these subjects, Reich is certainly correct that simple mathematics will not solve the distribution problem, and that we need more data on current selection policies, the incidence, and the kinds of research that are being performed with aged subjects.

Degree of risk and intrusiveness. The National Commission and the proposed regulations define three types of research: that involving not greater than minimal risk (which is defined as "the risk that is normally encountered in the daily lives, or in the routine medical or psychological examination, of normal persons"); greater than minimal risk; and greater than minimal risk but only by "a minor increase."

To define the "minimal risk" of an experiment as the "risk of daily living" may be less true for many elderly subjects, in or out of institutions, than it is for younger subjects for several reasons. First, the elderly tend to reduce the risks of daily living to an absolute minimum. Motor vehicle accidents, power tool mishaps, exposure to the weather and other's germs—these are daily risks that no longer pertain to many elderly persons who have both consciously and unconsciously minimized their risks while maximizing their comforts. Those who live long enough to become elderly often do so by decreasing the number of risks in their lives, for they know they have little or no control over the magnitude of these risks. For although the risks of daily life for an elderly subject may now be fewer, they are quantitatively greater. A fall can mean a broken hip, permanent disability, and the loss of independence. A cold may lead to pneumonia, a splinter to serious infection.

Second, the desire for maximal comfort often supersedes the fear of dying. For example it is often difficult to persuade an elderly, critically ill nursing home patient to go to the hospital, leaving a known protective environment of peers, nurses, the familiar begonia on a radiator sill, a favorite aide, and the reliable routine of a final lifestyle—in short, home.

Still another factor is the cognitive difficulty some elderly subjects may have in weighing risks. If the mentally competent writer of this article finds it cognitively taxing to ascertain exactly how much risk is meant when a comparative adjective is used to quantitate a superlative in "greater than minimal risk," how will an eighty-two-year-old with slight but definite senile dementia fare?

For many elderly research subjects, intrusiveness in the form of bodily invasion or psychological trauma has a complex relationship to the actual degree of risk. How this risk is perceived to affect the subject's autonomy and comfort may be more decisive than the real probability of risk or the likely extent of injury. For example, the minimal risk of venesection (taking blood from a vein) was ostensibly the reason the residents of the Hebrew Home refused to participate in the digoxin study. I have no doubt that a drug study, even a potentially dangerous drug study, would have gleaned more volunteers simply because its discomforts would have been less apparent. Similarly, elderly subjects might permit unethical psychological studies that violated their personhood by allowing them to "fail, suffer ridicule, embarrassment, or an increased sense of inadequacy."[12] They might agree to participation not because they do not care, but because the differences in intrusiveness are too subtle, are minimized, or are explained too quickly.

Since they may translate "risk" to mean the risk of discomfort, not death, elderly subjects' interpretation of intrusiveness may appear unreasonable at times. Thus, while the principle that increased risk requires increased protection applies to research involving the elderly subject, it is not sufficient. Respect must also be given the elderly subject's altered value system and perception of risk, whether "accurate" or not. The elderly subject needs as much protection in refusing venesection as in refusing drugs or homologous cancer cell injections. For an elderly subject allowed to choose, the decision to participate or not may center on a harmless needle. He or she must be permitted to say "No" to harmless needles for "irrational" reasons.

Consequently, Recommendation (4) of the National Commission—(Sec. 46.507 of the proposed regulations) permitting greater than minimal risk but not much more—is unacceptable for geriatric research. It would allow such risk if "the anticipated knowledge (i) is of vital importance for the understanding or amelioration of the type of disorder or condition of the subjects, or (ii) may reasonably be expected to benefit the subjects in the future," and as long as the subject consents, or assents. If the subject objects, a guardian's permission or court order is needed. This is a call for progress at the possible expense of the individual, an obligatory sacrifice that society has no right to expect.

Hans Jonas, in writing about self-sacrifice for medical research, draws a clear distinction between moral value and moral obligation: "To have done so [self-sacrifice] would be praise-worthy; not to have done so is not blame-worthy. It cannot be asked of him; if he fails to do so he reneges on no duty."[9] It seems particularly brazen to conscript incompetent elderly patients to serve, at the end of their lives, as "volunteers" under the flag of "anticipated future knowledge."

Since the wording of Recommendation (4) has an "or" between clauses (i) and (ii), any researcher who can show the relevance of an experiment on senile dementia and who can convince an institutional review board (IRB) (not always an effective barrier)[13] need only obtain the permission of a guardian before subjecting a totally vegetative senile person to more than minimal risk. Whether or not such experimentation affects the subject's condition, such a category of increased risk for nonspecific research is treating an incompetent person as a means. According to the proposed regulations, DHHS is considering four alternatives for subjects incapable of assenting to this category of risk: barring their involvement altogether; adopting the National Commission's recommendations; requiring, in addition, the approval of the legally authorized representative and the court approval by the Secretary; or requiring, in addition to that of the representative and the court, approval by an advocate.[3] If provisions were made for a consent auditor who had to visit the subject and who had veto power, Recommendation (4) might be acceptable.

Senile dementia research. The difference of senile dementia research from other types of research is particularly important for any discussion of clinical geriatric research, and is at the heart of many of its ethical quandaries. First, senile dementia of the Alzheimer's type—the most common form among the elderly—is a medically, psychologically, epidemiologically, and financially devastating illness. Second, the research into this disease process—its initial questions; its methodology; and its severe medical, scientific, and ethical constraints—has special characteristics. Human subjects must be used at earlier stages of the research process than other types of investigation since there can never be an acceptable animal model. Although the use of toad bladders to understand human kidneys has proved feasible, the study of old, retarded chimps to understand senile dementia never will be. In this, of course, senile dementia is not unique; the study of schizophrenia and other mental disorders is similar and raises equally troublesome problems.

The crux of the problem, of course, is the compelling and unanimously perceived need to *do* research on senile dementia. For if we do no research on senile dementia for "ethical" reasons, we may "be in danger of protecting our patients to the extent that, while nothing bad may happen to them as the result of experimentation, nothing good will happen either."[14] Although there is a consensus for the need for such research, there is yet no ethical consensus how best to perform it.

If we conduct senile dementia research using the National Commission's recommendations, the principles will certainly apply (with the problems mentioned earlier) to older persons institutionalized with senile dementia. They will not apply, however, to older subjects who are mentally disabled but not institutionalized. (The term "mentally infirm" was changed to "mentally disabled" by the regulation writers.) We need more specific guidelines for conducting research using elderly persons as subjects, especially those possibly and definitely senile whether in or outside institutions. These are areas not presently addressed by the National Commission's report or the proposed regulations.

One solution would be to do research on elderly senile subjects of all degrees of disability using no special guidelines (other than those for nonsenile subjects currently published by DHHS). Such is the status of senile dementia research now, and indeed much pharmacological and therapeutic research is currently being reported. Unfortunately, since the present guidelines have such little application to elderly subjects in general and elderly institutionalized subjects in particular, the spectrum of ethical compassion encountered in such research is at least as broad as the spectrum of senile dementia being studied.

Other solutions are to limit senile dementia research to institutionalized, minimally demented subjects (yet how minimal is "minimal"?) and/or noninstitutionalized minimally demented subjects. A good argument can be made for soliciting noninstitutionalized mentally "normal" volunteers over the age of sixty-five for some types of senile dementia research on the grounds that if, when tested, they show the same, albeit earlier, qualitative cognitive deficits seen in senile dementia, then research primarily intended for therapy could be done with truly informed consent; would probably be more successful than in subjects with far advanced, apparently irreversible disease; and would be sparing of the truly burdened, institutionalized demented person. If any promising drugs or therapies emerge, they can then be tried, according to the National Commission's recommended guidelines, first on the institutionalized minimally disabled, then on the institutionalized moderately disabled, and so on following Jonas's "descending order" of consent.[9]

If such research is important, and appropriate populations can be identified, can informed consent be obtained? Here lies perhaps the most difficult problem.

Informed Consent

Although many writers disagree about its function and how—or if—it can be obtained, informed consent is now generally understood to require three conditions. First, the research subject must freely volunteer to participate. Second, the subject must be mentally competent. Third, the subject must be informed of the risks, benefits, discomforts, compensation—in short, all the likely consequences—of the experiment. Although these three conditions are necessary, I suggest that they are not sufficient for geriatric research. I therefore propose the following fourth condition: that the elderly research subject's actual understanding of the experiment be accurate and complete to the satisfaction of the researcher, or IRB, or other monitor.

Voluntariness and autonomy. Voluntariness, the first element of a truly informed consent, raises the larger issue of autonomy. The elderly patient, whether institutionalized or not, often leads a dependent life. Dependence on social services, relatives, neighbors, federal monies in the form of health insurance and social security—this pervasive web of dependence creates one of the characteristic Catch-22s in clinical geriatric research. Succinctly stated: "The aged cannot be singled out for special advantages without also being stigmatized as being incompetent or needy."[15]

The loss of autonomy for elderly people is usually the result of the simultaneous physical, mental, and environmental forces of attrition, which necessitate the assistance of others. Such age-related dependence may be due, in part, to the subtle adoption of specific role expectations and age-appropriate norms, that is, changes in attitudes and roles that occur as a function of, and simultaneously with, successive life-stages. Bernice Neugarten, a sociologist, has pointed out that as they go from middle to old age people often become passive, in part because they think they are supposed to act that way. Their willing compliance, reinforced by society's expectations about behavior in the elderly, further complicates the problem of voluntariness.

This age-related behavior may explain, along with approaching death, the apathy frequently encountered in the elderly. As Father Luke, age seventy-five, in *The View in Winter* puts it, "I care less. . . . In fact I'm just about to fly out to South Africa, and I don't much mind whether the aeroplane crashes or it doesn't."[16] The obvious implications for acquiescing to research rather than volunteering for it require special consideration, especially in institutions.

Institutionalization usually leads to less, not more, autonomy with important psychological consequences. There is, for example, a marked diminution in patients' sense of well-being when they are told that their nurses, not they, will make decisions about themselves and their environment. In addition, the institutionalized elderly must deal with a heightened interdependency—what may be called the "dining room effect." Peer pressures exerted by communal eating and social gathering in institutions can be enormous. One study concluded, "Influences of environment and peer group seem to have more bearing on the decision to volunteer than explanations of the experiment itself. The decision to participate is made within a social context."[17] Peer pressure; institutionalization; and physical, mental, and financial vulnerabilities often subtly erode elderly subjects' autonomy to the degree that they need special protection—not so much from their vulnerabilities but from the loss of liberty which is a consequence of their vulnerabilities.

No specific legal guidelines recognize the unique status of elderly research subjects, but relevant case law may provide some help. According to one such case, *Wyatt* v. *Stickney,* mentally ill and mentally retarded patients involuntarily confined in institutions have a constitutional right to treatment. Included in this right to treatment is an institutionalized mentally ill patient's "right not to be subjected to experimental research without the express and informed consent of the patient, if the patient is able to give such consent, and of his guardian or next-of-kin, after opportunities for consultation with independent specialists and with legal counsel."

Wyatt v. *Stickney* concerns research intended primarily for therapy and only that research performed on institutionalized subjects and only those institutionalized subjects who are confined involuntarily. The strictures of *Wyatt* v. *Stickney* apply only to a very small subset of clinical geriatric research, namely, the elderly, involuntarily confined person who is involved in research primarily for therapy.

Many elderly persons are institutionalized involuntarily, albeit de facto rather than de jure in most instances. This closet institutionalization makes their research status undefined, leaving them, therefore, at greater risk

since they fall in between the federal regulations and the court cases. Rushing in to protect the elderly, especially the institutionalized elderly, is the angel of paternalism.

Paternalism. The most insidious loss of liberty for an elderly subject, the one least likely to be detected and corrected, is paternalism. The elderly often *do* need help in providing for themselves and thereby set the stage for what Lionel Trilling called "the dangers which lie in our most generous wishes . . . to go on to make them [our fellow men] the objects of our pity, then of our wisdom, ultimately of our coercion."[18]

Such paternalist coercion may be protective or intrusive. The protective paternalists no doubt share the concept, popularized by Sir Isaiah Berlin, of a "negative" sense of personal liberty, and the intrusive paternalists a "positive" sense. "Negative" liberty embodies the notion that personal freedom is freedom from intervention. "Positive" liberty is based on man's concept of self-mastery—the freedom to assert one's individuality. Whereas the intrusive paternalists were the rule in geriatrics (e.g., the JCDH case) in the 1960s and 70s, the advent of medical ethics has witnessed the ascendancy of a new breed of paternalists, the custodial protectors of the elderly.

In clinical geriatrics, three negative effects of such custodial protection of subjects from research have been identified: harm to the subject, exclusion of the subject from research, and limitation of research in general.[19] Harm to the subject is a consequence of the subject's making a choice that is based on incomplete or selected information in an attempt to protect him or her. This protection presupposes the inability of *all* elderly subjects to possess information and arrive at a decision. Marcia Leader and Elizabeth Neuwirth warn researchers not to "fall into the trap of underestimating the older person's capacities to act with as much enlightened self-interest as any other adult citizen in deciding whether a particular research project is something which is desirable for him or her."[20]

The second negative effect of paternalism

is the revocation of what many elderly subjects desire and feel is their right to volunteer, to help others, to participate. Exactly when to allow a subject of limited competence to exert this right, even at the possible risk of his or her own health, is indeed complex. Joseph Goldstein argues in a paper prepared for the National Commission that "to deny such persons the right to decide whether to participate in research because he or she is incompetent is to reduce that person's individual autonomy beyond that which can be justified by the designation or the incarceration."[10] In a study examining two approaches to elderly subject recruitment for clinical research, Leader and Neuwirth found that their "first obstacle was anxiety about experimental research among those who direct senior citizens programs."[20] They learned that previous researchers had already discovered that a successful strategy for thwarting paternalistic protectors was to seek approval from "highest administrative levels first."

The third danger of overprotection, limitation of research, represents still another paradox in geriatric research. If we can only perform senile dementia research using demented patients, but should not allow them to participate because they are incompetent, then we are left in a quandary. We cannot ethically conduct senile dementia research using demented subjects because they are incompetent; but we cannot technically perform it using competent subjects because they are not demented. Consequently, as Neil Chayet, a lawyer, rightly complains, "If prohibition of research continues to be the protective device that is utilized, we may well 'protect' thousands of institutionalized mentally ill persons to death or to lives of misery."[21]

To complicate matters, paternalists of the intrusive sort are still extant. In a survey of 83 investigators conducting research at institutions for the mentally disabled and 68 investigators at other institutions, Arnold Tannenbaum and Robert Cooke found that 23 percent of the former (compared with 18 percent of the latter) admitted that they did not divulge certain information to their research subjects.[13] If such research was felt, by the investigators, to be in the best interest of the mentally disabled, the elderly, and mankind in general, even if not beneficial to the particular elderly subject participating in it, we have an example of paternalism in the "positive" sense of liberty. That is, this altruistic volunteering represents a "better" choice for them to make than a refusal, at least in the minds of the researchers. Whether it is the protective or the intrusive sort, paternalism is a dilemma for anyone taking care of the elderly. As Thomas Halper asks, "Granting the utility of a limited paternalism for the aged," how do we "confine it within its proper bounds?"[15]

The answer to Halper's question is that it is difficult, requires experience, good faith, and constant reassessment. One solution might be to apply B. F. Skinner's "principle of making the controller a member of the group he controls,"[22] which for geriatrics would mean having elderly people help make most of the research policies for elderly people, a situation that certainly does not exist now.

Another solution would be to consider Gerald Dworkin's suggestion that paternalism is permissible in certain instances.[23] He views paternalism as acceptable if it "preserves and enhances for the individual his ability rationally to consider and carry out his own decisions," that is, a kind of volitional insurance policy. It is exactly this type of paternalism that the elderly need. They are often debilitated, needing help and asking for it. To do good in this setting is to restore only that which necessitated their requesting help, that is, their lost autonomy.

The only paternalism acceptable for the elderly is one that places them in a protected milieu of autonomy, a milieu over which they may exercise as much control as is consistent with our objective assessment of their deficits and their subjective perception of their benefits, not vice versa.

Competence. Mental competence, the second condition of an informed consent, is often assumed rather than objectively tested.

Indeed, there is considerable controversy over whether or not it can be tested, ought to be tested, and by whom. Legally, competence for a specific capability—such as being able to participate in one's defense in a trial—is strictly judged as present or absent without gradations. As Lance Tibbles states, however, the all-or-none judgment of competency is "inappropriate" for the gradations of competency found in clinical geriatric practice. He suggests alternatives such as power of attorney.[24]

Several tests used to determine competency include evidencing a choice, reasonable outcome of choice, choice based on rational reasons, ability to understand, and actual understanding. What then are the implications for informed consent in clinical geriatric research when using these different criteria for competence? First, there is much evidence for a decline in cognitive abilities with normal aging; thus any elderly subject's comprehension of the proposed research becomes problematic. Researchers have substantiated significant differences, and often a decline, in the memory and learning of older subjects when compared with younger ones.[25] The effects of aging on intellectual ability are more controversial but also suggestive of deterioration.[26] Many of the experiments testing cognition in the elderly repeatedly found that novelty of information, rate of response, complexity of tasks to be performed, and organizational strategies were all important factors apparently responsible for the decreased performances of normal older subjects. Indeed, some of the older persons with decreased cognitive abilities were well-educated professionals of high socioeconomic status. Some researchers have found that bright, aged normals, when compared with young normals, manifested a conceptual deficit comparable with that found in a group of neurologically impaired patients.[27]

Problem-solving ability, which is what the giving of informed consent is all about in a true volunteer, also seems to change with normal aging, and often for the worse. A "vicious spiral" retards and undermines the problem-solving process in some aged subjects: when faced with the increased memory load of a new problem, a weakened elderly memory gets slower and makes more mistakes, leading to wrong decisions that require extra operations, slowing memory down even more, leading to more mistakes, and so on.[28] An analysis of the problem-solving performance of 100 successful professional people suggests that there is a *different*, rather than an impaired, performance.[29] Some of the differences were: how the older subject defined the problem to be solved; the relation of the problem to new goals; the self-recognized necessity for greater discipline; and a tolerance toward people around them. These observations suggest that, in this research group at least, there was not only an approach to problem-solving different from that found in younger subjects but that it was consciously different. It may be that the differences in this group of older subjects are adaptations to aging, not intellectual deterioration. In any case, as Patrick Rabbitt points out, it would be naive merely to "regard them as passive victims of a cognitive degeneration of which they are helplessly unaware."[28]

A second consideration in the obtaining of informed consent from an apparently competent elderly subject is the increased likelihood of occult, that is, latent dementia, especially senile dementia of the Alzheimer's type, which is often clinically latent in its early stages. The clinical spectrum of senile dementia and its definition are sufficiently varied and problematic that the detection of minimally but definitely impaired elderly persons can be difficult when attempted and nearly impossible when not. The implications for obtaining informed consent from possibly demented subjects over the age of sixty-five are obvious.

Another aspect of early senile dementia that affects informed consent is the frequent fluctuation of its severity. The interplay between the effects of senile dementia itself, associated psychiatric illness, and the influence of medication can cause swings in mental ability such that competence to understand a problem may be fair on Monday, yet hopeless on Tuesday. Consequently, it seems unwise to obtain informed consent from an elderly person in whom there is the question of even minimal senile dementia using the same process one would for a younger one. Robert Veatch, a philosopher, argues that the problem of intermittent competence requires that a "formerly competent patient's wishes clearly expressed while competent should be determinative when the patient is no longer competent."[30] In theory, this is a good suggestion, though primarily for therapeutic decisions. However, for some future, unspecified research primarily intended for knowledge, no matter how unobtrusive or benign, this plan is obviously not tenable.

A related problem is the question of who determines competency. Legally, it has traditionally been a physician, usually a psychiatrist. If all the parties involved agree to having a psychiatrist establish the competency of an elderly subject, which psychiatrist will it be? Many large institutions have salaried or fee-for-service psychiatrists. If one of these evaluates the competency of an elderly subject for an institutional research project, a "double-agent" problem emerges. This conflict of interest becomes especially dangerous since the subject, by virtue of his or her possible incompetency and the dependency of institutionalization, is not likely to have the option—or having it, to exercise it—of selecting a different psychiatrist. If a psychiatrist other than the resident one is mandated, the establishment of competency may become a cumbersome routine.

Finally it is imperative for anyone judging the competency of an elderly subject to remember the differences in goals and values that many older subjects integrate into problem solving (for our discussion, the giving of informed consent). Tibbles makes the point clearly: "A long life of frugality followed at 65 years of age by the spending of large sums on pleasures foregone in the past may not be a sign of incompetence. It may be a recognition of mortality."[24]

Information. The third condition of in-formed consent is that the subject be provided with information about the experiment. But, how much information? Who provides it? The recent trend has been to give the patient more information. This shift is due mainly to a closer scrutiny of the medical profession by lay critics and the general movement over the past 15 years toward judicial and legislative protection of consumers' and individuals' rights. Part of this trend has been the emphasis on disclosure of material information.

Materiality of information is one of the most dramatic issues distinguishing clinical geriatric research from that in other age groups. The widespread alterations in function and decreased reserve of most organ systems in the elderly dictate a reorientation of emphasis when describing possible consequences of a particular experiment. If an experimental drug has a 1 percent chance of leaving the subject with impaired hearing, that information is "more" material for the subject to know if she is an eighty-three-year-old wearing a hearing aid than a healthy thirty-nine-year-old.

Another issue in informed consent relevant to geriatrics is the format of the explanation and consent form. Lynn Epstein and Louis Lasagna showed quite clearly that "comprehension and consent to volunteer were inversely related to length of form."[31] Ralph Alfidi compared two forms, an inclusive one and a less detailed one.[32] Both offered more information if desired. He found no appreciable difference in consent rates. In conjunction with these studies and the literature on problem solving (that is, complexity of tasks and novel information), I suggest that consent forms for the elderly resemble Alfidi's less detailed one.

Of practical importance for clinical geriatric researchers, no matter which consent form is used, is the question of how much information we *can* give the geriatric subject. For example, if anything, the growing literature on pharmacokinetics in the elderly reveals to us just how much we do not know.[33] Much of the experimental data concerning the differences between young and old subjects with cardiovascular disease, malnutrition, and surgery of all types lie buried in a literature antedating the advent of geriatrics as a discipline, with the result that all adults, both under and over sixty-five, are lumped together simply as "adults."

Perhaps the most controversial aspect of how much information should be provided to a subject is the question of intentional selection of information by the researcher or physician, commonly referred to as the therapeutic privilege. Although *Canterbury* v. *Spence* and *Cobbs* v. *Grant,* the 1972 cases that helped define the role of information in informed consent, involved mentally competent patients, some writers have stated that therapeutic privilege is no less inappropriate for mentally incompetent subjects. Goldstein argues that the patient's right of self-decision "is effectively safeguarded if the authorities provide him with a real opportunity (not with an obligation) to possess what information he and a reasonable person might require in order to exercise a choice."[10]

The real risk of therapeutic privilege, and therefore at the heart of the controversy, is manipulation. Such persuasion is usually toward therapy or participation. However, a physician can also manipulate the subject toward refusal by exaggerating risks or understating benefits. Whether motivated by paternalism or not, the physician-as-manipulator with his or her specialized knowledge is an almost insuperable adversary when invested with the respect and power usually imputed him or her, especially by elderly subjects. And if, as one recent study has found, older women react more positively to persuasive information despite their understanding less of it, such manipulation can become a science with almost guaranteed results.[34]

Assessment. I propose that a fourth stipulation be added for the obtaining of informed consent in clinical geriatric research, that is, the assessment of the subject's actual understanding of the experiment. One method proposed for assessing actual understanding is the two-part consent form. Such a consent form has been proposed for all sub-

jects of human research, the second part being a "questionnaire to check how well they understand the information that has been presented to them."[35] This questionnaire, it was proposed, would be an integral part of the consent process. It would be the embodiment, in practice, of the "actual understanding" criterion for informed consent.[36]

There is certainly ample evidence for the need of such a process. One useful paper demonstrated that prisoners volunteering to participate in a malaria experiment understood its risk "no better or worse" than those who did not volunteer.[17] Bradford Gray has shown that although they signed an informed consent form, 39 percent of the pregnant women in an experiment concerning labor induction said they only learned of their status as research subjects from Gray's interview after the experiment had already begun.[37]

There is also evidence for the efficacy of a two-part process. Roger L. Williams and his colleagues discovered an improvement in potential subjects' understanding of the experiment after a discussion of it with a physician for 20 minutes as compared with those subjects whose knowledge of the experiment consisted of details gleaned only from the hearsay of previous participants.[38]

However, the range of correct answers for both groups was wide and the informed group did "better" than the hearsay group in that only 12 of 20 informed subjects (as compared with 7 of 20 hearsay subjects) answered correctly the question: "Is it possible that you could develop a serious and even permanent illness as a result of participating in a study at this project?" When subjects scored less than 14 (of 20 questions), they were not accepted for participation. Moreover, those who scored between 14 and 19 were reinformed until "the physician was satisfied that comprehension of the material was complete."

In addition to assessing the comprehension and informing the subject of those areas he or she misunderstood, the two-part consent form helps protect the investigator. It also furnishes the investigator with responses concerning the perception of the experiment by the subjects, their perception of the explanation, and thus possible ways to improve both. Finally, it allows the subject more time to make an important decision.

Although dividing the consent process for elderly subjects into two or more interviews, held at different times, would improve the likelihood of a valid informed consent, it also allows more occasion for influence by private physicians, family, and other peer members who have already been approached by the interviewer. Interaction among subjects may lead to support during participation.[39] However, in the setting of an institution, such support would probably most often take the form of subtle peer pressures to refuse to participate. In a sense, that first moment of privacy in the first interview may be the institutionalized elderly subject's freest moment, the first and last chance to make a truly autonomous decision.

Some mechanism like the two-part consent form is essential for geriatric subjects. Their comprehension may be different, if not lessened, because of age. A deficient recent memory may convert a valid consent on Monday into a fiction on Tuesday; and a fluctuating mental status due to senile dementia or medication, or both, may make unethical an experiment that is separated from the consent process by more than an hour. Although older subjects have less time to live, they often need more time to consent.

Proxy consent. The difficult problem of proxy consent when a subject is unable, for whatever reason, to make decisions about care, experimental or otherwise, has been extensively reviewed. The question of proxy consent for elderly subjects suffering from a clinically wide range of significant cognitive deficits has not, unfortunately, received the same attention.

The proxies for elderly subjects are often their grown children or other close relatives. Such a proxy may have a lifetime of emotions invested in the subject or, worse, a hope of inheriting material goods. If there

are no close relatives, there is frequently no one at all. Like his or her cardiac reserve, the elderly person's reserve of interested others grows small with age.

It is therefore especially important, when considering proxy consent for an elderly subject, to avoid the protective paternalism of a relative (prohibiting what in fact the subject might have willed), and the exploitative paternalism of a researcher convincing an apathetic guardian or all-too-eager heir of the subject's noble role as martyr. What are some of the possible solutions to this problem?

One is to have the still competent subject appoint an agent who will be empowered with the authority to make any future medical decisions that occur after the subject is no longer able to decide them. Such is the gist of Leslie Libow's penultimate will[40] and the much publicized Michigan House Bill No. 4058.[41]

Another solution would be to appoint as proxy a consent auditor—a suggestion proposed by the National Commission. Unfortunately there are problems both with the consent auditor's assuming this role and with the very concept. First, who exactly is the consent auditor and who would it be for the institutionalized elderly? The National Commission is vague about his or her identity, how the person would be selected, and who would pay his or her salary. If salaried by the institution, the person would again face the double-agent problem. If salaried by the government, is this agreeable to all? If the consent auditor does become a federal employee, what would be the relationship to Veterans Administration institutions, one of the largest potential research sources of those institutionalized elderly most often needing a proxy? And most important, what would be the consent auditor's real power in the consent process—a vote or a veto? Should he or she be old, that is, a peer of the research subject? If so, who will assess his or her competence tactfully? These questions need answers before the consent auditor audits anything.

Of further interest is the almost complete

lack of discussion in the proxy consent literature about the proxy. Proxy consent, so often equated with the decision that a reasonable, competent subject would have made, or with the decision that someone (usually a relative) who knows the subject predicts he or she would have made, is merely shifting all the informed consent issues one step back, still begging all the fundamental questions of informed consent. Is the proxy informed? Has his or her actual understanding of the information been assessed? What is his or her motivation, a prime consideration for the proxy of many geriatric subjects?

NOTES

1. "The Jewish Chronic Disease Hospital Case," in Jay Katz (ed.), *Experimentation With Human Beings*, Russell Sage Foundation, New York, 1973, p. 9.

2. National Commission for the Protection of Human Subjects of Biomedical and Behavioral Research, *Report and Recommendations: Research Involving Those Institutionalized as Mentally Infirm*, DHEW Publication (OS) 78–0006, Washington, 1978.

3. DHEW, "Protection of Human Subjects: Proposed Regulation of Research Involving Those Institutionalized as Mentally Disabled," *Federal Register*, vol. 43, no. 223, p. 53950, November 17, 1978.

4. D. G. Fowles, *Some Prospects for the Future Elderly Population*, Washington, D.C.: DHEW Publication (OHDS) 78–20288, January 1978.

5. R. Goldman, "The Social Impact of the Organic Dementias of the Aged," in K. Nandy (ed.), *Senile Dementia: A Biomedical Approach*, Elsevier North-Holland Inc., New York, 1978, p. 3.

6. W. Reichel, "Demographic Aspects of Aging," in W. Reichel (ed.), *Clinical Aspects of Aging*, Williams and Wilkins Co., Baltimore, 1978, p. 435.

7. United States Bureau of the Census, *Current Population Reports*, Series P 25, no. 704, July 1977.

8. D. C. Martin, J. D. Arnold, T. F. Zimmerman, et al., "Human Subjects in Clinical Research: A Report of Three Studies," *New England Journal of Medicine*, vol. 279, p. 1426, 1968.

9. Hans Jonas, "Philosophical Reflections on Experimenting With Human Subjects," in Paul A. Freund (ed.), *Experimenting With Human Subjects*, George Braziller, New York, 1969, p. 1.

10. Joseph Goldstein, "On the Right of the 'Institutionalized Mentally Infirm' to Consent to or Refuse to Participate as Subjects in Biomedical and Behavioral Research," prepared for the National Commission, Appendix to *Research Involving Those Institutionalized as Mentally Infirm*. DHEW Publication (OS) 78–0007, Washington, 1978, p. 2.

11. W. T. Reich, "Ethical Issues Related to Research Involving Elderly Subjects," *Gerontologist*, vol. 18, p. 326, 1978.

12. B. M. Ashley, "Ethics of Experimenting with Persons," in Joseph C. Schoolar and Charles M. Gaitz (eds.), *Research and the Psychiatric Patient*, Brunner/Mazel, New York, 1975, p. 15.

13. A. S. Tannenbaum and R. A. Cooke, "Report on the Mentally Infirm," prepared for the National Commission, Appendix to *Research Involving Those Institutionalized as Mentally Infirm*. DHEW Publication (OS) 78–0007; B. H. Gray, R. A. Cooke, and A. S. Tannenbaum, "Research Involving Human Subjects," *Science*, vol. 201, p. 1094, 1978.

14. L. E. Hollister, "The Use of Psychiatric Patients as Experimental Subjects," in Frank J. Ayd, Jr. (ed.), *Medical, Moral and Legal Issues in Mental Health Care*, Williams and Wilkins Co., Baltimore, 1974, p. 28.

15. T. Halper, "Paternalism and the Elderly," in S. F. Spicker, K. M. Woodward, and D. D. Van Tassel (eds.), *Aging and the Elderly*, Humanities Press, Atlantic Highlands, N.J., 1978, p. 321.

16. R. Blythe, *The View in Winter: Reflections on Old Age*, Harcourt Brace Jovanovich, New York, 1979, p. 252.

17. Martin et al., "Human Subjects in Clinical Research"; see also E. M. Brody, "Environmental Factors in Dependency," in A. N. Exton-Smith and J. G. Evans (eds.), *Care of the Elderly: Meeting the Challenge of Dependency*, Grune & Stratton, New York, 1977, p. 81.

18. Lionel Trilling, "Manners, Morals, and the Novel," in *The Liberal Imagination*, Secker and Warburg, London, 1951, p. 221.

19. Makarushka and McDonald, "Informed Consent, Research, and Geriatric Patients," *Gerontologist*, vol. 19, p. 61, 1979.

20. M. A. Leader and E. Neuwirth, "Clinical Research and the Noninstitutional Elderly: A Model for Subject Recruitment," *Journal of the American Geriatric Society*, vol. 26, p. 27, 1978.

21. Neil L. Chayet, "Informed Consent on the Mentally Disabled: A Failing Fiction," *Psychiatric Annals*, vol. 6, p. 82, 1976.

22. B. F. Skinner, *Beyond Freedom and Dignity*, Bantam Books, New York, 1971, p. 164.

23. Gerald Dworkin, "Paternalism," *Monist*, vol. 56, p. 64, 1972.

24. Lance Tibbles, "Medical and Legal Aspects of Competency as Affected by Old Age," in *Aging and the Elderly*, p. 127.

25. F. I. M. Craik, "Age Differences in Human Memory," in J. E. Birren and K. W. Schaie (eds.), *Handbook of the Psychology of Aging*, Van Nostrand Reinhold Co., 1977, p. 384; D. Arenberg and E. A. Robertson-Tchabo, "Learning and Aging," in *Handbook of the Psychology of Aging*, p. 421.

26. J. Botwinick, "Intellectual Abilities," in *Handbook of the Psychology of Aging*, p. 580.

27. J. L. Mack and N. J. Carlson, "Conceptual Deficits and Aging: The Category Test," *Perception and Motor Skills*, vol. 46, p. 123, 1978.

28. P. Rabbitt, "Change in Problem Solving Ability in Old Age," in *Handbook of the Psychology of Aging*, p. 606.

29. J. E. Birren, "Age and Decision Strategies," in A. T. Welford and J. E. Birren (eds.), *Decision Making and Age: Interdisciplinary Topics in Gerontology*, S. Karger, Basel and New York, 1969.

30. Robert M. Veatch, "Three Theories of Informed Consent: Philosophical Foundations and Policy Implications," submitted to the National Commission (February 3, 1976), Recommendation 13.

31. L. C. Epstein and L. Lasagna, "Obtaining Informed Consent: Form or Substance," *Archives of Internal Medicine*, vol. 123, p. 682, 1969.

32. R. J. Alfidi, "Informed Consent: A Study of Patient Reaction," *Journal of the American Medical Association*, vol. 216, p. 1325, 1971.

33. *Pharmacological Intervention on the Aging Process*, J. Roberts, R. C. Adelman, and V. J. Cristofalo (eds.), Plenum Press, New York and London, 1978.

34. A. R. Herzog, "Attitude Change in Older Age: An Experimental Study," *Journal of Gerontology*, vol. 34, p. 697, 1979.

35. R. Miller and H. S. Willner, "The Two-Part Consent Form: A Suggestion for Promoting Free and Informed Consent," *New England Journal of Medicine*, vol. 290, p. 964, 1974.

36. Loren H. Roth, Alan Meisel, and Charles W. Lidz, "Tests of Competency to Consent to Treatment," *American Journal of Psychiatry*, vol. 134, p. 279, 1977.

37. Bradford H. Gray, "An Assessment of Institutional Review Committees in Human Experimentation," *Medical Care*, vol. 13, p. 318, 1975.

38. R. L. Williams, K. H. Rieckmann, G. M. Trenholme, et al., "The Use of a Test to Determine That Consent Is Informed," *Military Medicine*, vol. 142, p. 542, 1977.

39. D. Axelsen and R. A. Wiggins, "An Application of Moral Guidelines in Human Clinical Trials to a Study of a Benzodiazepine Compound as a Hypnotic Agent among the Elderly," *Clinical Research*, vol. 25, p. 1, 1977.

40. L. S. Libow and R. Zicklin, "The Penultimate Will: Its Potential as an Instrument to Protect the Mentally Deteriorated Patient," *Gerontologist*, vol. 13, p. 440, 1973.

41. Arnold S. Relman, "Michigan's Sensible 'Living Will,'" *New England Journal of Medicine*, vol. 300, p. 1270, 1979.

106.

Research on Children: National Commission Says, "Yes, if..."

James J. McCartney

The National Commission for the Protection of Human Subjects of Biomedical and Behavioral Research was mandated to establish guidelines to protect vulnerable populations, including children, from exploitation as research subjects. The impetus to include children in the Commission's mandate was partially a response to experiments performed at Willowbrook State Hospital in Staten Island, New York. There some newly admitted mentally retarded children were deliberately exposed to viral hepatitis to

Source: *Hastings Center Report*, vol. 8, October 1978.

study whether the disease could be better controlled in the institution. In its deliberation and debate, the Commission reached a middle ground between a total prohibition of research involving children at one extreme and an unqualified endorsement of research at the other.

The Mandate

The 1974 Congressional mandate to the Commission with regard to research involving children focused on the requirements for informed consent. The Commission was asked

> to determine the nature of the consent obtained from [children] or their legal representatives before such persons were involved in such research; the adequacy of this information given them respecting the nature and purpose of the research, procedures to be used, risks and discomforts, anticipated benefits from the research, and other matters necessary for informed consent; and the competence and the freedom of the persons to make a choice for or against involvement in such research.[1]

The Commission realized at a very early stage that protection of children in the context of research entails much more than adequate informed consent of the child or his representative. Thus the mandate was interpreted quite broadly to include issues of protection from harm, equitable selection of subjects, and benefits that might accrue to various classes of children through research endeavors. Its recommendations reflect concern not only for the ethical principle of respect for persons, but also for the principles of respect for vulnerable populations, beneficence, and justice.

In order to prepare for its debate the Commission (1) visited a school for the retarded; (2) commissioned several essays; (3) sponsored a national conference focusing on issues relating to the involvement of minority children as research subjects; (4) conducted public hearings at which numerous professional organizations, public interest groups, and individuals presented their views; and (5) surveyed institutional review board practices in reviewing research on children.[2]

Recommendations

The question of permitting research on children was debated longer and more thoroughly than any other item on the Commission's agenda. Preliminary discussion began in July 1976; the final version of the report and recommendations was not sent to the Secretary of Health, Education and Welfare until September 6, 1977. The recommendations went through at least ten drafts before they were finally accepted by the Commission, which never agreed unanimously on a "deliberations and conclusions" section, ultimately presenting two versions.[3]

The recommendations (pp. 28–29) include (1) a statement encouraging research involving children because of its importance for the health of all children; (2) general conditions that must apply for all such research; (3) approval of minimal risk research involving children; (4) approval of more than minimal risk research under certain conditions when it is "presented by an intervention that holds out the prospect of direct benefit for the individual subjects, or by a monitoring procedure required for the well being of the subjects"; (5) approval of research under certain stringent conditions that might not be beneficial to individual subjects when the risk to subjects "represent a minor increase over minimal"; (6) procedures for referral of difficult or exceptional cases to a National Ethics Advisory Board; (7) mechanisms for assuring that the permission of parents and the assent of children (when applicable) is free and informed; and (8) alternate criteria and mechanisms for inclusion in or exclusion from research of certain classes of children.[4]

All the recommendations were accepted unanimously except recommendation 5, which deals with research that carries more than minimal risk and is nonbeneficial to the subject. For reasons that will be explained later, Commissioner Robert E. Cooke (President, Medical College of Pennsylvania), and the late Robert H. Turtle (attorney, Washington, D.C.) voted against this recommendation and presented dissenting statements.[5]

In its protracted discussion and debate, the Commission broke substantial new conceptual and ethical ground. After determining quite early that at least some research involving children was ethically justifiable, the discusion began more and more to stress the importance of research involving children, especially in overcoming iatrogenic problems in newborn intensive care such as retrolental fibroplasia.[6] These initial convictions were quickly formulated into recommendation 1, which survived essentially intact throughout the debate.[7]

The Commission then had the more difficult task of determining the ethically justifiable limits of that research. Cooke pointed out that although research involving children is desirable and important, independent ethical justifications and limitations must still be set forth before researchers can legitimately proceed.[8] Thus most of the Commission's debate was concerned with the problem of ethical line-drawing, and all recommendations after the first deal with one or more aspects of the Commission's ethical principles: respect for persons, beneficence, and justice.

Respect for Persons

The Commissioners were greatly influenced by Cooke's early observation that the crucial issue regarding infants and very young children was not assuring informed consent in order to protect individual autonomy, since children are not autonomous in any real sense until late in childhood, if even then. Rather, he argued that the Commission had to make sure that mechanisms of proper protection were established for those unable to protect themselves.[9] This dual aspect of respect for persons, that is, pres-

ervation of individual autonomy and protection of the defenseless, has subsequently been developed by the Commission in the *Belmont Report*, its general statement of the ethical principles underlying research.[10]

Included under the same rubric of respect for persons is the importance of the family as a social unit, and the significance of parental rights in making decisions on behalf of their children. These themes continually reappeared during the course of the debate, with Cooke and Turtle contending that the whole family should become involved in the research project as a protective mechanism and that only children belonging to loving families should be allowed to participate in research.[11] Additionally, Karen Lebacqz (associate professor of Christian ethics, Pacific School of Religion) pointed out that parents are allowed to make many potentially risky decisions for their children, for example, allowing them to participate in contact sports. She argued that, within limits, society views these decisions as parental prerogatives and the Commission should not deny these prerogatives in a research context.[12]

In contrast to Cooke and Turtle's position, Patricia King (associate professor of law, Georgetown University Law Center) emphasized that children are on a sliding scale from nonautonomy to full autonomy. She stressed that mature minors should be treated as adults and allowed to participate in research even if they do not come from a loving family. She reminded the Commission that as children grow older more concern must be shown for the agreement of the children themselves to participate in research.[13] Acknowledging this developing autonomy, the Commission ultimately required that assent for participation in research must be given by children themselves after the age of seven. At any age a child's objection to research is held to be binding unless the intervention holds out a prospect of direct benefit to the child and is available only in the context of research.[14]

Since children are not fully autonomous, the Commission wished to avoid the language of informed consent in its deliberations. Instead it speaks of parental *permission* for research on a child and uses the term *assent* when speaking of the agreement of a child to participate in research. Conceptually this language moves away from the notion that the parent is giving proxy consent, that is, consent in the name of and on behalf of another. The view of parents as proxies for their children has led to many ethical quandaries in past discussions of the involvement of children in research.[15] When the Commission speaks of permission, it understands that parents or guardians are acting in their own right as the loving protectors and providers of their children and not as agents attempting to discern what these children would decide on their own if they could decide.[16]

Acknowledging Cooke's and Turtle's concerns, the Commission established mechanisms for increasingly involving the family unit as the research became more serious, including the requirement that one or both parents be present during the conduct of certain types of research in order to intervene if necessary.

Beneficence

Applying the principle of beneficence (which the Commission regards as including avoidance of risk of harm to others, or nonmaleficence) to research involving children proved to be the most difficult task the Commission faced. Most of the redrafts and hours of debate were attempts to deal with the implications of this principle when applied to research involving children. Basic differences and disagreements among the Commissioners about the importance and scope of this principle ultimately led to the two dissenting votes on recommendation 5.

One difficulty centered on making a clear distinction between what has traditionally been called "therapeutic" and "nontherapeutic" research. The Commission believed that research involving children could certainly be justified, even if there were substantial risk, if it were in the context of a treatment

intended to be beneficial for the health or well-being of the child. This type of procedure is customarily called therapeutic research. However, Lebacqz and Robert Levine, M.D., of Yale University and a special consultant to the Commission, insisted that research in the context of treatment could be used to justify too much.

They wished to drop the terms "therapeutic" and "nontherapeutic," and to define more precisely the meaning of the ideas behind these terms. Cooke and Kenneth J. Ryan (Chief of Staff, Boston Hospital for Women, and Chairman of the Commission) initially opposed this approach, but at the November 1976 meeting Ryan changed his mind.[17] Gradually a consensus grew that these terms would at least have to be carefully explicated, and eventually the Commission voted to eliminate them completely. In its final report, the Commission speaks of "research . . . by an intervention that holds out the prospect of direct benefit for the individual subjects, or by a monitoring procedure required for the well-being of the subjects" and contrasts this with "research . . . by an intervention that does *not* hold out the prospect of direct benefit for the individual subjects, or by a monitoring procedure *not* required for the well-being of subjects"[18] (italics added). For the sake of simplicity in its recommendations, the Commission would have done better to define the former description as therapeutic research and the latter as nontherapeutic research in its definitions section rather than to discard the terms completely. In an attempt to be as precise as possible, the Commission seems to have slipped into a verbal jargon that most will find quite confusing and difficult to understand and apply.

Research Beneficial to Subjects

Research intended to be beneficial to individual subjects was accepted in principle very early. Once the Commission emerged from the conceptual quagmire of terminology, it was relatively easy for it to develop a recommendation. The two specific requirements for conducting beneficial research upon children are (1) that research risks must be justified by the anticipated benefits to subjects, and (2) that the relations of anticipated benefits to these risks is at least as favorable to the subjects as that presented by available alternative approaches. In other words, children cannot be volunteered for a research project, even if it is believed to be for their benefit, if there is a proved safer way to treat them. The Commission also insisted that its general requirements for research involving children, listed in recommendation 2, be met.[19] Finally the Commission mentions in all its more specific recommendations (3, 4, 5, and 6) that provisions must be made for the assent of the children and permission of their parents whether the research benefits the subjects under study or not.[20]

Minimal Risk

Acceptance of minimal risk research was not so much an ethical problem as a theoretical dilemma. It was apparent early in the debate that most Commissioners felt that they could approve research involving children even when not for their benefit as long as the risks presented by research were minimal.[21]

But what was meant by minimal risk? One thing that the Commission always intended to include in the term was research that presented no more than "mere inconvenience."

Joseph V. Brady (professor of behavioral biology, Johns Hopkins University) and Eliot Stellar (professor of physiological psychology, University of Pennsylvania) were quick to point out that most behavioral research falls into this category, and for a while the Commission considered a recommendation approving research that entailed no more than mere inconvenience. However, this recommendation was eventually included within one approving any research that entailed no more than minimal risk.

Some Commissioners wished to define minimal risk research as that which does not involve any risks to children greater than those normally encountered in their daily lives or in routine medical or psychological examinations. Eventually this definition prevailed. Cooke, however, felt the definition was too restrictive and argued long and hard that some interventions not considered routine or customary should nevertheless be considered as generating only minimal risk because he wished the Commission "not to depart from minimal risk as the barrier to allowing research." He pointed out that "what is minimal in the circumstances of a normal infant is not minimal to the circumstances of a child with leukemia. . . ."[22] He summarized his position thus:

> I'm saying that this Commission could come out and say that they are against subjecting nonassenting subjects to more than minimal risk unless it's for the benefit of that particular subject but that minimal depends a great deal on the circumstances, on the life situations.[23]

Ultimately, the Commission rejected this point of view, defined minimal risk quite conservatively, and adopted recommendation 5 (allowing nonbeneficial research when there is a minor increase above minimal risk) to take care of Cooke's concern. Ironically, he wound up voting against this recommendation because he felt that it justified too much.

However, the Commission would have been well advised for other reasons to heed his advice to frame their definition of minimal risk as a sliding scale. As defined in the Commission's report, minimal risk uses the standard of "what healthy children normally encounter in their daily lives, or in routine medical or psychological examinations" as a measurement of acceptable nonbeneficial research procedures. But "healthy children" is in fact a very relative term. Healthy ghetto children may be subject to a probability of harm in their everyday life far greater than their affluent suburban counterparts. Yet the Commission provides no acknowledgment of this problem or any guidance for institutional review boards in dealing with sociocultural health differences among children who are potential research subjects. Perhaps if Cooke's approach to minimal risks had been accepted, the Commission would have seen this deficiency and dealt with it. Once having accepted a seemingly narrow definition of minimal risk, the Commission allows this type of research as long as the general requirements of recommendations 2 and the assent and permission provisions of recommendations 7 and 8 are followed.[24]

National Review

Originally, the Commission intended to ban nonbeneficial research that involved more than minimal risk. However, at the January 1977 meeting, Levine suggested that the Commissioners consider a mechanism for adjudicating cases in which more than minimal risk research might be considered because of a national epidemic or emergency. The mechanism he alluded to was the National Ethics Advisory Board, whose establishment the Commission had recommended in its fetal research report.[25] This board would consider cases that local institutional review boards felt they did not have the power to approve but which might be important enough to warrant approval. The Commission approved this policy in recommendation 6. In deference to objections of the late David W. Louisell (professor of law, University of California at Berkeley), the Commission also required public review and intervention any time the National Ethics Advisory Board considered a case. The Commission further provided standards upon which the National Ethics Advisory Board must base its decisions.[26]

Minor Increase above Minimal Risk

Having adopted the mechanism of national review and having defined minimum risk so narrowly, some Commissioners became worried that much useful research would be required to undergo national scrutiny before it could be approved. Brady, for example,

believed that the Commission should attempt to reduce the number of cases that might be sent to the National Ethics Advisory Board.[27] Donald W. Seldin (professor of internal medicine, University of Texas at Dallas), the Commissioner most in favor of encouraging research involving children, not surprisingly argued vigorously for a recommendation that would allow research entailing a minor increase over minimal risk, even when there were no guarantees that individual subjects would benefit from these research interventions. It was sufficient for him if the class to which they belonged was helped or benefited in a significant way. Seldin's adversary in this debate was Cooke, who viewed this recommendation as opening Pandora's box by allowing some children to be harmed for the benefit of others. Turtle agreed with Cooke on this point, but interestingly enough, Louisell, opposed in principle to any sort of utilitarian argument, believed he could go along with the recommendation as long as the increased risk was indeed slight and if the official Commission commentary to the recommendation specified examples of these minor increases over minimal risk.[28] This recommendation was ultimately accepted by the Commission with the dissenting votes of Turtle and Cooke.[29]

Justice

The third and final set of issues that the Commission dealt with can be grouped under the ethical principle of justice. One of the general requirements of the Commission for research involving children was that subjects be selected equitably. The Commission proscribed overutilization of any one group of children based solely upon administrative convenience or availability of a population living in conditions of social or economic deprivation. Thus studies such as those at Willowbrook would now be banned. In other words, the Commission believed that the burdens as well as the benefits, no matter how large or small, of participation in research should be equitably distributed among all segments of our society.[30] Besides this general requirement of equitable treatment, included in recommendation 2, the Commission singles out in its last two recommendations certain especially vulnerable subject groups, for example, wards of the state, and provides special protective mechanisms for them.[31]

A final issue with regard to the principle of justice is Turtle's dissenting statement to recommendation 5, contending that in approving this recommendation, the Commission is "potentially subjecting sick children to greater risks than other children without regard to foreseeable benefit."[32] The section of recommendation 5 to which he objects most strongly is part B:

> Such intervention or procedure (minor increase above minimal risk and non-beneficial) presents experiences to subjects that are reasonably commensurate with those inherent in their actual or expected medical, psychological, or social situations, and is likely to yield generalizable knowledge about the subjects' disorder or condition.[33]

In his dissent, Turtle argued both that sick children cannot be deemed to be a morally separate class for purposes of relaxing protective measures and mechanisms, and that sick children, if capable of being placed in a morally relevant separate class, would require even greater protection than that afforded to children in general. In other words, even though a child becomes accustomed to certain types of medical interventions because of an illness, Turtle believes it is unjust to utilize these techniques on the child in the context of research when there is little or no chance of benefiting that individual child upon whom the research is being performed.

Ryan, in rebutting Turtle, pointed out that the Commission was talking only about "minor" or "slight" additional risk over that normally encountered, and that recommendation 5 contemplated research only in the nature and treatment of *disorders* that specifically afflict children. Ryan contended

that such research cannot by its very nature be conducted on normal subjects.[34] I believe Turtle's criticisms, though not his conclusions, are ethically sound. It is unjust to discriminate between two classes solely on the basis of one class being more accustomed to a certain type of invasive procedure than another. The Commission offers no justification for making an implicit but morally relevant distinction between healthy and diseased children in this regard. It has not adequately justified its recommendation that when nonbeneficial research presents a minor increase over minimal risk, the only subjects that can be accepted are those who are accustomed to the invasions or procedures the research protocol will utilize. Ryan's contention that under the circumstances only diseased children could be involved in this type of research is fallacious because many important studies need healthy controls, who now appear to be banned from slightly risky research unless it could be shown that they themselves benefited directly in some way or were accustomed to the interventions or procedures they would have to undergo as experimental control subjects.

Although agreeing with Turtle's criticisms, one need not adopt his conclusion that all slightly risky research not beneficial to individual subjects should be proscribed. The Commission could have emphasized the slight nature of the additional risk they were willing to accept and have concluded that this research was ethically the same as minimal risk research. It then might have recommended that parents have the prerogative of enrolling their children for this type of research as long as the children themselves did not object. Ryan took this position early in the debate, but the Commission's argument over commensurability with usual experience clouded over the fact that they were still talking about only slightly risky research. The Commission has agreed that it is ethically allowable to put some children at risk for the benefit of others when the risk is minimal. They could have said the same thing about slightly more than minimal risk for all children regardless of commensurability with experience as long as they focused a bit more precisely on what "a minor increase over minimal risk" actually means. In this way the Commission would have avoided charges of discrimination, and Turtle's objections would have had to be grounded in some ethical principle other than justice.

Cooke is correct in arguing that recommendation 5 as it now stands is vague, despite the attempt of the Commission in its commentary to spell out what it means by these interventions or procedures.[35] Despite the amount of time and energy expended upon it, recommendation 5 still remains the weakest section of the report, and will no doubt engender confusion when institutional review boards attempt to interpret it.

The Department of Health, Education and Welfare recommended in the *Federal Register* of July 21, 1978, that the guidelines be issued as regulations with three major modifications: (1) the objection of children to participation in research is not held as binding; (2) no specific age is set after which the assent of the child is mandatory; rather institutional review boards are asked to consider age on a case-by-case basis; (3) the Secretary may appoint an ad hoc panel to consider difficult research protocols, rather than necessarily relying upon the National Ethics Advisory Board.[36] These proposed rules are open for public comment and criticism for 60 days, after which time, with appropriate modification, they will be incorporated into the *Code of Federal Regulations* (45 CFR 46).

Conclusion

The Commission on the whole has done a creditable service for both the public and the research community. Their deliberations on research involving children reflect a pervasive desire to achieve consensus and to accommodate the desires and special interests of everyone who participated in the debate. That the Commission adopted a moderate position was no accident; it reflects a concern often expressed by various commissioners that the Commission, while

its primary task remains the protection of human subjects, go on record as emphasizing that scientific research is important and can in most cases be performed ethically.

The Commission's Recommendations for Research on Children

Recommendation 1: Since the Commission finds that research involving children is important for the health and well-being of all children and can be conducted in an ethical manner, the Commission recommends that such research be conducted and supported, subject to the conditions set forth in the following recommendations.

Recommendation 2: Research involving children may be conducted or supported provided an Institutional Review Board has determined that: (A) the research is scientifically sound and significant; (B) where appropriate, studies have been conducted first on animals and adult humans, then on older children, prior to involving infants; (C) risks are minimized by using the safest procedures consistent with sound research design and by using procedures performed for diagnostic or treatment purposes whenever feasible; (D) adequate provisions are made to protect the privacy of children and their parents, and to maintain confidentiality of data; (E) subjects will be selected in an equitable manner; (F) the conditions of all applicable subsequent recommendations are met.

Recommendation 3: Research that does not involve greater than minimal risk to children may be conducted or supported provided an Institutional Review Board has determined that : (A) the conditions of Recommendation (2) are met; and (B) adequate provisions are made for assent of the children and permission of their parents or guardians, as set forth in Recommendations (7) and (8).

Recommendation 4: Research in which more than minimal risk to children is presented by an intervention that holds out the prospect of direct benefit for the individual subjects, or by a monitoring procedure required for the well-being of the subjects, may be conducted or supported provided an Institutional Review Board has determined that:

(A) such risk is justified by the anticipated benefit to the subjects;

(B) the relation of anticipated benefit to such risk is at least as favorable to the subjects as that presented by available alternative approaches;

(C) the conditions of Recommendation (2) are met; and

(D) adequate provisions are made for assent of the children and permission of their parents or guardians, as set forth in Recommendations (7) and (8).

Recommendation 5: Research in which more than minimal risk to children is presented by an intervention that does not hold out the prospect of direct benefit for the individual subjects, or by a monitoring procedure not required for the well-being of the subjects, may be conducted or supported provided an Institutional Review Board has determined that:

(A) such risk represents a minor increase over minimal risk;

(B) such intervention or procedure presents experiences to subjects that are reasonably commensurate with those inherent in their actual or expected medical, psychological or social situations, and is likely to yield generalizable knowledge about the subject's disorder or condition;

(C) the anticipated knowledge is of vital importance for understanding or amelioration of the subject's disorder or condition;

(D) the conditions of Recommendation (2) are met; and

(E) adequate provisions are made for assent of the children and permission of their parents or guardians, as set forth in Recommendations (7) and (8).

Recommendation 6: Research that cannot be approved by an Institutional Review Board under Recommendations (3), (4) and (5), as applicable, may be conducted or supported provided an Institutional Review Board has determined that the research presents an opportunity to understand, prevent or alleviate a serious problem affecting the health or welfare of children and, in addition, a national ethical advisory board and, following opportunity for public review and comment, the secretary of the responsible federal department (or highest official of the responsible federal agency) have determined either (a) that the research satisfies the conditions of Recommendation (3), (4) and (5), as applicable, or (B) the following:

(I) the research presents an opportunity to understand, prevent or alleviate a serious problem affecting the health or welfare of children;

(II) the conduct of the research would not violate the principles of respect for persons, beneficence and justice;

(III) the conditions of Recommendation (2) are met; and

(IV) adequate provisions are made for assent of the children and permission of their parents or guardians, as set forth in Recommendations (7) and (8).

Recommendation 7: In addition to the determinations required under the foregoing recommendations, as applicable, the Institutional Review Board should determine that adequate provisions are made for: (A) soliciting the assent of the children (when capable) and the permission of their parents or guardians; and, when appropriate, (B) monitoring the solicitation of assent and permission, and involving at least one parent or guardian in the conduct of the research. A child's objection to participation in research should be binding unless the intervention holds out a prospect of direct benefit that is important to the health or well-being of the child and is available only in the context of the research.

Recommendation 8: If the Institutional Review Board determines that a research protocol is designed for conditions or a subject population for which parental or guardian permission is not a reasonable requirement to protect the subjects, it may waive such requirement provided an appropriate mechanism for protecting the children who will participate as subjects in the research is substituted. The choice of an appropriate mechanism should depend upon the nature and purpose of the activities described in the protocol, the risk and anticipated benefit to the research subjects, and their age, status and condition.

Recommendation 9: Children who are wards of the state should not be included in research approved under Recommendations (5) or (6) unless such research is: (A) related to their status as orphans, abandoned children, and the like: or (B) conducted in a school or similar group setting in which the majority of children involved as subjects are not wards of the state. If such research is approved, the Institutional Review Board should require that an advocate for each child be appointed, with an opportunity to intercede that would normally be provided by parents.

Recommendation 10: Children who reside in institutions for the mentally infirm or who are confined in correctional facilities should participate in research only if the conditions regarding research on the institutionalized mentally infirm or on prisoners (as applicable) are fulfilled in addition to the conditions set forth herein.

NOTES

1. United States Government, *Public Law 93-348.*

2. National Commission for the Protection of Human Subjects of Biomedical and Behavioral Research (hereafter referred to as National Commission), *Report and Recommendations: Research Involving Children* [DHEW Publication No. (OS) 77-0004], 1977; and *Appendix to Report and Recommendations: Research Involving Children* (DHEW Publication No. (OS) 77-0005), 1977.

(The former publication will subsequently be referred to as *Children* and the latter as *Appendix.*)

3. *Children*, pp. 123-44.

4. Ibid., pp. 1-20.

5. Ibid., pp. 145-53.

6. See National Commission, *Transcript of the Meeting Proceedings* (hereafter referred to as *Proceedings*), July 1976, pp. 289-297, for the Commission's discussion of this issue.

7. *Children*, p. 1.

8. *Proceedings*, August 1976, pp. 268-270.

9. Ibid., July 1976, pp. 304-306.

10. National Commission, *The Belmont Report: Ethical Guidelines for the Protection of Human Subjects of Research* (DHEW Publication (OS) 78-0010), 1978.

11. *Proceedings*, September 1976, pp. 139-142.

12. Ibid., August 1976, pp. 262-263.

13. *Proceedings*, March 1977, pp. II-2 to II-8, and II-11 to II-13.

14. *Children*, pp. 12-17.

15. See, for example, the paper of William G. Bartholeme, "The Ethics of Non-Therapeutic Clinical Research on Children" in *Appendix*, pp. 3-1 to 3-54.

16. *Proceedings*, September 1976, p. 247.

17. Ibid., November 1976, pp. 2-15 to 2-82.

18. *Children*, pp. 5-8.

19. Ibid., pp. 2-3.

20. Ibid., pp. 5-11.

21. *Proceedings*, November 1976, p. 2-137.

22. Ibid., May 1977, p. 36.

23. Ibid., p. 42.

24. *Children*, p. 5.

25. *Proceedings*, January 1977, p. 76; National Commission, *Report and Recommendations: Research on the Fetus* [DHEW Publication (OS) 76-127], 1975, pp. 74-75.

26. *Children*, pp. 10-11.

27. *Proceedings*, January 1977, p. 178.

28. Ibid., April 1977, pp. II-4 to II-111, and May 1977, pp. 5 to 69 and II-5 to II-64.

29. *Children*, pp. 7-8.

30. *Children*, p. 3.

31. Ibid., pp. 19-20.

32. Ibid., pp. 146-147.

33. Ibid., p. 8.

34. Ibid., pp. 153-154.

35. Ibid., pp. 145-146.

36. United States Government, *Federal Register* (July 21, 1978) 43:31786-94.

Fetal Research, Morality, and Public Policy
Richard A. McCormick

Morality and Fetal Experimentation

By the term "experimentation" as used here, I understand all procedures not directly beneficial to the subject involved. (There is little moral problem and should be little policy problem where procedures are experimental but represent the most hopeful therapy for an individual.) By the term "nonviable fetus" I understand a fetus incapable of extrauterine survival. (Attention in this study will be restricted to the nonviable fetus because I shall suppose that in all decisively relevant moral and policy respects touching experimentation, the viable fetus should be treated as a child.)

The nonviable fetus, as an experimental subject, could be further subdivided as follows:

in utero	*ex utero*
-no abortion planned	-spontaneous abortion
-abortion planned	-living
-dead	
-during abortion	-induced abortion
	-living
	-dead

The literature on morality and fetal experimentation (to be reported below) is very sparse.[1] What does exist has drawn attention to the analogies with experiments on children. However, at least two things must be noted about this analogy. First, whether the question of fetal experimentation approximates, and indeed is, in most crucial respects identical with experimentation on children, depends on one's assessment of fetal life. If one regards the fetus as "disposable maternal tissue" or as "potential human life" only, then the questions are sharply different and will yield a different moral conclusion, and ultimately a different public policy. If, however, the nonviable fetus is viewed as "protectable humanity" or a "person"

with rights, then the problems are quite similar. Second, the nonviable fetus (whether abortion is contemplated or not) is in a dependency relationship, its health and growth being linked more or less to maternal health. This relationship can be read in a variety of ways in terms of its ethical yield. But one thing all would agree on is that whatever fetal experimentation is judged to be warranted, it must take account of maternal health.

Thus while there are possible differences in these two problems (experiments on children and fetuses), there are important continuities. If one judges all experimentation on living children (even if they are dying) to be an abuse and immoral, and at the same time regards the nonviable fetus as a person in its own right (even though within a dependency symbiosis), it is safe to say that one will condemn (morally) all experimentation on living fetuses in whatsoever condition they be. Contrarily, if one morally justifies some experimentation on children, it is quite possible, though not inevitable, that one could and would extend this justification to fetuses.

There are two identifiable schools of (moral) thought where experimentation on children is concerned. The first is associated with Paul Ramsey[3] and is supported by William E. May. The second is the position of Curran,[4] O'Donnell[5] and myself.[6] Ramsey argues that we may not submit a child to procedures that involve any risk of harm or to procedures that involve no harm but simply "offensive touching." . . .

Thomas O'Donnell accepts the moral validity of vicarious consent where the "danger is so remote and discomfort so minimal that a normal and informed individual would be presupposed to give ready consent."[5] Charles Curran has drawn a similar conclusion. . . .[4]

I have attempted to argue for a position

Source: *Hastings Center Report*, vol. 5, June 1975.

that would allow experimentation on children where there is no discernible risk or discomfort.[6] The position departs from Ramsey practically only if he disallows any give and play with the term "discernible risk." More importantly, it is at one with Ramsey's analysis in rejecting any utilitarian evaluation of children's lives that would submit their integrity to a quantity-of-benefit calculus far beyond any legitimately constructed consent. The heart of my argument is this: if we analyze proxy consent where it is accepted as legitimate—in the _therapeutic_ situation—we will see that parental consent is morally legitimate because, life and health being goods for the child, he would choose them because he _ought_ to choose the good of life. In other words, proxy consent is morally valid precisely insofar as it is a reasonable presumption of the child's wishes, a construction of what the child would wish could he do so. The child would so choose because he _ought_ to do so, life and health being goods definitive of his flourishing.

Once proxy consent in the therapeutic situation is analyzed in this way, the question occurs: are there other things that the child _ought_, as a human being, to choose precisely because and insofar as they are goods definitive of his well-being? As an answer to this question I have suggested that there are things we _ought_ to do for others simply because we are members of the human community. These are not precisely works of charity or supererogation (beyond what is required of all of us) but our personal bearing of our share that all may prosper. They involve no discernible risk, discomfort, or inconvenience, yet promise genuine hope for general benefit. In summary, if it can be argued that it is good for all of us to share in these experiments, and hence that we _ought_ to do so (social justice), then a presumption of consent where children are involved is reasonable, and proxy consent becomes legitimate.

The moral reasoning outlined above yields a conclusion that is shared, at a practical level, by Curran,[6] Beecher,[7] Ingelfinger,[8] the _Helsinki Declaration_,[7] the _Archives of Disease in Childhood_,[8] and others. Yet it has built into it rational limits and controls not always present in merely practical statements.

With this as a background we now turn to fetal experimentation itself. What one judges to be morally appropriate and acceptable where fetal experiments are concerned depends above all on his evaluation of the fetus. Here there are two general schools of thought. The first would regard the fetus as a nonperson or as "potential human life." These terms are used in the moral, not the legal, sense though it is clear that one who is not a person morally should not be considered such legally. At any rate, one who is not a _moral_ person, who is morally a nonperson—and therefore not the subject of rights and claims—seems to present little problem where experimentation is concerned. One who holds this position ought to conclude, if his moral reasoning is consistent, that experimentation on the fetus is legitimate and desirable, or if there are to be restrictions they are rooted in values other than the fetus itself in its present state.

The second general school of thought is that the fetus is, indeed, protectable, a protectable humanity, and an appropriate subject of rights. Within this school of thought, three distinct tendencies or subdivisions are identifiable.

1. The fetus is protectable humanity but to be valued less than a viable fetus or a born infant. This school would probably tolerate experiments if the benefits are great, but no literature has made this conclusion explicit.

2. The fetus is a fellow human being and must be treated, where experimentation is concerned, exactly as one treats the child. Just as the child may not be exposed not only to harm and risk, but also to "offensive touching," so the fetus may not be exposed to any risk or even to "offensive touching." This would seem to be the position of Ramsey.[1] Concretely at one point the nonviable fetus is to be likened to an unconscious patient; at another point the nonviable liv-

ing fetus (after instances of spontaneous or induced abortion) is to be likened to a dying patient; prior to an induced abortion the fetus is to be likened to the condemned. Since it is immoral to experiment on the unconscious, and, without their consent, on the condemned or dying, it is immoral to experiment on the fetus—and this would apply even to "offensive touching." In logic Ramsey ought to conclude that *no* experimentation on living fetuses is morally warranted.

3. The fetus is a fellow human being and ought to be treated, where experimentation is concerned, exactly as one treats the child. However, experiments on children, where no discernible risk or discomfort is involved, are morally legitimate if appropriate consent is obtained and if the experiments are genuinely necessary (trials on animals are insufficient) for medical knowledge calculated to be of notable benefit to fetuses or children in general. This is an extension to the fetus of the moderate position on children outlined above. It is, I believe, a defensible moral position—but the way the position is defended is utterly crucial (I shall return to this below) if sufficient protection of human subjects is to be assured.

The position just outlined is the one I would attempt to defend and the one I would propose to the Commission as the basis for its policy proposals. But since the fetus can be in a variety of postures or situations, this general approach must be carefully applied to this variety of postures. I emphasize here that I am discussing for the present a *moral* position (not immediately what public policy ought to be) and one that reflects *my own views*.

For purposes of clarity and precision, let me now return to the definition of those terms with which I began this section.

The Fetus in Utero

1. *No abortion planned.* Theoretically, if there is no discernible risk of discomfort to the fetus and to the mother, and appropriate proxy consent is obtained, such

experimentation could be defended as morally legitimate—on the same grounds that identical experiments on children could be defended. Practically, however, one must question the necessity of experimentation here (a factual matter). If fetal material is otherwise available, experimentation here would be inappropriate precisely as unnecessary.

2. *Abortion planned.* Here a preliminary general reflection is in order. It applies to the fetus prior to abortion, during abortion, and after abortion (whether the fetus be living or dead). It is the issue of cooperation. If one objects to most abortions being performed in our society as immoral, is it morally proper to derive experimental profit from the products of such an abortion-system? Is the progress achieved through such experimentation not likely to blunt the sensitivities of Americans to the immorality (injustice) of the procedure that made such advance possible, and thereby entrench attitudes injurious and unjust to nascent life? This is, in my judgment, a serious moral objection to experimentation on the products of most induced abortions (whether the fetus be living or dead, prior to abortion or postabortional). It is especially relevant in a society where abortion is widely done and legally protected.

However, I have no confidence that a society that does not share the underlying judgment on most abortions and is so highly pragmatic as to be insensitive to the issue of cooperation will be impressed by this moral consideration—factors that must be taken into account where public policy (feasibility) is concerned. That is, public policy must root in the deepest moral perceptions of the majority, or at least, in principles the majority is reluctant to modify. Since there is such profound division on the moral propriety of abortion, the moral notion of cooperation in an abortion system will not function at the level of policy.

a. *Prior to abortion.* One cannot approach the position of the fetus without a further distinction. *If the planned abortion is moral-*

ly legitimate, we might say that the fetus is in the situation of the tragically but justly condemned individual. In this instance, if the proposed experimentation will involve no discernible risk to the fetus, I believe that proxy consent (of the mother) would be a defensible construction of fetal wishes. If, however, the proposed experimentation will involve discernible risks to the fetus, then proxy consent is an invalid construction. *If the planned abortion is not morally legitimate,* we might say that the fetus is in the situation of an unjustly condemned individual. In my judgment, this is the case with most abortions now being planned and performed. In this instance, the full moral weight of the cooperation issue strikes home—but once again, not at the policy level, as stated above. Second, there is the issue of consent and its validity. The consent requirement is premised on the fact that the parents are the ones who have the best interests of the child (here the fetus) at heart. But does such a premise obtain when an abortion (presumably immoral) is being planned? Does a mother planning an abortion in the circumstances described have the best interests of the fetus at heart? I think not. Third, there is the possible change of mind of the mother. Allowing experimentation prior to abortion—that is, experimentation that is potentially risky or harmful to the fetus—prejudices the freedom of the woman to change her mind about the abortion, and thus constitutes an infringement on fetal rights for this reason alone, if for no other. To those who do not share my evaluation of fetal life, these considerations will, of course, seem marginally relevant at best.

b. During abortion. Once again, a distinction. *If the abortion is morally legitimate,* then granted appropriate proxy consent, experimentation could be legitimate if it left the fetus in no worse position during its dying than it is in as a result of the abortion. If, however, the experimentation leaves the fetus in a worse position, for example, in pain, then it is equivalent to illegitimate experimentation on the dying. *If the abortion is not morally legitimate,* then experimentation on the fetus raises two of the points

mentioned above (in section *a*): cooperation and invalidity of consent. The question of "discernible risk" seems meaningless morally, since it seems meaningless to speak of exposing to risk one who has already been inserted into a lethal situation.

The Fetus ex Utero

1. Spontaneous abortion. The fetus may be either living or dead. If it is dead, there should be no moral objection to experimentation. If the fetus is living, the same conclusion obtains, providing experimentation imposes no pain: for the fetus may be legitimately constructed to consent to experiments involving no discernible risk, and he is in a situation (lethal) where the distinction between no discernible risk and discernible risk is meaningless.

2. Induced abortion. The fetus may be living or dead. If the fetus is still living and the abortion was morally legitimate, then experimentation seems morally legitimate if it induces no pain or discomfort. For if the fetus may be constructed to consent to experiments where no discernible harm is involved, and if he is in a situation (lethal) where the difference between discernible harm or risk is meaningless, then he may be legitimately constructed to consent—given appropriate proxy consent. If the fetus is still living and the abortion was morally illegitimate, then the above issues (cooperation, consent) could intrude to prevent any morally legitimate proxy consent.

Summary

Within the paramaters of *my* evaluation of fetal life, fetal experimentation would be clearly justified, with appropriate safeguards, distinctions, and consent, where the abortion is spontaneous or has been justifiably (morally) induced. Where it has been induced without moral justification, I believe there are moral objections of various sorts against experimentation. However, since these objections are premised on the moral character of the abortion, and since this is a difficult (at times) determination in itself, and since the ultimate judgment will hardly be shared by a majority, these objections will be extremely difficult, indeed impossible, to formulate in policy proposals on fetal experiments. Moreover, one can question whether restriction on fetal experiments rooted in such considerations is the best way to highlight the moral illegitimacy of the abortion.

Where experimentation is morally justified, it is so because of the legitimacy and sharp limitations of proxy consent, extrapolated from the legitimacy of proxy consent where children are concerned. I wish to emphasize this point here. If proxy consent (with the clear limitations on the validity of this consent) is not the basis for the moral legitimacy of experimentation on fetuses, then the integrity of the individual will be "protected" not by soundly reasoned constructions of what the fetus—or any human being—would consent to because it *ought*, but by a very unpredictable and highly utilitarian assessment of its value and worth as over against great (alleged) scientific and medical benefits for others. Such an assessment does not provide but erodes—in a highly technological, pragmatic society—individual protection. Thus the DHEW's original but tentative version of *Protection of Human Subjects, Policies and Procedures*[10] stated: "The investigator must also stipulate either that the risk to the subjects (children) will be insignificant, or *that although some risk exists, the potential benefit is significant and far outweighs that risk.*" In such thought and language is the germ—and even more—of the subordination of the individual to the collectivity. That germ is in the conclusion, to be sure; but it is far more insidiously present and threatening in the very way of thinking, in the form of moral reasoning undergirding it. We call it utilitarianism. And whatever the policy proposals this Commission recommends, it will have only gotten mired in the cultural status quo if its conclusions root in a utilitarian assessment of the value and integrity of man, fetal or otherwise.

Avoidance of this trap will not be easy.

For if notable medical benefits do not justify *all* experimentation, they are the only things that justify *any* experimentation. And once that is said the tendency will be to give medical benefits the preference. Furthermore, if fetal individuality and dignity do no prohibit *all* experiments, they certainly prohibit *some*. It is the first task of this Commission to discover the form and structure of moral reasoning on which alone the proper protective balance can be based and spelled out in policy proposals. That form and structure centers around proxy consent, its legitimation and limitations.

Abortion Policy and Experimentation Policy

I raise this issue prior to an explicit consideration of policy proposals because I presume that in matters of law or policy consistency is, at least to some extent, a desideratum. From a *moral* point of view fetal experimentation and abortion are in some respects separable issues. That is, even though a particular abortion is judged to be morally justifiable, one could maintain that experimentation on the living abortus is illegitimate experimentation on the dying. And that is a different question from the morality of the abortion itself. There are those who would convert such separability as follows: even though the abortion was illegitimate, it does not follow that experimentation on the abortus is also illegitimate. (I do not believe the matter is that simple, as noted above.)

However, there is a point at which these issues converge, particularly in the popular mind. This convergence is best seen at the *policy* level. Under existing abortion law (*Roe* v. *Wade*, *Doe* v. *Bolton*) fetal life enjoys no protection during the first two trimesters of pregnancy, and even in the third the compelling interest of the state in protecting fetal life is qualified by considerations of maternal health so broadly defined that it would be difficult to convict anyone of an illegal interruption of pregnancy anytime during pregnancy. The rationale for this policy is the predominance of maternal interests, especially privacy, over "potential human

life." Now clearly, if fetal life is so totally
unprotected *with regard to its very existence
and survival,* and on the grounds that it is
only "potential human life," then any policy
restrictive of fetal experimentation must
find other grounds (other than present fetal
humanity and rights) for its restrictiveness—
at least if legal consistency is to be preserved.
For it is patently ridiculous to stipulate
that fetal life may be *taken* freely because
it is only "potential human life," and yet
to prohibit experimentation on this same
"potential human life," especially when great
medical benefits may be expected from
such experimentation. For such a prohibition would imply that the privacy or other
interests of one woman are of more value
than the survival and health of perhaps thousands of fetuses and infants.

I see no way out of this impasse where
the Commission for the Protection of Human
Subjects is concerned—except to say that
perhaps even legal inconsistency has its values. But the only value perceptible to
this commentator in such inconsistency
is that it may be a first step toward reassessment of the Court's "potential human life."
That may be a salutary step, but it reflects what appear to be the only two options open to this Commission: to reaffirm,
by implication, the Court's philosophy in
Roe v. *Wade,* or to establish proposals (restrictive in character) that are at some point
inconsistent with this philosophy. This latter alternative is, in my judgment, the
way to go.

Policy on Fetal Experimentation

In attempting to develop sound (feasible)
policies on fetal experimentation, I suggest
that the Commission must keep two points
in mind: moral pluralism and cultural pragmatism. A word about each.

Moral pluralism. Fetal life is variously
evaluated, as the abortion decision shows.
Even though abortion and experimentation
are separable, they are closely related as
I have pointed out. Therefore, the Commis-

sion is in a very delicate position and is faced
potentially with another *Roe* v. *Wade* decision. In a sense the Commission cannot
win in its conclusions. If it allows fetal experimentation without sufficient grounding
and controls, it will alienate and galvanize
those identified with right-to-life positions.
If it disallows fetal experiments without
sound and consistent reasoning, it will alienate and galvanize the "liberal" and research
communities. If it tries to walk a middle path
with a utilitarian sliding scale of costs and
benefits, most ethicists in the country will be
up in arms.

The only way out of this bind (and one
which avoids utilitarian costs-benefits theory)
is tied to the notion of proxy consent. In
other words, that measure of proxy consent
regarded as valid for children should be the
measure of acceptable fetal experimentation.
Where children are concerned, proxy consent is legitimate when the experimentation
involves no discernible risks, discomforts,
or inconvenience—in human judgment. Beyond that the individual must be free to
consent for himself. Analogously with the
fetus. If the experimentation involves no
discernible risk—or in cases where the nonviable fetus is dying, no pain—proxy consent may be regarded as legitimate. (There
is a moral problem, of course, with the
legitimacy of proxy consent where the fetus
is about to be aborted or has been aborted.
However, since the moral legitimacy of
the abortion itself is a highly disputed point
in our society, the legitimacy of proxy consent in these cases cannot be decisive at
the level of policy. To wit, it is not presently feasible.)

This practical policy structure (centering
on permissibility and controls grounded in
proxy consent) has the advantage of speaking
to all segments of a divided community.
To those convinced of fetal humanity and
protectability, it says: nothing more or
less is allowed on the fetus than on the child.
To the "liberal" and research community,
it states the legitimacy and need of fetal experimentation. To the ethical community

it states that the legitimacy and control of fetal experimentation is neither capricious not utilitarian in character, but soundly and rationally based in and controlled by an intelligible principle.

Cultural pragmatism. Our culture is one where: (1) technology, even medical, is highly esteemed; (2) moral judgments tend to collapse into pragmatic cost-benefit calculations; (3) youth, health, pleasure, and comfort are highly valued and tend to be sought and preserved at disproportionate cost; (4) maladaptations, such as senility, retardation, age, or defectiveness, are treated destructively rather than by adapting the environment to their needs. These factors suggest that the general cultural mentality is one that identifies the quickest, most effective way as the good way. Morality often translates into efficiency. This mentality constitutes the atmosphere in which the Commission's policies must be shaped. They are, I believe, calculated to be threatening and inimical to a careful implementation of proxy consent at the fetal-research level. Therefore, I believe that the Commission will best serve the community if it bends toward more protection of individuals, rather than toward more freedom for experimental research. The culture will bend this latter way, and the proposals ought to be conceived as a balancing influence, not simply a reinforcing one.

If the above reflections are accurate, the task of the Commission (once it has accepted the proxy-consent rationale for experimentation on fetuses) is twofold: first, to spell out insofar as is possible what degree of risk may be regarded, in broad human terms, as equivalent to "no discernible risk"; and second, to detail the procedural demands that will best assure that this determination is realized in individual protocols.

Proposals. The following points are suggested as an attempt to bring this twofold task to the level of concrete proposals:

1. *The experiment must be necessary.* Use of animals and dead fetal tissue is not sufficient; the experiment is not repetitive (of work being done elsewhere); proportionate benefits are reasonably anticipated.

The onus of showing necessity is on the experimental researcher.

2. *There must be no discernible risk for the fetus or mother* or, if the fetus is dying, there must be no added pain or discomfort. (This would prohibit all experiments that are aimed at determining what harm might come to the fetus, and all experiments that prolong the dying process of the fetus.)

The onus of showing no discernible risk is on the experimental researcher.

3. *The above demands must be secured by prior approval and adequate review* of all fetal experiments. The reviewing group ought to include at least some members outside of the research community. (There is a tendency, as the literature shows, for researchers to minimize risk not only in terms of prospective benefits, but also in terms of the ability to "handle complications" that may arise.)

If these policies appear to some to be too restrictive, it must be recalled that we shall only know whether they are unduly restrictive if they are tried. It is always possible to liberalize; it is much more difficult to retrench—and retrenchment occurs only after rights have been exposed or violated. Where the rights of others are even and only *possibly* at stake, the part of wisdom and humanity is to try the less obvious, perhaps the more arduous, but more conservative (of rights) way.

NOTES

1. See especially, Paul Ramsey, *The Ethics of Fetal Research*, Yale, New Haven, 1975; LeRoy Walters, "Ethical Issues in Experimentation on the Human Fetus," *Journal of Religious Ethics*, vol. 2, p. 33, 1974.

2. Paul Ramsey, *The Patient as Person*, p. 27, Yale, New Haven; 1970.

3. William E. May, "Experimentation on Human Subjects," *Linacre Quarterly*, vol. 41, p. 238, 1974.

4. Charles E. Curran, "Human Life," *Chicago Studies*, vol. 13, p. 293, 1974.

5. T. J. O'Donnell, "Informed Consent" *Journal of the American Medical Association*, vol. 227, p. 73, 1974.

6. Richard A. McCormick, "Proxy Consent in the Experimentation Situation," *Perspectives in Biology and Medicine*, vol. 18, p. 2, 1974.

7. H. K. Beecher, *Research and the Individual*, Little, Brown, Boston, 1970: see also W. J. Curran and H. K. Beecher, "Experimentation in Chil-

dren," *Journal of the American Medical Association*, vol. 210, p. 77, 1969.

8. F. J. Ingelfinger, "Ethics of Experiments on Children," *New England Journal of Medicine*, vol. 288, p. 791, 1973.

9. *Archives of Disease in Childhood*, vol. 48, p. 751, 1973.

10. *Federal Register*, vol. 38, p. 31738, 1973.

108.
Prison Research: National Commission Says, "No, Unless..."

Roy Branson

At least 3,600 United States prisoners were used during 1975 alone as the first humans on whom the safety of new drugs was tested—about 85 percent of the total of such tests, according to the Pharmaceutical Manufacturer's Association, whose 131 member firms develop most of the nation's prescription drugs.[1] The drug companies testify that they need to use prisoners, but are such experiments ethical? Because of the continuing controversy over this question, Congress specifically required its consideration in its 1974 mandate to the National Commission for the Protection of Human Subjects of Biomedical and Behavioral Research.

The Department of Health, Education and Welfare is still considering what regulations to write (see below) but last October, one year after it began its deliberations on the subject, the Commission gave its answer to the question of whether prisoners should be used in what has been called nontherapeutic biomedical research. In essence, the Commission said, no, unless. . . . Such research on prisoners should not be conducted unless (a) there are "compelling" reasons to involve prisoners, (b) conditions of equity are satisfied, and (c) there is a high de-

gree of voluntariness on the part of prisoners and "openness" in the prison. Research on incarceration and the nature of prisons, as well as research intended to improve the health of an individual prisoner, can be conducted if specified safeguards are followed.

The Commission did not reach this conclusion easily. Although its five recommendations were issued unanimously, the final decision was reached only after considerable debate and disagreement. It is instructive to look not only at the results of the Commission's work but also at the way they arrived at their conclusions, to see how they related ethical concerns to specific policy recommendations.

Gathering the Data

One of the Commission's first and most frustrating tasks was to determine the extent and nature of experimentation with prisoners. Although it was unable to gather exhaustive and unchallengeable data, the Commission did collect the most extensive information amassed so far. The total number of prisoners used in drug experiments during 1975 was probably higher than 3,600,

Source: *Hastings Center Report*, vol. 7, February 1977.

since companies representing only three-quarters of the industry's total research and development expenditures responded to the survey conducted by the pharmaceutical industry. Of the 51 firms reporting, 16 indicated use of prisoners in eight state and six county or municipal prisons. The Commission staff itself conducted a survey by letter; seven states reported that biomedical research was being conducted in their prisons and five states made the same statement for behavioral research. All behavioral programs were labeled therapeutic; no state reported any nontherapeutic research involving behavioral modification.[2]

Besides the initial tests of drugs, performed primarily by drug companies, the Commission determined that the federal government has funded a wide variety of biomedical and behavioral experiments. From 1970 to 1975 five of the six agencies within the Public Health Service supported research using prisoners—124 biomedical studies and at least 19 behavioral projects. The Department of Defense sponsored numerous studies that used prisoners for research on infectious diseases, and Commission members were startled by published reports that the Atomic Energy Commission (now the Energy and Development Administration) had funded research involving radiation of male prisoners' genitals.[3]

By contrast, another study for the Commission by the pharmaceutical industry concluded, after polling physicians active in research outside the United States, that "in none of the countries surveyed was it found that prisoners are used as volunteer subjects for medical projects, and we know of no countries other than the United States where this is done"[4] The countries surveyed included seven European countries (Belgium, France, Germany, Italy, the Netherlands, Spain, and Sweden), five English-speaking nations (Australia, Canada, New Zealand, South Africa, and the United Kingdom), four Latin American countries (Brazil, Colombia, Mexico, and Peru), and Japan. Virtually no country outside the United States conducts its clinical pharmacological

studies on healthy subjects in or out of prison, and unlike the United States, almost all nations will accept data generated from studies in other countries.[5]

Ever since 1962, following the thalidomide tragedy, the Food and Drug Administration has been required by federal statute to demand that drugs be tested for safety and efficacy on animals and normal subjects before being released for use on patients. The initial controlled experiments on humans are called Phase 1 drug tests. Phase 2 testing is research on substances that have gone through previous trials and are considered safe; Phase 3 is all follow-up testing. Aware of quite different regulations overseas, the Commission, as part of its Deliberations and Conclusions, suggests that Congress and the FDA study "whether present requirements for Phase 1 drug testing in normal volunteers should be modified."[6]

As the Commission approached its hearing, controversy continued to embroil various branches of both federal and state government. The National Prison Project of the American Civil Liberties Union had already filed a complaint in the U.S. District Court for the District of Maryland on behalf of seven prisoners involved in viral diarrhea, malaria, shegella, and typhoid experiments, some of which had been sponsored by the federal departments of Defense and DHEW. The complaint asked the court to declare for the first time in the United States that "the use of prisoners in nontherapeutic biomedical experimentation of this type is unconstitutional per se because of the impossibility of truly voluntary consent."[7] The same month the Commission received its first staff report, the House Subcommittee on Courts, Civil Liberties, and the Administration of Justice held hearings on a bill to prohibit medical research in federal prisons and prisons of states that receive certain kinds of federal support.

Eight states had prohibited the use of state prisons for biomedical experimentation—six by departmental policy, one by moratorium and one by legislation (Oregon). After the Commission's hearings began, the Federal Bureau of Prisons announced an indefinite moratorium on nontherapeutic biomedical experimentation conducted in any federal prison, and the Board of Directors of the American Correctional Association (the established professional organization of correctional officials at all levels of the United States government) officially adopted a statement saying: "The American Correctional Association has long viewed with concern the use of prisoners as subjects of medical pharmacological experimentation. . . . It now urges that efforts to eliminate such practices be undertaken by responsible bodies at the Federal, State and local levels." The statement concluded: "The authority which authorizes or permits prisoners to become subjects of human experimentation ignores his historic obligation as a custodian to protect and safely keep those for whom he assumes a legal responsibility."[8]

Hearing Appeals to Utility

When the Commission moved from surveys of the extent and nature of experimentation with prisoners to its hearings and deliberations, it heard a variety of ethical appeals. Utilitarian arguments for research with prisoners were urged in familiar risk-benefit language: low risk to prisoners, great benefits to society. The Pharmaceutical Manufacturer's Association argued that as far as Phase 1 drug tests were concerned, "few other populations are practical or available candidates for these sorts of controlled studies."[9] It testified that "to the best of our knowledge, not a single prisoner has died or been permanently injured as a result of a drug firm sponsored test"; indeed, "the record shows serious toxicity rarely occurs in these industry sponsored studies."[10] While the risks are minimal, the benefits are extensive. Eliminating prisoners from such research might well "delay the development of new drugs which will benefit everyone, including the prisoners themselves."[11]

The Commission was not persuaded. In sharp contrast to fetal research, the Com-

mission could not discover any scientific necessity of using prisoners in research that was not intended for or had a reasonable probability of improving the health of the subject. The benefits to society of drug research did not have to come specifically from experiments on healthy prisoners.

The Commission learned that several research programs had successfully used free populations for initial drug trials on humans. Some of these experiments relied on groups of free-living volunteers entering isolation wards for periods up to 30 days, an interval sufficient for conducting most of the Phase 1 drug tests required by the FDA. Dr. John Arnold, a researcher who had used prisoner subjects for 29 years, was adamant that his new policy of depending on free-living volunteers was superior, even from a strictly scientific viewpoint. Given the pervasive, unmonitored use of drugs in prisons, it was easier to control the relevant variables on free volunteers.[12]

After listening to all the evidence, except for research into the nature of prisons and the "causes, effects and processes of incarceration," the Commission agreed, in its Deliberations and Conclusions, on "the paucity of evidence of any necessity to conduct research in prisons."[13]

The Commissioners were concerned that certain experiments had involved considerable risk, but they agreed that overall, even within prisons, "the risks of research, as compared with other kinds of occupations, may be rather small."[14] However, the Commission insisted forcefully that degree of risk must be kept separate from the question of adequate conditions for giving consent. Even a minimally risky experiment must use volunteers who are in a position to give an adequately free and informed consent. And no matter how small, the burdens of research must be equitably distributed.

While the Commission was not interested in deciding the issue of prisoner research by calculating its scientific benefits to society, several Commissioners were impressed, at least initially, with the possibility that adopting standards for prisons housing research could lead to the improvement of prisons. The Commissioner selected by the other members as their Chairman, Kenneth J. Ryan, Chairman of Obstetrics and Gynecology, Harvard Medical School and Chief of Staff, Boston Hospital for Women, articulated this attitude in his remarks opening the preliminary deliberations of prisoner research in January 1976.

The Commissioners could decide that research should never be done in prison. But, Ryan said, "I see this as the opportunity of getting a tremendous amount of public good with respect to prison work." He believed that "if allowing research gets the public into prisons, and allows them the kind of opportunity for true rehabilitation . . . to develop people in the best sense of that word, then I think that it is an ethical means. I think it is a morally defensible means."[15] Halfway through the next meeting, he introduced the first outline of a possible Commission recommendation. Drafted with the aid of three of the staff, it recommended approval of prisoner research in correctional facilities certified by an appropriate review committee, which would be guided by enumerated standards.

However, the defense of the accreditation system as a means of accomplishing the good of improving prisons aroused increasing opposition. Some of the Commissioners reminded their colleagues that they had not been given a mandate to reform prisons. Nor did they have expertise in setting standards for openness in prisons. And even if acceptable standards could be devised, it would clearly be difficult to monitor and enforce standards within not only the experimental setting, but the entire prison.

Protecting Prisoners' Rights

Still, the accreditation idea persisted, defended on the nonutilitarian grounds of protecting prisoners' rights. This argument was perhaps put most eloquently by Donald Seldin, Chairman of the Department of Internal Medicine, University of Texas, Southwestern Medical School, one of the Com-

mission's strongest advocates of preserving the possibility of research with prisoners. He placed the right to be a research subject within the entire web of individual human rights.

> We can dismiss rights in some sort of gesture of saying this is just a marvelous hypothesis . . . but rights are not figments. Rights are claims to humanity, they are claims to the status of an individual as a human being. They are things that are threatened everywhere.[16]

Seldin's point was reinforced by the one site visit the entire Commission and many of the staff made to the State Prison of Southern Michigan at Jackson. Jackson, a maximum-security facility, is the largest penitentiary in the United States. Its 5,000 inmates include a pool of 800 prisoners available for research, and the prisoners said they had freely chosen to participate. In fact, there were complaints about exclusion from research.

The most extensive survey ever conducted of the attitudes of prisoner subjects of experiments, carried out for the Commission by the Survey Research Center of the University of Michigan, buttressed the impressions left by the Jackson State Prison visit. Interviews with 181 prisoner subjects in four prisons found that 87 percent would be "very willing" to participate in another research project. Compared with the 45 prisoners in two prisons who were not subjects of experiments, participants were better-educated (56 percent with twelve grades or better) and spent more hours working in other prison jobs than did nonparticipants.[17]

However, Seldin's arguments did not go unchallenged. One of the lawyers on the Commission, Robert Turtle, a Washington, D.C., attorney, doubted that, in addition to the general right of humane conditions of incarceration, a prisoner has a specific right to participate in medical research. Even if human beings in prison theoretically have such a right, all the attorneys, along with other Commissioners, raised the question of whether prisons actually permit a truly free exercise of that right.

Patricia King, Associate Professor of Law at the Georgetown University Law Center, and probably the Commission's most adamant opponent of prisoner experimentation, considered prisons total institutions that by their very purpose and character made a sufficiently free consent to research impossible. "I, personally, do not believe that theoretically one can ever remove enough of the constraints from a prison to afford self-determination because by the time you removed them all you would not have a prison."[18]

Even Commissioners who believed that in principle inmates of prisons could freely consent to be research subjects thought actual prison conditions raised grave doubts prisoners could give a sufficiently free consent. While some prisoners might be strong enough to give a sufficiently free consent, in an inherently coercive environment it would be impossible to know which few they were. In a prison like Jackson, the Commissioners pointed out, better-educated, more aggressive prisoners might very well move into a position that paid by far the most money. The Commissioners noted that when prison participants in research were asked in the Commission's survey why they had volunteered, 70 percent said it was to get money, a reason given almost three times as often as any other. After all, in some prisons research paid ten times as much as any other available activity. And money for cigarettes and toiletries was not the only need. Some prisoners were concerned about the financial demands of relatives outside prison and their own life after release.

When the Commission wrote out its ethical considerations in its Deliberations and Conclusions, it ignored the ethical principle of utility. Instead, it began with "the principle of respect for persons, which requires that the autonomy of persons be promoted and protected."[19] Without using the langauge of rights, the Deliberations acknowledged the force of the arguments made by Seldin and others. "It seems at first glance that the principle of respect for persons requires that prisoners not be deprived of the opportunity to volunteer for research." But the full Commission preferred another interpretation. "When persons seem regularly to engage in activities which, were they stronger or in better circumstances, they would avoid, respect dictates that they be protected against those forces that appear to compel their choices." Prisoners are such persons. "It has become evident to the Commission that, although prisoners who participate in research affirm that they do so freely, the conditions of social and economic deprivation in which they live compromise their freedom."[20]

While questions of autonomy occupied a high percentage of the Commission's debates, several members insisted that whether or not prisoners could give a genuinely free consent was not the only issue. While David Louisell, Professor of Law, University of California at Berkeley, first raised the problem of prisoners carrying an "undue burden" of medical research, particularly Phase 1 drug tests, Robert Cooke, Vice-Chancellor for Health Sciences at the University of Wisconsin, pressed the question most persistently. "Providing we have accreditation, providing we have the cells with self-locking doors that only the prisoner has the combination for . . . providing all those things, is the Commission willing to have an undue burden fall on prisoners?"[21] Turtle believed that quite apart from respect for personal autonomy, a clear issue of distributive justice was involved.[22]

The entire Commission came to agree. In autonomy, the other ethical principle adopted by the Commission in its Deliberations and Conclusions was "the principle of justice, which requires that persons and groups be treated fairly."[23] The Commission was concerned "that prisoners not be unjustly excluded from participation in research," but also at "the possibility that prisoners as a group bear a disproportionate share of the burdens of research or bear those burdens without receiving a commensurate share of the benefits that ultimately derive from research."[24]

Taking respect for persons and justice as

its two basic ethical principles, and finding that "the actual conditions of imprisonment in our society led the Commission to believe that prisoners are, as a consequence of being prisoners, more subject to coerced choice and more readily available for the imposition of burdens which others will not willingly bear," the Commission reached its summary conclusion that it must be "inclined toward *protection* as the most appropriate expression of respect for prisoners as persons and toward *redistribution* of those burdens of risk and inconvenience which are presently concentrated upon prisoners."[25] (Italics supplied)

Debating Specific Recommendations

Discussion of the ethical principles was, of course, woven through debates concerning the Recommendations. What prolonged the Commission's deliberations for several months was not conflict over what scientific data to accept or which ethical principles to adopt. Varying assessments of the nature and conditions of prisons deeply divided the Commission and complicated the task of expressing ethical concerns in the language of specific recommendations to the Secretary of DHEW.

The March, April, and May meetings of the Commission followed a similar pattern. A document drafted by the staff, recommending to the Secretary of DHEW, or the head of the responsible federal department, the establishment of a scheme to accredit prisons as sites of prisoner experiments, would gain support from a significant minority of the Commission—the two psychologists on the Commission, Joseph Brady, Professor of Behavioral Biology, Johns Hopkins University School of Medicine, and Eliot Stellar, Professor of Physiological Psychology and Provost of the University of Pennsylvania, together with Seldin. They would repeat their position that prisoners wanted to continue participating in research and their rights should be protected.

Their general position that prisoner experimentation should be permitted to continue was seconded by the staff. In ad-

dition to the delicate and influential responsibility of preparing the many drafts of recommendations, the staff, which had gained the confidence of the Commission and its chairman during the intense discussion on fetal experimentation, often joined the Commission's formal deliberations. Some staff members spoke more frequently than individuals on the Commission. Their questions, suggestions, and arguments reflected a sense that the Commission would be ignoring empirical data and a possibility of supporting the prisoner's opportunity for free choice if it halted prisoner research.

But the recommendations drafted by the staff also elicited opposition from a sizable minority—notably the three lawyers on the Commission—King, Louisell, and Turtle—along with Cooke. They pointed out specific problems with the proposed standards for accreditation.[26] King and Louisell repeatedly raised what they considered to be the well-nigh insurmountable problem of remuneration. Justice demanded that rates for prisoners be comparable with the typical $20 a day paid to free volunteers, so as to avoid exploitation; but respect for prisoners' freedom, and a desire to avoid coercing them, required that money paid for experimentation be roughly equivalent to the 25 or 50 cents a day often given prisoners for nonresearch activities. The various arrangements suggested to circumvent the problem would still be liable to manipulation by either prison officials or prisoner leaders.

Finally, midway through the May meeting, the Chairman of the Commission took dramatic action. Ruefully noting that his earlier position in favor of using requirements for prisoner experimentation to help reform prisons had been dismissed as a "naive hope," Ryan switched sides.[27] It had been impossible for the Commission to agree on standards. A thorough look at the evidence indicated that there was no "compelling reason" (he was the first Commissioner to employ the phrase) to use prisoners in nontherapeutic research. It was quite possible that the most realistic action for the Commission was to "just say research should not occur in prisons because of these conditions which we can document from the vast material that we have and then leave to the people who are supposed to be concerned about humanity for prisoners to redress these areas and only then might someone want to reintroduce research."[28] He also said that in the present political environment if the Commission were to have any impact it ought to come to a unanimous decision.

Finding Compromise Wording

From then on, the Commissioners trained in ethics became central to shaping the consensus that until then had eluded the Commission. The day of the Chairman's shift, they made it clear in a crucial straw vote that they would not join Ryan, Cooke, and all three lawyers on the Commission, to form what would have been a sizable majority in favor of an outright ban. Karen Lebacqz, Assistant Professor of Christian Ethics at the Pacific School of Religion, and Albert Jonsen, Associate Professor of Bioethics at the University of California, San Francisco, did not make direct ethical appeals to explain their reluctance. Instead, their thinking seemed more influenced by their understanding of the role of the Commission and their assessment of the empirical condition of prisons.

On this and other occasions, they expressed their preference for the National Commission to set as a priority the outlining of general principles. Recommendations for such concrete, specific actions as bans and moratoria were to be considered secondarily and adopted only if necessary. They also could not accept the proposition that prisons are so inherently coercive that prisoners in principle cannot give a sufficiently free consent to participate in research. Such a position would unwarrantedly raise questions about the ability of prisoners freely to consent to a broad range of activities. They did not believe that they had seen enough evidence about existing American prisons for them to say that respect for persons and their autonomy dictated that they recommend all prison facilities should be banned as sites for research.

However, the ethicists did feel the force of both the lack of scientific necessity to use prisoners in experimentation and the fact that prisoners, whose own health was not being improved, comprised a disproportionately large share of the humans on whom drugs were initially tested. The morning after the Chairman's change of position, Jonsen proposed a statement, warmly applauded by Lebacqz, that supported the Commissioners who would place the burden of proof on those who would argue for use of prisoners in experimentation.

At June's climactic session, Lebacqz suggested wording for conditions in addition to the often-debated standards for openness of prisons—conditions which would allow Cooke and the lawyers to accept the accreditation scheme that had persistently and ardently been advocated by Seldin and the psychologists. Asked by Cooke to strengthen a written amendment she had proposed, Lebacqz suggested that the lack of scientific necessity be recognized by making it necessary for an investigator to demonstrate that the proposed research fulfilled a "compelling need," and that the problems of undue burdens on prisoners be met with a requirement of fairness.[29] Jonsen perceived that a single recommendation (ultimately the critical third one) could take the form of saying that no research could be undertaken unless it met the two conditions suggested by Lebacqz, and the further condition of prison openness. Virtually half a day was devoted to debating the word "compelling." Although Lebacqz herself wavered in her support of the word, once it had been suggested, King and Turtle, in particular, made it clear that inclusion of "compelling" would be necessary if they were to vote with the majority in favor of some form of accreditation. It took no less than six straw ballots (including an early but short-lived unanimously favorable vote) before a permanent, unanimous vote was reached in favor of a recommendation that included the necessity of showing a compelling reason for using prisoners as research subjects. Once the entire third recommendation was approved, the other recommendations were easily and unanimously adopted.

Evaluating the Recommendations

The Commission's report made a significant contribution by clarifying terms commonly used in biomedical research and ethics. The Commission uses the single word "research," without modifiers. It felt free to avoid defining and distinguishing biomedical and behavioral research and constructing recommendations for each because the Commission was able to draw a firmer distinction than ever before between what has typically been called therapeutic and nontherapeutic research. Building on the work of Robert Levine, Professor of Medicine at Yale University School of Medicine and Special Consultant to the Commission, the Commission employed a circumlocution that specified both intent and probable effect. Instead of "therapeutic research," it used the words "research on practices, both innovative and accepted, which have the intent and reasonable probability of improving the health or wellbeing of the individual prisoner."[30] Although stylistically cumbersome, the greater exactness achieved by the formulation allowed the Commission to say that either biomedical or behavioral research of this sort could be allowed; any other kind would fall under the restrictions specified. The more precise language it adopted will no doubt affect the Commission's recommendations on topics other than prisoner research. It might even allow Congress to shorten the Commission's name.

What will be the effect of this report? More than one Commissioner said that prisons like Jackson State Prison should not qualify as sites for prisoner research. Certainly the negative wording of the crucial third recommendation—"research involving prisoners should not be conducted or supported, unless . . ."—puts the burden of proof on

researchers. It is also true that after the decisive June vote, Chairman Ryan was quoted by the *Washington Post* as saying that "I'm not aware of any prison that could now meet our standards,"[31] and the *New York Times* predicted that the recommendations would "probably result in a moratorium on most medical research conducted in prisons in the United States."[32] The ACLU lawyers at the National Prison Project agree.

However, the ultimate impact of the report will be determined by the way in which Congress, the state governments, the courts, and most particularly, officials at DHEW interpret the Commission's words "compelling" and "equity." Stephen Toulmin, Professor of Social Thought and Philosophy at the University of Chicago, serving as a consultant and staff member, predicted at one point what that understanding would be. Having already called the tone of the recommendation "chilling," he believed that the compelling and equity requirements would "between them guarantee that there will be no prison research."[33] But as Brady said on two occasions, calling for greater specification, "one man's 'compelling' is another man's 'eh.'"[34] But when Lebacqz and King suggested the wording of the third recommendation should be expanded to make it clear that the compelling reason for using prisoners as subjects would be the scientific inability to use populations other than prisoners, Brady objected. He, in turn, conjectured that a compelling reason for using prisoners would be the demands of an equitable distribution of research subjects. Cooke, King, and Turtle quickly questioned such a use of the equity provision in Recommendation 3.[35]

Still, the Deliberations and Conclusions refer not only to burdens but also to the benefits experienced by prisoners who participate in research. Appeals to the equitable distribution of the benefits of involvement in research might make it easier for some experiments to meet the "compelling" requirement. What "benefits" might mean with reference to the research in Recom-

mendation 3—that which does not have the
intent or reasonable probability of improving the health of the prisoner—is never made
clear in the Deliberations. In neither the more
binding Recommendations nor the accompanying comments are there specifications
of any kind regarding either "compelling" or
"equity."

Anyone who is confident that the Commission has given sufficiently precise direction to DHEW might note the comments,
during the June meeting, of the Commission's
Staff Director, Michael Yesley, a lawyer
with government experience. "As an old regulations drafter I have a problem with 'depending on social and scientific importance,'
and 'depending on fairness,' because using
those words I could draft a regulation that
would exclude nearly all Phase 1 research.
I could, as easily, draft a regulation that
would include nearly all Phase 1 research. So,
you can use the words, but if you do, they
have to be specified in the comment."[36]

Finally, it is impossible to have written
a paper for the National Commission, and to
still remain neutral regarding its conclusions
on the subject. The discussion of ethical
principles in the Commission's Deliberations
and Conclusions appears to be reasonable,
given the limitations of space. Both respect
for persons and their autonomy and justice
are fundamental principles relevant to
prisoner research. The Commissioners also
correctly avoided saying that all prisoners are, in principle, incapable of making a
sufficiently free consent research.

However, the Commission does appear to
have been overly sanguine in its assessment
of the present empirical conditions of American prisons. There has been, after all, sufficient experience and testimony concerning
the problems prisons in fact have in maintaining sufficient openness to convince not
only the civil libertarians at the ACLU
National Prison Project, but such presumably well-informed and nonradical bodies as
the Federal Bureau of Prisons and the American Correctional Association to call for a
halt to at least nontherapeutic drug research.

With a population as relevantly different

from the free-living majority as prisoners
are, in the degree of freedom it enjoys and in
its vulnerability to exploitation, justice would
not be violated if prisoners did not participate in experimentation. Apart from studies
of incarceration and penal institutions, the
benefits of research not intended to contribute to the improvement of the health of
prisoners could be made available to prisoners through means other than research involving them as subjects.

If a majority of the Commission actually
intended to achieve what its Chairman
says their Recommendations will accomplish—the cessation of research with prisoners not intended to improve their health—
they could have more certainly gained their
objective if they had recommended a halt
to present research until such time as it could
be demonstrated that American prisons
had achieved sufficient openness to resume.
Instead, the Commission, attempting to
avoid a minority report, unanimously approved an accreditation system employing
terms and requirements that are so unclear
that the force of its Recommendations remains uncertain.

Commission Recommendations

Recommendation 1: Studies of the possible causes, effects and processes of incarceration and studies of prisons as institutional
structures or of prisoners as incarcerated
persons may be conducted or supported, provided that (A) they present minimal or no
risk and no more than mere inconveniences
to the subjects, and (B) the requirements
under recommendation (4) are fulfilled.

Recommendation 2: Research on practices, both innovative and accepted, which
have the intent and reasonable probability of
improving the health or well-being of the
individual prisoner may be conducted or supported, provided the requirements under
recommendation (4) are fulfilled.

Recommendation 3: Except as provided
in recommendation (1) and (2), research
involving prisoners should not be conducted
or supported, and reports of such research

should not be accepted by the Secretary, DHEW, in fulfillment of regulatory requirements, unless the requirements under recommendation (4) are fulfilled and the head of the responsible federal department or agency has certified, after consultation with a national ethical review body, that the following three requirements are satisfied:

(A) The type of research fulfills an important social and scientific need, and the reasons for involving prisoners in the type of research are compelling.

(B) The involvement of prisoners in the the type of research satisfies conditions of equity; and

(C) A high degree of voluntariness on the part of the prospective participants and of openness on the part of the institution(s) to be involved would characterize the conduct of the research; minimum requirements for such voluntariness and openness include adequate living conditions, provisions for effective redress of grievances, separation of research participation from parole considerations, and public scrutiny.

Recommendation 4: (A) The head of the responsible federal department or agency should determine that the competence of the investigators and the adequacy of the research facilities involved are sufficient. . . .

(B) All research involving prisoners should be reviewed by at least one human subjects review committee or institutional review board comprised of men and women of diverse racial and cultural backgrounds that includes among its members prisoners or prison advocates and such other persons as community representatives, clergy, behavioral scientists and medical personnel not associated with the . . . research or institution. . . .

Recommendation 5: In the absence of certification that the requirements under recommendation (3) are satisfied, research projects covered by that recommendation that are subject to regulation by the

Secretary, DHEW, and are currently in progress should be permitted to continue not longer than one year from the date of publication of these recommendations in the Federal Register [Jan. 14, 1977] or until completed, whichever is earlier.

NOTES

1. "Survey—Use of Prisoners in Drug Testing, 1975" Pharmaceutical Manufacturer's Association, Report to the National Commission, March 1976.

2. "Research Involving Prisoners: Report and Recommendations," Draft Paper, National Commission for the Protection of Human Subjects of Biomedical and Behavioral Research, April 1976, pp. 25, 26. (Hereafter referred to as National Commission.)

3. Ibid., pp. 22, 23; cf. "Research Involving Prisoners: Report and Recommendations," Draft paper, National Commission, May 1976, p. 3; cf. "Proceedings," National Commission, March 1976, p. 192.

4. Marvin E. Jaffe, and C. Stewart Snoddy, "An International Survey of Clinical Research in Volunteers," report for the National Commission, February 10, 1976, p. 4.

5. "Only Italy requires long-term (1 to 3 months) controlled safety studies on normal, healthy volunteers before initiating studies in patients. Only France and Japan require that data on new drugs be generated from tests of indigenous populations, but not necessarily normal subjects.

"There has been a nontherapeutic survey not involving drugs that included prisoners in countries outside the United States: an inquiry into the incidence of the XYY chromosome anomaly." From "Report and Recommendations: Research Involving Prisoners," National Commission, October 1, 1976, pp. 70–72.

6. Ibid., p. 12.

7. Complaint before United States District Court for the District of Maryland, American Civil Liberties Union, National Prison Project.

8. "Position Statement: The Use of Prisoners and Detainees as Subjects of Human Experimentation," Officially adopted, Board of Directors, American Correctional Association, St. Louis, Missouri, February 20, 1976.

9. "Proceedings," National Commission, January 9, 1976, p. 134.

10. Ibid., pp. 132, 133.

11. Ibid., pp. 135.

12. John Arnold, Report on U.S. Alternatives to Prisoner Research, summarized in "Report and Recommendations: Research Involving Prisoners," National Commission, October 1, 1976, pp. 63–65.

13. Ibid., p. 12.

14. Ibid., p. 7.

15. "Proceedings," National Commission, January 10, 1976, pp. 273, 274.

16. "Proceedings," National Commission, May 1976, p. 92.

17. "Research in Prisons: A Preliminary Report to the Commission for the Protection of Human Subjects of Biomedical and Behavior Research," Survey Research Center, Institute for Social Research, The University of Michigan, March 8, 1976, pp. 87, 64, 75–80.

18. "Proceedings," National Commission, April 11, 1976, p. 588.

19. "Report and Recommendations: Research Involving Prisoners," National Commission, October 1, 1976, p. 5.

20. Ibid., p. 6.

21. "Proceedings," National Commission, April 11, p. 563.

22. Ibid., p. 565.

23. "Report and Recommendations: Research Involving Prisoners," National Commission, October 1, 1976, p. 5.

24. Ibid., p. 7.

25. Ibid., p. 8.

26. "Proceedings," April 11, 1976, p. 552.

27. "Proceedings," May 1976, p. 106.

28. Ibid., p. 113.

29. "Proceedings," National Commission, June 12, pp. 295, 298.

30. "Report and Recommendations: Research Involving Prisoners," National Commission, October 1, 1976, p. 15. See Recommendation 2.

31. *Washington Post,* June 14, 1976, section C, p. 4.

32. *New York Times,* June 14, p. 62.

33. "Proceedings," National Commission, June 12, p. 374.

34. Ibid., p. 374; cf. "Proceedings," National Commission, July 1976, p. 220.

35. "Proceedings," National Commission, July 1976, p. 221, 222.

36. "Proceedings," National Commission, June 12, p. 309.

Allocation of Resources

As an economic issue, the question of the delivery of health care exists on two levels—the macro and the micro. On the macro level, the question is how much should be expended for medical research, kidney dialysis, cardiac care, preventive medicine, etc. In allocating and distributing resources at the macro level, both competing medical and nonmedical needs, such as food, housing, and education, must be taken into consideration. On the micro level, the question is how to distribute to given individuals the resources already allocated for specific medical projects.

Four of the pieces in this section deal with the allocation at the macro level. The two technologies considered at this level are heart transplants and kidney dialysis. Knox's piece raises the interesting point that an evaluation of medical programs from a strictly cost-benefit basis, which considers only safety and effectiveness, is no longer considered sufficient by the Department of Health and Human Services. The question of the "quality" of life that is being maintained by various technologies must also be weighed into the ratio. Moreover, the scarcity of funds for health care implies that technologies can no longer be evaluated on an individual basis but must be compared with other possible uses of the same resources. Also, in allocating funds, the DHHS will be considering equity in the populations served. As a result of these new parameters, the future of heart transplants, along with other new technological advances, is called into question. Continuing the same debate, Leaf's piece, and the correspondence which follows, discusses the decision by the Massachusetts General Hospital not to embark on a limited program of heart transplants. The underlying moral issue here is the justifiability of a basically utilitarian ethic—to choose that alternative which will produce the greatest good for the greatest number. The question is whether this should be the pervading ethic of the medical profession.

The piece by Kolata on dialysis raises similar issues from a different perspective. Kidney dialysis has been federally funded since 1972. The hope was that no one suffering from kidney disease would be denied life because of the inability to afford a dialysis machine. With the increased funding, however, came numerous problems—not least of which is the fact that the quality of life being maintained is not always considered worthwhile and an appropriate use of the public's funds. As Kolata states, the program is a "study of national health insurance in a microcosm," and the success of a program even this self-contained is not clear.

Rescher's well-known piece addresses the allocation issue at the micro level. The question is how resources should be distributed to individuals when it is not possible to care for all. Whether it be dialysis machines, beds in the intensive care unit, nursing care, or drugs, the issue is essentially the same. Various criteria of selection are possible, ranging from ability to pay to social contribution. Rescher proposes a two-stage selection process, utilizing different criteria at each stage. Behind Rescher's entire discussion, however, is the question whether the individual personal physician should ever utilize selection criteria or whether the role of personal physician demands an unbending loyalty to the welfare of each individual patient, to the exclusion of considering others. Should such allocation questions ever be decided at the level of the attending physician, or should they be considered only at the hospital level? Furthermore, if policies along these lines are established, should they be made known so that they can be subjected to public scrutiny? The essays by Pellegrino and Fried in the section on Institutional Responsibility discuss this issue.

The articles in this section are also closely related to the more general pieces in the Right to Health Care section under Conceptual Foundations (See Cases *5, 8 to 13, 19, 20, 29, 58, 62, 63, 65, 67, 68, 70*.)

109.

Heart Transplants: To Pay or Not to Pay
Richard A. Knox

The reigning imperative of American medicine has been: *If it works, do it.* Or as many physicians might put it: *If it helps, how can it be withheld?* Up to now, the government has taken a similar stance, asking only three questions about a new medical technology before deciding whether to pay for it out of Medicare and Medicaid funds: Is it safe? Is it effective? Does it have wide acceptance in the medical community?

No longer. Using heart transplantation as a starting point, the government has embarked on a new and utterly uncharted course. Patricia Roberts Harris, Secretary of Health and Human Services (HHS), announced on June 12 that HHS will require new technologies to pass muster on the basis of their "social consequences" before "financing their wide distribution." This assessment will be a sort of environmental impact statement for medical innovation, encompassing such boundless issues as a new procedure's cost-effectiveness and cost-benefit ratios, its ethical implications,

and its "long-term effects on society." Voluminously detailed regulations embodying the requirement and setting forth its rationale are being drafted now. It will be the first time in the 15-year history of Medicare the government has attempted to define what is meant by the statutory requirement that the program pay only for "reasonable and necessary" medical care— including such controversy-fraught issues as "necessary for whom?" and "reasonable under what circumstances?"

As she announced plans for developing the all-encompassing new reimbursement tests, Harris declared that heart transplantation—a technology that holds symbolic first place in any ranking of therapies for aggressiveness, intensity, and derring-do—will be "the prototype" for such assessment. Beginning in the fall, the department plans to launch an unprecedentedly broad assessment of the operation and its ramifications. Harris said the study will embrace "the patient selection process,

Source: *Science*, vol. 209, August 1, 1980.

the long-term social, economic, and ethical consequences of the procedure, and the potential for national expansion of the heart transplantation procedure." She put the cost of the study at $2 million "at the outside" and said it would take 2 years, but HHS staffers say it will probably cost more and take longer.

As part of its venture into technology assessment, HHS will examine closely the data on the 200 or so heart transplants that have taken place in the United States during the past 11 years. And it will look at data on patients who receive transplants during the next couple of years. Although HHS may decide ultimately not to pay for the heart transplantation under Medicare, it will support certain qualified patients as part of the present study, which will, perforce, be centered at Stanford University Medical Center, the world's most active heart transplant unit. Other medical centers may also be part of the HHS study.

One question Harris said the department wants to answer is how much additional life a heart transplant buys, at what cost, but it also wants to analyze the quality of life posttransplantation.

Other "unanswered questions" that are likely to be reflected in the study design include:

• Characteristics of patients who have been selected for transplantation to see if there is any implicit discrimination by social class, education, economic resources, or age.

• What resources are necessary to perform heart transplants well, and whether the operation should be regionalized, which would be unprecedented.

• Prospects for advances in immunosuppression, preservation of donor hearts, and the artificial heart as a substitute for or stopgap measure for end-stage heart patients—any of which could drastically alter the demand and cost sides of the equation.

• The all-inclusive costs of heart transplantation, including but not limited to medical expenses. One controversial HHS staff

analysis recently estimated the total first-year cost of a national heart transplantation program at $212.2 million to $3.2 billion, depending on whether 2,000 or 30,000 transplants were done.

• The potential trade-offs. For instance, how does heart transplantation compare with other heroic medical care in terms of costs and benefits? Does transplantation imply diverting funds from other programs, such as immunization of the elderly against pneumonia?

Obviously an ambitious if not hopelessly broad undertaking, the study reflects a once-burned-twice-shy attitude traceable to Medicare's 8-year-old End-Stage Renal Disease program, which was launched with serious consideration of questions such as these (*Science*, May 2, 1980).

Ever since South African surgeon Christian Barnard sewed the heart of a 25-year-old woman into 53-year-old Louis Washkansky in December 1967, transplantation of the human heart has never been just another operation. Pressures have been building in the past 2 years, however, to put it into that category. Those pressures emanate mainly from Stanford University Medical Center, where Norman E. Shumway (who trained Barnard) quietly nursed the controversial operation through its nadir in the early 1970s and gradually improved its dismal early success rates through rigorous patient selection, better diagnosis of the early signs of rejection, and finetuning of immunosuppression.

Today the two dozen end-of-the-road patients who receive new hearts at Stanford annually have a 65 percent chance of living at least a year after the operation—versus a 100 percent chance of dying within about 6 months otherwise. One Stanford patient is doing well 11 years posttransplant; a few survivors have had two and three new hearts. Actuarial projections put overall 5-year survival currently at somewhat better than 50 percent.

Such relative success with such hopeless patients, of whom there may be 30,000 to 75,000 a year,* has long since convinced Shumway and heart surgeons across the nation that the time has come to disseminate this bold technology—at a measured rate.

That, in fact, is the rub. There has never been a mechanism in this country to regulate the diffusion rate of new medical technology once past the strictly investigational stage, other than the skepticism or enthusiasm of the doctors involved. Thus, the last decade has seen a lot of post hoc hand-wringing over kidney dialysis, coronary artery surgery, and computerized tomography. About a year ago, Congress set up a National Center for Health Care Technology (NCHCT) to serve as an early warning system for new medical technologies, but gave it only $3.2 million to do its mammoth task and provided no way to link its recommendations to the all-important reimbursement mechanism.

Meanwhile, the looseness of the Medicare reimbursement system, in which it is up to nongovernmental regional intermediaries to ask Baltimore headquarters whether a new procedure is "reasonable and necessary" and thus covered by the program, nearly gave the whole heart transplant show away by inadvertence. A year ago HHS officials discovered that Blue Cross of Northern California, the regional Medicare intermediary, had paid for 23 transplants and 21 posttransplant cases at Stanford since 1973 under the assumption that the procedure was approved—that is, no longer experimental. The department clumsily tried to shut off reimbursement, but soon an uninsured dying patient appeared at Stanford's door. The university hospital's trustees, beset with other financial headaches, decided they could not subsidize the operation. A Stanford attorney told the Los Angeles *Herald-Examiner* that the man "may be the patient to force the issue."

The department succumbed to the adverse publicity and political pressures from California Senator S. I. Hayakawa and said Medicare would pay for this patient and for others for heart transplants on a "tentative" and temporary basis at Stanford, saying it would have a final decision in early 1980.

As it turned out, last November's decision to think twice about heart transplantation led to 7 months of wide-ranging and often sharp debate within HHS in which the secretary became engrossed to an extraordinary degree. The first thing Harris wanted, naturally, was advice from the medical experts. She got it, and pretty quickly as these things go, but from her perspective it wasn't very helpful.

The experts, an ad hoc panel of 18 cardiologists and cardiac transplant surgeons, assembled by the National Heart, Lung, and Blood Institute (NHLBI) at the behest of the National Center for Health Care Technology, concluded they could make no "generalized or unqualified statement" about the safety, efficacy, and reasonableness of heart transplantation. The procedure is safe, effective, and reasonable at Stanford, they concluded, for the carefully culled population defined by Shumway's group.

In a January 21 consensus memo written by NHLBI Deputy Director Peter Frommer, the committee recommended that Medicare pay for heart transplants at Stanford and other U.S. centers that meet comparable standards of expertise, resources, and commitment, and for patients who fit the Stanford selection criteria or "acceptable equivalents." They also identified "several dangers which must be forcefully resisted or carefully avoided," though they didn't say how. These included proliferation of other centers not as well-equipped as Stanford and loosening of patient selection criteria (for example, to encompass older patients or those with multiple organ failure).

---

*A 1979 Ad Hoc Task Force on Cardiac Replacement estimated that there were about 32,000 candidates for a heart transplant in 1979. A member of the Stanford team, cardiologist John Speer Schroeder, estimated in an article in the *Journal of the American Medical Association* (May 11, 1979) that there are 75,000 patients a year "who might be suitable candidates for cardiac transplantation."

Frommer who, like NHLBI director Robert I. Levy, is an advocate of controlled expansion of heart transplantation, also tried to allay some of the anxieties he was hearing from HHS headquarters. It's highly unlikely that cardiac transplantation will become a runaway technology, he argued, because the supply of donor hearts will be so limited for the foreseeable future. Only about 1000 usable donor hearts might be "harvested" annually, Frommer estimated. Because of this foreseen shortage and the probability that many U.S. hospitals with the capacity to transplant hearts probably won't want to, Frommer predicted there would be no more than 10 to 20 groups taking up the technique "for at least the next 5 years." If all these centers eventually geared up to Stanford's arduous two-a-month rate, that would still mean only 250 to 500 heart transplants a year.

As the debate progressed, a special point of contention was the way the NHLBI–NCHCT recommendation brushed over ethical questions about how to choose the lucky 250 or 500 or 1000 or 2000 recipients from a potential pool of 15 to 120 times that size.

Noting that these issues have been discussed extensively in the past, Frommer said that to say that no one should benefit from a technology so scarce and expensive that it can be extended to only a fraction of those who might benefit "is analogous to arguing that if not everyone can fit into the only lifeboat from a sinking ship, it is unethical for anyone to get in."

This argument does not satisfy some within HHS who are troubled by Stanford's screening criteria, which require:

• A stable, rewarding family and/or vocational environment to return to posttransplant.

• A spouse, family member, or companion able and willing to make a long-term commitment to provide emotional support before and after the transplant.

• Financial resources to support travel to and from the transplant center accompanied by a family member for final evaluation: living expenses near the center before, during, and after the transplant (a period of up to 10 months); and all pretransplant medical care, which can run more than $8000. Contraindications at Stanford are a history of alcoholism, job instability, antisocial behavior, or psychiatric illness.

Hanft told the NCHCT advisory board that the Stanford criteria "raise questions of distributive justice." One HCFA official added recently: "If it turns out that all these patients are white middle-class males under the age of 50, that isn't the population that the department is concerned about."

Lois K. Christopherson, the Stanford social worker who does the initial screening of heart transplant patients, defends the criteria and says that in reality they produce candidates with a wide spectrum of socioeconomic and educational characteristics—though this has never been analyzed systematically in the nearly dozen years of the transplant program. The point, Christopherson says, is to find patients with a fierce will to live and strong coping skills, since having a heart transplant is an arduous lifelong process. "The coping skills to deal with financial problems are the same coping skills that make for long-term survival."

At least one Stanford observer, however, acknowledges the potential for selection of heart recipients based on unstated grounds of "social worth." Stanford Medical Center Chaplain Ernle Young, whose office is decorated with smiling pictures of successful heart transplant recipients and their families, worries about "a subtle temptation for the transplant team to select recipients on the basis of other than the publicly stated medical and sociopsychological criteria."

Addressing such sensitivities, nine of NHLBI's heart transplant experts decided at a meeting on May 27 that these thorny patient selection questions might be sidestepped if the criteria were stated in more explicitly medical language. "For the purposes of HCFA," says a memo summarizing the discussion, "these criteria must be stated more generally and exclusively in terms of enhancing the likelihood of successful medical outcome."

While the memos were flying and the HHS legal department was vacillating about selective reimbursement, an event in Arizona this spring nearly toppled all the resource allocation arguments that some were trying to pile up against the reimbursement gate.

In early March, Administrative Law Judge Walter McCormies of the Social Security Administration ruled that Medicare must pay a $30,533.68 claim for the heart transplant of Norman E. "Dutch" Tarr, a 50-year-old retired Air Force master sergeant who lives in Tucson. Tarr was one of the first patients in the heart transplant program set up at the University of Arizona Health Sciences Center by Jack Copeland, a Shumway trainee.

Blue Cross of Arizona, the Medicare intermediary locally, denied the University of Arizona's claim for Tarr's transplant because the operation "is considered experimental or investigational."

Charles E. Buri of the Arizona Attorney General's office countered successfully before Judge McCormies that "experimental" had nothing to do with it. The only test, Buri asserted, was whether a heart transplant was "reasonable and necessary" treatment for Tarr. It didn't hurt Buri's case to have Tarr at the hearing, looking fit nearly a year after his transplant—living proof that the operation was at least "necessary" for him.

Norman Tarr's case, which was supported by Arizona Senators Barry Goldwater and Dennis DeConcini and by Congressman Morris K. Udall, exactly illustrates the dilemma the government faces as it tackles heart transplantation and other potentially life-saving but very expensive technologies. Confronted with a dying patient, resource allocation arguments tend to appear bureaucratic, if not academic, to politicians and perhaps to some nonpoliticians as well.

To prevent more Norman Tarrs from determining the outcome of the process that Harris has set in motion, HHS has declared that any potential Medicare beneficiary now in the heart transplant selection "pipeline" will be covered retroactively as participants in the study. (So far HHS officals can identify only one such patient.)

A larger question remains. The government has no power to prevent any doctor or hospital from doing a heart transplant. In fact, the Mayo Clinic plans to begin doing heart transplants this fall despite the recent government decision, and whether or not it receives patient care funds under the study.

Moreover, government funds are not the only funds available for heart transplants. Some private insurance companies pay for the operation, as do some but by no means all Blue Cross plans. And HHS can do nothing about entire towns raising the money to pay for some patient's new heart, just as they used to pay for dialysis in the days before Congress placed that burden on the Medicare trust funds.

110

MGH Trustees Say No to Heart Transplants (I)
Alexander Leaf

*On February 1 of this year the trustees of
the Massachusetts General Hospital, after
months of deliberation, announced that they
had decided against allowing the hospital's
cardiac surgical service to begin a limited program of heart transplantation. This decision, which made headlines all over the country, is likely to be quoted and debated for
a long time to come. It raises important issues
about the allocation of scarce and costly
health-care resources in this country. In Great
Britain the National Health Service has recently lifted an embargo on payments for
heart transplantations that it had imposed
in 1973, but the new program will be limited
to two designated centers, each of which
will do eight or 10 transplant procedures a
year. Of course, this policy concerns only
government payments under the NHS and
does not control decisions in the private
sector.*

*In the following article, Dr. Alexander
Leaf, Chief of the Medical Service at Massachusetts General Hospital, discusses some
of the implications of the trustees' action.
For commentaries on heart transplantation from other perspectives, readers are referred to an earlier editorial in the* Journal
(1978, 298:682-4) and a recent one in
Lancet *(1980; 1:687-8.).*

Ed.

This, of course, is not the first time that
a hospital's trustee committee has made a
decision that importantly affected medical
resources and practice in a hospital and
community. Being fiscally and legally responsible, the trustees are the final authority in our private, nonprofit hospitals.
Nevertheless, the recent decision by the
trustees of the Massachusetts General Hospital that their institution would not engage in human heart transplantation sets a
precedent. Their decision demonstrates
two important principles: that physicians
may not make independent final decisions regarding what professional services
they provide, and that with the rapid
proliferation of expensive medical technology, there is a clear responsiblity to evaluate new procedures in terms of the greatest
good for the greatest number.

Since the preservation of useful, meaningful life is the goal of the medical profession,
the decision to pass up the opportunity to
save even one life by cardiac transplantation
was very difficult to make. It is this ethical
issue that today sparks divergent views
not only among the staff of the MGH but
among physicians and the public in general.
As one trustee stated, "It would have been
easier to say 'Yes' to the request to do
heart transplantations."

The request to do heart transplantations
came from the chief of the General Surgical Services. He noted that he was bringing
to the General Executive Committee of service chiefs a request for permission to
carry out a surgical procedure. Previously,
new therapeutic modalities could be introduced at will by each clinical service, depending on its own assessment of the value
of the procedure. Recognizing that heart
transplantation would require the collaboration and resources of many services and departments in the hospital, he requested
approval from his peers to proceed with the
operation. A previous request in 1974
had been considered but regarded as premature. In the interval, further experimental work by his cardiac surgical colleagues
and by transplantation immunologists, as
well as the Stanford experience, made the
procedure clinically feasible, he argued,
and his request was to do only six cases a

Source: *New England Journal of Medicine*, vol. 302, no. 19, May 8, 1980, pp. 1087–88.

year. His arguments won support from nearly all the service chiefs, and all agreed that the excellent record of the hospital's cardiac surgeons and the immunologic research of the kidney-transplant unit warranted doing the procedure at the MGH.

The debate over heart transplantation centered about three basic issues: the therapeutic efficacy of the procedure, the possible scientific fallout from conducting the procedure, and the effects of the procedure on the allocation of costly and limited resources.

The possibility of saving even six lives a year was weighed against the potential impact of this procedure, now and in the foreseeable future, on the incidence of cardiovascular deaths in our society. Estimates of the number of potential candidates for this operation nationwide vary from a few thousand to over 40,000 a year. No one knows the real figure, of course, and with some four million Americans suffering from clinically manifest heart disease, the number of potential candidates would clearly depend on the evolving surgical and medical indications for the procedure. But the availability of donor hearts must also be considered. The number obtainable will be considerably lower than the number needed. The situation contrasts with that of kidney transplants. Nature has generously provided us with two kidneys, only one of which is necessary for normal life, and technology has provided renal dialysis—a procedure that allows the recipient to be kept alive almost indefinitely, until the appropriate live or cadaver kidney can be procured for transplantation. Such abundance of donor organs and leeway to temporize is not available for heart transplantation.

Most important is the fact that the problem of tissue rejection has not been solved. The surgical technology involved in heart transplantation is less demanding than that in some other procedures currently performed, but the limitations on success are now immunologic rather than surgical. Although there has been steady improve-

ment in the management of tissue rejection, the problem is far from solved. It was chiefly this consideration that led to the conclusion that for the present, human heart transplantation cannot be considered routine clinical therapy. To conclude otherwise would be to raise false hopes among the many patients who suffer from heart disease and to create serious public-relations problems when applicants would have to be denied inclusion in the program.

To assess what potential scientific knowledge might accrue from establishing a heart-transplantation program, the trustees turned to the hospital's committee on research. The committee interrogated a number of expert immunologists and clinical cardiac physiologists within and outside the hospital. Most thought that there was little likelihood that a new clinical transplantation program would add appreciably to understanding of tissue rejection. There was already so much motivation to solve this problem in relation to transplantation of kidney and other tissues that a further clinical program was not needed. Many laboratories around the world are intensely pursuing the problem. New important knowledge about cardiovascular function did not seem a likely consequence of the procedure either. All witnesses indicated, however, that important scientific advances might emerge unexpectedly from the serious study of almost any problem.

Another major concern is the impact on overall patient care that the assumption of a heart-transplantation program would entail. Such a program would commit costly and scarce resources to a procedure that at best would benefit a very few patients; these are the same resources that public demand has kept available for the benefit of many. A heart-transplantation program would further load the already overburdened intensive-care facilities with prospective transplant recipients as well as postoperative patients. Many of the former would die while awaiting a donor heart. To deny many patients the services of the hospital for procedures and care known to improve survival and the quality of life in an effort to help a few through the very difficult and resource-consuming procedure of heart transplantation was considered by the trustees to be unjustified at present.

Thus, the unproved ability of the procedure to benefit a large number of the many patients at risk, the unsolved problem of tissue rejection, and the diversion of limited resources to a procedure that at present has little impact on the all-too-common health problem that it addresses presumably weighed heavily in the final decision of the trustees. The lack of evident scientific fallout from this clinical procedure must have been a secondary consideration and would not have carried weight if clinical benefits from the procedure were clearly available.

The very success of technology is responsible for the considerations involved in this decision. Before we had the capability for such demanding procedures, we were not confronted as a profession by the need to make these hard choices. We are now in the era when the decision to act in one way reduces or forecloses our options to do other things that we may want to do or have to do. In recent years we have often been admonished that with resources becoming limited, we as a profession must set our priorities or others will do it for us. Not all will agree with the decision of the trustees, and some will argue that only the profession should be involved in such determinations. If one considers that the medical profession has historically been fostered and supported to serve a societal need and not to supply physicians with a privileged status, one can find little argument with the course that MGH trustees thoughtfully and responsibly followed.

111.

MGH Trustees Say No to Heart Transplants (II)

Percy L. Miller   Willard Rosegay   Muir Gray
Francis D. Moore

Percy L. Miller

To the Editor: The Sounding Board by Leaf in the May 8 issue of the *Journal* is a well-presented cri de coeur. The issue discussed will preoccupy us for many years to come, i.e., cost/benefit ratio, or how many people will fit into the lifeboat?

There is no dissent from the statement, "Being fiscally and legally responsible, the trustees are the final authority in our private, nonprofit hospitals." The precedent setting by the board of MGH, however, extends its authority, as well as the already implied authority for triage, over the professional services to be provided by physicians. In the past, the board would have sought the means to support the professional services to be provided in the hospital.

It is conceivable that cardiac transplantation will never be a procedure in which the benefits outweigh the costs, unless one happens to be the recipient of a cardiac transplantation that has been, in every respect, successful. However, unless enough transplantations are performed in institutions in every way qualified to do them, the summit will never be attained, and we shall not know what lies ahead—a bottomless chasm or an easy descent into a broad, verdant valley.

Source: *The New England Journal of Medicine*, vol. 303, no. 17, October 23, 1980.

Willard Rosegay

To the Editor: Dr. Leaf is to be lauded
for his careful evaluation of the MGH trustees' decision against heart transplantation.
It is this type of reasoned restraint that will
allow our medical-care system, as we know it
today, to survive.

Muir Gray

To the Editor: I was very impressed by
the courage of the MGH trustees not only in
making the decision to say "no to heart
transplants," but also in publishing their decision and their reasons. I support their
decision, but I wish to point out the weakness in the "greatest good for the greatest
number" principle that the trustees advance
as their main reason.

The Utilitarian principle[1,2] has many
good aspects, but it has one serious drawback: some people must suffer so that others
may enjoy some "good." Would the MGH
trustees put to death a small number of people a month or two before they were due
to die of disease, for "the benefit of many"?

Of course, it can be argued that letting
people die is not the same as killing them;
however, I have been persuaded by the
arguments of Glover[3] that the distinction between active and passive euthanasia, or
between death by commission and by omission, is not ethically defensible, although
it needs to be maintained for the sanity and
emotional survival of those who must allocate limited resources or those who practice clinical medicine. There is no single
ethical principle on which such allocation
decisions can be made.[4] It is important
to emphasize (as the MGH trustees have done)
that there is always an ethical aspect to such
decisions, for the ethics of resource allocation will be an increasingly important topic.

NOTES

1. J. Bentham, "An Introduction to the Principles of Morals and Legislation," in M. Warnock (ed.),
Utilitarianism, p. 35, Fontana, New York, 1962.

2. M. Warnock (ed.), *Utilitarianism*, p. 257,
Fontana, New York, 1962.

3. J. Glover, *Causing Death and Saving Lives*,
Penguin, New York, 1977.

4. J.A.M. Gray, "Choosing Priorities," *Medical
Ethics*, vol. 5, p. 73, 1979.

Francis D. Moore

To the Editor: Dr. Leaf attempted to justify retrospectively the trustees' decision
against cardiac transplantation at the Massachusetts General Hospital. A week or two
later, I read in the press (*Boston Globe* and
New York Times, June 11) that government funding bureaus are also looking un-
kindly at the procedure.

Transplantation of single organs, such as
the heart or liver, will always be infrequent
as compared with transplantation of a
paired organ, such as the kidney. But for patients who need these precious organs, there
is no substitute.

In a nation of this size, there should be
four to five centers where heart and liver
transplantation can be performed competently. The historical position of Boston in
transplant surgery, immunology, cardiology,
and hepatology, along with its record of
close collaboration between the laboratory
and the clinic and between disciplines (medicine, surgery, and pathology), recommends
it as a center to supplement the remarkably fruitful work in California and New York
on heart transplantation and in Colorado
and Cambridge (England) on liver transplantation. Several hospitals in Boston should
share this responsiblity, working together
without competition. The models of the
Boston Inter-Hospital Organ Bank and the
Joint Center for Radiation Therapy should
prove that this cooperative effort can be
made. There are only four, or possibly five,
other centers in the country that could
join Boston in shouldering this responsibility.

Although the costs of this type of episodic
transplantation activity seem high, the procedure will not lead to repetitive readmission.
In all major teaching hospitals in Boston

(including the MGH) patients with much rarer and more costly diseases are undergoing only occasionally effective treatment every day. Why was the cardiac transplantation singled out for the negative vote?

It seems an unfortunate precedent when a group of trustees (even very distinguished ones) sitting in a board room decide against treatment that needs exactly the sort of aggressive, sophisticated clinical exploration characteristic of the MGH since that bright October day in 1846, now so frequently celebrated.

As the final decade of the 20th century nears, are we really beginning to lose compassion for those suffering from rare illnesses, merely because such illnesses are costly?

112.
Dialysis after Nearly a Decade   Gina Bari Kolata

On the Saturday morning of September 30, 1972, the Senate hurriedly passed an amendment to the Social Security bill, thereby extending Medicare coverage to patients with kidney failure. Thus began the End Stage Renal Disease (ESRD) program, an extraordinary experiment in health care delivery, the wisdom of which has been questioned but the continuation of which is a certainty. The program is a study of national health insurance in a microcosm, and a number of physicians and close observers say they question the government's ability to administer even a program this comparatively small and self-contained.

The program now reaches about 50,000 patients and costs the government $1 billion a year in medical bills. Many patients who would have died of kidney failure are now alive, but all are not necessarily well. The "new" dialysis population includes patients with serious chronic illness such as cancer and heart disease and senile patients who are delivered to dialysis centers three times a week from their nursing homes. For some patients, the dialysis machine has become the equivalent of the respirator, sustaining life when hope of regaining health is gone. In light of the enormous costs of the program, some of the benefits are questionable.

The impetus for the ESRD program began in the 1960s, when it first became possible to save the lives of patients whose kidneys had failed. But dialysis was new, experimental, and costly, with limited facilities that could not possibly accommodate the numbers of individuals who could benefit. Although kidney transplants were sometimes done they were often unsuccessful; about 40 percent of the patients died within a year.

The more common way to save these patients was to dialyze their blood with artificial kidney machines.

In the early 1960s dialysis was highly publicized as a heroic and dramatic procedure. Blood is circulated from a vein in the patient's arm through an artificial kidney machine, where it is cleansed of toxins before returning through a tube to the patient's arm. The cost of dialysis, however, was near $40,000 a year for each patient. As was pointed out in newspaper and magazine articles at the time, someone had to choose which patients should be offered dialysis and which allowed to die. In Seattle, an anonymous committee of seven community members made these decisions. In Boston, Constantine Hampers recalls, "We [the doctors] used to sit around and decide who would go on dialysis. I felt terrible about making those decisions and tended to blot them out of my mind." Today, Hampers is chairman of the board of National

Source: *Science*, vol. 208, May 2, 1980.

Medical Care, a company that provides dialysis services at outpatient centers.

In 1972, when the amendment to provide federal funds for dialysis or kidney transplants was being debated, the senators were all too aware of the ethical problems that arise when doctors or lay committees have to decide how to allocate scarce medical resources. The only thing standing in the way of more machines was money—not technology. Vance Hartke (D–Ind.), who sponsored the amendment, asked, "How do we explain that the difference between life and death in this country is a matter of dollars?" Senator Lawton Chiles (D–Fla.) said, "in this country, with so much affluence, to think that there are people who die this year merely because we do not have enough money."

The decision to start the ESRD program was founded on humanitarian motives. But like other programs in which it was "only a question of money," it has come back to haunt the government with a set of perplexing problems, not the least of which is a tremendous growth in costs.

In 1979, 48,000 dialysis patients were treated at a cost to the government of about $1 billion, up from $250 million in 1972. (A few thousand patients receive kidney transplants each year, but most of them are given kidneys from cadavers, more than half of which are rejected within 1 year. So the ESRD program is essentially a dialysis program.) Although end stage renal disease patients constitute only 0.2 percent of the total Medicare population, they account for 5 percent of the Medicare funds. Yet, when inflation is taken into account, the costs of dialysis per patient, now about $28,000 a year, have decreased since the program began. The number of patients being kept alive after kidney failure, however, has increased more than eightfold since 1972 and is expected to continue rising to about 70,000 patients by 1990. High as it is, the $1 billion figure understates the true costs to the government. As Richard Rettig of the Rand Corporation points out, a substantial number—there are no good

data available on just how many—of the patients also collect federal disability payments.

When the government began paying for dialysis, the patient population changed. The average age of patients in 1972 was between 37 and 43, and fewer than 20 percent were over the age of 50. Now the average age is more than 50. According to Christopher Blagg, director of the Northwest Kidney Center in Seattle, it used to be unheard of for elderly and very sick patients to be dialyzed.

John Sadler of the University of Maryland Medical School in Baltimore was one of the physicians who lobbied for the ESRD program. Looking back, he sees that he and his colleagues were naïve. "We had [in 1972] what was in many ways an idealized population. A large fraction of the patients were in a productive period of their lives. They were young and [apart from their kidney failure] had little else wrong with them." Sadler and others agreed that most such kidney patients could be rehabilitated to lead productive lives.

All too often now, rehabilitation has proved to be impossible or has been neglected. "We have patients who have never worked, patients who are retired, and patients for whom a low paying job can't compete with the disability payments available to them," says Sadler. In the days before the ESRD program, when resources were scarce, they were spent on patients who could benefit from them medically in the most complete sense—not only by having blood detoxified but by being made well to resume useful lives. Now, with payment for all, the program is getting a lot of people whose lives can't be rehabilitated by dialysis alone, and that may account for the "failure" to rehabilitate.

Rettig, who has closely followed the politics and economics of the ESRD program, says that whether there is any effort to rehabilitate patients who are capable of working depends largely on the dialysis unit and the physician in charge. For example, one patient from a central Ohio dialysis center spoke at a seminar Rettig conducted and revealed that he was the only one of the approximately 40 patients at the center who was working. "Moreover," Rettig recalls, "this patient said that the other patients found it amazing to think that it was possible to return to work." A patient from a Washington, D.C., center who works full time says that his center's directors discouraged patient rehabilitation when they moved back the starting time for the evening dialysis shift from 7:00 to 5:30 p.m. When he complained that he didn't even finish work until 5:30 and the center is more than 10 miles from his office, he says he was told that he was being unreasonable.

The picture that Sadler, Rettig, and others paint of dialysis patients hardly resembles that envisioned by the Senate when it debated the amendment that established the ESRD program. In 1972 Senator Hartke said, "Sixty percent of those on dialysis can return to work but require retraining and most of the remaining 40 percent need no retraining whatsoever. These are people who can be active and productive but only if they have the life-saving treatment they need so badly."

According to doctors who treat them, dialysis patients are often deeply unhappy. Edmund Lowrie, director of the Kidney Center in Boston, says that when patients are tested with the Minnesota Multiphasic Personality Inventory, their scores show that many are depressed and have a tendency toward hypochondria. "They feel captured by the medical profession," Lowrie says.

Alan M. Goldstein, a clinical psychologist at the John Jay College of Criminal Justice in New York, says that dialysis patients have a suicide rate seven times higher than the national average. This is comparable with the rate for patients with other chronic diseases, he explains. Some kill themselves outright, but others do so indirectly by missing medical appointments and failing to follow the strict diet required of those on dialysis.

In the early days of dialysis, suicide was essentially nonexistent, according to Belding Scribner of the University of Washing-

ton in Seattle. But in 1964, Scribner predicted that as dialysis became less of an extraordinary treatment the number of suicides would increase. "Now dialysis is perceived as a burden rather than a way of saving lives," he points out. Before the ESRD program, patients with kidney failure expected to die and were so glad to be alive when they were given dialysis that suicide was virtually inconceivable. Also, of course, the early patients were carefully selected— they were young and had positive attitudes toward life, Scribner explains.

Now that dialysis is taken for granted, its burdensome aspects are brought into sharp focus. It is impossible for dialysis patients ever to forget that their kidneys have failed, for they must adhere to a rigid diet that is low in sodium, low in potassium, and low in fluids. Some patients, for example, are allowed only a pint of fluid each day. Sandra Madison, head nurse at the Kidney Center, explains that if patients break their diet regularly, they can develop life-threatening potassium or fluid imbalances. She has seen patients gain as much as 20 pounds in the 2 or 3 days between dialysis sessions because they ignored their fluid restrictions. Dialysis then can be extremely uncomfortable, causing severe cramps, weakness, and nausea. "The body does not easily adjust to extremes," Madison says.

Dialysis itself takes a toll on patients, whether or not they break their diets. The patients are not physiologically normal; they are anemic, prone to bone degeneration, and male patients often are impotent. Then there is the inconvenience of dialysis. It takes an average of 4 hours for a dialysis treatment and patients must be dialyzed three times a week. Although some patients are dialyzed at home with the help of a trained family member or friend, most go to dialysis centers such as the proprietary ones run by National Medical Care. But the staffs at the centers sometimes have strained relationships with the patients and the patients say they have inadequate avenues of complaint.

Lowrie explains that the close long-term

relationships between patients and staffs
at dialysis centers often led to difficult situations. The patients develop close ties with
the doctors, nurses, and technicians, but
in some cases these ties are not helpful. Lowrie says, "There are rules of behavior. A
professional cannot show aggression. The patient is unbridled and can be unkind, to
say the least. It can be hard to maintain a
professional distance."

The patients, on the other hand, often
tell a different story. Some say they dislike
and distrust their doctors but have no choices
because they have nowhere else to go for
dialysis. Dialysis facilities are centralized and
to switch from one center to another often
requires commuting a long distance, which
can be especially difficult for sick patients.
Some patients claim their doctors are insensitive to their complaints and tell them
bluntly that if they are unhappy, they
can leave. Others say that they are afraid
of their doctors since their very lives depend
on the doctors' good graces. Doctors such
as Lowrie, Sadler, and Blagg say these complaints are familiar and hard to deal with,
especially since emotionally upset patients
sometimes selectively hear or misinterpret what their doctors say.

Since the ESRD program is federally
sponsored, patients feel that Congress
is a recourse. Yet they say that when they
complain to their senators or representatives or to federal officials, they get only
polite responses that, essentially, brush
off their concerns. For example, a Washington, D.C., man has an entire file of letters
he wrote to various officials about what
he thinks is substandard medical care in the
center where he is dialyzed. In no case
did he get an adequate response, he says.

A government official, who wishes not
to be named, agrees that patients have
a hard time being heard. "It's not that the
patients have not complained to the right
person. There *is* no right person to complain to."

A number of physicians believe that the
government is remiss in not keeping tabs
on the quality of care. There is no way to
pick out centers with abnormally high

mortality rates, for example, since even such
minimal data are not available.

Sadler, who has long been politically involved in the design of the ESRD program, says the government "has a total
disregard for quality of care." The government has data in its own computers that
provide at least a gross estimate of the minimum quality of care, but that information
is never retrieved, according to Sadler. He
says that the government, in its bills for services, has data on such things as the number of times patients are hospitalized each
year, the number of times they receive
blood transfusions, and the number of times
they are dialyzed outside their usual setting
(in a hospital, for example, if they usually are dialyzed in an outpatient center). "We
have told the government for the past 8
years how to measure quality of care," Sadler says. He can only conclude that the
federal bureaucracy is not set up to deal
with this matter.

Blagg, another of the political doctors,
agrees with Sadler. "The government talks
about quality of care but it hasn't done
anything yet to measure it," he says. Blagg
thinks that Sadler's suggested measures
are reasonable.

In addition to their concerns about patient rehabilitation, patient complaints, and
the lack of even the most minimal information on quality of care, physicians and
other health care specialists say they are disturbed by the increasing number of terminally ill or incompetent patients who are
dialyzed. In other countries, England, in particular, doctors do not refer such patients
for dialysis. But in this country, where Congress intended that dialysis be available
to all those who need it, it has become legally and morally difficult to refuse patients.

Blagg and Scribner, for example, tell of a
woman patient of theirs who, at age 67
and after 12 years of dialysis, began having
severe convulsions. She spent more than
3 months in a hospital at a cost of more than
$50,000 while in a stupor from repeated
seizures and high doses of anticonvulsant
medications.

Her family wanted her dialysis to be discontinued but Scribner and Blagg were strongly advised by the state attorney general not to stop the dialysis treatments. The legal argument was that only the woman herself could request that her dialysis be terminated. She, of course, could not make that request because of her mental condition. This quandary was resolved, Blagg says, when the patient died.

Then there is the highly publicized case of Earle Spring, a nursing home patient in Springfield, Massachusetts. Spring is senile, although he has lucid periods, and his family has requested that his dialysis be terminated. But the Massachusetts courts have ruled that the decision on whether to terminate Spring's dialysis must be made on the basis of what he would want if he were capable of communicating. At present, the final decision has not been made and Spring continues to be dialyzed.

Spring and the patient of Scribner and Blagg are extreme cases, although, according to Scribner and others, incompetent patients are growing in number. But there is still another class of patients for whom the value of dialysis has been questioned. These are patients who, in addition to kidney failure, have underlying severe chronic diseases.

Sadler is quite candid in describing what he says to these patients, who, he explains, include patients with disseminated cancer, patients with debilitating heart disease, and others such as blind, depressed diabetics. "I sit down and say, 'Dialysis will correct your uremia but, because you have a progressive disease, the struggle to survive will be difficult and death also will be a struggle.'" Usually, Sadler says, the patients ask him some questions, then conclude that they do not want dialysis.

It is Sadler's opinion and that of others, including Hampers, that the current federal policy of offering dialysis to everyone is unwise and a waste of resources. Hampers suggests that, difficult as it may be, the government could appoint a committee to set up guidelines for deciding whom to treat. Scribner points out, however, that the setting up of such a committee would be impossible. It would have ramifications far beyond that of dialysis and the government would not want to get into the business of deciding whose lives are worth saving and at what cost.

A number of physicians and health care specialists say they are deeply disappointed in the way the government has run the ESRD program. Both physicians and patients tend to become frustrated when faced with bureaucratic entanglements that seem to be routine. Typical of the complaints that are voiced is Blagg's statement that "There has been and still is no effective leadership for the program at the federal level." Scribner says, "The government has failed completely. No one is in charge." Says Rettig, "The data system is a shambles." And says Lowrie, "The government has been totally unable to manage the program."

Worse yet, say these specialists, there is no indication that the situation will change. Since its inception, the program has been plagued with bureaucratic reorganization, high personnel turnovers, and a lack of efficient organization.

Philip Jos, who was until very recently the director of the Office of ESRD in the Social Security Administration, responds by saying that these criticisms must be put into perspective, that so far over 100,000 individuals have benefited from the program. Moreover, according to Jos, the government has been responsive to the community's views and has not been reluctant to change its policies when necessary. "Notwithstanding the problems of the program, when one fairly views its accomplishments a judgment that it represents a complete failure of program management by the government is unsupportable," he says.

113.
Allocation of Exotic Medical Lifesaving Therapy
Nicholas Rescher

The Problem

Technological progress has in recent years transformed the limits of the possible in medical therapy. However, the elevated state of sophistication of modern medical technology has brought the economists' classic problem of scarcity in its wake as an unfortunate side product. The enormously sophisticated and complex equipment and the highly trained teams of experts requisite for its utilization are scarce resources in relation to potential demand. The administrators of the great medical institutions that preside over these scarce resources thus come to be faced increasingly with the awesome choice: *Whose life to save?*

A (somewhat hypothetical) paradigm example of this problem may be sketched within the following set of definitive assumptions: We suppose that persons in some particular medically morbid condition are "mortally afflicted": It is virtually certain that they will die within a short time period (say ninety days). We assume that some very complex course of treatment (e.g., a heart transplant) represents a substantial probability of life prolongation for persons in this mortally afflicted condition. We assume that the facilities available in terms of human resources, mechanical instrumentalities, and requisite materials (e.g., hearts in the case of a heart transplant) make it possible to give a certain treatment—this "exotic (medical) lifesaving therapy," or ELT for short— to a certain, relatively small number of people. And finally we assume that a substantially greater pool of people in the mortally afflicted condition is at hand. The problem then may be formulated as follows: How is one to select within the pool of afflicted patients the ones to be given the ELT treatment in question: how to select those "whose lives are to be saved"? Faced with many candidates for an ELT process that can be made available to only a few, doctors and medical administrators confront the decision of who is to be given a chance at survival and who is, in effect, to be condemned to die.

As has already been implied, the "heroic" variety of spare-part surgery can pretty well be assimilated to this paradigm. One can foresee the time when heart transplantation, for example, will have become pretty much a routine medical procedure albeit on a very limited basis, since a cardiac surgeon with the technical competence to transplant hearts can operate at best a rather small number of times each week and the elaborate facilities for such operations will most probably exist on a modest scale. Moreover, in "spare-part" surgery there is always the problem of availability of the "spare parts" themselves. A report in one British newspaper gives the following picture: "of the 150,000 who die of heart disease each year [in the U.K.], Mr. Donald Longmore, research surgeon at the National Heart Hospital [in London] estimates that 22,000 might be eligible for heart surgery. Another 30,000 would need heart and lung transplants. But there are probably only between 7,000 and 14,000 potential donors a year."[1] Envisaging this situation in which at the very most something like one in four heart-malfunction victims can be saved, we clearly confront a problem in ELT allocation.

A perhaps even more drastic case in point is afforded by long-term hemodialysis, an ongoing process by which a complex device— an "artificial kidney machine"—is used

Source: *Ethics*, vol. 79, no. 3, p. 173, April 1969.

periodically in cases of chronic renal failure to substitute for a nonfunctional kidney in "cleaning" potential poisons from the blood. Only a few major institutions have chronic hemodialysis units, whose complex operation is an extremely expensive proposition. For the present and the foreseeable future the situation is that "the number of places available for chronic hemodialysis is hopelessly inadequate."[2]

The traditional medical ethos has insulated the physician against facing the very existence of this problem. When swearing the Hippocratic Oath, he commits himself to work for the benefit of the sick in "whatsoever house I enter."[3] In taking this stance, the physician substantially renounces the explicit choice of saving certain lives rather than others. Of course, doctors have always in fact had to face such choices on the battlefield or in times of disaster, but there the issue had to be resolved hurriedly, under pressure, and in circumstances in which the very nature of the case effectively precluded calm deliberation by the decision maker as well as criticism by others. In sharp contrast, however, cases of the type we have postulated in the present discussion arise predictably, and represent choices to be made deliberately and "in cold blood."

It is, to begin with, appropriate to remark that this problem is not fundamentally a medical problem. For when there are sufficiently many afflicted candidates for ELT then—so we may assume—there will also be more than enough for whom the purely medical grounds for ELT allocation are decisively strong in any individual case, and just about equally strong throughout the group. But in this circumstance a selection of some afflicted patients over and against others cannot *ex hypothesi* be made on the basis of purely medical considerations.

The selection problem, as we have said, is in substantial measure not a medical one. It is a problem *for* medical men, which must somehow be solved by them, but that does not make it a medical issue—any more

than the problem of hospital building is a medical issue. As a problem it belongs to the category of philosophical problems—specifically a problem of moral philosophy or ethics. Structurally, it bears a substantial kinship with those issues in this field that revolve about the notorious whom-to-save-on-the-lifeboat and whom-to-throw-to-the-wolves-pursuing-the-sled questions. But whereas questions of this just-indicated sort are artificial, hypothetical, and far-fetched, the ELT issue poses a *genuine* policy question for the responsible administrators in medical institutions, indeed a question that threatens to become commonplace in the foreseeable future.

Now what the medical administrator needs to have, and what the philosopher is presumably *ex officio* in a position to help in providing, is a body of *rational guidelines* for making choices in these literally life-or-death situations. This is an issue in which many interested parties have a substantial stake, including the responsible decision maker who wants to satisfy his conscience that he is acting in a reasonable way. Moreover, the family and associates of the man who is turned away—to say nothing of the man himself—have the right to an acceptable explanation. And indeed even the general public wants to know that what is being done is fitting and proper. All these interested parties are entitled to insist that a reasonable code of operating principles provides a defensible rationale for making the life-and-death choices involved in ELT.

The Two Types of Criteria

Two distinguishable types of criteria are bound up in the issue of making ELT choices. We shall call these *criteria of inclusion and criteria of comparison,* respectively. The distinction at issue here requires some explanation. We can think of the selection as being made by a two-stage process: (1) the selection from all possible candidates (by a suitable screening process) of a group to be taken under serious consideration as candidates for therapy, and then (2) the actual singling out, within this group, of the particular individuals to whom therapy is to be given. Thus the first process narrows down the range of comparative choice by eliminating *en bloc* whole categories of potential candidates. The second process calls for a more refined, case-by-case comparison of those candidates that remain. By means of the first set of criteria one forms a selection group; by means of the second set, an actual selection is made within this group.

Thus what we shall call a "selection system" for the choice of patients to receive therapy of the ELT type will consist of criteria of these two kinds. Such a system will be acceptable only when the reasonableness of its component criteria can be established.

Essential Features of an Acceptable ELT Selection System

To qualify as reasonable, an ELT selection must meet two important "regulative" requirements: it must be *simple* enough to be readily intelligible, and it must be *plausible,* that is, patently reasonable in a way that can be apprehended easily and without involving ramified subtleties. Those medical administrators responsible for ELT choices must follow a modus operandi that virtually all the people involved can readily understand to be acceptable (at a reasonable level of generality, at any rate). Appearances are critically important here. It is not enough that the choice be made in a *justifiable* way; it must be possible for people—*plain* people—to "see" (i.e., understand without elaborate teaching or indoctrination) that *it is justified,* insofar as any mode of procedure can be justified in cases of this sort.

One "constitutive" requirement is obviously an essential feature of a reasonable selection system: all its component criteria—those of inclusion and those of comparison alike—must be reasonable in the sense of being *rationally defensible.* The ramifications of this requirement call for detailed consideration. But one of its aspects should

be noted without further ado: it must be *fair*—it must treat relevantly like cases alike, leaving no room for "influence" or favoritism, etc.

The Basic Screening Stage: Criteria of Inclusion (And Exclusion)

Three sorts of considerations are prominent among the plausible criteria of inclusion/exclusion at the basic screening stage: the constituency factor, the progress-of-science factor, and the prospect-of-success factor.

The constituency factor. It is a "fact of life" that ELT can be available only in the institutional setting of a hospital or medical institute or the like. Such institutions generally have normal clientele boundaries. A veterans' hospital will not concern itself primarily with treating nonveterans, a children's hospital cannot be expected to accommodate the "senior citizen," an army hospital can regard college professors as outside its sphere. Sometimes the boundaries are geographic—a state hospital may admit only residents of a certain state. (There are, of course, indefensible constituency principles—say race or religion, party membership, or ability to pay; and there are cases of borderline legitimacy, e.g., sex. [4]) A medical institution is justified in considering for ELT only persons within its own constituency, provided this constituency is constituted upon a defensible basis. Thus the hemodialysis selection committee in Seattle "agreed to consider only those applicants who were residents of the state of Washington.... They justified this stand on the grounds that since the basic research ... had been done at ... a state-supported institution—the people whose taxes had paid for the research should be its first beneficiaries." [5]

While thus insisting that constituency considerations represent a valid and legitimate factor in ELT selection, I do feel there is much to be said for minimizing their role in life-or-death cases. Indeed a refusal to recognize them at all is a significant part of medical tradition, going back to the very oath of Hippocrates. They represent a departure from the ideal arising with the institutionalization of medicine, moving it away from its original status as an art practiced by an individual practitioner.

The progress-of-science factor. The needs of medical research can provide a second valid principle of inclusion. The research interests of the medical staff in relation to the specific nature of the cases at issue is a significant consideration. It may be important for the progress of medical science—and thus of potential benefit to many persons in the future—to determine how effective the ELT at issue is with diabetics or persons over sixty or with a negative Rh factor. Considerations of this sort represent another type of legitimate factor in ELT selection.

A very definitely *borderline* case under this head would revolve around the question of a patient's willingness to pay, not in monetary terms, but in offering himself as an experimental subject, say by contracting to return at designated times for a series of tests substantially unrelated to his own health, but yielding data of importance to medical knowledge in general.

The prospect-of-success factor. It may be that while the ELT at issue is not without *some* effectiveness in general, it has been established to be highly effective only with patients in certain specific categories (e.g., females under forty of a specific blood type). This difference in effectiveness—in the absolute or in the probability of success— is (we assume) so marked as to constitute virtually a difference in kind rather than in degree. In this case, it would be perfectly legitimate to adopt the general rule of making the ELT at issue available only or primarily to persons in this substantial-promise-of-success category. (It is on grounds of this sort that young children and persons over fifty are generally ruled out as candidates for hemodialysis.)

We have maintained that the three factors of constituency, progress of science, and prospect of success represent legitimate criteria of inclusion for ELT selection. But it remains to examine the considerations which legitimate them. The legitimating factors are in the final analysis practical or pragmatic in nature. From the practical angle it is advantageous—indeed to some extent necessary—that the arrangements governing medical institutions should embody certain constituency principles. It makes good pragmatic and utilitarian sense that progress-of-science considerations should be operative here. And, finally, the practical aspect is reinforced by a whole host of considerations—including moral ones— in supporting the prospect-of-success criterion. The workings of each of these factors are of course conditioned by the ever-present element of limited availability. They are operative only in this context; that is, prospect of success is a legitimate consideration at all only because we are dealing with a situation of scarcity.

The Final Selection Stage: Criteria of Selection

Five sorts of elements must, as we see it, figure primarily among the plausible criteria of selection that are to be brought to bear in further screening the group constituted after application of the criteria of inclusion: the relative-likelihood-of-success factor, the life-expectancy factor, the family role factor, the potential-contributions factor, and the services-rendered factor. The first two represent the *biomedical* aspect, the second three the *social* aspect.

The relative-likelihood-of-success factor. It is clear that the relative likelihood of success is a legitimate and appropriate factor in making a selection within the group of qualified patients that are to receive ELT. This is obviously one of the considerations that must count very significantly in a reasonable selection procedure.

The present criterion is of course closely related to the prospect-of-success factor above. There we were concerned with prospect-of-success considerations categorically and *en bloc*. Here at present they come into play in a particularized case-by-case comparison among individuals. If the therapy at issue is not a once-and-for-all proposition and requires ongoing treatment, cognate considerations must be brought in. Thus, for example, in the case of a chronic ELT procedure such as hemodialysis it would clearly make sense to give priority to patients with a potentially reversible condition (who would thus need treatment for only a fraction of their remaining lives).

The life-expectancy factor. Even if the ELT is "successful" in the patient's case he may, considering his age and/or other aspects of his general medical condition, look forward to only a very short probable future life. This is obviously another factor that must be taken into account.

The family role factor. A person's life is a thing of importance not only to himself but to others—friends, associates, neighbors, colleagues, etc. But his (or her) relationship to his immediate family is a thing of unique intimacy and significance. The nature of his relationship to his wife, children, and parents, and the issue of their financial and psychological dependence upon him, are obviously matters that deserve to be given weight in the ELT selection process. Other things being anything like equal, the mother of minor children must take priority over the middle-aged bachelor.

The potential-future-contributions factor (prospective service). In "choosing to save" one life rather than another, "the society," through the mediation of the particular medical institution in question—which should certainly look upon itself as a trustee for the social interest—is clearly warranted in considering the likely pattern of future *services to be rendered* by the patient (adequate recovery assumed), considering his age, talent, training, and past record of performance. In its allocations of ELT, society "invests" a scarce resource in one person as against another and is thus entitled to look to the probable prospective "return" on its investment.

It may well be that a thoroughly egalitarian society is reluctant to put someone's

social contribution into the scale in situations of the sort at issue. One popular article states that "the most difficult standard would be the candidate's value to society," and goes on to quote someone who said: "You can't just pick a brilliant painter over a laborer. The average citizen would be quickly eliminated."[6] But what if it were not a brilliant painter but a brilliant surgeon or medical researcher that was at issue? One wonders if the author of the *ober dictum* that one "can't just pick" would still feel equally sure of his ground. In any case, the fact that the standard is difficult to apply is certainly no reason for not attempting to apply it. The problem of ELT selection is inevitably burdened with difficult standards.

Some might feel that in assessing a patient's value to society one should ask not only who if permitted to continue living can make the greatest contribution to society in some creative or constructive way, but also who by dying would leave behind the greatest burden on society in assuming the discharge of their residual responsibilities.[7] Certainly the philosophical utilitarian would give equal weight to both these considerations. Just here is where I would part ways with orthodox utilitarianism. For —though this is not the place to do so—I should be prepared to argue that a civilized society has an obligation to promote the furtherance of positive achievements in cultural and related areas even if this means the assumption of certain added burdens.[8]

The past services-rendered factor (retrospective service). A person's services to another person or group have always been taken to constitute a valid basis for a claim upon this person or group—of course a moral and not necessarily a legal claim. Society's obligation for the recognition and reward of services rendered—an obligation whose discharge is also very possibly conducive to self-interest in the long run—is thus another factor to be taken into account. This should be viewed as a morally necessary correlative of the previously considered factor of *prospective* service. It would be morally indefensible of society in effect to say: "Never mind about services you rendered yesterday—it is only the services to be rendered tomorrow that will count with us today." We live in very future-oriented times, constantly preoccupied in a distinctly utilitarian way with future satisfactions. And this disinclines us to give much recognition to past services. But parity considerations of the sort just adduced indicate that such recognition should be given *on grounds of equity*. No doubt a justification for giving weight to services rendered can also be attempted along utilitarian lines. ("The reward of past services rendered spurs people on to greater future efforts and is thus socially advantageous in the long-run future.") In saying that past services should be counted "on grounds of equity"—rather than "on grounds of utility"—I take the view that even if this utilitarian defense could somehow be shown to be fallacious, I should still be prepared to maintain the propriety of taking services rendered into account. The position does not rest on a utilitarian basis and so would not collapse with the removal of such a basis.[9]

As we have said, these five factors fall into three groups: two biomedical factors, a familial factor, and two social factors. With the biomedical factors the need for a detailed analysis of the medical considerations comes to the fore. The age of the patient, his medical history, his physical and psychological condition, his specific disease, etc., will all need to be taken into exact account. These biomedical factors represent technical issues: they call for the physicians' expert judgment and the medical statisticians' hard data. And they are ethically uncontroversial factors—their legitimacy and appropriateness are evident from the very nature of the case.

Greater problems arise with the familial and social factors. They involve intangibles that are difficult to judge. How is one to develop subcriteria for weighing the relative social contributions of (say) an architect or a librarian or a mother of young children? And they involve highly problematic issues.

(For example, should good moral character be rated a plus and bad a minus in judging services rendered?) And there is something strikingly unpleasant in grappling with issues of this sort for people brought up in times greatly inclined towards maxims of the type "Judge not!" and "Live and let live!" All the same, in the situation that concerns us here such distasteful problems must be faced, since a failure to choose to save some is tantamount to sentencing all. Unpleasant choices are intrinsic to the problem of ELT selection; they are of the very essence of the matter.[10]

But is reference to all these factors indeed inevitable? The justification for taking account of the medical factors is pretty obvious. But why should the social aspect of services rendered and to be rendered be taken into account at all? The answer is that they must be taken into account not from the *medical* but from the *ethical* point of view. Despite disagreement on many fundamental issues, moral philosophers of the present day are pretty well in consensus that the justification of human actions is to be sought largely and primarily—if not exclusively—in the principles of utility and of justice.[11] But utility requires reference of services to be rendered and justice calls for a recognition of services that have been rendered. Moral considerations would thus demand recognition of these two factors. (This, of course, still leaves open the question of whether the point of view provides a valid basis of action: Why base one's actions upon moral principles?— or, to put it bluntly—Why be moral? The present paper is, however, hardly the place to grapple with so fundamental an issue, which has been canvassed in the literature of philosophical ethics since Plato.)

More Than Medical Issues Are Involved

An active controversy has of late sprung up in medical circles over the question of whether nonphysician laymen should be given a role in ELT selection (in the specific context of chronic hemodialysis). One physician writes: "I think that the assessment of the candidates should be made by a senior doctor on the [dialysis] unit, but I am sure that it would be helpful to him—both in sharing responsibility and in avoiding personal pressure—if a small unnamed group of people [presumably including laymen] officially made the final decision. I visualize the doctor bringing the data to the group, explaining the points in relation to each case, and obtaining their approval of his order of priority."[12]

Essentially this procedure of a selection committee of laymen has for some years been in use in one of the most publicized chronic dialysis units, that of the Swedish Hospital of Seattle, Washington.[5] Many physicians are apparently reluctant to see the choice of allocation of medical therapy pass out of strictly medical hands. Thus in a recent symposium on the "Selection of Patients for Haemodialysis,"[13] Dr. Ralph Shakman writes: "Who is to implement the selection? In my opinion it must ultimately be the responsibility of the consultants in charge of the rental units . . . I can see no reason for delegating this responsibility to lay persons. Surely the latter would be better employed if they could be persuaded to devote their time and energy to raise more and more money for us to spend on our patients."[14] Other contributors to this symposium strike much the same note. Dr. F. M. Parsons writes: "In an attempt to overcome . . . difficulties in selection some have advocated introducing certain specified lay people into the discussions. Is it wise? I doubt whether a committee of this type can adjudicate as satisfactorily as two medical colleagues, particularly as successful therapy involves close cooperation between doctor and patient."[15] And Dr. M. A. Wilson writes in the same symposium: "The suggestion has been made that lay panels should select individuals for dialysis from among a group who are medically suitable. Though this would relieve the doctor-in-charge of a heavy load of responsibility, it would place the burden on those who have no personal knowledge and have

to base their judgments on medical or social reports. I do not believe this would result in better decisions for the group or improve the doctor-patient relationship in individual cases."[16]

But no amount of flag waving about the doctor's facing up to his responsibility—or prostrations before the idol of the doctor-patient relationship and reluctance to admit laymen into the sacred precincts of the conference chambers of medical consultations—can obscure the essential fact that ELT selection is not a wholly medical problem. When there are more than enough places in an ELT program to accommodate all who need it, then it will clearly be a medical question to decide who does have the need and which among these would successfully respond. But when an admitted gross insufficiency of places exists, when there are ten or fifty or one hundred highly eligible candidates for each place in the program, then it is unrealistic to take the view that purely medical criteria can furnish a sufficient basis for selection. The question of ELT selection becomes serious as a phenomenon of scale—because, as more candidates present themselves, strictly medical factors are increasingly less adequate as a selection criterion precisely because by numerical category-crowding there will be more and more cases whose "status is much the same" so far as purely medical considerations go.

The ELT selection problem clearly poses issues that transcend the medical sphere because—in the nature of the case—many residual issues remain to be dealt with once *all* the medical questions have been faced. Because of this there is good reason why laymen as well as physicians should be involved in the selection process. Once the medical considerations have been brought to bear, fundamental social issues remain to be resolved. The instrumentalities of ELT have been created through the social investment of scarce resources, and the interests of the society deserve to play a role in their utilization. As representatives of their social interests, lay opinions should function to complement and supplement medical views once the proper arena of medical considerations is left behind.[17] Those physicians who have urged the presence of lay members on selection panels can, from this point of view, be recognized as having seen the issue in proper perspective.

One physician has argued against lay representation on selection panels for hemodialysis as follows: "If the doctor advises dialysis and the lay panel refuses, the patient will regard this as a death sentence passed by an anonymous court from which he has no right of appeal."[18] But this drawback is not specific to the use of a lay panel. Rather, it is a feature inherent in every *selection* procedure, regardless of whether the selection is done by the head doctor of the unit, by a panel of physicians, etc. No matter who does the selecting among patients recommended for dialysis, the feelings of the patient who has been rejected (and knows it) can be expected to be much the same, provided that he recognizes the actual nature of the choice (and is not deceived by the possibly convenient but ultimately poisonous fiction that because the selection was made by physicians it was made entirely on medical grounds).

In summary, then, the question of ELT selection would appear to be one that is in its very nature heavily laden with issues of medical research, practice, and administration. But it will not be a question that can be resolved on solely medical grounds. Strictly social issues of justice and utility will invariably arise in this area—questions going outside the medical area in whose resolution medical laymen can and should play a substantial role.

The Inherent Imperfection (Nonoptimality) of Any Selection System

Our discussion to this point of the design of a selection system for ELT has left a gap that is a very fundamental and serious omission. We have argued that five factors must be taken into substantial and explicit account:

1. *Relative likelihood of success.* Is the chance of the treatment's being "successful" to be rated as high, good, average, etc.?[19]

2. *Expectancy of future life.* Assuming the "success" of the treatment, how much longer does the patient stand a good chance (75 percent or better) of living—considering his age and general condition?

3. *Family role.* To what extent does the patient have responsibilities to others in his immediate family?

4. *Social contributions rendered.* Are the patient's past services to his society outstanding, substantial, average, etc.?

5. *Social contributions to be rendered.* Considering his age, talents, training, and past record of performance, is there a substantial probability that the patient will—*adequate recovery being assumed*—render in the future services to his society that can be characterized as outstanding, substantial, average, etc.?

This list is clearly insufficient for construction of a reasonable selection system, since that would require not only *that these factors be taken into account* (somehow or other) but—going beyond this—would specify *a specific set of procedures for taking account of them.* The specific procedures that would constitute such a system would have to take account of the interrelationship of these factors (e.g., 2 and 5), and to set out exact guidelines as to the relevant weight that is to be given to each of them. This is something our discussion has not yet considered.

In fact, I should want to maintain that there is no such thing here as a single rationally superior selection system. The position of affairs seems to me to be something like this: (1) It is necessary (for reasons already canvassed) to *have* a system, and to have a system that is rationally defensible, and (2) to be rationally defensible, this system must take factors 1 through 5 into substantial and explicit account. But (3) the exact manner in which a rationally defensible system takes account of these factors cannot be fixed in any one specific way on the basis of general considerations. Any of the variety of ways that give factors 1 through 5 "their due" will be acceptable and viable. One cannot hope to find within this range of workable systems some one that is *optimal* in relation to the alternatives. There is no one system that does "the (uniquely) best"—only a variety of systems that do "as well as one can expect to do" in cases of this sort.

The situation is structurally very much akin to that of rules of partition of an estate among the relations of a decedent. It is important *that there be* such rules. And it is reasonable that spouse, children, parents, siblings, etc., be taken account of in these rules. But the question of the exact method of division—say that when the decedent has neither living spouse nor living children then his estate is to be divided, dividing 60 percent between parents, 40 percent between siblings versus dividing 90 percent between parents, 10 percent between siblings—cannot be settled on the basis of any general abstract considerations of reasonableness. Within broad limits, a *variety* of resolutions are all perfectly acceptable—so that no one procedure can justifiably be regarded as "the (uniquely) best" because it is superior to all others.[20]

A Possible Basis for a Reasonable Selection System

Having said that there is no such thing as *the optimal* selection system for ELT, I want now to sketch out the broad features of what I would regard as *one acceptable* system.

The basis for the system would be a point rating. The scoring here at issue would give roughly equal weight to the medical considerations in comparison with the extramedical considerations (family role, services rendered, and services to be rendered), also giving roughly equal weight to the three items involved here. The result of such a scoring

procedure would provide the essential *starting point* of our ELT selection mechanism. I deliberately say "starting point" because it seems to me that one should not follow the results of this scoring in an *automatic* way. I would propose that the actual selection should only be guided but not actually be dictated by this scoring procedure, along lines now to be explained.

The Desirability of Introducing an Element of Chance

The detailed procedure I would propose—not of course as optimal (for reasons we have seen), but as eminently acceptable—would combine the scoring procedure just discussed with an element of chance. The resulting selection system would function as follows:

1. First the criteria of inclusion above would be applied to constitute a *first phase selection group*—which (we shall suppose) is substantially larger than the number *n* of persons who can actually be accommodated with ELT.

2. Next the criteria of selection are brought to bear via a scoring procedure of the type described. On this basis a *second phase selection group* is constituted which is only *somewhat* larger—say, by a third or a half—than the critical number *n* at issue.

3. If this second phase selection group is relatively homogeneous as regards rating by the scoring procedure—that is, if there are no really major disparities within this group (as would likely if the initial group was significantly larger than *n*)—then the final selection is made by *random* selection of *n* persons from within this group.

This introduction of the element of chance—in what could be dramatized as a "lottery of life and death"—must be justified. The fact is that such a procedure would bring with it three substantial advantages.

First, as we have argued above, any acceptable selection system is inherently non-optimal. The introduction of the element of chance prevents the results that life-and-death choices are made by the automatic application of an admittedly imperfect selection method.

Second, a recourse to chance would doubtless make matters easier for the rejected patient and those who have a specific interest in him. It would surely be quite hard for them to accept his exclusion by relatively mechanical application of objective criteria in whose implementation subjective judgment is involved. But the circumstances of life have conditioned us to accept the workings of chance and to tolerate the element of luck (good or bad): human life is an inherently contingent process. Nobody, after all, has an absolute right to ELT—but most of us would feel that we have "every bit as much right" to it as anyone else in significantly similar circumstances. The introduction of the element of chance assures a like handling of cases over the widest possible area that seems reasonable in the circumstances.

Third (and perhaps least), such a recourse to random selection does much to relieve the administrators of the selection system of the awesome burden of ultimate and absolute responsibility.

These three considerations would seem to build up a substantial case for introducing the element of chance into the mechanism of the system for ELT selection in a way limited and circumscribed by other weightier considerations, along some such lines as those set forth above.[21]

It should be recognized that this injection of *man-made* chance supplements the element of *natural* chance that is present inevitably and in any case (apart from the role of chance in singling out certain persons as victims for the affliction at issue). As F. M. Parsons has observed: "any vacancies [in an ELT program—specifically hemodialysis] will be filled immediately by the first suitable patients, even though their claims for therapy may subsequently prove less than those of other patients refused later."[22]

Life is a chancy business and even the most rational of human arrangements can cover this over to a very limited extent at best.

NOTES

1. Christine Doyle, "Spare-Part Heart Surgeons Worried by Their Success," *Observer*, May 12, 1968.

2. J. D. N. Nabarro, "Selection of Patients for Haemodialysis," *British Medical Journal*, March 11, 1967, p. 623. Although several thousand patients die in the U.K. each year from renal failure—there are about thirty new cases per million of population—only 10 percent of these can for the foreseeable future be accommodated with chronic hemodialysis. Kidney transplantation—itself a very tricky procedure—cannot make a more than minor contribution here. As this article goes to press, I learn that patients can be maintained in home dialysis at an operating cost about half that of maintaining them in a hospital dialysis unit (roughly an $8,000 minimum). In the United States, around 7,000 patients with terminal uremia who could benefit from hemodialysis evolve yearly. As of mid-1968, some 1,000 of these can be accommodated in existing hospital units. By June 1967, a worldwide total of some 120 patients were in treatment by home dialysis. (Data from a forthcoming paper, "Home Dialysis," by C. M. Conty and H. V. Murdaugh. See also R. A. Baillod et al., "Overnight Haemodialysis in the Home," *Proceedings of the European Dialysis and Transplant Association*, vol. VI, 1965, p. 99.

3. For the Hippocratic Oath see *Hippocrates: Works*, Loeb, ed., London, 1959, vol. 1, p. 298.

4. Another example of borderline legitimacy is posed by an endowment "with strings attached," e.g., "In accepting this legacy the hospital agrees to admit and provide all needed treatment for any direct descendant of myself, its founder."

5. Shana Alexander, "They Decide Who Lives, Who Dies," *Life*, vol. LIII, November 9, 1962, p. 107.

6. Lawrence Lader, "Who has the Right to Live?" *Good Housekeeping*, January 1968, p. 144.

7. This approach could thus be continued to embrace the previous factor, that of family role.

8. Moreover a doctrinaire utilitarian would presumably be willing to withdraw a continuing mode of ELT such as hemodialysis from a patient to make room for a more promising candidate who came into view at a later stage and who could

not otherwise be accommodated. I should be unwilling to adopt this course, partly on grounds of utility (with a view to the demoralization of insecurity), partly on the nonutilitarian ground that a "moral commitment" has been made and must be honored.

9. Of course, the difficult question remains of the relative weight that should be given to prospective and retrospective service in cases where these factors conflict. There is good reason to treat them on a par.

10. This in the symposium on "Selection of Patients for Haemodialysis," *British Medical Journal*, March 11, 1967, pp. 622–24. F. M. Parsons writes: "But other forms of selecting patients [distinct from first come, first served] are suspect in my view if they imply evaluation of man by man. What criteria could be used? Who could justify a claim that the life of a mayor would be more valuable than that of the humblest citizen of his borough? Whatever we may think as individuals none of us is indispensable." But having just set out this hard-line view he immediately backs away from it: "On the other hand, to assume that there was little to choose between Alexander Fleming and Adolf Hitler . . . would be nonsense, and we should be naive if we were to pretend that we could not be influenced by their achievements and characters if we had to choose between the two of them. Whether we like it or not we cannot escape the fact that this kind of selection for long-term hemodialysis will be required until very large sums of money become available for equipment and services [so that *everyone* who needs treatment can be accommodated]."

11. The relative fundamentality of these principles is, however, a substantially disputed issue.

12. J. D. N. Nabarro, op. cit., p. 622.

13. *British Medical Journal*, March 11, 1967.

14. Ibid., p. 624. Another contributor writes in the same symposium, "The selection of the few [to receive haemodialysis] is proving very difficult —a true 'Doctor's Dilemma'—for almost everybody would agree that this must be a medical decision, preferably reached by consultation among colleagues" (Dr. F. M. Parsons, ibid., p. 623).

15. "Selection of Patients for Haemodialysis," op. cit. (note 10 above), p. 623.

16. Dr. Wilson's article concludes with the perplexing suggestion—wildly beside the point given the structure of the situation at issue—that "the final decision will be made by the patient." But this contention is only marginally more ludicrous than Parson's contention that in selecting patients for hemodialysis "gainful employment in a well

chosen occupation is necessary to achieve the best results" since "only the minority wish to live on charity."

17. To say this is of course not to deny that such questions of applied medical ethics will invariably involve a host of medical considerations—it is only to insist that extramedical considerations will also invariably be at issue.

18. M. A. Wilson, "Selection of Patients for Haemodialysis," op. cit., p. 624.

19. In the case of an ongoing treatment involving complex procedure and dietary and other mode-of-life restrictions—and chronic hemodialysis definitely falls into this category—the patient's psychological makeup, his will-power to "stick with it" in the face of substantial discouragements —will obviously also be a substantial factor here. The man who gives up, takes not his life alone, but (figuratively speaking) also that of the person he replaced in the treatment schedule.

20. To say that acceptable solutions can range over broad limits is *not* to say that there are no limits at all. It is an obviously intriguing and fundamental problem to raise the question of the facets that set these limits. This complex issue cannot be dealt with adequately here. Suffice it to say that considerations regarding precedent and people's expectations, factors of social utility, and matters of fairness and sense of justice all come into play.

21. One writer has mooted the suggestion that: "Perhaps the right thing to do, difficult as it may be to accept, is to select [for hemodialysis] from among the medical and psychologically qualified patients on a strictly random basis" (S. Gorovitz, "Ethics and the Allocation of Medical Resources." *Medical Research Engineering*, vol. V, p. 7, 1966) Outright random selection would, however, seem indefensible because of its refusal to give weight to considerations which, under the circumstances, *deserve* to be given weight. The proposed procedure of superimposing a certain degree of randomness upon the rational-choice criteria would seem to combine the advantages of the two without importing the worst defects of either.

22. "Selection of Patients for Haemodialysis," op. cit., p. 623. The question of whether a patient for chronic treatment should ever be terminated from the program (say if he contracts cancer) poses a variety of difficult ethical problems with which we need not at present concern ourselves. But it does seem plausible to take the (somewhat antiutilitarian) view that a patient should not be terminated simply because a "better quali-

fied" patient comes along later on. It would seem that quasi-contractual relationship has been created through established expectations and reciprocal understandings, and that the situation is in this regard akin to that of the man who, having under- taken to sell his house to one buyer, cannot afterward unilaterally undo this arrangement to sell it to a higher bidder who "needs it worse" (thus maximizing the overall utility).

IV.   APPENDIXES

Medical Cases

The following section contains 74 "case studies." Although placed in an Appendix, the cases can have the central function of stimulating the kinds of small group discussion which are vital to the success of a clinical ethics course. Medical faculty and students will be familiar with the format of a case presentation as a method for developing discussion.

Students should be asked to read the cases selected by the faculty to supplement the readings. They should be assigned the open-ended task of analyzing the ethical features of the case. More specifically, students should then be asked to formulate specific questions applicable to that case. One major difference between these cases and the standard medical history is the relative absence of detailed clinical data. It is important that students (and faculty) not be lured into the seductive belief that, if there were only more specific and complete data, the medical and ethical decisions would be obvious. The cases contain varying amounts of data, but in all cases students should be encouraged to begin their analysis on "what's available." Of course, in many cases more information could make a relevant difference to significant ethical features. A useful exercise is to ask the students to consider hypothetical alternatives to the case as described, alternatives in which either further information is available or some of the facts are changed. For example, in a case concerned primarily with communication in which the physician did *not* inform the patient of a diagnosis, one can ask not only "what if she had told the patient," but more importantly, "what should she have told the patient?" or "Should she have told the patient part of the story?"

In order to facilitate access to the cases, we have labeled each one with relevant headings chosen from the section headings employed in this text. The italicized headings indicate the main issues we think each case raises, and other headings refer to secondary issues. In reality cases do not neatly fall into single categories and there has been no attempt here to create cases that perfectly illustrate specific issues. Most of the cases have been supplied to us by medical and philosophical colleagues from a variety of institutions and cover a diverse range of topics. The cases themselves are not listed in any topical ordering; however, there is an index to cases which lists, for each topic in the book, cases which raise the topic as a primary or secondary issue. And we have cross-referenced the cases by number at the end of each of the section introductions. (Italicized numbers refer to cases which present the section topic as a primary issue.)

There is no standard format for the cases. Some include bits of medical history, some are quite brief presentations of the outcome of a situation, and some follow the chronology of a sequence of events in which a patient's case evolves, engendering different sets of problems (see Case 28). Although the language is for the most part nontechnical, there is sufficient medical information presented in many cases to require an occasional trip to the dictionary by the general undergraduate. Some abbreviations, e.g., GYN for gynecology service, are rather obvious, as is "meds" for medicines.

Some of the cases are documents that can serve as a further source of information for class discussion. Case 57 contains a sample of an actual consent form and Case 58 is a historical review of the economic history of the dialysis program in the United States.

It must be stressed that successful employment of the cases will require that they be used in such a manner that students are led to raise questions not only about the course of events in the cases as presented, but about the imaginable alternative courses of actions that could have been open to the characters in the case. Some cases end quite abruptly. One must ask of them, "What were the alternatives to this course of events?" "What other information about the patients would have made a difference?" Asking such questions about what could have been is the basic way of engaging students and faculty into motivated discussions on what should have been.

Finally, in some instances the case history as presented may present students with a situation that seems patently "wrong." There may seem to be little to discuss. It is then essential to ask the students to explain the basis for their judgments. Since this is a reader dedicated to the philosophical approach toward clinical ethics, it is the fundamental goal of the case exercises to lead students to develop *reasons* as part of an analysis of a well-conceptualized clinical situation understood as ethical. And there is no better method for achieving this than the development of imagined possibilities in response to a confrontation with realities of clinical life.

INDEX TO CASES

Italic numbers refer to cases in which the topic is a primary issue.

III. *Issues in Clinical Ethics*

A. Informed Consent and Refusal of Treatment, *1, 14, 17, 21, 33, 44, 51, 55, 59, 64, 68. See also* I.A., Informed Consent.

Italicized words and phrases indicate primary issues raised by each case.

CASE 1. *Informed Consent* / Paternalism / Rights / Roles and Norms: Clinical Authority / *Refusal of Treatment*

One evening, the psychiatric resident on duty at a city hospital was called to see a patient who had come into the emergency room. The patient, H.G., presented with a slashed Achilles tendon, the result of a knife fight. A surgical consult determined that if the tendon were sutured within 24 to 36 hours, the patient would recover completely. If it were not treated, the patient would have a mild debilitation, with a chronic limp. The emergency room physician attempted to admit H.G. and prepare him for surgery. But H.G. refused to be treated. He stated that he believed that hypodermic syringes contained poison and that the doctors would try to kill him.

During the history and physical exam, H.G. admitted that he was periodically receiving psychiatric treatment, but he was presently on no medications. The psychiatrist who examined him felt that if he were given antipsychotic medication for a short period, he would become more reasonable and consent to treatment. However, H.G. repeated his delusion about the syringes and stated that he knew he could go to another hospital where they wouldn't try to kill him. He would not voluntarily consent to any medication or surgery.

H.G. did not appear to be dangerous to himself or to others. He left the hospital AMA (against medical advice) within an hour after his arrival.

CASE 2. *Psychiatric Issues (Involuntary Commitment)*

Alfred Fuller was found guilty of the murder of an elderly woman. Fuller had already been convicted of manslaughter and had served seven years of a ten-year sentence. He was an alcoholic and was proven to be intoxicated during both these killings. The parole on his first conviction had been conditional on his not drinking. The trial leading to his present conviction revealed that he had bludgeoned a 70-year-old woman to death after he had forcibly handled her in a sexually sadistic manner. A psychiatrist testified that Fuller was an alcoholic, a sexual psychopath with ambiguous gender preference and sadistic propensity.

The state of venue for the trial had a mandatory death penalty for repeat homicide offenders. This legislation was presently going through a lengthy appeals process. The court decided not to hold Fuller on "death row," and instead had him declared criminally insane and sentenced him to an irrevocable life sentence. He was subsequently committed to an institution for the criminally insane. Once at the institution, a battery of diagnostic tests were planned for Fuller. He refused to submit to these and to any future treatment.

CASE 3. *Informed Consent/Professional-Patient Communication*

A chief resident of surgery was trying to convince his patient that she ought to undergo a surgical procedure he felt would be extremely beneficial to her, and which carried minimal risk. He had earlier explained to her that there was a 10 percent mortality rate for this particular surgery—a ratio he thought was quite favorable. In the course of their conversation he emphasized that he could not understand why she would not undergo a surgical procedure with a 90 percent survival rate. His patient looked at him with surprise, quickly agreed that a 90 percent survival rate was an acceptable risk, and consented to the surgery.

Months later the chief resident was still moved by this patient's change of mind and he decided to conduct a survey of the third-year medical class at his affiliate university medical school. Two hundred students were first asked the following: "Disability A can be remedied by surgical procedure X; this procedure has a 10 percent mortality rate. Disability A can also be treated with therapy Y with 30 percent less recovery than the full recovery expected were surgery performed. Which would you select?" A week later the same group was asked the following: "Disability B can be remedied by surgical procedure W; this procedure has a 90 percent survival rate. Disability B can also be treated by therapy Z with 30 percent less recovery than the full recovery expected were the surgery performed. Which would you select?"

Eighty of the students who initially selected therapy decided upon surgery when asked the second question.

CASE 4. *Informed Consent*/Professional-Patient Communication/*Human Experimentation*

A noted cancer researcher had done work involving the injection of tissue-cultured cancer cells into human subjects and then measuring the speed with which the injected substance was rejected by the body. Earlier phases of the work had established that healthy persons would reject the tissue culture in 4 to 6 weeks and that individuals already ill with advanced cancer would reject them in a longer period ranging from 6 weeks to several months. To test the hypothesis that the slower rate of rejection in the cancer patients was in fact attributable to their cancer and not to their general debility that accompanies any chronic illness, it was necessary to perform the experiment on subjects who were severely ill with nonmalignant diseases. A chronic disease hospital was the obvious place to look for patients with the required characteristics.

This research was considered by the scientific community to be among the most significant work on malignant diseases at the present time. The researcher had no trouble gaining approval from the director of the Jewish Chronic Disease Hospital to use several patients there for the experiment. Nineteen patients with nonmalignant chronic diseases and three cancer patients were selected for the experiment. The consent form explained that they would be given an injection as a test to discover their immunity to disease. It further stated that a lump would form at the site of the injection and in a few weeks it would go away. All twenty-two patients consented on these terms to participate and were subjected to the experiment.

Source: *Science*, vol. 151, no. 11, p. 663, February 1966.

CASE 5. *Aggressiveness of Care/Allocation of Resources*

Dr. XP was a seventy-seven-year-old retired male orthopedic surgeon who was admitted to the hospital with congestive heart failure, cardiomegaly (enlarged heart), mild cirrhosis, and chronic renal failure. Prior to admission he had been living a restricted life, bedridden for the most part although managing some assisted ambulation at home. He had been admitted earlier in the year for the renal failure which required dialysis acutely, but he was sent home managed on diet and diuretics.

During the current admission, his heart failure could not be controlled with medications; dialysis was again instituted with the patient's full understanding. Because of his poor cardiorespiratory status and the onset of numerous premature ventricular beats, the patient was transferred to the ICU for cardiac monitoring and the intravenous administration of carefully titrated antiarrhythmic drugs which as a matter of hospital procedure could not be administered on floor units. Despite aggressive therapy, the patient's medical and mental condition deteriorated over the next few days until he was responsive only to pain. However, his arrhythmia was controlled.

There was great concern among the house staff about how to respond to a further crisis in the patient's current condition. He remained stable, but responsive only to pain. The ICU was full; a forty-eight-year-old taxi driver with an anteroseptal myocardial infarction was in the emergency room and needed a monitored ICU bed. Dr. XP was transferred to the floor, which necessitated discontinuing the monitor and the IV antiarrhythmics. He suffered a cardiac arrest within 10 hours. Resuscitation was unsuccessful.

CASE 6. *Confidentiality*/Roles and Norms: Doctors' Roles/*Transplantation*

For three years, Dr. Foti had been the attending physician for five-year-old Marian, who, for that period, had been a chronic renal dialysis patient at University Hospital. Dr. Foti had decided to attempt a renal transplant for her, though her prognosis was questionable. It was reasonably certain that she would not be as susceptible to infection were she to have the transplant.

Tissue typing was performed. The mother was not histocompatible and the father was very compatible with his daughter. He was also found to have renal circulation anatomically advantageous for transplantation. In a private meeting with the father, Dr. Foti imparted the results of the typing and explained that his daughter's prognosis with a transplant was hazy. The possibility of a cadaver transplant was possible but quite remote. The father was overtly nervous and after some silence said he did not want to donate. "Her chances for recovery are not good," he reasoned, "a cadaver donor may show up; my daughter has suffered too much already, and I'm just too frightened." He asked Dr. Foti not to tell the family about their meeting and beseeched the doctor to tell his wife he was not histocompatible. If his wife knew, he claimed, she would blame him for his daughter's death and desert him. Though Dr. Foti was much unsettled by the father's decision and request, he decided to tell the wife that the father would be a "medically inappropriate donor."

CASE 7. Ideals and Models of the Physician-Patient Relationship/*Professional Accountability*

A resident moonlighting as a house physician in a small community hospital was called by the nurses on the floor to see a patient having respiratory problems. The patient, a 67-year-old female non-insulin-dependent diabetic, was being treated for gallstones. She had a nasogastric tube attached to suction and was on intravenous fluids (glucose in half strength normal saline). The attending physician, a seventy-year-old general practitioner, was managing the case, although a surgeon had been consulted for the anticipated surgery. The resident examined the patient, who was lethargic, breathing rapidly and deeply, despite having clear lungs. He made a diagnosis of diabetic ketoacidosis based on his physical assessment and blood tests which revealed a blood sugar of 868 (normal about 100) and a pH of 7.10 (normal 7.35 to 7.45). While studying the chart, the resident noted that the admission blood sugar from 3 days ago was 420, and that from 1 day previous it was 730. The attending had not seen the patient for 2 days and had instituted no insulin coverage. The resident began appropriate therapy, called the attending, and requested transferring the patient to the ICU. From his discussion with the attending, who refused to move the patient to the ICU, the resident became aware that the attending did not appreciate the seriousness of the situation, nor did he understand the requisite therapy and careful monitoring for diabetic ketoacidosis. The resident, who was off-duty in 15 minutes, wrote orders as detailed as possible, signed the case out to the incoming house physician, and explained the situation to the nurses, telling them to call the house physician and attending with all lab results and any changes in the patient's status. He learned later that the patient died while still in a general floor bed about 2 hours after he left.

CASES 8, 9, 10, and 11. *Right to Health Care/Allocation of Resources*

The next four cases are to be taken as a series. They indicate the wide disparity in the distribution of health resources as a function of the patient's economic position. Each patient seeks medical assistance for his symptoms of duodenal ulcer.

Case 8. This patient came to the ER, and because of his assumed unreliability was hospitalized. The upper GI series documented a duodenal ulcer (DU), and he was begun on an appropriate regimen of diet and antacids. As soon as his symptoms disappeared three days later, he signed out of the hospital against medical advice, was given an outpatient clinic appointment which he failed to keep, and took none of his medications. Four months later recurrent symptoms led to rehospitalization. Overall, his symptoms had not improved; he had failed to follow his doctor's advice, and the outcome of his care must be judged unsatisfactory, despite the $700 cost for his care covered by Medicaid.

Case 9. The schoolteacher was enrolled in a prepaid health plan and consulted his physician in his office. He was immediately begun on therapy and the duodenal ulcer diagnosed the following day by UGIS (upper GI series). On the prescribed regimen, the patient was free of symptoms after 3 days, although the symptoms recurred intermittently over the next 4 months. The patient continued to follow his doctor's regimen, and a repeat UGIS showed chronic scarring of duodenal ulcer. His symptoms were not so severe as to require surgery. Although there was only partial improvement in symptoms, the patient's compliance and understanding of his illness were good, and the outcome was satisfactory. The cost to the patient was $100, his monthly health plan payment being $25.

Case 10. The construction worker developed symptoms of duodenal ulcer at a time of uncertainty in the construction industry. He had no insurance, so he went to the emergency room of his local hospital. The attending physician advised him to be admitted to the hospital for tests, but the prospect of paying for these discouraged him, and he chose instead to "see it through." The staff did convince him to have both his upper GI series done and to come in for another appointment in 2 weeks. As the time for his appointment approached, his symptoms had gone and he decided to skip the appointment and so save his money. After 4 months he remained free of symptoms while off his medication. Because he was unaware of his diagnosis, his outcome must be regarded as unsatisfactory despite the cost of his UIGS and ER visit which he paid out of his pocket.

Case 11. The executive visited his fee-for-service physician, who hospitalized him. Although he was free of symptoms after 3 days, his physician kept him in the hospital another 7 days. The patient kept his monthly appointments and took the medications his physician had prescribed. Although he was without symptoms at 4 months, his UGIS still showed chronic change at the site of his duodenal ulcer. His hospital bill was paid in full by his comprehensive insurance coverage, but he had to pay for his follow-up visits and follow-up x-rays. The total cost of his care, including 4 months of insurance premiums, was $2300.

CASE 12. Informed Consent/*Allocation of Resources/Aggressiveness of Patient Care*

An 86-year-old retired secretary was first seen in the Medical Care Group (MCG) of Washington University in the spring of 1975 complaining of lack of memory. She had been in a hospital only once for some unknown cause as a young woman. She gave a history of labile blood pressure, nervousness, and memory loss. The latter had been severe enough to lead her to assign power of attorney to a third party who made her financial and other decisions. Despite this, she was able to communicate directly with the examining physician and to give an adequate history. She had no living relatives and lived by herself in a home for the aged. She went to the theater occasionally and sometimes received visiting friends. Positive physical findings included a blood pressure of 170/82 mm Hg, bilateral carotid bruits, a grade 2/6 systolic murmur along the left sternal border, and a very firm, 7- to 8-cm pulsatile mass in the upper mid-abdomen with an overlying harsh, systolic bruit. Laboratory data were unremarkable except that a roentgenogram of the abdomen confirmed the presence of a large, mid-abdominal aortic aneurysm.

A surgeon was contacted and the patient's problems were discussed by telephone. The surgeon believed that an 86-year-old woman with labile hypertension was not a candidate for aortic aneurysm replacement. The patient's guardian was informed of this view and accepted it; the patient was not included in this decision.

Nothing more was heard from the patient until the evening of October 24, 1975, when a call was received from the nursing home stating that the patient had experienced sudden, severe back pain, that she had become cold, sweaty, and weak, and that she had collapsed to the floor. The patient was brought to the emergency room by ambulance. The blood pressure was 70/40 mm Hg and increased to 140/80 mm Hg following the intravenous infusion of saline solution. The patient was alert and able to converse. The abdomen was firm and tender with a very large palpable mass in the upper abdominal quadrant; the stool was guaiac positive. The hematocrit value had fallen to 25 percent. The diagnosis of rupturing abdominal aortic aneurysm was made. In the emergency room, the situation was discussed with the patient, who elected to have surgery even though it was made clear that the chances for success were small. The guardian was not available.

The patient was taken to the operating room and a 7-cm graft was placed in the abdominal aorta after the removal of a large, ruptured aneurysm. The patient was in the surgical intensive care unit for approximately 30 hours, during which time progressive obtundation and, despite apparent graft function, mottling of the lower extremities and progressive acidosis developed. She died the morning of October 27, 1975.

Source: Reprinted with permission from "Decisions Regarding the Provision or Withholding of Therapy," *Journal of the American Medical Association,* vol. 61, p. 915, December 1976.

CASE 13. Informed Consent/*Allocation of Resources*/*Aggressiveness of Patient Care*

A 90-year-old man presented for his first and only visit to MCG on August 14, 1975, complaining of weight loss and anorexia for 2 months. The patient lived alone and had taken care of himself for many years, although he had only minimal vision and very poor hearing. In June 1975 he noticed a decrease in appetite and subsequently lost approximately 20 pounds. He had not had nausea, vomiting, or a change in bowel habits. He had been hospitalized elsewhere in 1954 and was told that he had a "lump" in the large intestine which should be removed, but he chose not to have surgery.

Physical examination showed an elderly man with an irregular pulse of 76/min, normal temperature and respirations, a weight of 109 pounds, and a blood pressure of 180/90 mm Hg. There were bilateral dense cataracts, and both ears showed severe chronic otitis media. The heart was slightly enlarged with a grade 4/6 crescendo-decrescendo systolic murmur at the aortic area and along the left sternal border. All pulses were palpable. Examination of the abdomen revealed a hard, 10- by 15-cm mass in the midline below the umbilicus. Rectal examination disclosed a markedly enlarged prostate and a negative stool guaiac. The neurologic examination was within normal limits, and the patient was oriented and mentally clear.

Upon admission to the hospital, a catheter inserted into the bladder yielded 1,600 ml of bloody urine which was removed in several stages; the midline abdominal mass disappeared. The hematocrit value was 34.5 percent. Urinalysis showed numerous red blood cells. The serum creatinine was 1.9 mg/100 ml and the albumin 3.4 g/100 ml, but the results of all other routine serum chemistry studies were normal. Cystoscopy showed grade 4 trabeculation of the bladder; an intravenous urogram and retrograde studies did not reveal any abnormalities. The patient was scheduled for a transurethral prostatectomy.

The night after cystoscopy the patient's temperature rose to 38.5°C and he felt chilly, but the findings on physical examination and urinalysis were unchanged. The next morning, left pleuritic chest pain developed, the arterial oxygen tension (pO_2) was 55 mm Hg and, upon repeat, 53 mm Hg. A ventilation-perfusion lung scan showed defects in the lower field of both lungs compatible with pulmonary emboli, and the patient was given heparin. Over the next two days he continued to complain of pleuritic chest pain, but he was not dyspneic and his heparin therapy proceeded without difficulty. Because of the past history of a colonic mass, a barium enema was performed on August 21; it revealed only diverticulosis. By August 24, however, the patient had not had a bowel movement, and abdominal distention and cramping abdominal pain had developed. Increased infiltrates in the lower lobe of the left lung and upper lobe of the right lung were evident on a chest film, and hyponatremia was present. Repeat x-ray examination of the abdomen showed a large impaction of retained barium in the colon extending to the cecum. Repeated enemas and laxatives relieved only part of the obstruction. Following preoperative anesthesiology evaluation the patient was classified as a grade 4 risk, unacceptable for transurethral prostatectomy, and surgery was canceled.

The fever continued, the chest infiltrates increased, and the abdominal pain became so severe that the patient required meperidine. He began to state repeatedly that he wanted no additional therapy and that he wished to die; he refused all further diagnostic procedures. By August 29 he was coughing steadily and had bilateral, diffuse pulmonary rales. New infiltrates had appeared in the middle and upper lobes of the right lung. It was believed that he had pneumonia. After considerable discussion, it was decided to treat the patient with penicillin. On August 30 the abdominal pain increased, the hematocrit value decreased suddenly from 30 to 22 percent, and the stools became guaiac positive. It was believed that retroperitoneal and gastrointestinal hemorrhage had developed secondary to anticoagulation, and heparin therapy was discontinued. After further discussion, it was decided not to give the patient any blood transfusions but to continue the administration of fluids and penicillin. By September 3 the patient was semicomatose. He had bilateral diffuse rales and persistent anemia with a hematocrit value of 18 percent. The abdomen had become less distended; the patient occasionally was roused from his stupor, but he refused to accept any fluids or other personal ministrations. He died on September 7, 1975.

Source: Reprinted with permission from "Decisions Regarding the Provision or Withholding of Therapy," *Journal of the American Medical Association,* vol. 61, p. 915, December 1976.

CASE 14. Informed Consent/Paternalism/Rights/Ideals and Models of the Physician-Patient Relationship/Roles and Norms: Clinical Authority, Doctors' Roles, Patients' Roles/Institutional Responsibility/*Refusal of Treatment/Psychiatric Issues (Involuntary Commitment)*

A 22-year-old black male was arrested for swinging a stick at officers. He was charged with menacing, disorderly conduct, and resisting arrest and assault. During the arrest, he was shot in the shoulder and thigh. Friends observed that he had been acting strangely lately. Although he was studying to be a computer operator, he had dropped out and had taken to locking himself in his room or wandering about the city. The patient told the court-appointed attorney that he loved the police, the charges were unwarranted, and that they had not respected him as a man.

After hospitalization for his shotgun wounds, the patient appeared in court. His speech and mannerisms were so incoherent, the judge committed him for mental observation. He was diagnosed as paranoid schizophrenic, and found incompetent to understand or participate in the proceedings against him, and committed to a state mental hospital until found competent to stand trial.

While hospitalized, the doctors prescribed Stelazine for treatment. The patient refused to take the drug, coherently arguing that the drug would alter his mind and he could handle things for himself. He was warned that taking the medication would probably gain his release from the hospital, but he still refused, saying he did not want it under any circumstances.

Doctors in the case believe his condition to be deteriorating. Under the law, he can be confined for 2/3 of his probable criminal sentence, or 4 years and 8 months. The patient's doctors believe that he will continue to refuse the medication, and that forced medication would improve his condition. The patient's lawyer, citing the patient's good record, believes that if the patient stood trial, he would receive a lesser sentence and could not be confined for so long a period. There appears to be no rule of law established on whether, or when, forced medication is permissible.

Source: Reprinted with permission from the Program on Human Values and Ethics, University of Tennessee, Center for the Health Sciences, Memphis, Tenn.

CASE 15. Informed Consent/*Paternalism*/Rights/Roles and Norms: Patients' Roles/*Aggressiveness of Patient Care*

J.P. was a sixty-year-old black male with an admittedly sketchy past history due to ineffective follow-up. However, he was apparently diagnosed as having chronic renal disease, secondary to hypertensive renovascular disease, approximately 2 years prior to his last admission. During the 9 months prior to this admission, the patient had been hospitalized four separate times for management of his renal disease and associated medical problems.

Throughout his known contact with the health care system, the patient had expressed and demonstrated a certain disregard for recommended therapeutic modalities. He refused to be compliant with a diet, intermittently took prescribed medicines, and almost consistently missed appointments. His laissez-faire approach to his chronic disease was interrupted only when his family brought him to emergency rooms for acute problems—GI distress, profound weakness, lethargy, and even seizures.

With the progress of his renal disease, the option of dialysis was discussed with him and he usually refused with apparent understanding of the implications. However, during the last of these four hospitalizations, he tentatively agreed to peritoneal dialysis in the future if it meant saving his life. Nevertheless, soon thereafter the patient was brought to the emergency room again with significant metabolic derangement and still refused dialysis. He was treated symptomatically before being released.

On his last admission, the patient was a lethargic, incoherent, severely wasted individual with physical findings consistent with uremia, including a pericardial friction rub. Laboratory examination revealed the presence of metabolic acidosis with severe derangement of AM electrolytes, anemia, and evidence of a urinary tract infection with possible sepsis. The patient was unable to discuss therapeutic options and the family could not be reached. Contact was made with a neighbor, who confirmed that the patient had not been compliant with his complicated pharmacological regime of at least ten different agents. Apparently, the patient had progressively deteriorated since his discharge 8 weeks earlier.

Source: Reprinted with permission from the Program on Human Values and Ethics, University of Tennessee, Center for the Health Sciences, Memphis, Tenn.

CASE 16. Informed Consent/Paternalism/*Rights*/Right to Health Care/*Institutional Responsibility*

A male inmate patient suffering from glaucoma, and taking regular medication for this condition, had not had his intraocular pressure checked for over a year. There was no one in the institution who could check intraocular pressure; so the prison physician arranged for a clinic visit at a community hospital. Prison regulations, however, required that inmates submit to a pre-exit rectal search. The inmate patient refused to submit to this search, and was therefore not permitted to go for the pressure check.

Source: Presented at conference on Conflict Resolution in Prison Health Care presented by the Department of Social Medicine, Montefiore Hospital and Medical Center, March 26, 1979, under a grant from the National Science Foundation entitled Legal and Ethical Issues in the Delivery of Health Care in Detention and Correctional Institutions.

CASE 17. Informed Consent/Paternalism/*Rights*/Sanctity of Life/Roles and Norms: Doctors' Roles, Patients' Roles/Professional-Patient Communication/*Refusal of Treatment*/Aggressiveness of Patient Care

R.B. was a 15-year-old-boy, the only child of parents now in their 50s. He was a sophomore in high school, academically above average, and interested in sports, having earned positions on both the football and track teams.

His present illness began early in September, when he injured his right leg in football practice. In the next two days after that injury, he continued to have pain just below the knee of the right leg. After two days of continued pain, the coach recommended whirlpool baths but felt that he could continue practice. The pain continued for another week in spite of this program and he mentioned it to his father, who said that he probably had a bruise and that it would improve. However, the pain persisted for still another week, and at that time the football coach called the parents and recommended that he be taken to the family physician for further studies. The parents were able to get an appointment toward the end of the next week and the family physician found local tenderness and some swelling. He obtained a roentgenogram at the local hospital and the following day asked the parents to come to his office for a discussion. At that time he told them that it looked as if there was a tumor in the bone just below the right knee. Because of these findings, he referred the patient to the St. Jude Children's Research Hospital.

On further study at this institution, the boy was found, indeed, to have a tumor in the right fibula which was interpreted as being most likely osteosarcoma. There was no evidence of tumor involvement in the lungs or in other bones. The rest of the physical and laboratory findings supported the impression of clinically localized osteosarcoma. A recommendation of an above-the-knee amputation of the right leg was made, to be followed by a period of adjuvant chemotherapy according to the current protocol study, lasting for a period of 10 to 12 months. The protocol study included randomization to receive or not receive immunotherapy with irradiated tumor cells during the course of treatment.

The parents and the boy were understandably upset about this proposal. The boy in particular was concerned about the amputation and asked if there were alternative methods of treatment. He told the parents he did not want to have the leg removed and would refuse treatment. His parents were undecided but finally went along with the boy's wishes. In spite of long conversations, the parents remained adamant. It was recommended that they return home, talk with their family physician, family, and pastor about this decision. After an additional week of discussion and continued contact with this hospital, the decision was finally made to allow amputation and treatment.

The amputation went without incident, and the boy was fitted immediately with a walking prosthesis. Chemotherapy, according to protocol, was begun after receiving permission from the boy and the parents. After 4 months, however, the boy decided against any further chemotherapy. He had lost his hair with treatment and had episodes of vomiting, especially in association with the administration of methotrexate. He was missing school and was particularly concerned and distressed about the fact that his friends were beginning practice for track. In talking with both parents, the physicians had been able to convince the father of the need for continued treatment but the mother said that she would not allow any further treatment if the boy did not want it. The boy had expressed to her his conviction that he had been cured and needed no further treatment. The father reluctantly concurred with the mother about this decision, although it was clear that actually he had withdrawn from the situation shortly after the initial surgery and it was the mother who was truly determining the response to the son's decision.

Source: Reprinted with permission from the Program on Human Values and Ethics, University of Tennessee, Center for the Health Sciences, Memphis, Tenn.

CASE 18. *Informed Consent* /Rights/Ideals and Models of the Physician-Patient Relationship/Roles and Norms: Clinical Authority, Doctors' Roles/Professional-Patient Communication/*Institutional Responsibility/Professional Accountability*

Wallace: This is John Perry. He is 66. Tomorrow morning he will undergo surgery for a hernia repair. The man who is examining him is the chief resident, Dr. Tom Penn. He will do the surgery. But Mr. Perry doesn't know that.

Doctor: Okay? Deep breath.

Wallace: Perry is in Strong Memorial Hospital in Rochester, New York—a teaching hospital run by the medical school at the university here. Medical students—interns who want to be surgeons—look on an appointment to Strong as a plum, for only the best of them are chosen. Most patients here, like John Perry, are private. Most of them have Blue Cross, Blue Shield. Their private doctors are among the best in town, and they are good teachers.

Doctor: Okay, fine. Wrinkle your forehead.

Wallace: Perry is under the impression that he will be operated on by Dr. Charles Rob, Chief of Surgery at Strong. He has confidence in him. Perry has been in the hospital in recent years, after a heart attack, and for an operation on his leg. He thinks that Tom Penn will just be standing by at tomorrow morning's surgery.

Dr. Tom Penn: Mr. Perry, I'd like to get you to sign the operative consent.

Perry: Uh-hmm.

Dr. Penn: In signing this, what you'll be doing—it says, "I, John Perry, authorize Dr. Charles Rob" to treat you for a right inguinal hernia. One other part of the consent I'd like you to understand, and that is this portion here, which entails the authorization of the exercise of professional judgment by Dr. Rob, who's your operating surgeon. Do you understand that, or have any questions?

John Perry: Yes, I do. No, I have no questions.

Dr. Penn: Fine. And have you . . .

Wallace: At no time is Perry told that Penn, not Rob, will do the cutting.

Dr. Penn: In order to be a surgeon, I have to do the surgery. I have to get experience by actually doing the surgery. And I think that this is the best way to get that experience.

Dr. Rob: Dr. Penn is in the final year of five years of surgical training. He's got to the stage now when he should do operations, particularly an operation like a hernia, which is not a big one, supervised and controlled, and do the thing himself.

Wallace: Dr. Rob told us residents get enough training to satisfy the American Board of Surgery, which certifies surgeons. Without that certification today, it's almost impossible to get a surgical post at any hospital. (*To Dr. Penn.*) In the case of Mr. Perry, you did—you performed that operation.

Dr. Penn: I performed the operation, yes.

Wallace: Beginning to end.

Dr. Penn: That's right.

Wallace: You handled the scalpel.

Dr. Penn: That's right.

Wallace: You did all the work.

Dr. Penn: That's right.

Wallace: Where was Dr. Rob?

Dr. Penn: Dr. Rob was across the table from me.

Wallace: But you actually did the job?

Dr. Penn: That's right. He was assisting me, yes.

Wallace (to Perry): Are you aware of the fact that, when you came into this hospital for surgery, you signed a release form? Do you know what you signed?

Perry: Yes, I did.

Wallace: All right. Now, I have a copy of that form here. And it says, "I"—your name, and so forth—"hereby authorize Dr. Rob, and/or such assistants as may be selected by him"—

Perry: That's true. But they don't operate. They assist. He's the surgeon.

Wallace: You're sure?

Perry: I'm positive.

Wallace: You're positive it was Rob who did the—

Perry: Oh, yes, I know that.

Wallace: How do you know?

Perry: Because I know him well enough, and I'm a registered male nurse, so that I know what his procedures are.

Wallace: What if I were to tell you that it wasn't Rob who did the surgery; that it was Penn who did the surgery?

Perry: I'd be surprised. But that's never been the case. It's never been the case. He's too well known for that. He's famous, that guy.

Wallace: Who? Rob?

Perry: Yes. England, United—all over the United States. He goes all over. He's the chief of the whole bloody works.

Wallace: Uh-hmm. (*To Dr. Penn.*) Did you tell Perry that you were going to do the surgery?

Dr. Penn: No, I did not.

Wallace: Did Dr. Rob tell Perry that you were going to do the surgery?

Dr. Penn: I can't say that I—I personally heard Dr. Rob tell him, but I know—do know that it is a practice of his that he informs his patients that he will be assisted by his resident staff.

Wallace: But actually you were doing the surgery, and he was assisting you.

Dr. Penn: That's not unusual in—even in the biggest of operations.

Wallace: Dr. Penn—

Dr. Charles Rob: Yeah.

Wallace: —performed that hernia operation.

Dr. Rob: With me helping him.

Wallace: Well actually, he handled the knife all the way.

Dr. Rob: That is correct. That is what we—we—I mean. I was there. I held the retractors. I was fully there. But Dr. Penn did the cutting.

Wallace: Should not the patient have the right to know? The AMA says—and I—I've got to come back to that—

Dr. Rob: I agree.

Wallace: —to have another physician operate on one's patient without that patient's consent and without his knowledge of the substitution is a fraud and deceit and violation of basic ethical concept. The patient, as a human being, is entitled to choose his own physician, and he should be permitted to acquiesce in or refuse to accept the substitution. Well—

Dr. Rob: Well, we—

Wallace: —Perry didn't have an opportunity to refuse or acquiesce to the substitution of Penn for Rob.

Dr. Rob: Well, I think he did—because twice I personally told him that the operation was going to be performed by the resident, with me helping him.

Wallace (to Perry): You understood—

Perry: That it was Dr. Rob.

Wallace: And Dr. Rob told you today—

Perry: That he had done it.

Wallace: —that he held the knife, he did the surgery?

Perry: And that it was very successful.

Wallace: Uh-hmm. And that Penn was just—

Perry: I imagine that he was just standing by—(*indistinct*) circulating.

Source: Sixty Minutes, CBS Television Network, August 13, 1978.

CASE 19. Active and Passive Euthanasia / Sanctity of Life / *Roles and Norms: Clinical Authority / Aggressiveness of Patient Care* / Allocation of Resources

An 80-year-old man was brought into the hospital in respiratory distress. His medical history indicated that he had suffered two strokes in the past: a partial one on the right side and a later severe one which left him completely paralyzed and aphasic. For the past two years, he has been totally dependent on others for his care. He has been completely noncommunicative, except for partial physical withdrawal from pain stimuli, but it is not clear whether he cannot understand others or cannot express himself.

On admission, the patient was found to be in congestive heart failure, which responded adequately to medical care. The family was contacted for permission to insert a gastrostomy tube for feeding. The house staff wanted the procedure performed because, since he was not in any acute life-threatening distress, they felt constrained to do something for him. The family consented to the feeding procedure, but wished that nothing more be done for him.

**CASE 20. Active and Passive Euthanasia/Rights/Sanctity of Life/Roles and Norms: Doctors'
Roles, Patients' Roles/*Aggressiveness of Patient Care*/*Allocation of Resources***

A 70-year-old man found on the floor of a hotel room was brought to the hospital by a
paramedic. At the time of admission he was in a stuporous, lethargic state though able to speak.
He quickly became comatose. His initial lab results showed low sugar and malnutrition
which was believed to be the result of alcohol abuse. He was placed in the ICU on the remote
possibility that the cause was something else. The hope was that his condition would improve in a few days, permitting him to be moved to the ward.

Once in the ICU he deteriorated quickly. He did not respond to pain, though his EEG test
showed some activity. The physician in charge met with the house staff and related the prognosis for the patient. "He will contract an infection, probably pneumonia. There is no family
to contact. When the infection takes, no antibiotics will be administered, for the patient
has no chance to recover."

**CASE 21. *Informed Consent (Competency)*/Paternalism/Rights/Roles and Norms: Clinical
Authority/*Psychiatric Issues (Involuntary Commitment)***

A 26-year-old divorced unemployed black male was brought to the emergency room September 15, 1975, having been unconscious on a sidewalk. On examination, he was comatose, had a cardiac arrhythmia, and pressure necrosis of the skin of his right ear, right arm,
and chest. He was admitted to the ICU and after his medical condition stabilized, he was
transferred to Plastic Surgery for skin grafting.

A psychiatric consultation was requested when it was determined he had made a suicide
attempt by drug overdose. Pertinent past psychiatric history included three previous suicide
attempts—two by drug overdose and one by jumping out a third-story window. He had four
psychiatric hospitalizations for the treatment of paranoid schizophrenia and had signed out
against medical advice on each hospitalization, most recently 6 weeks prior to this admission.
He was being followed in a mental health clinic where he received the medications he had
taken in this suicide attempt.

On examination, the patient was sullen, mute, and withdrawn. He was oriented, seemed
to be responding to auditory hallucinations, and thought that someone wanted to kill him. His
behavior was impulsive and unpredictable. He was begun on antipsychotic medication and
a private duty nurse was assigned. Several hours later, he struck the nurse and eloped from the
unit. He was later returned by his relatives and transferred to the psychiatric unit. On the
third day of psychiatric hospitalization, he insisted that he wanted to leave and signed an official notice indicating that five days hence he would leave the hospital against his doctor's
advice.

CASE 22. *Informed Consent*/Paternalism/*Experimentation*

Many patients have undergone technically successful corrective cardiac surgery but cannot be weaned from the bypass machinery. A protocol was submitted to an Institutional
Review Board (IRB) to investigate the safety and efficacy of a left-ventricular assist device
that would facilitate the weaning process and would remain in place through the immediate
postoperative period. The investigator estimated that about 10 percent of patients on a

bypass cannot be weaned easily; 8 percent respond to what is now considered standard therapy; and only the remaining 1 or 2 percent would be candidates for this device. It would be impossible to predict, however, which patients would need it prior to the corrective surgery.

The IRB found, after considerable discussion with expert consultants, that it could assume three facts: (1) this device showed acceptable promise of effectiveness; (2) any patient in this situation would be sure to die unless this device worked; (3) no device had been developed elsewhere which could be predicted to be more effective.

The IRB was thus confronted with a protocol involving an investigative device which, if successful, would be the only means of saving patients' lives. The question of concern was what form of consent would be appropriate and by whom it should be given.

Source: Reprinted with permission from "Consent to the Use of An Investigational Cardiac Assist Device," *Hastings Center Report,* vol. 1, no. 1, p. 6, March 1979.

CASE 23. Informed Consent/Paternalism/*Active and Passive Euthanasia*/Ideals and Models of the Physician-Patient Relationship/Roles and Norms: Clinical Authority, Doctors' Roles/Professional-Patient Communication/*Aggressiveness of Patient Care*

Mrs. Hagstrom, age 73, was admitted to the hospital because of shortness of breath. She had had severe high blood pressure for several years. Vigorous out-patient treatment with all available drugs had been unsuccessful in controlling the pressure. During the few weeks prior to her admission to the hospital, she had developed shortness of breath and weakness.

Initial evaluation in the hospital revealed heart failure and kidney failure, both caused by the high blood pressure. The heart failure was successfully treated; thus the shortness of breath disappeared. She remained weak. She developed persistent nausea, attributable to the kidney failure. Clonidine, a new drug for controlling high blood pressure, was begun. The pressure was partially controlled, but Mrs. Hagstrom became more nauseated and developed severe light-headedness when standing, a common side effect of clonidine. She complained to her physician about the side effects, and asked for reassurance that the drug was working. Her physician decided to discontinue the drug and accept the risks of higher blood pressure. Mrs. Hagstrom was discharged.

She remained very weak and nauseated and a week later was readmitted to the hospital. Despite vigorous treatment, she experienced swelling of the legs—a symptom of heart failure. On the tenth day Mrs. Hagstrom had a fever, was coughing up thick phlegm, and was short of breath. The physician diagnosed pneumonia. Later, that evening, she suffered congestive heart failure and was brought to the medical ICU. The physician told the house staff not to vigorously treat the pneumonia. Mrs. Hagstrom died the next day.

Source: Reprinted with permission of Dr. Gordon Mosser, Share-Health Plan, St. Paul, Minnesota.

CASE 24. *Roles and Norms: Doctors' Roles*/Professional-Patient Communication/*Institutional Responsibility*

John M. was born prematurely with respiratory distress syndrome. He was immediately placed on a respirator. In the first two months in the ICU he developed several other lung complications with tremendous strain on the heart. These difficulties subsided, but for six additional months he had to be isolated to prevent his contracting pneumonia.

His parents are from Rumania; they emmigrated to the United States via Israel. They visited John very infrequently, and the mother never stayed longer than two hours. She is immature, constantly cowering in front of the father, and she is frightened by "all the tubes" in the ICU. She rarely handles John, though the father usually does.

The nurses, though never the attending physicians, have tried repeatedly to wean John from the respirator. He had become a "mascot" to the nurses on the floor. They have brought him toys and have played with him when they had the time.

After one year in the ICU, at a cost of $320 a day, a medical student was brought in to relate to John, because the nurses noted that he never smiled. He was found to be absorbed in self-stimulatory behavior, revealing severe social retardation.

The medical student succeeded in eliciting a social smile from John, as well as some mimicking with his mouth. The nursing staff is not sure what will happen once the student leaves.

CASE 25. Informed Consent/Ideals and Models of the Physician-Patient Relationship/ Roles and Norms: Clinical Authority/*Professional-Patient Communication*/Institutional Responsibility

January 1972 was the first hospital admission for baby G.R., a 2½-month-old-child who was admitted for the evaluation and diagnosis of ambiguous genitalia. At birth there was some confusion regarding the gender of G.R., though the parents were told they had a son with underdeveloped genitalia. Chromosome studies were performed and they revealed a true mosaic: 46 XY and 45 XO with an 80/20 distribution. If the child was held from an anterior position one would see a phallus, two unfused labial-scrotal folds, and a palpable gonad in the left inguinal canal. A lateral view of the phalus revealed two openings: a false one and one that urine came out of. Tests on the sinogram revealed geographs of a normal bladder, a normal external sphincter, a vagina, and a uterus. The medical opinion was that if G.R. were reconstructed into a male he would not function urologically or sexually, and if G.R. were reconstructed into a female she would be able to function urologically and sexually though not reproductively. There was controversy as to whether the gonad, which was abdominal, was actually an ovary. As such the decision was placed to parents with the attendings pressing for a girl.

G.R.'s mother was a 20-year-old known drug addict involved in a methadone program. The father was a known alcoholic who had a lengthy criminal record and an active child abuse case pending on him. The mother agreed to the female solution but the father, having been told earlier he had a son, refused to let anyone "touch his little boy." The maternal grandmother also agreed to reconstructing G.R. into a female and said the father was "a crazy man who refused to work and who frequently beat up G.R.'s elder sister." After a month of procrastination the father agreed to the surgery.

In surgery a true testicle and true ovary were found, making G.R. a one-in-a-million true hermaphrodite. The child could have been reconstructed to either male or female. Reconstruction of G.R., now named Sherene, into a female was successful. Sherene was returned to her parents two weeks later.

CASE 26. Informed Consent/Paternalism/Rights/Sanctity of Life/Ideals and Models of the Physician-Patient Relationship/*Roles and Norms: Clinical Authority, Doctors' Roles*/Institutional Responsibility/*Aggressiveness of Patient Care*

A 67-year-old female was admitted to the hospital under cardiac arrest. She had a long history of high blood pressure, smoking, cardiac instability, respiratory insufficiency, and pancreatitis. During the initial two weeks of her hospitalization, it was extremely difficult to maintain her stability. Both the intern and the resident, who believed in very aggressive medical management, worked day and night keeping her alive. Eventually the patient stabilized, came out of the coma she was initially in, and, although she still required a respirator, began to sit up in her bed and in a nearby chair.

She was being prepared to be moved out of the ICU when she had another cardiac arrest. She stabilized again, though now had a flail chest, resulting from rigorous cardioplumonary resuscitation, and a mild fever. Three days after her transferral out of the ICU she arrested again and required six cardioversions. She rebounded immediately from this incident and recovered mental status within one hour of this arrest.

The new resident at this time nevertheless felt her situation to be hopeless and stated to the house staff, "We're not going to be able to save this person's life." As predicted, she arrested again the next day, was again resuscitated, and was placed on alternate antiarrhythmic medications.

CASE 27. Informed Consent/Active and Passive Euthanasia/Rights/The Concept of a Person/Sanctity of Life/Ideals and Models of the Physician-Patient Relationship/*Roles and Norms: Clinical Authority, Doctors' Roles, Patients' Roles*/Professional-Patient Communication/*Aggressiveness of Patient Care*

Jenny was the product of an uncomplicated pregnancy, labor, and mid-forceps vaginal delivery. She did well until one week of age when she developed a heart murmur which became so intense that she required an oxygen hood at 2 weeks of age. Jenny was started on digitalis, and a chromosome study was performed. The child was found to have Down's syndrome.

The parents were informed and were asked for consent to place a cardiac catheter in Jenny in order to document her heart disease and thus devise a treatment. The reaction was disbelief and they demanded another chromosome study, though they reluctantly agreed to the catheterization. They also said that if there was any surgery that could be performed for her benefit, it ought to be done.

The catheter revealed serious heart disease, and Jenny was not responding to the medical management. After considering palliative surgery, the surgeons rejected it, because of the extreme mortality risk and questionable prognosis.

The purpose of such surgery would be to get Jenny to the age (about 1 to 2 years) when a definitive, corrective, operative procedure could be performed. If the child made it to this age, the prognosis would be good. If the palliative surgery were not performed, the surgeons believed Jenny would die in a few weeks of congestive heart failure. Corrective surgery was out of the question at her present age.

The repeated chromosome study confirmed Down's syndrome, and the parents were informed of this. The surgeons chose not to inform the parents that they decided against palliative surgery and simply told them that nothing more could be done for their child.

CASE 28. Informed Consent/Paternalism/*Ideals and Models of the Physician-Patient Rela-tionship*/Roles and Norms: Clinical Authority, Doctors' Roles/*Professional-Patient Communication/Abortion*

Thirteen-year-old D.H. was 4½ months pregnant, though she had only become aware of her pregnancy during the last month. When her mother was told, she immediately decided that D.H. would not keep the baby. D.H. stressed to her mother her desire to keep the baby and pointed out that her boy friend (the baby's father) was very supportive. Argu-ments made by her mother concerning D.H.'s age, her position in school, and the family's reputation had D.H. submitting, but she still felt strongly about keeping the baby.

Before adolescents are seen by the GYN residents in the clinics, they speak with counselors in the Teen Family Health Clinic. The counselors are there to listen and give some advice, but they do not become part of any major decisions. These sessions are particularly important if the patient is pregnant. D.H. identified one woman in this clinic as someone she felt close to and who she felt understood her need and desire to have the baby. For unclear reasons, this wish was not communicated adequately to the GYN residents. When D.H. and her mother went to the gynecologist, D.H. maintained her position of wanting to keep the baby but Mrs. H. overrode her daughter and persuaded the resident that an abortion would be in every-one's best interest. The resident decided to listen to Mrs. H. He could have carried out the patient's wishes but chose not to. He felt that a 13-year-old girl had no business being preg-nant in the first place. In this respect, he had made his decision almost before hearing the two sides presented by the patient and her mother.

Accordingly, then, a Laminaria tent was inserted into the patient's cervix and D.H. went home with her mother. The next day, D.H.'s conviction to have her baby was as strong as ever and she returned to the hospital to speak with the teen counselor. This time, D.H. con-vinced her and the gynecologist of her desire to carry the pregnancy through, and the Lam-inaria tent was removed. For two days D.H. did well physically, although she had many arguments with her mother—but there was nothing Mrs. H. could do, since D.H. had taken matters into her own hands. On the third day following the removal, D.H. began to experience abdominal cramps, and on the fourth day she felt the gush of "water" which brought her into the emergency room.

The gynecology resident who removed the Laminaria did not explain to D.H. that it was probably too late to prevent an abortion. He felt there was a slight chance the aborting process would be stopped by stopping the cervical dilatation. He also decided to spare her the knowledge that she was responsible for the abortion, since she wanted the baby so badly. When D.H. came into the hospital, she was seen by GYN, who diagnosed an inevitable abortion with premature rupture of membranes and admitted her to Pediatrics. D.H. was led to believe that she was now having a miscarriage which was not connected in any way to the manipulations with the Laminaria. The Pediatrics staff collaborated in this deception with the GYN. The Pediatric intern felt that D.H. would be spared a lot of postabortion guilt if she thought that the miscarriage had been spontaneous and unrelated to the Laminaria insertion.

After this entire episode, D.H. was sad about having lost the baby but comfortable in the knowledge that it had been a spontaneous, not induced, abortion. She was also optimistic about finishing school before she got pregnant again.

CASE 29. Paternalism/*Active and Passive Euthanasia*/Sanctity of Life/*Roles and Norms: Clinical Authority, Doctors' Roles*/Professional-Patient Communication/Institutional Responsibility/Allocation of Resources

A two-year-old child with acute leukemia was brought to the hospital from Venezuela because the parents were not happy with the treatment the child was receiving. For the first three weeks the child was placed on chemotherapy but, having failed the initial induction, he continued to deteriorate. Chemotherapy was stopped but the patient was still in the ICU and Hematology was still drawing bloods.

The chief resident of Pediatrics wanted the child out of the ICU. He directed the residents not to do anything "heroic" for the child (no resuscitation) and to administer only pain killers. The parents, he reasoned, would find a private ward room more conducive to grieving, and to keep the patient in the ICU would be a poor utilization of resources. Hematology, on the contrary, wanted the patient kept in the ICU because they believed the parents were not ready to accept the child's imminent death, which a removal from the ICU would surely signal.

The chief resident was angered that he had accepted the patient in the first place. He had initially thought it was too late to help the child, but, not wanting to produce any guilt for the parents, he had agreed to treat him. Now the chief resident had placed his residents in an awkward position with Hematology by ordering them not to treat the child. He went to Hematology and agreed with them to keep the patient in the ICU though still only pain killers would be administered.

The patient died 24 hours later. During this time Hematology had continued to draw bloods and record vital signs in order to monitor the admittedly dying patient.

CASE 30. *Rights*/Institutional Responsibility/*Abortion*

A mother of four children now pregnant with another came to the Valley Abortion Center in Phoenix to have an abortion. A doctor at the center estimated the woman to be 19 weeks pregnant.

Her family history revealed significant parenting difficulties with her four children. Her husband was a salesman and would often be absent from home for two months at a time. Two of her four boys were frequently truant from elementary school. The eldest boy was currently in an institution for problem adolescence. She and her husband decided they could not handle another child.

At the abortion center she was injected with a saline solution and sent home. Three days later she went into labor at night. Because the abortion center was closed at night, the woman was told to report to Doctors Hospital in the city "to deliver the fetus." There she gave birth to a girl weighing 2 pounds, 9 ounces.

A statement made by the hospital read, "The child is making satisfactory progress and should be able to be discharged in about three to four weeks. The baby's natural parents will be taking her home to join several other children in the family."

CASE 31. Informed Consent/Paternalism/*Rights*/Ideals and Models of the Physician-Patient Relationship/Roles and Norms: Doctors' Roles/*Psychiatric Issues (Involuntary Commitment)*

Manfred Munro, age 49, appeared before Judge Johnson because his wife had petitioned the court for his civil commitment. Immediately before the hearing Mr. Munro had been examined by Dr. Smith, a general practitioner, and by Dr. Jones, a psychiatrist.

Mrs. Munro testified that she and her husband were living apart. She described very strange behavior by her husband recently. She quoted him as saying that "no one works anymore" and that "nobody's driving cars anymore." She reported that he had denied that the children attended school and had thrown out their report cards. She said that he had planned to give away the children's bicycles and other toys and that he had given away some food from their freezer. He was a carpenter, she said, but had not worked for many months. She said that he behaved normally when taking Stelazine (trifluoperazine, a major tranquilizer) but that he had stopped taking it. She stated that he had been hospitalized three times previously for mental breakdowns.

Mr. Munro stated that he had thrown out some old papers recently, clearing out the house; he was unaware of having thrown out the children's report cards. He said that he had not given away the children's bicycles and did not plan to do so. He had given some "tough old buck roast" in the family's freezer to a friend. He denied saying that "no one works anymore." He said that he no longer wished to work as a carpenter and that he was trying to choose a new line of work. He described his love of family life and made a plea for reconciliation with his wife and children.

A psychologist at the state mental hospital had administered three psychological tests to Mr. Munro a few days before the hearing. The psychologist testified that Mr. Munro probably had "some type of organic [that is, physical] problem affecting his brain . . . [causing] behavior that he may not be completely aware of at the time."

Drs. Smith and Jones both testified that Mr. Munro, in their opinions, required hospitalization for further observation and treatment for his mental illness.

Mr. Munro objected to their conclusions. He stated that confinement in the state hospital, with which he was quite familiar, would not help him. He stated that he was not sick. He noted that he had broken no laws. He said that he did not want to go to the hospital.

Judge Johnson stated that by reason of paranoid schizophrenia, the diagnosis made by Dr. Jones, he was committing Mr. Munro to the state hospital.

Source: Reprinted with permission of Dr. Gordon Mosser, Share-Health Plan, St. Paul, Minnesota.

CASE 32. *Definition of Death*/The Concept of a Person/Sanctity of Life/Professional-Patient Communication/*Aggressiveness of Patient Care*/Transplantation

The patient was an 11-year-old black male brought to the hospital by his uncle after having been shot in the head by his brother. The patient was taken to the pediatric ICU, suffered a short cardiac arrest, and was resuscitated. The initial x-rays were mislabeled and indicated a bullet entrance on the left side of the head, with a visible exit wound on the right. Upon closer examination in the ICU and with new x-rays it was determined that the bullet wound was on the right side only. An implication of the first films would have been that the bullet had cornered the midbrain, possibly causing significant irreversible damage. A cerebral angiogram was taken.

The patient was intubated and placed on a respirator. An IV was started with D5 solution with electrolytes. There was a marked improvement in his condition during the first day with growing response to verbal commands, half-open eyes, response to deep pain, and leg raising motor control exhibited in response to commands. An intracranial screw was inserted to measure the intracranial pressure (ICP), which began to drop toward normal range during the second day. On the second day the patient was removed from the respirator. By the end of the day, respiratory difficulties required support of a respirator again. The patient then began to show increased intracranial pressure and a lack of responses to anything except deep pain. On the fourth day the patient was taken for CT scan. At that time he suffered cardio-respiratory arrest and was resuscitated. There was no improvement in response, and on the fifth day he exhibited hypothermy (low temperature), no neurological signs, and flat EEG in two readings. On the fifth day the residents, in consultation with the neurologists, decided that the patient's brain had failed, assuming midbrain damage due to cerebral edema and the high pressure. The ICP screw was removed. On the sixth day the parents were reached by telephone for consent to do an EEG and cerebral flow study to determine brain death. The parents requested that support be maintained until they could consult with their pastor. Support was maintained during the next several days, although the ICP screw was not replaced. There was no ICP monitoring and therefore no care for further deterioration of ICP. During the period a resident approached the mother to discuss the possibility of donating kidneys for transplant. The mother became very angry and insisted on the maintenance of her son. On the eleventh day the patient suffered a cardiac arrest with flat EKG and was declared dead.

CASE 33. Informed Consent/Paternalism/Active and Passive Euthanasia/Rights/Sanctity of Life/Roles and Norms: Clinical Authority, Doctors' Roles, Patients' Roles/Refusal of Treatment/Aggressiveness of Patient Care

M.H. was a middle-aged man with metastatic carcinoma of the colon. The cancer had been diagnosed two years previously, and despite chemotherapy during this time, there was metastasis to the liver. M.H. was told his diagnosis from the outset and informed his private physician and family that he wanted to die at home with no heroic measures.

One week prior to his last hospital admission, M.H. became deeply jaundiced and developed an upper GI bleed. He believed his condition was the result of his cancer and did not want to come to the hospital. He wanted to stay home and die. His family, however, coerced him into going to the hospital. Although it is not clear why they did this, the house staff believe the family panicked when he started bleeding from the rectum and vomiting blood. They had not realized this could happen and that this was how he might die. Throughout all this, the patient was alert and conscious.

Upon arrival at the hospital, it was determined that the upper GI bleed was caused by medication and was not a direct result of the cancer. The patient was treated for approximately one day and then refused all medication. He claimed he wanted to leave the hospital, despite the fact that he was bleeding. He actually took out his IV and signed release papers. Although his private physician was willing to let M.H. die of intestinal bleeding, the house staff was not. Following numerous attempts by the house staff to explain to the patient that the bleeding was probably just intercurrent and would stop in a few days following treatment, M.H. agreed to stay in the hospital. His bleeding finally stopped on the second day, at which time, however, he developed an altered mental status which was believed to be a result of the cancer.

All treatment was then stopped, except analgesics. It was decided not to resume chemotherapy. On the sixth day, the patient died of liver failure.

CASE 34. Informed Consent/Roles and Norms: Clinical Authority/*Psychiatric Issues (Psychosurgery)*/Experimentation

Mrs. A is a 49-year-old married, white female with two children. She has always been a very fastidious woman who has kept her house immaculate for as long as her husband could remember. Over the past ten years she has become increasingly concerned about cleaning her house. At first she would require that everyone entering the house remove their shoes. Eventually this was insufficient and her husband had to take a shower upon entering the house. It was not unusual for this patient to be seen scrubbing her sidewalk while on her hands and knees. After a few years of this behavior the family became quite upset and convinced her to seek psychiatric treatment. At first she was treated by psychoanalytically oriented psychotherapy. Much time was spent searching through her past history to establish the roots of what later became obsessive-compulsive behavior. After three years of this treatment, the family, unable to discern any change in her overall behavior, decided to have her treated in behavioral therapy which she underwent for a year and a half, again with minimal benefits. In fact, her obsessions about dirt reached the stage where she was afraid to step outside the house and be confronted by various particles of dirt on the streets. Finally, in desperation they took her to another psychiatrist who recommended a neurosurgeon for evaluation of possible psychosurgery. The psychiatrist indicated that this was likely the last resort of treatments, and that it often resulted in significant improvement. On the other hand, he described in detail some of the negative features of psychosurgery. The neurosurgeon emphasized instead the positive features of the procedure—that a "cure" was possible. At times the neurosurgeon almost guaranteed the results of the operation. After much debate in the family, it was agreed that psychosurgery was the last hope; so the patient, influenced strongly by family pressure, consented to a lobotomy. The procedure was successful in that the patient's obsessions were brought under control. The family noted, however, that she had considerable difficulty with her memory and that much of the time she appeared lethargic and apathetic.

CASE 35. Informed Consent/*Paternalism/Professional-Patient Communication*

L.D., a 17-year-old Hispanic female, came to the Gynecology (GYN) clinic complaining of severe dysmenorrhea (painful menstruation). She was accompanied by her mother, Mrs. D. The doctor who took care of L.D. was a male resident in his second year of training.

At first, Mrs. D. was unwilling to leave the examining room and answered all the questions directed toward her daughter. She appeared very domineering and L.D. behaved in a childlike, submissive fashion. After Mrs. D. was finally persuaded to leave, the patient was able to tell her own story.

Menarche (onset of menstruation) was at age 12 and had always been accompanied by severe cramping on the first two days. The cramps caused her to miss school and other activities because she was forced to remain in bed. Home remedies had been tried to no avail— nausea, vomiting, and diarrhea were usually associated with her periods as well. In addition, the menstrual cycle was irregular, with anywhere from 3 to 5 weeks between periods. L.D. does well in school and aspires to be a nurse. Unknown to her mother, she has a 20-year-old boyfriend who has just started to pressure her into having sex with him. At this point she is still a virgin and admittedly ignorant of sexual matters and contraception.

When it became time for L.D. to be examined internally (for the first time), she grew anxious and tense. The resident had an extremely difficult time because L.D. would not relax and cooperate. He felt that he did not do a good GYN exam but reported that no abnormalities were detected on physical exam.

After discussing this case with an attending physician (male) who had many years of experience and had seen similar cases, the resident prescribed a form of the birth control pill for 6 months. This "pill" would regulate the menstrual cycle and relieve the cramps. However, the resident deliberately misled L.D. and her mother—he said the pills were "pain relievers." They would take care of the cramping; in addition her periods would come with greater regularity and the flow would be lighter.

The resident felt justified in his decision to prescribe the "pill" and to deceive his patient because of the following: (1) the patient's dysmenorrhea and irregularity would resolve; (2) in the event that L.D. had sex she would be protected; (3) he assumed Mrs. D. would refuse to permit her daughter to take birth control pills; (4) the "pill" could not hurt L.D. for 6 months. She would realize that menstruation was not always associated with pain and would probably not suffer from dysmenorrhea after the prescription ran out. (This reflects the common feeling that there is a significant psychological and emotional basis for dysmenorrhea, as opposed to an organic basis, especially in young girls.) There was no attempt by the resident to discuss normal female physiology, contraception, or sex with either L.D. or her mother.

CASE 36. Informed Consent/Right to Health Care/*Roles and Norms: Clinical Authority*/ *Allocation of Resources*

This is one of several hospital admissions for a 47-year-old blind black male with a history of chronic schizophrenia and diabetes with a $2°$ neuropathy, retinopathy, and renal failure. The patient has a history of drug and alcohol use. He lives by himself in a welfare hotel. He was admitted to orthopedics for treatment of a foot ulcer and osteomyelitis which would probably eventually need amputation. On admission he was found to have markedly reduced renal function and was in a state of metabolic acidosis. A renal consult was called, and suggested that he should be treated with dialysis. The patient refused dialysis even when told that he would die without it. (He also refused to have blood taken, threw things around, and refused to leave the hospital.) A psychiatrist saw the patient and felt that although he was schizophrenic, his decision had been made rationally.

On 9/6 the patient's attitude toward dialysis changed and so he was transferred to medicine for management of his acidosis and the dialysis. As his acidosis was managed his renal function improved so that the renal consult no longer felt that dialysis was necessary.

On 9/13 the patient was transferred back to orthopedics for debridement of his osteomyelitis. The debridement was performed without any complications and the patient stayed on the orthopedic service. They failed to manage his acidosis, and his renal failure became more severe. The patient was not following the prescribed diet and was becoming more fluid overloaded. His mental status also seemed to have worsened as manifested by his eating habits and refusal of meds and phlebotomy. He still desired dialysis but the renal team, after consulting with their attending, felt that he was not a candidate for chronic dialysis and therefore it was useless to dialyze him acutely. The renal group believed he could not comply (follow diet and get to and from hospital). There was also no family support and there were a limited number of machines. The patient's mental status declined further with periods of somnolence and extreme agitation. Furthermore his renal failure continued to progress. The patient's mental status declined further after the following days. He became hostile and somewhat violent and it was felt he could no longer be managed on a medical floor; therefore, on 9/28 he was transferred to psychiatry, where he was treated with thorazine. During this phase of his illness, the patient wished very strongly to have dialysis, but the decision by the renal group remained unchanged. While on psychiatry the patient remained agitated and on at least one occasion pulled out his urethral catheter. His condition was stable by 10/2, and so he was transferred back to medicine for better management of his renal failure. The impression of the intern and psychiatrist at this time was that the patient was well medicated on his increased doses of thorazine and that he would be cooperative if dialysis was offered to him. The attending, social worker, medical attending, and psychiatrist intervened and convinced the renal group that they could provide enough ancillary support for him—that the patient should get dialysis, and so a fistula was created. Currently he is awaiting hemodialysis and is presently on diuretics. Also the patient informed orthopedists that he would not consent to the amputation if required.

CASE 37. *Informed Consent* / Roles and Norms: Clinical Authority, Doctors' Roles / *Professional-Patient Communication* / Professional Accountability

A 75-year-old man was admitted to a rehabilitation institute for therapy consequent upon amputation of his left leg above the knee. The patient had made excellent progress, setting a near record for recovery (6 weeks).

Approximately 8 weeks earlier, the patient had been examined by internists for abdominal aneurysm which had been noted as enlarged since his last full examination a year before, at age 73. Although surgery had not been recommended upon its initial discovery, its growth during the subsequent 2 years led two consultants to recommend surgery. The patient collaborated with this internist and consented to surgery. Although the operation was a success, the patient threw a clot to the lower left leg. Irreversible gangrene developed, and an above-the-knee amputation was performed. The decision to amputate was made by the patient upon recommendation of the physicians. The patient then informed his family in a meeting with the physician present. The patient is a determined, optimistic individual who worked until the Friday before his hospital admission and who intends to travel and do some work after a vacation with his younger son. He has a wife (they celebrated their fiftieth wedding anniversary a year earlier) and two sons, ages 42 and 46.

When discussing the "good luck" of developing a blood clot and his relationship to his physician, whom he called a "great guy, a really nice person," the patient indicated annoyance at recounting the events leading up to the amputation. He then stated with well-controlled but visible anger that this was a black mark in his life, that the physician had never mentioned that there was any risk of blood clots and complications as he experienced, and that if this had been mentioned he never would have consented to this operation. From earlier remarks it was clear that the patient had been informed that despite his age this was a good time to operate, given his good physical condition and continued vigorous work life. Apparently, his physician had suggested that there would be possible complications later in life which would not pose a problem if they operated at this time. This resentment at being misinformed, as explicitly stated, was labeled by him as a black mark in an otherwise successful and happy life. He stated that he preferred not to speak about it again.

One of the patient's sons is a lawyer. It is clear from the way in which the patient stated that "information" had not been discussed with him when he was making this decision, and that if it had been, he would not have made the same decision, that he had discussed this with his son. Despite this he maintains a relationship with the same internist, and thinks highly of his medical skill and character.

CASE 38. Informed Consent/Paternalism/*Roles and Norms: Clinical Authority, Doctors' Roles*/Professional Accountability/*Aggressiveness of Patient Care*

R.S. was an adopted boy, 2 years of age, who was brought to the hospital for first admission at 1½ months with large body masses diagnosed upon examination as large liver and spleen. Further examination was postponed to allow for a period of growth and development. The mother returned in August with the child at age 4 months. Tentative diagnosis of polycystic kidney disease was made, based upon abnormal IVP, although this was not supported by other clinical evidence; e.g., there was not hypertension and other systems were normal. The prognosis for polycystic disease is inevitably very poor. The parents were advised about the tentative nature of the diagnosis, but for over one month they prepared for a poor diagnosis. In October, results of an angiogram supported a firm diagnosis of bilateral Wilms tumor, with a prognosis of 90 percent chance of cure.

Chemotherapy was initiated and resulted in a significant reduction of the mass, although the left kidney could not be saved. How much of the right kidney would have to be removed by the surgeons was unknown. No further improvement was expected without surgical intervention to remove the remaining tumor. The boy would then receive chemotherapy follow-up treatment for two years. If enough of the right kidney could be saved, the boy would not need any dialysis. If not, this would be the youngest patient on dialysis at the hospital. The parents did not want any possibility of dialysis.

The parents' injunction against dialysis placed two constraints on the surgeons. Concerning the outcome, the right kidney was to remain regardless of the extent of tumor involvement. Regarding operating method, it meant the surgeons could not use the preferred method of clamping of the vessels leading to the kidney before removing the tumor. This procedure usually requires the patient to go on dialysis for a period following the operation until kidney function returns, approximately one month. There was no guarantee that kidney function would return, but the procedure might permit the surgeons to remove more tumor.

The surgeons initially agreed to operate on these terms, but there was the feeling that if complications developed, the clamping procedure should be used despite the parents' preference. Also, it remained the possibility that the entire right kidney would have to be removed.

The parents were a middle-class couple with a five-year-old normal boy. They had a friend on dialysis as well as other friends who had suffered from amputation. They had spent many hours with the pediatricians reviewing all aspects of the case. The surgeons had virtually refused to operate but were persuaded to cooperate. The pediatrician described the parents as very concerned with R.S.'s future quality of life and would not permit the possibility of a life on dialysis.

The operation was postponed one week because of an apparent lung infection diagnosed as probable pneumonia, and antibiotics were started. There was the possibility, however, that this could have been a metastasized lung tumor. An episode of respiratory distress in early January led to R.S. being trached and placed on a respirator. Therefore, the surgeons preferred to wait for any infection to clear, but the pediatricians preferred operating as soon as possible. R.S. was operated on at the beginning of February, wtih some remaining lung problem still believed to be pneumonia. The operation was successful, leaving a functioning right kidney. During the next month the pneumonia cleared, revealing two lesions on the lungs, indicating metastatic spread. The parents then refused any further chemotherapy, since physicians could not guarantee a significantly improved survival rate. R.S. is now under the care of a pediatrician.

CASE 39. Confidentiality/Concept of a Profession/Rights/Roles and Norms: Doctors' Roles, Patients' Roles/*Reproductive Technologies*

Mary and Bruce were not married, though they lived together. They had decided to have a child now and were concerned that Mary had not become pregnant earlier, as she had never used any contraception before. They went to her obstetrician-gynecologist requesting an infertility work-up for Mary. The physician said he would do this only after a sperm count on Bruce was obtained. Though it took some convincing, Bruce finally agreed.

The test showed Bruce to have an extremely low sperm count. He was very distressed by the information and refused to believe it, claiming that there must have been some mistake. A week after the results were given to them, Mary came to the physician and asked him to artificially inseminate her with donor sperm and requested that he keep this confidential as she intended to let Bruce believe it was his child. She pleaded with the physician, stating that her relationship with Bruce would end if Bruce was unable to impregnate her.

CASE 40. Informed Consent/*Paternalism*/Right to Health Care/Roles and Norms: Doctors' Roles/Institutional Responsibility/Reproductive Technologies

Neil White came in for his appointment at the urology clinic of a large city hospital. He stated that he wanted a vasectomy (sterilization by surgical interruption of part of the spermatic ducts). The urologist, Dr. Baker, looked at his record and saw that Neil was 24 years of age, single, and childless. Dr. Baker turned to Neil and said, "I wouldn't touch you with a ten-foot pole. There are no benefits you could get from such surgery. You are too young and you have never had children. Come back in ten years and I will reconsider."

Neil said there *were* considerable benefits he could derive from a vasectomy. First, he wanted no children. Parenthood, he felt, was an unparalleled lifelong commitment. It was definitely not a life he wanted. He had held this view for several years. Second, "The purpose of contraception," he said, "is to prevent pregnancy until the day one wants children. Contraception in its current mechanical and chemical forms is fraught with danger and anxiety—especially for some. I know that a woman can easily get infections; the Pill has known and probably unknown risks; and abortions are nasty business. I can't justify imposing these risks on any woman I care for. Stopping all of this would have profound benefits for me."

Dr. Baker was impressed by Neil's remarks. The young man seemed to know what he wanted and was intelligent. Nonetheless Dr. Baker still felt that Neil was too young to make such an irreversible decision. Though some research has been successful, vasectomy is still considered irreversible. "You aren't married," Dr. Baker replied, "and you don't know what your future wife or mate might want. I will not perform the operation at this point of your life." At this point Dr. Baker informed Mr. White of the hospital rule that childless candidates for sterilization must have an interview with a hospital psychiatrist.

Although Neil could not afford surgery at any other hospital, he refused to talk with a hospital psychiatrist. He resented any suggestion that his thinking was irrational or immature.

CASE 41. Active and Passive Euthanasia / Rights / *Sanctity of Life / Roles and Norms: Clinical Authority, Doctors' Roles* / Professional Accountability / Aggressiveness of Patient Care

A 71-year-old man had always been in vigorous and excellent health. He had last seen a physician 15 years before and was told he had high blood pressure. On the night of admission to the hospital, while watching television with his wife, he suddenly fell forward unconscious.

He was brought to the emergency room in deep coma, and was noted to have shallow respirations, and was consequently intubated, placed on a respirator, and admitted to the medical service.

On admission to hospital, he was in deep coma, and had no corneal reflexes, or doll's eyes. His breathing was supported by a respirator and when it was removed momentarily, he was apneic. Blood pressure was 300/230. His blood pressure was rapidly controlled by the use of parenteral antihypertensive agents, and two hours later his clinical condition had not changed.

No further laboratory studies were performed.

He was seen in consultation by a neurologist, who believed he had sustained a large intracerebral bleed, and that neurologic function was absent. The neurologist suggested a "stress test" of removing the patient from the respirator in order to determine whether he would survive. The intern did this and asked the nurse to "wait here until he dies."

Following death, the intern and students practiced endotracheal intubation and subclavian punctures on the body.

The following morning, during sedate social service rounds, the conference room erupted. The nurses were angry and emotionally overwrought about the events of the previous night concerning this patient.

The two medical students became very upset and one of them began to cry. When asked why he was crying, he replied that he was upset with his actions in practicing on the dead body, but he was even more deeply concerned that he hadn't paused to reflect on the appropriateness of his action at the time. He was crying, he said, because he felt that the attitudes inculcated in medical school had now allowed him to do things unreflectingly that he would have hesitated to do in the past.

The intern said he refused to discuss the matter in the context of social service rounds, and he argued that the nurses were questioning an appropriate medical decision, and he didn't feel compelled to defend medical decisions in front of nurses. He said that he and the neurologist agreed on a course of action. He said that the patient was old, and had not followed previous medical advice to have his high blood pressure treated.

The resident and the other intern volunteered that when they were medical students they always practiced techniques on dead patients, and they saw nothing wrong in continuing this procedure. They asked, wasn't it better to perfect techniques on the dead so that the next living patient might be saved?

The attending physician became angry, particularly toward the first intern, who refused to discuss the case. The attending suggested that the diagnosis of intracerebral hemorrhage had not been verified, that a differential diagnosis existed, and that the intern had acted precipitously and perhaps negligently.

CASE 42. Informed Consent/Paternalism/*Aggressiveness of Patient Care*

David Doe, age 67, was admitted to the hospital because of intermittent confusion. For 15 years prior to admission, he had had chronic bronchitis with emphysema. He used a portable oxygen tank at all times. Four months prior to admission a spot was seen on his chest x-ray. (The x-ray showed a coin lesion.) His physician suspected cancer. Because of the high risk of respiratory failure in Mr. Doe, no attempt was made to obtain a sample of tissue from the area of the spot. (Bronchoscopy was not performed.) This procedure would have been useful for establishing a definite diagnosis. On subsequent x-rays the spot enlarged rapidly. This sequence indicated that the problem was indeed a cancer. There is no effective treatment for lung cancer except surgery; because of his emphysema Mr. Doe could not have survived surgery.

Examination revealed that Mr. Doe was quite confused and intermittently sleepy. A scan of the brain showed that the cancer had spread to several areas there. Over the first 21 hospital days he developed severe headache and became stuporous. On the twenty-second day he developed a fever. A new chest x-ray showed a white area which had not been present previously, indicating pneumonia. Antibiotics would have offered a reasonably good chance of curing the pneumonia. Mr. Doe's physician decided not to use antibiotics and informed the patient's family of his decision. Mr. Doe continued to have a fever and continued to have a headache until his death on the twenty-fourth day.

Source: Reprinted with permission of Dr. Gordon Mosser, Share-Health Plan, St. Paul, Minnesota.

CASE 43. Informed Consent/Sanctity of Life/*Abortion*/Genetic Counseling and Screening

Mrs. Polly Peters, age 34, consulted her gynecologist because she suspected that she was pregnant. She had noted breast tenderness and frequent urination. A pregnancy test was positive.

Mrs. Peters had previously delivered five children. The youngest three of these had cystic fibrosis, a hereditary disease resulting in recurrent pneumonia and bronchitis, usually causing death by age 20. After the birth of their fifth child, Mrs. Peters and her husband had begun practicing birth control to avoid conceiving another child who might have cystic fibrosis. Mrs. Peters was unable to use birth control pills safely because of her history of blood clotting in her leg veins, a problem whose recurrence would have been made more likely by taking the pills. She chose to use an intrauterine device.

Nevertheless she had become pregnant. The intrauterine device was safely removed. She was advised that she stood an increased risk of suffering a miscarriage because the pregnancy had begun in the presence of an intrauterine device. The possibility of her producing another child with cystic fibrosis was discussed with her.

Because of their moral convictions, Mr. and Mrs. Peters decided that they did not wish to have an abortion performed. Mrs. Peters finished a normal pregnancy and delivered a boy with cystic fibrosis.

Shortly after the birth, the couple decided that Mrs. Peters should be sterilized. Surgical sterilization was carried out soon after.

Source: Reprinted with permission of Dr. Gordon Mosser, Share-Health Plan, St. Paul, Minnesota.

CASE 44. Informed Consent / Paternalism / *Rights* / Ideals and Models of the Physician-Patient Relationship / *Refusal of Treatment* / Aggressiveness of Patient Care

Axel Anderson, age 62, was admitted to the hospital because of anemia caused by iron deficiency. A recent test had shown occult blood in his feces. He had become deficient in iron by losing small amounts of blood into his bowel.

Physical examination was essentially normal except for the findings of mild chronic bronchitis with emphysema. Routine chemical tests revealed mild impairment of liver function, probably caused by alcohol. A barium enema examination of the large intestine revealed an "apple-core" defect, the characteristic x-ray finding of a colon cancer. The cause of the blood loss was thus explained.

Mr. Andersen's physician advised surgical exploration of the abdomen and removal of the probable cancer. Mr. Andersen refused. When asked why he did not want the surgery, he acknowledged that he understood he very likely had a cancer and that it might be small, confined to a small area, and curable by surgery. He would elaborate no further. He remained willing to discuss the issue, unwilling to undergo surgery, and unable (or unwilling) to specify his reasons.

The physician saw Mr. Andersen several times in his office for the purpose of discussing the cancer problem and trying to persuade him to undergo the surgery. After a time, however, he decided that he was only pestering Mr. Andersen. He began to see him only infrequently for the purpose of assessing the anemia and providing transfusions when needed.

Source: Reprinted with permission of Dr. Gordon Mosser, Share-Health Plan, St. Paul, Minnesota.

CASE 45. *Paternalism* / Ideals and Models of the Physician-Patient Relationship / Roles and Norms: Clinical Authority, Doctors' Roles, Patients' Roles / Professional Accountability / *Placebos*

Michael Marks, age 55, was admitted to the hospital because of shortness of breath. For 15 years he had suffered from chronic bronchitis with emphysema, complicated by intermittent brief lung infections. He also suffered from chronic pain in his shoulder muscles. This pain had been thoroughly investigated on a previous hospital admission; no cause was found.

Mr. Marks was admitted to the intensive care unit because of his precarious respiratory function. He did not require the use of a respirator. He repeatedly and loudly called out to the nurses, disturbing other patients, asking for codeine injections by name. His physician was reluctant to give him narcotics because of his respiratory status. Narcotics suppress the brain's respiratory drive center. Instead he ordered injections of salt water.

Mr. Marks received several injections at three-hourly intervals. He no longer complained of pain and slept apparently well.

Source: Reprinted with permission of Dr. Gordon Mosser, Share-Health Plan, St. Paul, Minnesota.

CASE 46. *Definition of Death* / The Concept of a Person / *Aggressiveness of Patient Care*

John Jones, age 64, was admitted to the hospital because of stupor. His landlady had found him in his boardinghouse room. He had been brought to the hospital by emergency ambulance.

On admission his blood pressure was severely elevated at 270/150 mm of mercury. Except for the depressed mental status, the physical examination was otherwise normal.

On treatment with diazoxide, a rapidly acting drug for blood pressure control, the pressure fell to 180/110 mm of mercury, still elevated but not in itself threatening a catastrophe. Within an hour Mr. Jones fell into a coma and ceased breathing. His respiration was maintained with a mechanical ventilator. A lumbar puncture was performed to obtain a sample of cerebrospinal fluid; it was bloody, indicating that he was bleeding somewhere in the brain. An electroencephalogram or brain wave test showed generalized poor function of the cerebrum, the outermost part of the brain. X-rays were taken of the two major arteries supplying blood to the brain in an attempt to identify the site of the bleeding. (In other words, Mr. Jones underwent bilateral carotid angiography.) The site of bleeding was shown to be deep within the brain and not amenable to surgical treatment.

On the fourth hospital day, Mr. Jones had no response to loud noises, pinching, or any other external stimuli. He had no spontaneous movement. Neurological testing indicated that his brainstem was not functioning. (His brainstem reflexes were absent.) He did not breathe without assistance from the respirator. His electroencephalogram was flat, indicating no detectable function of the brain. Twenty-four hours later these findings were unchanged. He was pronounced dead, and then the respirator was turned off.

Source: Reprinted with permission of Dr. Gordon Mosser, Share-Health Plan, St. Paul, Minnesota.

CASE 47. *Informed Consent*/Paternalism/*Confidentiality*/Rights/Ideals and Models of the Physician-Paitent Relationship/Roles and Norms: **Clinical Authority, Doctors' Roles/Professional-Patient Communication**

An obstetrician/gynecologist has been caring for a 41-year-old Catholic woman for approximately 15 years. He has delivered all her children and feels quite familiar with both the woman and her husband, who has been present for all the births. The couple has been married for about 18 years.

One day, the husband calls the physician and states that on a recent business trip to Honolulu he made a terrible "mistake." He does not know how he could have allowed it to happen, but he has learned that the woman he was with had gonorrhea and is currently being treated by a physician. He believes he has contracted it also. He is calling the gynecologist to ask him to check his wife for gonorrhea without her knowing and, if necessary, treat her.

The gynecologist is not sure what to do. He knows that Catholic law in addition to marriage law explicitly prohibits adultery. He decides that the marriage is a good one and should not be unnecessarily destroyed by one fling. The woman had coincidentally just come in about two weeks before for a check-up and a pap test. The gynecologist takes advantage of this and calls up the woman. "You know your pap smear—well everything is OK. There is no cancer. But you know that infection you had last year? Well, the smear indicates it has returned. It could wait until your next visit in 6 months, but you know how I am. I think you should come in now." The woman visits the doctor; he examines her and, without her knowing, does a culture to test for gonorrhea. He sends it off to the Board of Health, as he is rerequired to do (without any identification). He then tells the woman that instead of treating the infection locally, as he did in the past, he would like to get rid of it once and for all, and he gives her appropriate antibiotic therapy.

CASE 48. Informed Consent/*Paternalism*/Ideals and Models of the Physician-Patient Relationship/Abortion/*Genetic Counseling and Screening*

A sixteen-year-old girl is one of two sisters whose two brothers have Duchenne's muscular dystrophy, an X-linked disorder which is a progressive, degenerative muscle disease. The patients are incapacitated and confined to a wheelchair, usually between 9 and 12 years. Respiratory difficulties appear in the late teenage years, and death occurs by early adulthood.

Both girls were evaluated for carrier status. The results of muscle function studies were equivocal and the patient was told to proceed as if she were a carrier. It was clear that this girl did not understand the full implications of the diagnosis. She had limited intelligence. The family was on welfare and the parents had little education. Her mother also had limited intelligence, and the father was not seen. The patient and her sister were scheduled to return for additional counseling. They did not show up.

A few months later the patient was seen on a home visit by a social worker associated with the neuromuscular clinic, and it was discovered that she was pregnant, and that she did not intend to live with the father. She returned at this time, with her sister, for further counseling, and it was again evident that she had an unrealistic concept of the severity of the disease and its implications.

At the time of this counseling session she was approximately 20 weeks past the last menstrual period, and with her mother's signed permission an amniocentesis was performed immediately. Prior to amniocentesis she had indicated that she was undecided about what to do in the event that the fetus was a male. Results of the amniocentesis indicated that she was carrying a male child. She refused termination of the pregnancy and refused any further personal contact. Her mother throughout assumed a passive role and overtly "went along."

CASE 49. Informed Consent/Ideals and Models of the Physician-Patient Relationship/ *Experimentation*

A ten-month-old black female was admitted to the hospital for evaluation of a neurological disorder characterized by cortical blindness, severe mental and motor retardation, macrocephaly, and spastic quadriparesis. The mother noted that at the age of three months the child did not respond as her older children had at that age. The child was quite limp, her eyes had unusual dancing movements, and it was thought from very early age that she was unable to see. Past history, including pregnancy, labor, and delivery, was totally unremarkable.

Examination at time of admission revealed a well-nourished markedly retarded infant. Her head circumference was 51 cm. There were widely separated fontanelles, blindness, unusual nystagmoid eye movements, increased tendon reflexes, and increased muscle tone.

All routine laboratory studies were within normal limits. Diagnostic x-ray studies (angiogram and ventriculogram) revealed increased ventricular size, small posterior fossa, and aqueductal stenosis. It was determined that the infant should undergo a ventriculoperitoneal shunt procedure in order to prevent progressive head enlargement. Prior to this surgery, which was successful, an experimental diagnostic study (indium cysternography) was performed on the infant for the purpose of assessing the prognosis of early shunt surgery for the prevention of progressive hydrocephalus in children.

Source: Reprinted with permission from the Program on Human Values and Ethics, University of Tennessee, Center for the Health Sciences, Memphis, Tenn.

CASE 50. Informed Consent/Paternalism/*Roles and Norms: Doctors' Roles/Professional-Patient Communication*/Aggressiveness of Patient Care

Dr. Anderson, Chief Resident of Geriatrics at University Hospital, was taking Mark Gold, a third-year medical student, with him to see Mrs. Rothko, a patient with a variety of medical problems including a weak heart and high blood pressure. When they walked into her private room Dr. Anderson said, "Good morning, Mrs. Rothko! This is a junior colleague of mine, Mark Gold; he'll be drawing some bloods from you today. After administering a brief physical exam, Dr. Anderson indicated Mark should draw the bloods. It took Mark five attempts before he successfully drew blood, resulting in significant discomfort to the patient. During these attempts the patient said "Doctor . . . ," trying to get Mark's attention, "Doctor, is everything all right?" Mark stammered, and Dr. Anderson interceded, "Yes, yes, this frequently happens."

Mrs. Rothko had had five cardiac arrests since her arrival at University Hospital and had stabilized moderately quickly after each. It was Dr. Anderson's opinion that she would not improve sufficiently, and he had ordered the house staff not to resuscitate her again. The hospital had been unsuccessful in contacting her family, who lived in another state, though they were still trying.

Just before Mark and Dr. Anderson left the room, Mrs. Rothko asked Dr. Anderson how she was doing. "You're coming along fine; don't you worry," he said comfortingly. When they left the room, Dr. Anderson explained to Mark that in light of her poor prognosis he didn't want to upset her and so make her inevitably more anxious. While Mark had some sympathy for this reasoning, he still felt the patient should be told more, though he was confused as to whether he ought to take the initiative himself.

A week later Mrs. Rothko suffered a cardiac arrest, was not resuscitated, and died. Her family had finally been contacted only hours before; they would arrive at the hospital any minute. Dr. Anderson told Mark that he was too busy to meet the family and told Mark he would have to explain the events himself. As Dr. Anderson rushed down a corridor to answer a page, Mark felt paralyzed; he had no idea how to inform the family.

CASE 51. Informed Consent/Paternalism/Rights/*Refusal of Treatment/Aggressiveness of Patient Care*

A 35-year-old Puerto Rican male was found on the street unconscious and was brought to the emergency room at a large hospital. He was believed to be an alcoholic suffering from withdrawal symptoms. Tests revealed he had a severe case of pneumonia. He was febrile, and the pneumonia was becoming more severe.

When he was approached for consent to treat the pneumonia, he made it clear he wanted no treatment whatsoever. His only family was a sister who could not be reached. The house staff questioned his competency and called in a psychiatrist. The psychiatric interview found him competent and aware of the severity of his illness.

No treatment was administered, and the patient experienced a rapid deterioration. When he became comatose, the house staff decided to treat him, but their efforts proved fruitless. The patient died within 30 hours after his admission to the hospital.

CASE 52. Roles and Norms: Doctors' Roles/Professional-Patient Communication/*Institutional Responsibility/Professional Accountability*

J.C. was born to a type B diabetic mother. At 10 hours of age the baby was noticed to have hypoglycemia as well as a feeding problem. These problems were resolved. Twenty days later he was transferred to the ICU where a cardiac catheterization was performed with a diagnosis of severe tetrology of Fallot. Four days later heart surgery was performed to relieve the baby's cyanosis. A shunt was inserted, though the baby was too small for total correction. When J.C. was returned to the ICU, the staff noticed that the left hand was blanched. This was caused by improper monitoring of an arterial catheter placed in a radial artery in order to monitor blood pressure and gases. J.C. was taken back to surgery to explore for a clot caused by the same catheter. The surgery was unsuccessful, and the chief resident had to partially amputate the second, third, fourth, and fifth fingertips. It is unclear whether J.C. will eventually have any use of the hand.

In addition, when the baby was prepped for surgery, a misunderstanding resulted in using iodine, instead of betadine. An interaction between the plastic taping on the surgical dressing and soap caused a chest burn which required skin grafting.

J.C.'s mother, a 20-year-old Catholic, visited the hospital infrequently and only after she was told the baby could not be discharged until she did so. The house staff wanted her to become used to handling and feeding the baby before discharging him. The father, who has not yet seen the baby, stated this was a ridiculous thing to have to do. The mother has canceled her last three appointments to see her assigned social worker. The baby's maternal grandfather and paternal grandmother are married and live with the mother and father, who are presently not married. The mother and the grandmother do not get along well. The grandmother, who has a history of seizures and is on phenobarbitol, visits the hospital, and on these occasions she is very vocal. She alternately accuses the hospital of malpractice and thanks them for saving the baby.

J.C. is being prepared for discharge.

CASE 53. Informed Consent/Confidentiality/Right to Health Care/Ideals and Models of the Physician-Patient Relationship/Roles and Norms: Patients' Roles/Abortion/ Genetic Counseling and Screening

Mrs. Roller was recently married and is having her first pregnancy. She went to her obstetrician when she was 6 weeks late with her menstruation. Upon having her pregnancy confirmed, she requested an abortion. She said her sister suffered from Down's syndrome and was currently in an institution. Her husband did not know about her sister, and Mrs. Roller wanted to keep it that way. She was terrified of the possibility of having a mongoloid child.

She was counseled, and amniocentesis was suggested in order to determine if the fetus was affected. The risks of this procedure were explained. Mrs. Roller felt the risks were high and reiterated her desire for an abortion, and further requested tubal ligation be performed at the same time. In addition, she asked that both procedures be kept secret from her husband.

CASE 54. *Confidentiality/Rights/Roles and Norms: Patients' Roles*

Mrs. O. was interviewed in the labor room by a nurse who was to fill in a chart on the wall containing the patient's name and the number of previous abortions and deliveries. Mrs. O. revealed that she had had three abortions prior to her present marriage and did not want her husband to know. Her husband was outside the labor room waiting to enter after the interview. If this information were put on the wall, the husband would surely see it. It is generally put there in order to provide the residents with immediate important information, should the need arise.

The nurse decided to put zeros on the form—meaning no abortions and no deliveries, and went out to explain to the residents what she had done.

CASE 55. *Informed Consent/Paternalism/Rights/Roles and Norms: Clinical Authority/ Refusal of Treatment*

A black 60-year-old female is married and has one daughter. She suffered from diabetes mellitus, which was under control. She also suffered from hypertension and was on medication for this. Recently, she pulled a corn off of her foot and subsequently developed an infection of the toe which spread quite rapidly to the knee. The patient was brought to the hospital, whereupon an amputation (probably around the ankle) was recommended. The patient refused the amputation, claiming that God gave her her foot and thus she placed her trust in God's wisdom regarding what happened to her foot.

The physician in charge spoke to her family in the hopes of having them change her mind. The family, on the contrary, agreed with the patient. A psychiatric consult was called in who found her "competent" but displaying a "primitive personality based on denial." Her affect was found to be strange, though no thought disorder was diagnosed.

The physician believes she will die without the amputation. The patient wants to go home, but she would die in a few weeks without antibiotics. She is not likely to take her medication at home, as she has systematically not taken her medication for hypertension in the past (she claimed it made her drunk), nor did she take her insulin regularly.

According to the house staff, she would rather be dead than have the amputation, though the staff comes in every day to try to convince her to have it. On these occasions, the patient either gives an anxious look and simply refuses, or else cites that a surgeon told her, when she first came into the hospital, that she would be dead in a day without the amputation and he was wrong; so the doctors are probably wrong now as well.

CASE 56. Informed Consent/Paternalism/*Roles and Norms: Clinical Authority*, Doctors' Roles/Professional-Patient Communication/*Placebos*

A female patient in her mid-fifties was admitted to a university hospital in preparation for surgery on a tumor in her cheek. She developed a fever and her chest x-rays were abnormal, though the house staff had difficulty diagnosing them; her liver function tests were also abnormal. She was transferred to medicine, where after two days her fever subsided. During this time arrangements were trying to be made by the Chest Service to perform a bronchoscopy, since no diagnosis could be made from the abnormal chest x-rays.

After two weeks there was still no diagnosis and the patient asked to leave the hospital. She was told that the surgery could not be performed because of the possibility of infection or tuberculosis and that she could not be sent to surgery until they could determine that she had neither. If she did have an infection, she was told she would be started on medication and after responding to the medication she could then have her surgery.

The hospital staff felt that if she could be kept in the hospital throughout the weekend, the Chest Service would be able to arrange the bronchoscopy. The patient made it clear she wanted to leave unless medication was started. The hospital staff decided to give her a placebo and tell her that the medication was started.

CASE 57. Informed Consent/Confidentiality/*Placebos/Experimentation*

This project, entitled *A Double Blind Comparison of Amitriptyline, Fluotracen, and Placebo in Hospitalized Depressed Patients* was submitted by the Director of Psychiatric Research, an experienced psychiatrist with extensive and well-recognized credentials in medical research. The investigators propose to test a new compound known as fluotracen with a reported activity as an antidepressant. Patients in the hospital because of depression would be evaluated for preexisting medical conditions that would preclude the use of the drugs and, if they met certain criteria, would then be enrolled in this study. Patients would be randomly assigned to receive either the new agent, a standard agent for the treatment of this disorder, or placebo. Patients who worsened on placebo would be removed from the trial and treated with the standard agent.

Subject Consent Form

Title of Protocol: A Comparison of Fluotracen, Amitriptyline, and Placebo in Hospitalized Depressed Patients

Co-Investigators: M. D.

I hereby agree to participate as a subject in the following project: A comparison of fluotracen, amitriptyline (ElavilR), and placebo in the treatment of depression.

I understand that the project will include the following experimental procedures: amitriptyline is a drug which has been approved for the treatment of depression. Fluotracen is considered experimental at the present time. The investigators have received approval from the Food and Drug Administration for this project. I understand that I will receive either fluotracen, amitriptyline, or placebo (an inactive substance).

I understand that the possible discomforts or risks are as follows: amitriptyline can cause dry mouth, blurred vision, constipation, or reduced blood pressure. Fluotracen can cause sleepiness, reduced blood pressure, and occasionally nausea. I understand that if I receive placebo there is the possibility that my depression may not improve. I understand that if my condition worsens while I am taking placebo I will be withdrawn from the study and treated in a standard manner.

I understand that the possible and desired benefits of this project are: if fluotracen does prove to be effective in the treatment of my condition, it may be a more desirable treatment than those currently available owing to a more rapid onset of action and a broader range of therapeutic effect.

I understand that the following alternative treatments are available: I could receive standard antidepressants (which include monoaminoxidase inhibitors) or electroconvulsive (shock) therapy.

The Institution will make available hospital facilities and professional attention at   Medical Center (or at an affiliated hospital should the research study have been conducted at the affiliated hospital) to a patient who may suffer physical injury resulting directly from the research. The expense for hospitalization and professional attention will be borne by the patient. Financial compensation from   Medical Center will not be provided.

I have been given the opportunity to ask further questions and know that I can do so during the course of the project. I understand that in comparison to the costs of medical care which I would normally bear, my participation in this study may: (a) greatly increase; (b) increase; (c) have no effect; (d) decrease; (e) greatly decrease my cost. (The researcher must circle one of the preceding.)

I am aware that I am under no obligation to participate in this project. I am also aware that I may withdraw my (ward's) participation at any time without prejudice to my medical treatment at   Medical Center.

I further understand that should I have any questions about my (ward's) treatment or any other matter relative to my (ward's) participation in this project, I may call the Office of Grants and Contracts at (212)   and I will be given an opportunity to discuss, in confidence, any questions with a member of the Human Subjects Review Committee. This is a committee which, as required by federal regulations and New York state law, is an independent committee composed of Medical Center physicians and staff as well as lay members of the community not affiliated with this institution. This committee has evaluated the potential risks and possible benefits of this study.

To the extent permitted by law, my participation in this study will be confidential.

Patient's Name _____ Date _____

          (Please Print)

Patient's Signature _____ Chart No. _____

Parent/Guardian's Name _____ /Signature _____

          (Please Print)

Witness _____ /Signature _____

Relationship of Witness to Patient _____

CASE 58. *Allocation of Resources*

It is a simple truth that in our system nearly all resources must be purchased. Receiving medical treatment for a serious disease requires the purchase of a physician's time; the use of expensive technological equipment; the consumption of drugs, bandages, and other medical supplies; possibly the rental of expensive facilities (hospital rooms, special care centers, etc.); and the purchase of the services of nearly 100 allied health professionals. We all know that regardless of programs in preventive medicine, serious illness and the need for these goods and services is independent of the person's ability to pay. But if these medical services are to be provided to those who are in need, someone must pay.

The first artificial kidney machine was built in 1940 by Dr. William J. Wolff in Holland. It was a crude prototype, and it was not until 1950 that operating prototypes based on Wolff's machine were constructed in the United States. They were extremely limited machines, and as late as 1960 no patient was able to use these machines longer than 6 months.

In January 1960 Dr. Belding Scribner and his colleagues at the University of Washington School of Medicine in Seattle developed a surgical procedure which made the repeated use of dialysis machines possible. He developed a semipermanent cannula apparatus. This began the era of chronic hemodialysis.

During the early period there were only a few centers for dialysis. In 1965 it was estimated that there were 58,788 deaths from kidney disease. The kidney centers attempted to use *psychosocial criteria* to decide which medically eligible patients would be admitted to the center. Even for those willing to pay there was not enough room.

In 1970, there were 3,100 persons on dialysis with almost 1,000 transplant patients out of an estimated suitable renal disease population of 7,500. Therefore, 3,000 persons died because of lack of facilities. The costs for dialysis, performed in a center, averaged $12,000, with individual costs as high as $66,000 per patient per year. The development of home-dialysis units in 1964 lowered costs further, although in-center training was required; training plus equipment averaged $12,000 with an annual cost of $3,000 to $5,000.

Despite the existence of insurance programs and wealthy donors, the costs of the expanding dialysis centers were beyond their income. At Seattle in 1970, the budget was $1,268,294, with an expected 10 percent or $230,000 deficit developed by indigent patients.

In 1969, a study by A.H. Katz and P.M. Proctor of 93 out of 120 centers reported that the mental status, prison record, employment record, poverty status, etc., were each used by most centers to exclude patients. Sixty-eight percent used "mental deficiency" and as many as 21 percent used poverty. Approximately 29 percent cited poor family environment and 17 percent required state residency. Most centers had admissions and selection committees.

In 1971, Ernie Crowfeather, a poor part-American Indian, died of end-stage renal disease.

Although nearly $100,000 in public funds had been expended to provide him with dialysis, his death helped focus national attention on the fact that a clearly identifiable group of people were losing their lives because of lack of funding for dialysis machines and centers. This issue was highlighted by a series of articles in *The New York Times* by Lawrence K. Altman, an NYU faculty member.

In 1972, Congress passed Public Law 92–603, which made end-stage renal patients "the first, and thus far only, victims of catastrophic illness singled out for special coverage of their treatment costs by the federal government." This law basically wrote a blank check to pay for dialysis and transplantation for renal disease for those who cannot pay. The estimated cost, based on known kidney disease patients and then current costs, was $35 to $75 million for the first year. The real cost for that year (1973–1974) was approximately $240 million.

With the availability of dialysis machines, the increasing longevity of chronic dialysis patients, and the utilization of dialysis for a variety of postoperative problems, the cost as of 1978 was estimated at *$1 billion.* The projections for 1984 were reaching *$3 billion.* The number of dialysis patients in 1978 was about 37,000 compared with the 6,000 to 7,000 patients in 1972. There are now 50,000 patients with an average age over 50.

Figures from the not-for-profit centers claim that in 1978 costs were averaging as low as $8,000 per patient compared with $24,000 in the profit-oriented proprietary centers. Recently the National Medical Care Corporation, a profit-based nationwide company which runs over 120 dialysis centers, has been able to earn a profit of $19 million/year on an average fee of $28,000/year, of which Medicare will pay 80 percent. The company claims that its profits are based upon efficiency. The not-for-profit university centers receive the same reimbursement rates.

It is reckoned that if one other group of terminal patients receives the same "blank check" benefits from the federal government, viz., coronary victims, the artificial heart program could cost as much as the entire current national budget for health care, i.e., *$213 billion.*

Source: Developed from R. Fox and J. Swazey, *The Courage to Fail*, University of Chicago Press, 1978; and "NMC Thrives Selling Dialysis," *Science*, vol. 208, April 25, 1980.

CASE 59. *Informed Consent (Competency)* / Paternalism / *Psychiatric Issues (Involuntary Commitment)*

Mrs. M.C., a 32-year-old, married housewife and mother of two children (aged 4 years and 2 months, respectively) was brought to the hospital in December of 1978 under an order (Form 1) for assessment at a psychiatric facility empowering the facility to hold the patient for a maximum of 120 hours. Her two-month-old baby had recently been admitted to hospital with a diagnosis of "failure to thrive." The pediatrician in charge of the child's care and the patient's husband suggested that Mrs. M.C.'s apparent preoccupation with concerns other than that of her household had contributed significantly to the infant's problems. The patient's husband stated that she spent a lot of time in front of the TV and was "getting messages of bringing world peace." Mrs. M.C. had had three previous hospital admissions in the last five years and was diagnosed as "schizo-affective reaction," "schizo-affective disorder," and "paranoid state," respectively.

On admission, the patient was angry for being brought into hospital against her will and stated that there was absolutely nothing wrong with her. She spoke of feeling well, and disclaimed hallucinations, thought insertion, and thought withdrawal. She disagreed with her husband and her physician that there was cause for concern about herself or the welfare of her children. She was accurately oriented in time, place, and person, and struck the examiner as being of average or slightly above average intelligence. The patient said little about "messages of world peace" as reported by her husband but enough to suggest that she did indeed suffer from a delusion of a grandiose kind involving her bringing peace to the world with the help of a TV announcer, whom she felt attracted to but did not know. She classified a bunch of keys, a pen knife, and a comb and labeled these as "personal objects." She gave brief concrete interpretations to two proverbs. It was deemed that she had very little insight into her illness which was diagnosed as being a paranoid state.

The patient had responded well to neuroleptics in the past and the intention was to treat her with thioridazine. However, she refused to take the medication, saying that she was a "conscientious objector" and she feared the "awful side effects."

It then became crucial in our dealing with this patient to determine whether or not she was mentally competent. She understood what we meant by a false belief and that we thought her belief about bringing world peace was false, yet she disagreed that it was in fact false. She understood too that our intentions in advising treatment for her were benevolent. She understood the potential side effects of the medication and that if she did not take the medication she would likely prolong her hospitalization, as she was an involuntary patient and would not be released until she was deemed no longer a danger to her baby. She understood that we were concerned about the care she had been giving her two-month-old child, but disagreed that such care had in fact been inadequate.

We decided that she was mentally competent.

In accordance with the Act, two other psychiatrists (one of whom was on the staff of the facility where the patient was detained) were consulted. Following notice to the patient and her husband, application was made to the Regional Review Board. The Board gave consent for treatment. The patient was started on fluphenazine decanoate by intramuscular injection and showed rapid improvement over the next four weeks when she was discharged. At that time the patient expressed herself as thinking that her previous ideas about bringing peace to the world were "silly." She has since been maintained on an injection of fluphenazine decanoate biweekly and is cooperating well with the treatment.

CASE 60. Rights/Abortion/*Reproductive Technologies*

Two women in their mid-twenties, Kay and Ono, contracted, albeit illegally, to be surrogate mothers for a couple who were unable to bear children. The arrangement was made surreptitiously through a lawyer. Kay and Ono wanted to write a book together and so needed to free themselves from their jobs for several months. They were artificially inseminated with sperm from the husband, and both were successfully impregnated. The terms of the contract were somewhat complex. The couple wanted a boy; if either Kay or Ono or both had boys, they would receive $30,000 to be divided between them. If they both had girls, the couple would take only one of the offspring, and Kay and Ono would receive only $15,000. Neither twins nor the possibility of dysfunction in the children were mentioned in the contract. Kay and Ono were to receive $5,000 up front and the cost of prenatal care. The remaining sum was to be paid once the child or children were delivered to the couple.

When Kay and Ono were four months pregnant they each had an amniocentesis to identify the sex of the fetuses. Kay was carrying a male and Ono a female; both were normal. Ono decided she did not want the child for herself and had an abortion, which was financed by the contracting couple.

Kay met with the couple weekly and they got along very nicely. Two days after Kay gave birth to her son, she informed the couple that she had changed her mind and now intended to keep the child.

CASE 61. Roles and Norms: Doctors' Roles/Professional-Patient Communication/*Abortion*/*Genetic Counseling and Screening*

Mr. and Mrs. Chu visited the Genetic Counseling Clinic at University Medical Center in the fall of 1977. The couple had been married for one year, and now Mrs. Chu was pregnant. Because she was 38 years old, they were concerned about the effects of maternal age on their child, and the Chinese-speaking couple decided to investigate the possibility of amniocentesis. When the couple met with the staff at the clinic, it was decided that it would be wise to have the procedure done, as a routine screening because of Mrs. Chu's advanced maternal age. Amniocentesis was performed during the fourth month of pregnancy, and an examination of the fetal karyotype revealed a positive test for Turner's syndrome.

Turner's syndrome is a disorder of phenotypic females who have only one instead of two X chromosomes. The genotype arises from nondysjunction of chromosomes, and it has an incidence of 1 in 25,000, with no correlation with maternal age. The syndrome is characterized by primary amenorrhea, sexual infantilism, short stature, gonadal dysgenesis, and multiple congenital abnormalities. Other findings include webbing of the neck, shieldlike chest, fishlike mouth, and deformed ears. Moreover, these patients often developed unexplained hypertension, renal and cardiac malformations, and keloid formations. Intelligence may be normal in those affected. Detection may occur at birth, or else at puberty when the secondary sexual characteristics do not develop as they should.

The disorder and its manifestations was explained to Mrs. Chu, who spoke some English. Following a family discussion, the couple returned to the medical center and told the staff that they would not terminate the pregnancy, although the findings were positive. Mr. Chu did not believe the diagnosis was completely accurate, and the couple did not want to let this child die if their next child would be more severely affected. It was obvious to the counselor that the couple did not understand what was involved; so she again explained the disorder, its effects, and its mode of transmission to the Chus. This time they appeared to understand, but stuck to their decision about going through with the pregnancy. At this time the staff felt comfortable with their decision, because it was evident that the couple wanted this child badly, and because they seemed to know what the disorder was all about.

Shortly thereafter, a young female obstetrical fellow learned of the Chu's decision, and she was very upset about it. The doctor approached the staff in the counseling clinic and told the counselors that these people needed to be recounseled, even if she had to do it herself. She felt very uncomfortable about the idea of this couple giving birth to an "abnormal" baby, and had the staff arrange another meeting with the family.

That week, the fellow in obstetrics, an obstetrical resident, the genetic counselor, Mrs. Chu, and a member of the staff who spoke Chinese all met together in the hospital. During this meeting the doctor described the syndrome to Mrs. Chu, but in addition presented her with many pictures of adults with cases of Turner's syndrome. The pictures portrayed patients who had the most extreme cases of the disease, with the worst congenital abnormalities possible, and none of them portrayed individuals with mild forms of the syndrome. In explaining the disorder to Mrs. Chu, the fellow used extremely descriptive terms in order to influence her decision. Furthermore, the doctor was quoted as saying the following to Mrs. Chu: "Remember, you are not in China now, this is America, a very sexual society" and "Do you know how you feel when you do not want to make love to someone, well this is how your daughter will feel for the rest of her life." Following the presentation, the genetic counselor was extremely upset over the amount of bigotry and prejudice which came out during the session, and had asked Mrs. Chu to call her at home that night so the two women could speak about what had happened during the meeting.

That evening, Mrs. Chu contacted the counselor. Although the counselor was very upset about the manner in which the doctor had described the disorder, and the prejudice and demeaning attitude of the fellow, Mrs. Chu was relatively calm. She said she was aware of what had been done, but maybe the cultural barrier prevented her from getting the same reaction to the doctor's behavior. In any event, she told the counselor that she now planned on getting an abortion, because now she knew what it was like to have a child with Turner's syndrome. She thanked the counselor for her help, and told her that she would stay in touch.

Mrs. Chu eventually had the abortion. Following the procedure, she contacted the counselor, who had learned that the fetus was born with a normal phenotype except for immature gonads, thus leaving an unconfirmed diagnosis based on appearance. The counselor asked Mrs. Chu how she was feeling. She responded by saying that she was feeling well but was upset that the medical staff did not let her see her daughter. Based on instructions from one of the doctors, the nurse in the operating room told Mrs. Chu that she could not see her baby. Mrs. Chu was told that "the fetus was born with a webbed neck and other severe abnormalities, and was too ugly to look at."

CASE 62. *Right to Health Care*/Roles and Norms: Patients' Roles/*Allocation of Resources*

A 4-year-old child fell from some playground equipment, sustaining a 2-cm superficial laceration to his eyebrow area which required five sutures. The child never lost consciousness, was alert and playful, and the remainder of his exam was entirely normal. The father, when given standard instructions for observing children carefully following head injuries, became very upset and insisted that x-rays and further tests be done to ensure that his child was all right. The emergency room doctor explained that no further tests were needed at this time. The father became irate, called the child's pediatrician, and threatened to sue if anything happened to the child after taking him home. The pediatrician elected to admit the child for observation, requesting skull and cervical spine x-rays. These were done as well as routine admission blood work. The bill for the uneventful admission was $800.

CASE 63. Informed Consent/*Institutional Responsibility*/*Allocation of Resources*

Toni D. is an 18-year-old black female who was born with amputations in her lower extremities and several fingers missing on both hands. She was admitted to a hospital rehabilitation program as a 17-year-old, for ambulation training with a new bilateral lower prosthesis. Her medical staff felt that she would not need to be an inpatient for long, but at the time of admission, no one was aware what profound effects her family life and eighteenth birthday would have on her ability to be discharged.

Besides her congenital amputations, Toni was born with a cleft palate, kyphoscoliosis, and numerous muscle deformities. She has spent most of her life in various hospitals and institutions, for surgery and rehabilitation training. Her outpatient clinic record is sporadic, with many missed appointments. She has a history of smoking marijuana and drinking. At the time of the present admission, she was not suffering from any acute medical problems.

Toni is single and, prior to admission, lived at home with her mother and an older sister in a four-room apartment on the seventeenth floor of their building. Neither she, her mother, nor the medical records made any mention of her father. Toni attends high school, and will most likely have to repeat part of eleventh grade because of poor school attendance. When questioned about what she would like to do following discharge, she responded by saying that she would like to hang out with her friends and smoke and drink, although she was hoping to find a summer job.

Toni has lived in hospitals and foster homes most of her life, and she has an extremely poor relationship with both her mother and sister. The staff psychologist described her as "an outgoing and talkative young woman who has the ability to relate warmly and with concern to others, but on the surface is impulsive and frequently verbally abusive to all." She gets along well with her roommates on the floor, but often relates to others by teasing. The nature of her disability, along with her history of familial rejection, results in her being very cautious and distrustful of others, and being very quick to fight for herself, often without good judgment. Toni refuses to cooperate with psychological testing, and the psychologist felt she "needed to benefit from a stable psychotherapeutic relationship and a consistent home environment following her discharge."

Hospital History and Chronology

3/16 Toni is admitted to the rehabilitation training with her new prosthesis.

3/18 Toni's mother, Mrs. D., meets with the social worker to complain about her housing, claiming that it is inadequate for her daughter since the elevators are frequently out of service, causing Toni to miss school. She makes it known that she does not want her daugher to come home to this housing, and the social worker registers the family in a program which helps find apartments for families in need. At this time, the doctors decide to grant Toni an extension of stay on the floor. Although some work is needed with the prosthesis, their major reason is that the mother refused to take Toni back home.

3/22 Toni celebrates her eighteenth birthday. She is no longer a minor, but the consequences of this do not seem important now.

4/3 Toni is cleared for discharge whenever transportation can be arranged with Medicaid.

4/8 Mrs. D. reaffirms her position of not wanting to care for her daughter. It is learned that both mother and daughter have lied about the elevator service in their building, and that at least one is always in service. Placement is now being actively sought for Toni.

4/9 Finding a home for Toni has become a grueling effort. Because of her age, she is too old for facilities for minors, and too young for agencies which place persons 21 years of age and older. The search is complicated by the nature of Toni's disability, and the fact that she

is being funded by Medicaid. Moreover, Toni's behavior on the floor has
become a major problem. She has begun
to try to sleep late in order to miss
therapy, she has begun leaving the hospital to go drinking, and she has become abusive to the staff.

4/21 An adult foster home agency accepts
Toni, but she refuses them, claiming
that the "group home" is not good
enough for her. Toni says that she
wants to stay in the hospital until she
can go home with her mother.

4/22 Mrs. D.'s open rejection of her daughter
is evident. The social worker has asked
the hospital administration to check
on the nature of the mother's legal responsibility in the affair, since it was
she who signed her daughter in "until
discharge" when she was a 17-year-old
minor.

4/25 The hospital administrators inform the
staff that since Toni is no longer a
minor, her mother is not legally responsible for her. At this time, the mother
refuses to allow Toni to return home,
and Toni refuses to move into a temporary placement facility. She is taking
up a needed bed in the hospital, and
staff resentment is increasing; they
joke about getting handcuffs for Toni,
as she is caught getting high in her
room. The housing search continues.

4/29 At a reevaluation conference about
Toni, the staff discussion did not center
on the therapy or medical aspects of
her case, but on how to discharge her.
Temporary housing is being sought
and the family is on a priority waiting
list, but the patient's behavior and
compliance are increasing problems.
Because Toni is an 18-year-old adult,
she is allowed "self-determination"
and can refuse to be placed in any situation which she does not like, and
she is rejecting agencies which will take
her on. In addition, she expresses ambivalence between returning home to
her mother and her self-independence,
while her feelings of rejection and
abandonment are being demonstrated
by her acting out and abusiveness toward the staff. To make matters worse,
the mother has had a representative
from the local political party pressure
the social worker, warning her not to
try to kick the young woman out on
the street by throwing her out of the
hospital with no place to go.

4/30 Arrangements are tentatively set to
transfer Toni to a local hospital. The
doctors are going to "close down her
files" and get her off their hands. A
general feeling of relief prevails with
the staff.

CASE 64. Informed Consent/*Paternalism*/Professional-Patient Communication/*Refusal of Treatment*

Johnny Cross is a seventy-year-old Bowery bum who occasionally resides at a men's shelter. He is an alcoholic who smokes heavily, has no family, and confesses to having no friends.
He was admitted to a city hospital with a bladder infection which caused him considerable
pain.

His physician, who has treated many old derelicts on the Bowery, was concerned that Mr.
Cross would not take his medication—antibiotics—if he were released. He had been informed
on several occasions that patients of his had been found dead in their rooms with untouched
bottles of medication at their bedside.

The physician decided not to let Mr. Cross leave with his medication as a "normal" patient,
and instead informed Mr. Cross that he would have to stay in the hospital a few days. Mr.
Cross was given heavy doses of antibiotics for three days in the hospital, recovered, and was
released.

During this period he suffered considerably from alcohol withdrawal, and sedatives had to be administered. Two days after his release a social worker reported to the physician at City Hospital that Mr. Cross was happily getting drunk on the Bowery.

CASE 65. *Informed Consent/*Rights*/Ideals and Models of the Physician-Patient Relationship/Roles and Norms: Doctors' Roles/*Allocation of Resources

During his internship, P.C. rotated onto a medical ward where he "inherited" the case of a 65-year-old female with a large, open sinus tract of the anterior abdominal wall which drained feculent material. A thorough perusal of the chart surprisingly failed to reveal an explanation for the lesion. Only by telephoning the private attending did P.C. learn that the patient had a large unresectable adenocarcinoma of the transverse colon at the base of the fistula with documented metastatic disease. She was very anemic, requiring periodic transfusions. Her mental functions were intact. At the time, her care consisted only of daily dressing changes and supportive nursing care. The husband was aware of the diagnosis, but the patient knew only that she had a large "sore" on her belly that stubbornly refused to heal. The husband and the attending physician had jointly decided on this course of action.

The intern, despite many discussions with the attending and husband, failed to convince them of the patient's right to know her diagnosis and prognosis. P.C. found it very difficult to make rounds on the patient, change her dressings, and ward off all her inquiries concerning various pains and the enlarging "sore."

One evening when P.C. was on call, the patient called him to her room and said pointedly, "Doctor, please tell me if I'm dying. This is cancer, isn't it?" P.C. found it impossible not to deal directly with the patient, and they had a long discussion about her disease, during which the woman decided that she wanted to leave the hospital to die at home. The intern arranged for home care with a nurse, and the patient was discharged the following week. The husband and the only other relatives (all over age 70) were extremely hostile to P.C. for telling the patient and for "saddling" them with the responsibility of caring for a dying loved one, even with a nurse's help. The attending seemed relieved at the patient's acceptance of her diagnosis.

CASE 66. *Informed Consent/Ideals and Models of the Physician-Patient Relationship/*Roles and Norms: Doctors' Roles*/Experimentation*

A 64-year-old female was being treated at a regional cancer research institute for adenocarcinoma of the colon. When the tumor was discovered, she underwent a colostomy and then a regimen of chemotherapy for disseminated disease at the time of surgery. She responded well to the chemotherapy for 6 months, but then failed to respond. Further tests showed additional involvement of the liver.

Because she was no longer responding to standard chemotherapy, the patient was now eligible for experimental drug treatment. Dr. Kahn was in the process of testing a new drug regimen. In his experimental design, he needed 21 subjects to receive the chemotherapy with significant toxicity (vomiting, nausea) and no positive benefits in order to determine with 95 percent confidence that the therapy would be effective in less than 20 percent of cancer patients with this form of cancer. Thus far, Dr. Kahn has had 19 patients participate in the drug trial, and none have shown positive benefits. He needs two more patients to complete the trial.

At the same research institute, Dr. Jenson has just received approval from the Institutional Review Board to begin a study of yet another experimental drug regimen. She is about to begin randomizing patients to her therapy.

Dr. Kahn and Dr. Jenson confer about which therapy to offer the patient.

CASE 67. Roles and Norms: Doctors' Roles, Patients' Roles/*Genetic Counseling and Screening/Reproductive Technologies*/Allocation of Resources

In the fall of 1975, Mr. and Mrs. Turner visited a genetic counseling clinic. The couple wished to learn more about the nature of Mr. Turner's illness, and to explore the possibility of artificial insemination for Mrs. Turner. Normally, issues such as these would be mundane for the clinic, but this September morning was unique; both Mr. and Mrs. Turner were disabled and wheelchair bound.

Mrs. Turner suffers from spastic, nonprogressive cerebral palsy, and experiences regurgitation after feeding due to a diaphragmatic hernia. An attractive woman in her twenties, she requires a part-time attendant and spends much of her time in a wheelchair. Mr. Turner, also in his twenties, suffers from progressive spinal muscular atrophy. Afflicted since childhood, he requires a full-time attendant and is unable to perform such activities as transferring or dressing himself. In addition, he has compromised pulmonary function and was given a prognosis of only 10 to 15 years' life expectancy.

The Turners visited the clinic to learn about the genetic component of Mr. Turner's disability, and to have spermatazoa studies done to see if he could serve as a donor for his wife. The couple hoped that there would be no genetic transmissibility which would pass any risk to the child. They were told that the genetic aspects of his disability were presently unknown. A sperm count was to be performed, but the couple was prepared to use the sperm of an anonymous donor if Mr. Turner's count was unacceptable.

During the interview with the counselor, the discussion did not focus on genetics but rather on the couple's ability to care for a child. When asked their reasons for wanting a baby, the Turners responded by saying that they love children and that "everybody has kids." Evidently they loved each other very much, but when questioned further it also became evident that their desire was not realistic. The couple had met in their housing project for the disabled, and had been married for only 9 months at this time. Neither was employed, and they described their daily lifestyle as "being centered around watching TV, since there was nothing else to do." They were supported by SSI and felt that they would be able to take care of a child if Mrs. Turner's attendant worked full time. With further discussion they admitted that they never spent any time with children, and it became obvious to the counselor that their desire to have a child stemmed from a wish to alleviate the boredom of their lives and to give some purpose to their existence. Further discussion centered around caring for children, genetic teaching and background, and a discussion of the risk of pregnancy to Mrs. Turner's health.

Two months later, the Turners again met with the staff at the clinic to discuss the results of the sperm studies and to find out about the possibility of artificial insemination for Mrs.

Turner. At this time, they learned that Mr. Turner's sperm count was low and abnormal; the staff found it likely that he was probably infertile and would be a poor sperm donor. In addition, several issues rose to the surface. The genetic counselor confronted Mr. Turner and asked him why he would want to bring a child into the world if it was likely that he might not live for more than 10 to 15 years. Despite failing lung capacity, increasing susceptibility to pneumonia, and his disability, he defended his wish to be a parent with emotional desires instead of rational reasoning. The couple was then asked if they thought they could possibly give adequate care to their child; they responded that it would be possible with the help of the attendants. They did not react to the thought that it might be exceedingly difficult for a child to be raised under such circumstances. Finally, the counselor told the Turners about a new problem which had developed.

The genetic counselor was unable to find a willing obstetrician who would perform the artificial insemination for Mrs. Turner. The doctors who had been contacted considered it to be "immoral and inhumane" to participate, stating that it would be "horrible to bring a child into a world with such a quality of life." The medical staff was not concerned with the possibility of genetic transmission from the husband's sperm; they based their decision on their feelings that this couple could not adequately raise a child. In addition, they cited the risk of worsening Mrs. Turner's hernia with a pregnancy and the fact that Medicaid would never consider reimbursing such a procedure. They felt that "no reliable or respectable doctor would do such a procedure." After informing the Turners of this news, the counselor said that she would continue to look for a doctor but that the Turners should carefully consider what they wanted to do in light of these developments.

Several weeks later Mr. and Mrs. Turner returned to the counseling clinic for the last time. The genetic counselor told the couple that they would have to approach the staff at the high-risk clinic at another hospital, because no one at this hospital would agree to do the procedure. The Turners again expressed a strong desire to have a child and said that they would look for an anonymous donor to supply the sperm for the insemination. After discussing the importance of reliable donor screening, the couple left the clinic, leaving the counselor hoping that they might become more realistic before going ahead with their plan.

CASE 68. Paternalism/Roles and Norms: Clinical Authority/*Refusal of Treatment/Allocation of Resources*

John Jonas, a fifty-five-year-old derelict, had been sitting outside for hours with no shoes on, in the dead of winter, while getting drunk. His feet were numb and white, and a colleague told him he was "frostbit." John walked two miles to the hospital emergency room. He was hospitalized, but still he developed gangrene from his extremely frostbitten feet. The attending physicians decided that they had to amputate or they would be putting John's life in danger. The patient refused the amputation, claiming he had to "keep his feet on."

The hospital went to court to have Mr. Jonas declared incompetent so that they could proceed with the amputation. The State Supreme Court ruled that Mr. Jonas was competent and could thus refuse the treatment.

Mr. Jonas spent 5 months in the hospital and lost two of his toes. The medical expenses totaled $35,000, for which Medicaid was billed. Typically huge bills of this sort are either partially paid and/or payment is subjected to a lengthy delay by Medicaid.

CASE 69. The Concept of a Profession/Ideals and Models of the Physician-Patient Relationship/*Psychiatric Issues*

Dr. Martin Bernard, a psychiatrist, was sued for malpractice by 20-year-old Catherine Morris, a former patient of his. Ms. Morris had been persuaded by her parents to submit to therapy for her sexual promiscuity and homosexual tendencies. She was under Dr. Bernard's care for 14 months. Concomitant with the discontinuance of her therapy her suit was filed. During the trial she claimed that her psychiatrist had "tricked" her into having repeated sexual intercourse with him. Dr. Bernard stated he never had claimed the sexual activity to be part of her therapy. While Ms. Morris admitted that sexual intercourse was never "stated" to be part of her therapy, she "believed" it was. Three witnesses, all female former patients of Dr. Bernard's, gave testimony strikingly similar to Ms. Morris'. It was further established that the sexual encounters took place in various hotel rooms in close proximity to Dr. Bernard's office.

In the course of the trial Ms. Morris "broke down" during cross examination and refused thereafter to submit to any further cross examination. The suit had to be dropped. In the period subsequent to the trial, Dr. Bernard's license to practice was renewed.

CASE 70. Institutional Responsibility/*Abortion/Allocation of Resources*

Marilyn Temple had missed two menstruations and was concerned that she was pregnant. She had come to the clinic for a pregnancy test—the same clinic where she had had four previous abortions. She had been dependent on Medicaid funding for all these abortions. Her physician called her in from the waiting room and told her the results were positive. He further explained that Medicaid no longer funded abortions unless the life of the mother were endangered or if the pregnancy was due to a rape. Marilyn was stunned; she said she could not come up with the fee ($175) and definitely did not want to carry her pregnancy to term. She explained she was learning a new job, which was just covering her living expenses, and was in a tentative position with her employer. The amount of time she would miss from work because of her pregnancy would simply place too much strain on her situation. The father was not available for assistance.

Her physician asked her why she had not been using any form of contraception as he had advised her to in the past. She said there were too many hazards and too much nuisance involved in contraception. She preferred not to use contraception and rather have abortions whenever she became pregnant. The physician asked her to come back in a month for a prenatal checkup; expenses deriving from these checkups, and the cost of delivering, he informed her, would be covered by Medicaid.

CASE 71. *Informed Consent*/Paternalism/*Ideals and Models of the Physician-Patient Relationship*/Roles and Norms: Doctors' Roles, Patients' Roles/Professional-Patient Communication

David Armstrong was nervous at this appointment with an orthopedic specialist. He is a forty-five-year-old stockbroker, who, during the last year, had developed a persistent pain in the bones of all his limbs. Nine months ago his family physician had diagnosed arthritis and placed him on a treatment of indomethacin, an antiarthritic drug. His pain increased and treatment was stopped.

Mr. Armstrong was a father of four and had managed to make a decent living for his family, though he was not able to save much. Two children were currently in college and two more were in the latter stages of high school. During the weeks his orthopedic specialists were performing tests, Mr. Armstrong had come upon a financial scheme that had some risks to it but could potentially give him "the big money I've been making for others all my life." He had decided to invest almost his entire savings on the project. It wouldn't pay off for possibly many years, but he had calculated his current income to be sufficient to carry his family through.

The orthopedic specialist met Mr. Armstrong with the results of the tests under his arm. Mr. Armstrong flashed through his mind the memory of his neighbor who had died from bone cancer. "Doctor, I have too much to be bothered by the intricacies of my health," he exclaimed. "You just do whatever it is that's best for me and stop the pain. I don't want to know the diagnosis . . . just treat me . . . I don't want to know." The specialist knew that "cancer" was the word Mr. Armstrong did not want to hear.

CASE 72. Ideals and Models of the Physician-Patient Relationship / Roles and Norms: Clinical Authority / Professional-Patient Communication / *Genetic Counseling and Screening*

Mrs. Schwartz, a 24-year-old Sephardic Jew, gave birth to a baby girl, Rachel. The baby was examined in the hospital nursery by a staff pediatrician and genetic counselor, and was diagnosed as having Down's syndrome. The father, a 28-year-old dentist, was informed of the diagnosis and immediately requested that his wife not be told until chromosome studies were completed. Mrs. Schwartz had still not seen her baby, and the pediatrician and genetics counselor encouraged him not to wait and to tell his wife as soon as possible. Reluctantly, he informed his wife's mother, who became visibly upset and exclaimed, "Who is going to marry our other granddaughter now?" (referring to Rachel's 3-year-old sister). Then, with assistance from the doctor and counselor, the mother was told of the diagnosis and its implications. Both Dr. and Mrs. Schwartz asserted that this was their baby and they would take her home.

The next morning, the genetics counselor met with the mother alone, who appeared to be much more talkative without the presence of her husband and parents. She reported that she and her husband now felt that they could not take the baby home. She cited the problems connected with the cultural milieu of their Sephardic community, and the effects this would have on their older daughter, on themselves, and on any future children. Furthermore, she said, her obstetrician had strongly advised them to place the baby immediately, claiming that it would be much easier to do this now than if the child were to go home for a while first, and that it would be wiser not to become attached to the baby at this point. The parents had refused to see the baby, and at this time it appeared that their way of reacting was to pretend that nothing had happened and to tell family and friends that the baby had died or was too seriously ill to bring home.

That afternoon, the genetics counselor spoke with the parents at length, with Dr. Schwartz doing most of the talking. He expressed a desire to "protect his wife and daughter." He told the counselor of their religious custom of having the younger daughter be maid of honor at the older sister's wedding, and his belief that this could not happen now. Furthermore, the parents mentioned that this would be a reflection on the family, and that they might not be able to supply the constant care that Rachel would require for life. They felt it was inevitable that Rachel would be placed.

The genetics counselor discussed Down's syndrome in detail with the parents, covering its cause, variability of conditions and implications, incidence and risk of recurrence, and the availability of amniocentesis for future pregnancies. She also stressed that any decision that they made was not irrevocable, binding, or permanent, and that perhaps they should defer a final decision until the initial shock had subsided. She assured the parents that their reactions were similar to those of other families. In addition, they spoke about the attitudes of other individuals who were encouraging them to place the baby immediately, including the obstetrician and the grandparents. Finally, they discussed the potential problems which might develop if the parents did not tell family and friends the truth, and how the burden of "keeping a secret" might in itself become a real problem. The father admitted that he had already been worried about telling people different stories by accident, and the counselor said that one problem would be their increasing anxiety over the truth becoming known.

The staff had arranged for Mrs. Schwartz to remain in the hospital longer than usual, and during this time the family had directed a social worker to find a placement for the baby. An agency placement was found, and the Schwartz couple began to tell their friends that "their daughter was born with a lung disease which would lead to death within a year, and that she had been placed in order to avoid the anguish which would someday come."

When Mrs. Schwartz left the hospital, the family was very grateful to the genetics counselor for her help and advice. However, in an opinion form about the genetic counseling service which Dr. Schwartz filled out several months later, he stated that he "felt harassed by the coercion" used by the counselor and the pediatrician in trying to influence his wife. This came as quite a shock to the counselor, who felt, if anything, that she had been the one telling the family that they did not have to make an immediate and permanent decision, in contrast to the obstetrician, who was advocating placement.

Fifteen months later, Mrs. Schwartz was again about to deliver a child at the hospital. She had had an amniocentesis at a different private hospital. Dr. Schwartz visited the genetics counselor who had been involved in Rachel's case, and explained why he had completed the evaluation questionnaire the way he did. He told the counselor that he found her to be coercive because she did not support the family's initial decision to place Rachel, while the obstetrician was not coercive because he had supported the family from the onset. Moreover, he told the counselor that he had visited Rachel and her family several times in order to check up on her welfare, but that this was done without his wife's knowledge in order to "protect her emotions."

CASE 73. The Concept of a Profession/Right to Health Care/*Roles and Norms:* Clinical Authority, *Doctors' Roles*

Mrs. Kent is an elderly woman married to a long-time shopkeeper. The two of them recently took membership in a Health Maintenance Organization. This health plan, her husband stressed, would keep their growing health care costs down. After her initial work-up by physicians at the HMO, results of a calcium test showed her to have a high-normal level. When she was informed of this, she requested that the test be repeated. The results again revealed a high-normal calcium level.

Though her physicians told her not to worry, that they would monitor her calcium levels periodically, Mrs. Kent wanted further tests conducted. A friend of hers, she explained, had cancer which manifested itself as hypercalcemia. She had been constipated and had had abdominal pain off and on for years. Her husband told the physician at the H.M.O. that she was often mentally confused.

Her physician knew that the costs for tests to locate or rule out a cancer at this stage would be very expensive, including, as it would, several days' stay in the hospital. He explained to Mrs. Kent that such testing would be premature. Mrs. Kent left exceedingly angry, exclaiming that her "usual physician would give me any tests I wanted."

CASE 74. Ideals and Models of the Physician-Patient Relationship / Roles and Norms: Doctors' Roles, Patients' Roles / *Abortion / Genetic Counseling and Screening*

A 29-year-old mother of three sons came to her obstetrician, who had delivered all her children, with symptoms of breast soreness, frequent urination, and two missed menstruations. A pregnancy test was performed, and the result was positive. Two weeks later, the woman returned to the obstetrician and requested an amniocentesis for gender identification. She explained that, although this pregnancy was planned, both she and her husband never wanted more than four children and wanted this child only if it were female. The obstetrician explained to her the risks of amniocentesis (approximately 1 percent chance of miscarriage or infection). As they talked, he questioned her decision to choose whether or not to have an abortion on the basis of the gender of the fetus. Although he was not generally opposed to abortion, he was not comfortable with the idea of "rejecting a child on the basis of sex." The woman argued that it was her husband's and her decision to make, and, since the risks were minimal, she still wanted the doctor to do the amniocentesis and, if the fetus were male, to perform the abortion.

Professional Codes and Statutes

1. Principles of Medical Ethics: American Medical Association
2. Code for Nurses: American Nurses Association
3. A Patient's Bill of Rights: American Hospital Association
4. Directive to Physicians: California Natural Death Act
5. Standards for Health Services in Prisons: American Medical Association
6. Policy for the Protection of Human Research Subjects: U.S. Department of Health and Human Services
7. A Bill to Provide that Human Life Shall be Deemed to Exist from Conception: 97th Congress, 1st Session, S.158
8. Constitution of the World Health Organization
9. The Nuremberg Code
10. Declaration of Helsinki: World Medical Association

1. PRINCIPLES OF MEDICAL ETHICS   American Medical Association

The medical profession has long subscribed to a body of ethical statements developed primarily for the benefit of the patient. As a member of this profession, a physician must recognize responsibility not only to patients, but also to society, to other health professionals, and to self. The following Principles adopted by the American Medical Association are not laws, but standards of conduct which define the essentials of honorable behavior for the physician.

I. A physician shall be dedicated to providing competent medical service with compassion and respect for human dignity.

II. A physician shall deal honestly with patients and colleagues, and strive to expose those physicians deficient in character or competence, or who engage in fraud or deception.

III. A physician shall respect the law and also recognize a responsibility to seek changes in these requirements which are contrary to the best interests of the patient.

IV. A physician shall respect the rights of patients, of colleagues, and of other health professionals, and shall safeguard patient confidences within the constraints of the law.

V. A physician shall continue to study, apply and advance scientific knowledge, make relevant information available to patients, colleagues, and the public, obtain consultation, and use the talents of other health professionals when indicated.

VI. A physician shall, in the provision of appropriate patient care, except in emergencies, be free to choose whom to serve, with whom to associate, and the environment in which to provide medical services.

VII. A physician shall recognize a responsibility to participate in activities contributing to an improved community.

Adopted by AMA House of Delegates at annual meeting, July 22, 1980.

2. CODE FOR NURSES   American Nurses Association

The Code for Nurses *is based on belief about the nature of individuals, nursing, health, and society. Recipients and providers of nursing services are viewed as individuals and groups who possess basic rights and responsibilities, and whose values and circumstances command respect at all times. Nursing encompasses the promotion and restoration of health, the prevention of illness, and the alleviation of suffering. The statements of the* Code *and their interpretation provide guidance for conduct and relationships in carrying out nursing responsibilities consistent with the ethical obligations of the profession and quality in nursing care.*

1. The nurse provides services with respect for human dignity and the uniqueness of the client unrestricted by considerations of social or economic status, personal attributes, or the nature of health problems.

2. The nurse safeguards the client's right to privacy by judiciously protecting information of a confidential nature.

3. The nurse acts to safeguard the client and the public when health care and safety are affected by the incompetent, unethical, or illegal practice of any person.

4. The nurse assumes responsibility and accountability for individual nursing judgments and actions.

5. The nurse maintains competence in nursing.

6. The nurse exercises informed judgment and uses individual competence and qualifications as criteria in seeking consultation, accepting responsibilities, and delegating nursing activities to others.

7. The nurse participates in activities that contribute to the ongoing development of the profession's body of knowledge.

8. The nurse participates in the profession's efforts to implement and improve standards of nursing.

9. The nurse participates in the profession's efforts to establish and maintain conditions of employment conducive to high-quality nursing care.

10. The nurse participates in the profession's effort to protect the public from misinformation and misrepresentation and to maintain the integrity of nursing.

11. The nurse collaborates with members of the health professions and other citizens in promoting community and national efforts to meet the health needs of the public.

Reprinted with permission. American Nurses Association, 1976.

3. A PATIENT'S BILL OF RIGHTS   American Hospital Association

The American Hospital Association Board of Trustees' Committee on Health Care for the Disadvantaged, which has been a consistent advocate on behalf of consumers of health care services, developed the Statement on a Patient's Bill of Rights, *which was approved by the AHA House of Delegates February 6, 1973. The statement was published in several forms, one of which was the S74 leaflet in the Association's S series.*

The American Hospital Association presents a Patient's Bill of Rights with the expectation that observance of these rights will contribute to more effective patient care and greater satisfaction for the patient, his physician, and the hospital organization. Further, the Association presents these rights in the expectation that they will be supported by the hospital on behalf of its patients, as an integral part of the healing process. It is recognized that a personal relationship between the physician and the patient is essential for the provision of proper medical care. The traditional physician-patient relationship takes on a new dimension when care is rendered within an organizational structure. Legal precedent has established that the institution itself also has a responsibility to the patient. It is in recognition of these factors that these rights are affirmed.

1. The patient has the right to considerate and respectful care.

2. The patient has the right to obtain from his physician complete current information concerning his diagnosis, treatment, and prognosis in terms the patient can be reasonably expected to understand. When it is not medically advisable to give such information to the patient, the information should be made available to an appropriate person in his behalf. He has the right to know, by name, the physician responsible for coordinating his care.

3. The patient has the right to receive from his physician information necessary to give informed consent prior to the start of any procedure and/or treatment. Except in emergencies, such information for informed consent should include but not necessarily be limited to the specific procedure and/or treatment, the medically significant risks involved, and the probable duration of incapacitation. Where medically significant alternatives for care or treatment exist, or when the patient requests information concerning medical alternatives, the patient has the right to such information. The patient also has the right to know the name of the person responsible for the procedures and/or treatment.

4. The patient has the right to refuse treatment to the extent permitted by law and to be informed of the medical consequences of his action.

5. The patient has the right to every consideration of his privacy concerning his own medical care program. Case discussion, consultation, examination, and treatment are confidential and should be conducted discreetly. Those not directly involved in his care must have the permission of the patient to be present.

6. The patient has the right to expect that all communications and records pertaining to his care should be treated as confidential.

7. The patient has the right to expect that within its capacity a hospital must make reasonable response to the request of a patient for services. The hospital must provide evaluation, service, and/or referral as indicated by the urgency of the case. When medically permissible, a patient may be transferred to another facility only after he has received complete information and explanation concerning the needs for and alternatives to such a transfer. The institution to which the patient is to be transferred

must first have accepted the patient for transfer.

8. The patient has the right to obtain information as to any relationship of his hospital to other health care and educational institutions insofar as his care is concerned. The patient has the right to obtain information as to the existence of any professional relationship among individuals, by name, who are treating him.

9. The patient has the right to be advised if the hospital proposes to engage in or perform human experimentation affecting his care or treatment. The patient has the right to refuse to participate in such research projects.

10. The patient has the right to expect reasonable continuity of care. He has the right to know in advance what appointment times and physicians are available and where. The patient has the right to expect that the hospital will provide a mechanism whereby he is informed by his physician or a delegate of the physician of the patient's continuing health care requirements following discharge.

11. The patient has the right to examine and receive an explanation of his bill regardless of source of payment.

12. The patient has the right to know what hospital rules and regulations apply to his conduct as a patient.

No catalog of rights can guarantee for the patient the kind of treatment he has a right to expect. A hospital has many functions to perform, including the prevention and treatment of disease, the education of both health professionals and patients, and the conduct of clinical research. All these activities must be conducted with an overriding concern for the patient, and, above all, the recognition of his dignity as a human being. Success in achieving this recognition assures success in the defense of the rights of the patient.

4. DIRECTIVE TO PHYSICIANS   California Natural Death Act

Directive made this _____ day of _____ (month, year).

I, _____ _____, being of sound mind, willfully and voluntarily make known my desire that my life shall not be artificially prolonged under the circumstances set forth below, do hereby declare:

1. If at any time I should have an incurable injury, disease, or illness certified to be a terminal condition by two physicians, and where application of life-sustaining procedures would serve only to artificially prolong the moment of my death and where my physician determines that my death is imminent whether or not life-sustaining procedures are utilized, I direct that such procedures be withheld or withdrawn, and that I be permitted to die naturally.

2. In the absence of my ability to give directions regarding the use of such life-sustaining procedures, it is my intention that this directive shall be honored by my family and physician(s) as the final expression of my legal right to refuse medical or surgical treatment and accept the consequences from such refusal.

3. If I have been diagnosed as pregnant and that diagnosis is known to my physician, this directive shall have no force or effect during the course of my pregnancy.

4. I have been diagnosed and notified at least 14 days ago as having a terminal condition by _____ , M.D. whose address is _____ , and whose telephone number is _____ . I understand that if I have not filled in the physician's name and

address, it shall be presumed that I did not have a terminal condition when I made out this directive.

5. This directive shall have no force or effect five years from the date filled in above.

6. I understand the full import of this directive and I am emotionally and mentally competent to make this directive.

Signed _____

City, County, and State of Residence _____

The declarant has been personally known to me and I believe him or her to be of sound mind.

Witness _____

Witness _____

(Note: This directive is legally binding under the law only if the patient is terminally ill at the time of signing and has completed Section 4; otherwise the directive is of informational value only.)

Contained in the California Natural Death Act, Assembly Bill No. 3060, signed into law September 1976. The California law recognizes only those directives executed exactly in this form. Key terms such as "terminal condition" and "life-sustaining procedure" are defined elsewhere in the law.

5. STANDARDS FOR HEALTH SERVICES IN PRISONS (Excerpts)
American Medical Association

The AMA's Standards for Health Services in Prisons *are the result of deliberations by the AMA Advisory Committee to Improve Medical Care and Health Services in Correctional Institutions, three special national task forces, and AMA staff. Equally important, several hundred correctional health care administrators and health care providers throughout the United States have contributed substantially to the prison standards. A "prison" is defined as an adult postconviction correctional facility, under the management of state or federal auspices, which has custodial authority over adults sentenced to confinement for more than a year.*

The standards reflect the viewpoint of organized medicine regarding the definition of "adequate" medical care and health services insisted upon by the courts. Many correctional facilities are under one form or another of legal action for failure to provide adequate health care. The trend in court decisions has been to respond positively to systems which are attempting to improve health care services, even though they have not met all minimum standards.

The health service program must function as part of the overall institutional program. The Standards *call for close cooperation and coordination between the medical staff, other professional staff, correctional personnel and facility administration.*

Treatment Philosophy

Written policy states that health care is rendered with consideration of the patient's dignity and feelings.

Discussion: Medical procedures are performed in privacy, with a chaperone present when indicated, and in a manner designed to encourage the patient's subsequent utilization of appropriate health services.

When rectal or pelvic examinations are indicated, verbal consent should be obtained from the patient.

Continuity of Care

Written policy and defined procedures require continuity of care from admission to discharge from the facility, including referral to community care when indicated.

Discussion: As in the community, health providers should obtain information regarding previous care when undertaking the care of a new patient; likewise, when the care of the patient is transferred to providers in the community, appropriate health information is shared with the new providers in accord with consent requirements.

Interim Health Appraisal: Mentally Ill and Retarded

Written policy and defined procedures require post-admission screening and referral for care of mentally ill or retarded inmates whose adaptation to the correctional environment is significantly impaired.

The health authority provides a written list of specific referral resources.

Discussion: Psychiatric problems identified either at receiving screening or after admission must be followed up by medical staff. The urgency of the problems determines the responses. Suicidal and psychotic patients are emergencies and require prompt attention.

Inmates awaiting emergency evaluation should be housed in a specially designated area with constant supervision by trained staff. Inmates should be held for only the minimum time necessary but no longer than 12 hours before emergency care is rendered.

All sources of assistance for mentally ill and retarded inmates should be identified in advance of need, and referrals should be made in all such cases.

Preventive Care

Written policy and defined procedures require that *medical preventive maintenance* is provided to inmates of the facility.

Discussion: Medical preventive maintenance includes health education and medical services, such as inoculations and immunizations, provided to take advance measures against disease, and instruction in self-care for chronic conditions.

Subjects for health education may include: personal hygiene and nutrition; venereal disease, tuberculosis and other communicable diseases; effects of smoking; self-examination for breast cancer; dental hygiene; drug abuse and danger of self-medication; family planning, including, as appropriate, both services and referrals; physical fitness; and chronic diseases and/or disabilities.

Confidentiality of Health Record

Written policy and defined procedures which affect the principle of confidentiality of the health record require that:

The active health record is maintained separately from the confinement record; and

Access to the health record is controlled by the health authority.

Discussion: The principle of confidentiality protects the patient from disclosure of confidences entrusted to a physician during the course of treatment.

Any information gathered and recorded about alcohol and drug abuse patients is confidential under federal regulations and cannot be disclosed without written consent of the patient or the patient's parent or guardian. (42 CFR Sec. 2.1 et seq.)

The health authority should share with the facility administrator information regarding an inmate's medical management and security. The confidential relationship of doctor and patient extends to inmate/patients and their physician. Thus, it is necessary to maintain active health record files under security, completely separate from the patient's confinement record.

Informed Consent

All examinations, treatments and procedures governed by informed consent practices applicable in the jurisdiction are likewise observed for inmate care. In the case of minors, the *informed consent* of parent, guardian or legal custodian applies when required by law.

Discussion: Informed consent is the agreement by the patient to a treatment, examination or procedure after the patient receives the material facts regarding the nature, consequences, risks and alternatives concerning the proposed treatment, examination or procedure. Medical treatment of an inmate without his or her consent (or without the consent of parent, guardian or legal custodian when the inmate is a minor) could result in legal complications.

Obtaining informed consent may not be necessary in all cases. These exceptions to obtaining informed consent should be reviewed in light of each state's law as they vary considerably. Examples of such situations are:

a. An emergency which requires immediate intervention for the safety of the patient.

b. Emergency care involving patients who do not have the capacity to understand the information given.

c. Public health matters, such as communicable disease treatment.

Physicians must exercise their best medical judgment in all such cases. It is advisable that the physician document the medical record for all aspects of the patient's condition and the reasons for medical intervention. Such documentation facilitates review and provides a defense from charges of battery. In cer-

tain exceptional cases, a court order for treatment may be sought, just as it might in the general community.

The law regarding consent by juveniles to medical treatment, and their right to refuse treatment, varies greatly from state to state. Some states allow juveniles to consent to treatment without parental consent, as long as they are mature enough to comprehend the consequences of their decision; others require parental consent until majority, but the age of majority varies among the states. The law of the jurisdiction within which the facility is located should be reviewed by legal counsel, and based upon counsel's written opinion, a facility policy regarding informed consent should be developed. In all cases, however, consent of the person to be treated is of importance.

Medical Research

Any research done on inmates is done in compliance with state and federal legal guidelines and with the involvement of an appropriate "Human Subjects Review Committee."

Discussion: This standard recognizes past abuses in the area of research on involuntarily confined individuals and stresses the very narrow guidelines under which any such research should be done.

6. POLICY FOR THE PROTECTION OF HUMAN RESEARCH SUBJECTS (Excerpts)
U.S. Department of Health and Human Services

§46.101 To What Do These Regulations Apply?

(a) Except as provided in paragraph (b) of this section, this subpart applies to all research involving human subjects conducted by the Department of Health and Human Services or funded in whole or in part by a Department grant, contract, cooperative agreement or fellowship.

Observations are recorded in such a man-

ner that the human subjects can be identified, directly or through identifiers linked to the subjects, (ii) the observations recorded about the individual, if they became known outside the research, could reasonably place the subject at risk of criminal or civil liability or be damaging to the subject's financial standing or employability, and (iii) the research deals with sensitive aspects of the subject's own behavior such as illegal conduct, drug use, sexual behavior, or use of alcohol.

(5) Research involving the collection or study of existing data, documents, records, pathological specimens, or diagnostic specimens, if these sources are publicly available or if the information is recorded by the investigator in such a manner that subjects cannot be identified, directly or through identifiers linked to the subjects.

(c) The Secretary has final authority to determine whether a particular activity is covered by these regulations.

§46.102 Definitions

(a) "Secretary" means the Secretary of Health and Human Services and any other officer or employee of the Department of Health and Human Services to whom authority has been delegated.

(b) "Department" or "HHS" means the Department of Health and Human Services.

(c) "Institution" means any public or private entity or agency (including federal, state, and other agencies).

(d) "Legally authorized representative" means an individual or judicial or other body authorized under applicable law to consent on behalf of a prospective subject to the subject's participation in the procedure(s) involved in the research.

(3) "Research" means a systematic investigation designed to develop or contribute to generalizable knowledge. Activities which meet this definition constitute "research" for purposes of these regulations, whether or not they are supported or funded under a program which is considered research for other purposes. For example, some "demonstration" and "service" programs may include research activities.

(f) "Human subject" means a living individual about whom an investigator (whether professional or student) conducting research obtains (1) data through intervention or interaction with the individual, or (2) identifiable private information. "Intervention" includes both physical procedures by which data are gathered (for example, venipuncture) and manipulations of the subject or the subject's environment that are performed for research purposes. "Interaction" includes communication or interpersonal contact between investigator and subject. "Private information" includes information about behavior that occurs in a context in which an individual can reasonably expect that no observation or recording is taking place, and information which has been provided for specific purposes by an individual and which the individual can reasonably expect will not be made public (for example, a medical record). Private information must be individually identifiable (i.e., the identity of the subject is or may readily be ascertained by the investigator or associated with the information) in order for obtaining the information to constitute research involving human subjects.

(g) "Minimal risk" means that the risks of harm anticipated in the proposed research are not greater, considering probability and magnitude, than those ordinarily encountered in daily life or during the performance of routine physical or psychological examinations or tests.

(h) "Certification" means the official notification by the institution to the Department in accordance with the requirements of this part that a research project or activity involving human subjects has been reviewed and approved by the Institutional Review Board (IRB) in accordance with the approved assurance on file at HHS. (Certification is required when the research is funded by the Department and not otherwise exempt in accordance with § 46.101 (b)).

§ 46.111 Criteria for IRB Approval of Research

(a) In order to approve research covered by these regulations the IRB shall determine that all of the following requirements are satisfied:

(1) Risks to subjects are minimized: (i) By using procedures which are consistent with sound research design and which do not unnecessarily expose subjects to risk, and (ii) whenever appropriate, by using procedures already being performed on the subjects for diagnostic or treatment purposes.

(2) Risks to subjects are reasonable in relation to anticipated benefits, if any, to subjects, and the importance of the knowl-

edge that may reasonably be expected to result. In evaluating risks and benefits, the IRB should consider only those risks and benefits that may result from the research (as distinguished from risks and benefits of therapies subjects would receive even if not participating in the research). The IRB should not consider possible long-range effects of applying knowledge gained in the research (for example, the possible effects of the research on public policy) as among those research risks that fall within the purview of its responsibility.

(3) Selection of subjects is equitable. In making this assessment the IRB should take into account the purposes of the research and the setting in which the research will be conducted.

(4) Informed consent will be sought from each prospective subject or the subject's legally authorized representative, in accordance with, and to the extent required by § 46.116.

(5) Informed consent will be appropriately documented, in accordance with, and to the extent required by § 46.117.

(6) Where appropriate, the research plan makes adequate provision for monitoring the data collected to insure the safety of subjects.

(7) Where appropriate, there are adequate provisions to protect the privacy of subjects and to maintain the confidentiality of data.

(b) Where some or all of the subjects are likely to be vulnerable to coercion or undue influence, such as persons with acute or severe physical or mental illness, or persons who are economically or educationally disadvantaged, appropriate additional safeguards have been included in the study to protect the rights and welfare of these subjects.

§ 46.116 General Requirements for Informed Consent

Except as provided elsewhere in this or other subparts, no investigator may involve a human being as a subject in research covered by these regulations unless the investigator has obtained the legally effective informed consent of the subject or the sub-

ject's legally authorized representative. An investigator shall seek such consent only under circumstances that provide the prospective subject or the representative sufficient opportunity to consider whether or not to participate and that minimize the possibility of coercion or undue influence. The information that is given to the subject or the representative shall be in language understandable to the subject or the representative. No informed consent, whether oral or written, may include any exculpatory language through which the subject or the representative is made to waive or appear to waive any of the subject's legal rights, or releases or appears to release the investigator, the sponsor, the institution or its agents from liability for negligence.

(a) Basic elements of informed consent. Except as provided in paragraph (c) of this section, in seeking informed consent the following information shall be provided to each subject:

(1) A statement that the study involves research, an explanation of the purposes of the research and the expected duration of the subject's participation, a description of the procedures to be followed, and identification of any procedures which are experimental;

(2) A description of any reasonably foreseeable risks or discomforts to the subject;

(3) A description of any benefits to the subject or to others which may reasonably be expected from the research;

(4) A disclosure of appropriate alternative procedures or courses of treatment, if any, that might be advantageous to the subject;

(5) A statement describing the extent, if any, to which confidentiality of records identifying the subject will be maintained;

(6) For research involving more than minimal risk, an explanation as to whether any compensation and an explanation as to whether any medical treatments are available if injury occurs and, if so, what they consist of, or where further information may be obtained;

(7) An explanation of whom to contact for answers to pertinent questions about the research and research subjects' rights, and whom to contact in the event of a research-

related injury to the subject; and

(8) A statement that participation is voluntary, refusal to participate will involve no penalty or loss of benefits to which the subject is otherwise entitled, and the subject may discontinue participation at any time without penalty or loss of benefits to which the subject is otherwise entitled.

(b) Additional elements of informed consent. When appropriate, one or more of the following elements of information shall also be provided to each subject:

(1) A statement that the particular treatment or procedure may involve risks to the subject (or to the embryo or fetus, if the subject is or may become pregnant) which are currently unforeseeable;

(2) Anticipated circumstances under which the subject's participation may be terminated by the investigator without regard to the subject's consent;

(3) Any additional costs to the subject that may result from participation in the research;

(4) The consequences of a subject's decision to withdraw from the research and procedures for orderly termination of participation by the subject;

(5) A statement that significant new findings developed during the course of the research which may relate to the subject's willingness to continue participation will be provided to the subject; and

(6) The approximate number of subjects involved in the study.

(c) An IRB may approve a consent procedure which does not include, or which alters, some or all of the elements of informed consent set forth above, or waive the requirement to obtain informed consent provided the IRB finds and documents that:

(1) The research is to be conducted for the purpose of demonstrating or evaluating: (i) Federal, state, or local benefit or service programs which are not themselves research programs, (ii) procedures for obtaining benefits or services under these programs, or (iii) possible changes in or alternatives to these programs or procedures; and

(2) The research should not practicably be carried out without the waiver or alteration.

(d) An IRB may approve a consent procedure which does not include, or which alters, some or all of the elements of informed consent set forth above, or waive the requirements to obtain informed consent provided the IRB finds and documents that:

(1) The research involves no more than minimal risk to the subjects;

(2) The waiver or alteration will not adversely affect the rights and welfare of the subjects;

(3) The research could not practicably be carried out without the waiver or alteration; and

(4) Whenever appropriate, the subjects will be provided with additional pertinent information after participation.

(e) The informed consent requirements in these regulations are not intended to preempt any applicable federal, state, or local laws which require additional information to be disclosed in order for informed consent to be legally effective.

(f) Nothing in these regulations is intended to limit the authority of a physician to provide emergency medical care, to the extent the physician is permitted to do so under applicable federal, state, or local law.

Code of Federal Regulations, Title 45, U.S. Code, Part 46, revised as of July 27, 1981.

7. A BILL TO PROVIDE THAT HUMAN LIFE SHALL BE DEEMED TO EXIST FROM CONCEPTION
97th Congress, 1st Session, S.158

S.158: A Bill to Provide That Human Life Shall be Deemed to Exist from Conception

Be it enacted by the Senate and House of Representatives of the United States of America in Congress assembled, That title 42 of the United States Code shall be amended at the end thereof by adding the following new chapter:

"CHAPTER 101

"Section 1. The Congress finds that present day scientific evidence indicates a significant likelihood that actual human life exists from conception.

"The Congress further finds that the fourteenth amendment to the Constitution of the United States was intended to protect all human beings.

"Upon the basis of these findings, and in the exercise of the powers of the Congress, including its power under section 5 of the fourteenth amendment to the Constitution of the United States, the Congress hereby declares that for the purpose of enforcing the obligation of the States under the fourteenth amendment not to deprive persons of life without due process of law, human life shall be deemed to exist from conception, without regard to race, sex, age, health, defect, or condition of dependency; and for this purpose 'person' shall include all human life as defined herein.

"Sec. 2. Notwithstanding any other provision of law, no inferior Federal court ordained and established by Congress under article III of the Constitution of the United States shall have jurisdiction to issue any restraining order, temporary or permanent injunction, or declaratory judgment in any case involving or arising from any State law or municipal ordinance that (1) protects the rights of human persons between conception and birth, or (2) prohibits, limits, or regulates (a) the performance of abortions or (b) the provision at public expense of funds, facilities, personnel, or other assistance for the performance of abortions.

"Sec. 3. If any provision of this Act or the application thereof to any person or circumstance is judicially determined to be invalid, the validity of the remainder of the Act and the application of such provision to other persons and circumstances shall not be affected by such determination.".

8. CONSTITUTION OF THE WORLD HEALTH ORGANIZATION

The States Parties to this Constitution declare, in conformity with the Charter of the United Nations, that the following principles are basic to the happiness, harmonious relations and security of all peoples:

Health is a state of complete physical, mental and social well-being and not merely the absence of disease or infirmity.

The enjoyment of the highest attainable standard of health is one of the fundamental rights of every human being without distinction of race, religion, political belief, economic or social condition.

The health of all peoples is fundamental to the attainment of peace and security and is dependent upon the fullest co-operation of individuals and States.

The achievement of any State in the promotion and protection of health is of value to all.

Unequal development in different countries in the promotion of health and control of disease, especially communicable disease, is a common danger.

Healthy development of the child is of basic importance; the ability to live harmoniously in a changing total environment is essential to such development.

The extension to all peoples of the benefits of medical, psychological and related knowledge is essential to the fullest attainment of health.

Informed opinion and active co-operation on the part of the public are of the utmost importance in the improvement of the health of the people.

Governments have a responsibility for the health of their peoples which can be fulfilled only by the provision of adequate health and social measures.

Accepting these principles, and for the purpose of co-operation among themselves and with others to promote and protect the health of all peoples, the Contracting Parties agree to the present Constitution and hereby establish the World Health Organization as a specialized agency within the terms of Article 57 of the Charter of the United Nations.

[Reprinted from *World Health Organization: Basic Documents,* 26th ed. (Geneva: World Health Organization, 1976), p. 1.]

9. THE NUREMBERG CODE

The great weight of the evidence before us is to the effect that certain types of medical experiments on human beings, when kept within reasonably well-defined bounds, conform to the ethics of the medical profession generally. The protagonists of the practice of human experimentation justify their views on the basis that such experiments yield results for the good of society that are unprocurable by other methods or means of study. All agree, however, that certain basic principles must be observed in order to satisfy moral, ethical and legal concepts:

1. The voluntary consent of the human subject is absolutely essential. This means that the person involved should have legal capacity to give consent; should be so situated as to be able to exercise free power of choice, without the intervention of any element of force, fraud, deceit, duress, over-reaching, or other ulterior form of constraint or coercion; and should have sufficient knowledge and comprehension of the elements of the subject matter involved as to enable him to make an understanding and enlightened decision. This latter element requires that before the acceptance of an affirmative decision by the experimental subject there should be made known to him the nature, duration, and purpose of the experiment; the method and means by which it is to be conducted; all inconveniences and hazards reasonably to be expected; and the effects upon his health or person which may possibly come from his participation in the experiment.

The duty and responsibility for ascertaining the quality of the consent rests upon each individual who initiates, directs or engages in the experiment. It is a personal duty and responsibility which may not be delegated to another with impunity.

2. The experiment should be such as to yield fruitful results for the good of society, unprocurable by other methods or means of study, and not random and unnecessary in nature.

3. The experiment should be so designed and based on the results of animal experimentation and a knowledge of the natural history of the disease or other problem under study that the anticipated results will justify the performance of the experiment.

4. The experiment should be so conducted as to avoid all unnecessary physical and mental suffering and injury.

5. No experiment should be conducted where there is an *a priori* reason to believe that death

or disabling injury will occur; except, perhaps, in those experiments where the experimental physicians also serve as subjects.

6. The degree of risk to be taken should never exceed that determined by the humanitarian importance of the problem to be solved by the experiment.

7. Proper preparations should be made and adequate facilities provided to protect the experimental subject against even remote possibilities of injury, disability, or death.

8. The experiment should be conducted only by scientifically qualified persons. The highest degree of skill and care should be required through all stages of the experiment of those who conduct or engage in the experiment.

9. During the course of the experiment the human subject should be at liberty to bring the experiment to an end if he has reached the physical or mental state where continuation of the experiment seems to him to be impossible.

10. During the course of the experiment the scientist in charge must be prepared to terminate the experiment at any stage, if he has probable cause to believe, in the exercise of the good faith, superior skill and careful judgment required of him that a continuation of the experiment is likely to result in injury, disability, or death to the experimental subject.

Reprinted from *Trials of War Criminals before the Nuremberg Military Tribunals under Control Council Law No. 10,* vol. 2, Government Printing Office, Washington, D.C., 1949.

10. DECLARATION OF HELSINKI   World Medical Association

Introduction

It is the mission of the medical doctor to safeguard the health of the people. His or her knowledge and conscience are dedicated to the fulfillment of this mission.

The Declaration of Geneva of the World Medical Association binds the doctor with the words, "The health of my patient will be my first consideration," and the International Code of Medical Ethics declares that, "Any act or advice which could weaken physical or mental resistance of a human being may be used only in his interest."

The purpose of biomedical research involving human subjects must be to improve diagnostic, therapeutic and prophylactic procedures and the understanding of the aetiology and pathogenesis of disease.

In current medical practice most diagnostic, therapeutic or prophylactic procedures involve hazards. This applies *a fortiori* to biomedical research.

Medical progress is based on research which ultimately must rest in part on experimentation involving human subjects.

In the field of biomedical research a fundamental distinction must be recognized between medical research in which the aim is essentially diagnostic or therapeutic for a patient, and medical research, the essential object of which is purely scientific and without direct diagnostic or therapeutic value to the person subjected to the research.

Special caution must be exercised in the conduct of research which may affect the environment, and the welfare of animals used for research must be respected.

Because it is essential that the results of laboratory experiments be applied to human beings to further scientific knowledge and to help suffering humanity, The World Medical Association has prepared the following recommendations as a guide to every doctor in biomedical research involving human subjects. They should be kept under review in the future. It must be stressed that the standards as drafted are only a guide to physicians all over the world. Doctors are not relieved from criminal, civil and ethical responsibilities under the laws of their own countries.

I. Basic Principles

1. Biomedical research involving human subjects must conform to generally accepted scientific principles and should be based on adequately performed laboratory and animal experimentation and on a thorough knowledge of the scientific literature.

2. The design and performance of each experimental procedure involving human subjects should be clearly formulated in an experimental protocol which should be transmitted to a specially appointed independent committee for consideration, comment and guidance.

3. Biomedical research involving human subjects should be conducted only by scientifically qualified persons and under the supervision of a clinically competent medical person. The responsibility for the human subject must always rest with a medically qualified person and never rest on the subject of the research, even though the subject has given his or her consent.

4. Biomedical research involving human subjects cannot legitimately be carried out unless the importance of the objective is in proportion to the inherent risk to the subject.

5. Every biomedical research project involving human subjects should be preceded by careful assessment of predictable risks in comparison with foreseeable benefits to the subject or to others. Concern for the interests of the subject must always prevail over the interests of science and society.

6. The right of the research subject to safeguard his or her integrity must always be respected. Every precaution should be taken to respect the privacy of the subject and to minimize the impact of the study on the subject's physical and mental integrity and on the personality of the subject.

7. Doctors should abstain from engaging in research projects involving human subjects unless they are satisfied that the hazards involved are believed to be predictable. Doctors should cease any investigation if the hazards are found to outweigh the potential benefits.

8. In publication of the results of his or her research, the doctor is obliged to preserve the accuracy of the results. Reports of experimentation not in accordance with the principles laid down in this Declaration should not be accepted for publication.

9. In any research on human beings, each potential subject must be adequately informed of the aims, methods, anticipated benefits and potential hazards of the study and the discomfort it may entail. He or she should be informed that he or she is at liberty to abstain from participation in the study and that he or she is free to withdraw his or her consent to participation at any time. The doctor should then obtain the subject's freely-given informed consent, preferably in writing.

10. When obtaining informed consent for the research project the doctor should be particularly cautious if the subject is in a dependent relationship to him or her or may consent under duress. In that case the informed consent should be obtained by a doctor who is not

engaged in the investigation and who is completely independent of this official relationship.

11. In the case of legal incompetence, informed consent should be obtained from the legal guardian in accordance with national legislation. Where physical or mental incapacity makes it impossible to obtain informed consent, or when the subject is a minor, permission from the responsible relative replaces that of the subject in accordance with national legislation.

12. The research protocol should always contain a statement of the ethical considerations involved and should indicate that the principles enunciated in the present Declaration are complied with.

II. Medical Research Combined with Professional Care (Clinical Research)

1. In the treatment of the sick person, the doctor must be free to use a new diagnostic and therapeutic measure, if in his or her judgment it offers hope of saving life, reestablishing health or alleviating suffering.

2. The potential benefits, hazards and discomfort of a new method should be weighed against the advantages of the best current diagnostic and therapeutic methods.

3. In any medical study, every patient—including those of a control group, if any—should be assured of the best proven diagnostic and therapeutic method.

4. The refusal of the patient to participate in a study must never interfere with the doctor-patient relationship.

5. If the doctor considers it essential not to obtain informed consent, the specific reasons for this proposal should be stated in the experimental protocol for transmission to the independent committee.

6. The doctor can combine medical research with professional care, the objective being the acquisition of new medical knowledge, only to the extent that medical research is justified by its potential diagnostic or therapeutic value for the patient.

III. Non-Therapeutic Biomedical Research Involving Human Subjects (Non-Clinical Biomedical Research)

1. In the purely scientific application of medical research carried out on a human being, it is the duty of the doctor to remain the protector of the life and health of that person on whom biomedical research is being carried out.

2. The subjects should be volunteers—either healthy persons or patients from whom the experimental design is not related to the patient's illness.

3. The investigator or the investigating team should discontinue the research if in his/her or their judgment it may, if continued, be harmful to the individual.

4. In research on man, the interest of science and society should never take precedence over considerations related to the wellbeing of the subject.

Adopted by the 18th World Medical Assembly, Helsinki, Finland, 1964, and as revised by the 29th World Medical Assembly, Tokyo, Japan, 1975. Reprinted by permission.

Legal Cases

1. ROE V. WADE

Majority Opinion, Blackmun, Justice

It is . . . apparent that at common law, at the time of the adoption of our Constitution, and throughout the major portion of the nineteenth century, abortion was viewed with less disfavor than under most American statutes currently in effect. Phrasing it another way, a woman enjoyed a substantially broader right to terminate a pregnancy than she does in most States today. At least with respect to the early stage of pregnancy, and very possibly without such a limitation, the opportunity to make this choice was present in this country well into the nineteenth century. Even later, the law continued for some time to treat less punitively an abortion procured in early pregnancy. . . .

Three reasons have been advanced to explain historically the enactment of criminal abortion laws in the nineteenth century and to justify their continued existence.

It has been argued occasionally that these laws were the product of a Victorian social concern to discourage illicit sexual conduct. Texas, however, does not advance this justification in the present case, and it appears that no court or commentator has taken the argument seriously. . . .

A second reason is concerned with abortion as a medical procedure. When most criminal abortion laws were first enacted, the procedure was a hazardous one for the woman. This was particularly true prior to the development of antisepsis. Antiseptic techniques, of course, were based on discoveries by Lister, Pasteur, and others first announced in 1867, but were not generally accepted and employed until about the turn of the century. Abortion mortality was high. Even after 1900, and perhaps until as late as the development of antibiotics in the 1940s, standard modern techniques such as dilation and curettage were not nearly so safe as they are today. Thus it has been argued that a state's real concern in enacting a criminal abortion law was to protect the pregnant woman, that is, to restrain her from submitting to a procedure that placed her life in serious jeopardy.

Modern medical techniques have altered this situation. Appellants and various *amici* refer to medical data indicating that abortion in early pregnancy, that is, prior to the end of first trimester, although not without its risk, is now relatively safe. Mortality rates for women undergoing early abortions, where the procedure is legal, appear to be as low as or lower than the rates for normal childbirth. Consequently, any interest of the state in protecting the woman from an inherently hazardous procedure, except when it would be equally dangerous for her to forgo it, has largely disappeared.

The third reason is the state's interest—some phrase it in terms of duty—in protecting prenatal life. Some of the argument for this justification rests on the theory that a new human life is present from the moment of conception. The state's interest and general obligation to protect life then extends, it is argued, to prenatal life. Only when the life of the pregnant mother herself is at stake, balanced against the life she carries within her, should the interest of the embryo or fetus not prevail. Logically, of course, a legitimate state interest in this area need not stand or fall on acceptance of the belief that life begins at conception or at some other point prior to live birth. In assessing the state's interest, recognition may be given to the less rigid claim that as long as at least *potential* life is involved, the state may assert interests beyond the protection of the pregnant woman alone.

Parties challenging state abortion laws have sharply disputed in some courts the contention that a purpose of these laws, when enacted, was to protect prenatal life. Pointing to the absence of legislative history to support the contention, they claim that most state laws were designed solely to protect the woman. Because medical advances have lessened this concern at least with respect to abortion in early pregnancy, they argue that with respect to such abortions the laws can no longer be justified by any state interest. There is some scholarly support for this view of original purpose. The few states courts called upon to interpret their laws in the late nineteenth and early twentieth centuries did focus on the state's interest in protecting the woman's health rather than in preserving the embryo and fetus. . . .

The Constitution does not explicitly mention any right of privacy. In a line of decisions, however, going back perhaps as far as *Union Pacific R. Co.* v. *Botsford* (1891), the Court has recognized that a right of personal privacy, or a guarantee of certain areas or zones of privacy, does exist under the Constitution. In varying contexts the Court or individual Justices have indeed found at least the roots of that right in the First Amendment, . . . in the Fourth and Fifth Amendments . . . in the penumbras of the Bill of Rights . . . in the Ninth Amendment . . . or in the concept of liberty guaranteed by the first section of the Fourteenth Amendment, . . . These decisions make it clear that only personal rights that can be deemed "fundamental" or "implicit in the concept of ordered liberty," . . . are included in this guarantee of personal privacy. They also make it clear that the right has some extension to activities relating to marriage, . . . procreation, . . . contraception, . . . family relationships, . . . and child rearing and education. . . .

This right of privacy, whether it be founded in the Fourteenth Amendment's concept of personal liberty and restrictions upon state action, as we feel it is, or, as the District Court determined, in the Ninth Amendment's reservation of rights to the people, is broad enough to encompass a woman's decision whether or not to terminate her pregnancy. . . .

Appellants and some *amici* argue that the woman's right is absolute and that she is entitled to terminate her pregnancy at whatever time, in whatever way, and for whatever reason she alone chooses. With this we do not agree. Appellants' arguments that Texas either has no valid interest at all in regulating the abortion decision, or no interest strong enough to support any limitation upon the woman's sole determination, is unpersuasive. The Court's decisions recognizing a right of privacy also acknowledge that some state regulation in areas protected by that right is appropriate. As noted above, a state may properly assert important interests in safe guarding health, in maintaining medical standards, and in protecting potential life. At some point in pregnancy, these respective interests become sufficiently compelling to sustain regulation of the factors that govern the abortion decision. The privacy right involved, therefore, cannot be said to be absolute. . . .

We therefore conclude that the right of personal privacy includes the abortion decision, but that this right is not unqualified and must be considered against important state interests in regulation.

We note that those federal and state courts that have recently considered abortion law challenges have reached the same conclusion. . . .

Although the results are divided, most of these courts have agreed that the right of privacy, however based, is broad enough to cover the abortion decision; that the right, nonetheless, is not absolute and is subject to some limitations; and that at some point the state interests as to protection of health, medical standards, and prenatal life, become dominant. We agree with this approach. . . .

The appellee and certain *amici* argue that the fetus is a "person" within the language and meaning of the Fourteenth Amendment. In support of this they outline at length and in detail the well-known facts of fetal development. If this suggestion of personhood is established, the appellant's case, of course, collapses, for the fetus' right to life is then guaranteed specifically by the Amendment. The appellant conceded as much on reargument. On the other hand, the appellee conceded on reargument that no case could be cited that holds a fetus is a person within the meaning of the Fourteenth Amendment. . . .

All this, together with our observation, *supra,* that throughout the major portion of the nineteenth century prevailing legal abortion practices were far freer than they are today, persuades us that the word "person," as used in the Fourteenth Amendment, does not include the unborn. . . . Indeed, our decision in *United States* v. *Vuitch* (1971), inferentially is to the same effect, for we there would not have indulged in statutory interpretation favorable to abortion in specified circumstances if the necessary consequence was the termination of life entitled to Fourteenth Amendment protection. . . .

As we have intimated above, it is reasonable and appropriate for a state to decide that at some point in time another interest, that of health of the mother or that of potential human life, becomes significantly involved. The woman's privacy is no longer sole and any right of privacy she possesses must be measured accordingly.

Texas urges that, apart from the Fourteenth Amendment, life begins at conception and is present throughout pregnancy, and that, therefore, the state has a compelling interest in protecting that life from and after conception. We need not resolve the difficult question of when life begins. When those trained in the respective disciplines of medicine, philosophy, and theology are unable to arrive at any consensus, the judiciary, at this point in the development of man's knowledge, is not in a position to speculate as to the answer.

It should be sufficient to note briefly the wide divergence of thinking on this most sensitive and difficult question. There has always been strong support for the view that life does not begin until live birth. This was the belief of the Stoics. It appears to be the predominant, though not the unanimous, attitude of the Jewish faith. It may be taken to represent also the position of a large segment of the Protestant community, insofar as that can be ascertained; organized groups that have taken a formal position on the abortion issue have generally regarded abortion as a matter for the conscience of the individual and her family. As we have noted, the common law found greater significance in quickening. Physicians and their scientific colleagues have regarded that event with less interest and have tended to focus either upon conception or upon live birth or upon the interim point at which the fetus becomes "viable," that is, potentially able to live outside the mother's womb, albeit with artificial aid. Viability is usually placed at about seven months (28 weeks) but may occur earlier, even at 24 weeks. . . .

In areas other than criminal abortion the law has been reluctant to endorse any theory that life, as we recognize it, begins before live birth or to accord legal rights to the unborn except in narrowly defined situations and except when the rights are contingent upon live birth. . . . In short, the unborn have never been recognized in the law as persons in the whole sense.

In view of all this, we do not agree that, by adopting one theory of life, Texas may override the rights of the pregnant woman that are at stake. We repeat, however, that the state does have an important and legitimate interest in preserving and protecting the health of the pregnant woman, whether she be a resident of the state or a nonresident who seeks medical consultation and treatment there, and that it has still *another* important and legitimate interest in protecting the potentiality of human life. These interests are separate and distinct. Each grows in substantiality as the woman approaches term and, at a point during pregnancy, each becomes "compelling."

With respect to the state's important and legitimate interest in the health of the mother, the "compelling" point, in the light of present medical knowledge, is at approximately the end of the first trimester. This is so because of the now established medical fact . . . that until the end of the first trimester mortality in abortion is less than mortality in normal childbirth. It follows that, from and after this point, a state may regulate the abortion procedure to the extent that the regulation reasonably relates to the preservation and protection of maternal health. Examples of permissible state regulation in this area are requirements as to the qualifications of the person who is to perform the abortion; as to the licensure of that person; as to the facility in which the procedure is to be performed, that is, whether it must be a hospital or may be a clinic or some other place of less-than-hospital status; as to the licensing of the facility; and the like.

This means, on the other hand, for the period of pregnancy prior to this "compelling" point, the attending physician, in consultation with his patient, is free to determine, without regulation by the state, that in his medical judgment the patient's pregnancy should be terminated. If that decision is reached, the judgment may be effectuated by an abortion free of interference by the state.

With respect to the state's important and legitimate interest in potential life, the "compelling" point is at viability. This is so because the fetus then presumably has the capability of meaningful life outside the mother's womb. State regulation protective of fetal life after viability thus has both logical and biological justifications. If the state is interested in protecting fetal life after viability, it may go so far as to proscribe abortion during that period except when it is necessary to preserve the life or health of the mother. . . .

To summarize and repeat:

1. A state criminal abortion statute of the current Texas type, that excepts from crimi-

nality only a *lifesaving* procedure on behalf of the mother, without regard to pregnancy stage and without recognition of the other interests involved, is violative of the Due Process Clause of the Fourteenth Amendment.

(a) For the stage prior to approximately the end of the first trimester, the abortion decision and its effectuation must be left to the medical judgment of the pregnant woman's attending physician.

(b) For the stage subsequent to approximately the end of the first trimester, the state, in promoting its interest in the health of the mother, may, if it chooses, regulate the abortion procedure in ways that are reasonably related to maternal health.

(c) For the stage subsequent to viability the state, in promoting its interest in the potentiality of human life, may, if it chooses, regulate, and even proscribe, abortion except where it is necessary, in appropriate medical judgment, for the preservation of the life or health of the mother.

2. The state may define the term "physician" . . . to mean only a physician currently licensed by the state, and may proscribe any abortion by a person who is not a physician as so defined. . . .

The decision leaves the state free to place increasing restrictions on abortion as the period of pregnancy lengthens, so long as those restrictions are tailored to the recognized state interests. The decision vindicates the right of the physician to administer medical treatment according to his professional judgment up to the points where important state interests provide compelling justifications for intervention. Up to those points the abortion decision in all its aspects is inherently, and primarily, a medical decision, and basic responsibility for it must rest with the physician. If an individual practitioner abuses the privilege of exercising proper medical judgment, the usual remedies, judicial and intraprofessional, are available.

Reprinted from 410 *United States Reports* 113, Decided January 22, 1973.

2. CANTERBURY V. SPENCE

Background

The appellant, Jerry W. Canterbury, sought medical treatment for severe back pain. He underwent a laminectomy (the excision of the posterior arch of the vertebra) for correction of a possible ruptured disk, without having been informed of a risk of paralysis due to the procedure. A day after the operation, he fell from his hospital bed after having been left without assistance while voiding. A few hours after the fall, the lower half of his body was paralyzed. Despite a second operation and extensive medical care, he remains paralyzed, with bowel and urinary incontinence. Mr. Canterbury sued the neurosurgeon, William T. Spence, for negligent performance of an operation and negligent failure to disclose a risk of serious disability inherent in the operation, and sued the hospital for negligent postoperative care. A lower court found for the defendants, and the case was accepted for review by the U.S. Court of Appeals.

Spottswood W. Robinson III, Circuit Judge

A physician is under a duty to treat his patient skillfully but proficiency in diagnosis and therapy is not the full measure of his responsibility. The cases demonstrate that the physi-

cian is under an obligation to communicate specific information to the patient when the exigencies of reasonable care call for it. Due care may require a physician perceiving symptoms
of bodily abnormality to alert the patient to the condition. It may call upon the physician
confronting an ailment which does not respond to his ministrations to inform the patient
thereof. It may command the physician to instruct the patient as to any limitations to be
presently observed for his own welfare, and as to any precautionary therapy he should seek
in the future. It may oblige the physician to advise the patient of the need for or desirability
of any alternative treatment promising greater benefit than that being pursued. Just as plainly, due care normally demands that the physician warn the patient of any risks to his well-
being which contemplated therapy may involve.

The context in which the duty of risk-disclosure arises is invariably the occasion for
decision as to whether a particular treatment procedure is to be undertaken. To the physician,
whose training enables a self-satisfying evaluation, the answer may seem clear, but it is the
prerogative of the patient, not the physician, to determine for himself the direction in which
his interests seem to lie. To enable the patient to chart his course understandably, some familiarity with the therapeutic alternatives and their hazards becomes essential . . .

Once the circumstances give rise to a duty on the physician's part to inform his patient,
the next inquiry is the scope of the disclosure the physician is legally obliged to make. The
courts have frequently confronted this problem but no uniform standard defining the adequacy of the divulgence emerges from the decisions. Some have said "full" disclosure, a norm
we are unwilling to adopt literally. It seems obviously prohibitive and unrealistic to expect
physicians to discuss with their patients *every* risk of proposed treatment—no matter how
small or remote—and generally unnecessary from the patient's viewpoint as well. Indeed, the
cases speaking in terms of "full" disclosure appear to envision something less than total
disclosure, leaving unanswered the question of just how much.

The larger number of courts, as might be expected, have applied tests framed with reference to prevailing fashion within the medical profession. Some have measured the disclosure
by "good medical practice," others by what a reasonable practitioner would have bared
under the circumstances, and still others by what medical custom in the community would
demand. We have explored this rather considerable body of law but are unprepared to follow
it. The duty to disclose, we have reasoned, arises from phenomena apart from medical custom and practice. The latter, we think, should no more establish the scope of the duty than
its existence. Any definition of scope in terms purely of professional standard is at odds
with the patient's prerogative to decide on projected therapy himself. That prerogative, we
have said, is at the very foundation of the duty to disclose, and both the patient's right
to know and the physician's correlative obligation to tell him are diluted to the extent that
its compass is dictated by the medical profession.

In our view, the patient's right of self-decision shapes the boundaries of the duty to reveal.
That right can be effectively exercised only if the patient possesses enough information to
enable an intelligent choice. The scope of the physician's communications to the patient,
then, must be measured by the patient's need, and that need is the information material to
the decision. Thus the test for determining whether a particular peril must be divulged is
its materiality to the patient's decision: all risks potentially affecting the decision must be un-
masked. And to safeguard the patient's interest in achieving his own determination on treatment, the law must itself set the standard for adequate disclosure.

Optimally for the patient, exposure of a risk would be mandatory whenever the patient
would deem it significant to his decision, either singly or in combination with other risks.

Such a requirement, however, would summon the physician to second-guess the patient, whose ideas on materiality could hardly be known to the physician. That would make an undue demand upon medical practitioners, whose conduct, like that of others, is to be measured in terms of reasonableness. Consonantly with orthodox negligence doctrine, the physician's liability for nondisclosure is to be determined on the basis of foresight, not hindsight; no less than any other aspect of negligence, the issue on nondisclosure must be approached from the viewpoint of the reasonableness of the physician's divulgence in terms of what he knows or should know to be the patient's informational needs. If, but only if, the fact-finder can say that the physician's communication was unreasonably inadequate is an imposition of liability legally or morally justified.

Of necessity, the content of the disclosure rests in the first instance with the physician. Ordinarily it is only he who is in position to identify particular dangers; always he must make a judgment, in terms of materiality, as to whether and to what extent revelation to the patient is called for. He cannot know with complete exactitude what the patient would consider important to his decision, but on the basis of his medical training and experience he can sense how the average, reasonable patient expectably would react. Indeed, with knowledge of, or ability to learn, his patient's background and current condition, he is in a position superior to that of most others—attorneys, for example—who are called upon to make judgments on pain of liability in damages for unreasonable miscalculation.

From these considerations we derive the breadth of the disclosure of risks legally to be required. The scope of the standard is not subjective as to either the physician or the patient; it remains objective with due regard for the patient's informational needs and with suitable leeway for the physician's situation. In broad outline, we agree that "[a] risk is thus material when a reasonable person, in what the physician knows or should know to be the patient's position, would be likely to attach significance to the risk or cluster of risks in deciding whether or not to forgo the proposed therapy."

The topics importantly demanding a communication of information are the inherent and potential hazards of the proposed treatment, the alternatives to that treatment, if any, and the results likely if the patient remains untreated. The factors contributing significance to the dangerousness of a medical technique are, of course, the incidence of injury and the degree of the harm threatened. A very small chance of death or serious disablement may well be significant; a potential disability which dramatically outweighs the potential benefit of the therapy or the detriments of the existing malady may summons discussion with the patient.

There is no bright line separating the significant from the insignificant; the answer in any case must abide a rule of reason. Some dangers—infection, for example—are inherent in any operation; there is no obligation to communicate those of which persons of average sophistication are aware. Even more clearly, the physician bears no responsibility for discussion of hazards the patient has already discovered, or those having no apparent materiality to patients' decision on therapy. The disclosure doctrine, like others marking lines between permissible and impermissible behavior in medical practice, is in essence a requirement of conduct prudent under the circumstances. Whenever nondisclosure of particular risk information is open to debate by reasonable-minded men, the issue is for the finder of the facts.

Two exceptions to the general rule of disclosure have been noted by the courts. Each is in the nature of a physician's privilege not to disclose, and the reasoning underlying them is appealing. Each, indeed, is but a recognition that, as important as is the patient's right to know, it is greatly outweighed by the magnitudinous circumstances giving rise to the privilege. The first comes into play when the patient is unconscious or otherwise incapable of consenting, and harm from a failure to treat is imminent and outweighs any harm threatened by the proposed treatment. When a genuine emergency of that sort arises, it is settled that the impracticality of conferring with the patient dispenses with need for it. Even in situations of that character the physician should, as current law requires, attempt to secure a relative's consent if possible. But if time is too short to accommodate discussion, obviously the physician should proceed with the treatment.

The second exception obtains when risk-disclosure poses such a threat of detriment to the patient as to become unfeasible or contraindicated from a medical point of view. It is recognized that patients occasionally become so ill or emotionally distraught on disclosure as to foreclose a rational decision, or complicate or hinder the treatment, or perhaps even pose psychological damage to the patient. Where that is so, the cases have generally held that the physician is armed with a privilege to keep the information from the patient, and we think it clear that portents of that type may justify the physician in action he deems medically warranted. The critical inquiry is whether the physician responded to a sound medical judgment that communication of the risk information would present a threat to the patient's well-being.

The physician's privilege to withhold information for therapeutic reasons must be carefully circumscribed, however, for otherwise it might devour the disclosure rule itself. The privilege does not accept the paternalistic notion that the physician may remain silent simply because divulgence might prompt the patient to forgo therapy the physician feels the patient really needs. That attitude presumes instability or perversity for even the normal patient, and runs counter to the foundation principle that the patient should and ordinarily can make the choice for himself. Nor does the privilege contemplate operation save where the patient's reaction to risk information, as reasonably foreseen by the physician, is menacing. And even in a situation of that kind, disclosure to a close relative with a view to securing consent to the proposed treatment may be the only alternative open to the physician.

No more than breach of any other legal duty does nonfulfillment of the physicians's obligation to disclose alone establish liability to the patient. An unrevealed risk that should have been made known must materialize, for otherwise the omission, however unpardonable, is legally without consequence. Occurrence of the risk must be harmful to the patient, for negligence unrelated to injury is nonactionable. And, as in malpractice actions generally, there must be a causal relationship between the physician's failure to adequately divulge and damage to the patient.

A causal connection exists when, but only when, disclosure of significant risks incidental to treatment would have resulted in a decision against it. The patient obviously has no complaint if he would have submitted to the therapy notwithstanding awareness that the risk was one of its perils. On the other hand, the very purpose of the disclosure rule is to protect the patient against consequences which, if known, he would have avoided by forgoing the treatment. The more difficult question is whether the factual issue on causality calls for an objective or a subjective determination.

Better it is, we believe, to resolve the causality issue on an objective basis: in terms of what a prudent person in the patient's position would have decided if suitably informed of all perils bearing significance. If adequate disclosure could reasonably be expected to have caused that person to decline the treatment because of the revelation of the kind of risk or danger that resulted in harm, causation is shown, but otherwise not. The patient's testimony is relevant on that score, of course, but it would not threaten to dominate the findings. And since that testimony would probably be appraised congruently with the factfinder's belief in its reasonableness, the case for a wholly objective standard for passing on causation is strengthened. Such a standard would in any event ease the fact-finding process and better assure the truth as its product.

Reprinted from 464 *Federal Reporter,* 2d Series 772, Decided May 19, 1972.

3. TARASOFF V. REGENTS OF THE UNIVERSITY OF CALIFORNIA

Tobriner, Justice

On October 17, 1969, Prosenjit Poddar killed Tatiana Tarasoff. Plaintiffs, Tatiana's parents, allege that two months earlier Poddar confided his intention to kill Tatiana to Dr. Lawrence Moore, a psychologist employed by the Cowell Memorial Hospital at the University of California at Berkeley. They allege that on Moore's request, the campus police briefly detained Poddar, but released him when he appeared rational. They further claim that Dr. Harvey Powelson, Moore's superior, then directed that no further action be taken to detain Poddar. No one warned plaintiffs of Tatiana's peril.

Plaintiff's complaints predicate liability on two grounds: defendant's failure to warn plaintiffs of the impending danger and their failure to bring about Poddar's confinement pursuant to the Lanterman-Petris-Short Act (Welf. & Inst. Code, § 5000ff.) Defendants, in turn, assert that they owed no duty of reasonable care to Tatiana and that they are immune from suit under the California Tort Claims Act of 1963 (Gov. Code, § 810ff.).

[1] We shall explain that defendant therapists cannot escape liability merely because Tatania herself was not their patient. When a therapist determines, or pursuant to the standards of his profession should determine, that his patient presents a serious danger of violence to another, he incurs an obligation to use reasonable care to protect the intended victim against such danger. The discharge of this duty may require the therapist to take one or more of various steps, depending upon the nature of the case. Thus it may call for him to warn the intended victim or others likely to apprise the victim of the danger, to notify the police, or to take whatever other steps are reasonably necessary under the circumstances.

Plaintiffs' first cause of action, entitled "Failure to Detain a Dangerous Patient," alleges that on August 20, 1969, Poddar was a voluntary outpatient receiving therapy at Cowell Memorial Hospital. Poddar informed Moore, his therapist, that he was going to kill an unnamed girl, readily identifiable as Tatiana, when she returned home from spending the summer in Brazil. Moore, with the concurrence of Dr. Gold, who had initially examined Poddar, and Dr. Yandell, assistant to the director of the department of psychiatry, decided that Poddar should be committed for observation in a mental hospital. Moore orally notified Officers Atkinson and Teel of the campus police that he would request commitment. He then sent a letter to Police Chief William Beall requesting the assistance of the police department in securing Poddar's confinement.

Officers Atkinson, Brownrigg, and Halleran took Poddar into custody, but satisfied that Poddar was rational, released him on his promise to stay away from Tatiana. Powelson, director of the department of psychiatry at Cowell Memorial Hospital, then asked the police to return Moore's letter, directed that all copies of the letter and notes that Moore had taken as therapist be destroyed, and "ordered no action to place Prosenjit Poddar in 72-hour treatment and evaluation facility."

Although, under the common law, as a general rule, one person owed no duty to control the conduct of another, nor to warn those endangered by such conduct, the courts have carved out an exception to this rule in cases in which the defendant stands in some special relationship to either the person whose conduct needs to be controlled or in a relationship to the foreseeable victim of that conduct. Applying this exception to the present case, we note that a relationship of defendant therapists to either Tatiana or Poddar will suffice to establish a duty of care; as explained in section 315 of the Restatement Second of Torts, a duty of care may arise from either "(a) a special relation . . . between the actor and the third person which imposes a duty upon the actor to control the third person's conduct, or (b) a special relation . . . between the actor and the other which gives to the other a right of protection."

Although plaintiffs' pleadings assert no special relation between Tatiana and defendant therapists, they establish as between Poddar and defendant therapists the special relation that arises between a patient and his doctor or psychotherapist. Such a relationship may support affirmative duties for the benefit of third persons. Thus, for example, a hospital must exercise reasonable care to control the behavior of a patient which may endanger other persons. A doctor must also warn a patient if the patient's condition or medication renders certain conduct, such as driving a car, dangerous to others.

Although the California decisions that recognize this duty have involved cases in which the defendant stood in a special relationship *both* to the victim and to the person whose conduct created the danger, we do not think that the duty should logically be constricted to such situations. Decisions of other jurisdictions hold that the single relationship of a doctor to his patient is sufficient to support the duty to exercise reasonable care to protect others against dangers emanating from the patient's illness. The courts hold that a doctor is liable to persons infected by his patient if he negligently fails to diagnose a contagious disease or, having diagnosed the illness, fails to warn members of the patient's family.

Since it involved a dangerous mental patient, the decision in *Merchants Nat. Bank & Trust Co. of Fargo v. United States* (D.N.D.1967) 272 F.Supp.-409 comes closer to the issue. The Veterans Administration arranged for the patient to work on a local farm, but did not inform the farmer of the man's background. The farmer consequently permitted the patient to come and go freely during nonworking hours; the patient borrowed a car, drove to his wife's residence and killed her. Notwithstanding the lack of any "special relationship" between the Veterans Administration and the wife, the court found the Veterans Administration liable for the wrongful death of the wife.

Defendants contend, however, that imposition of a duty to exercise reasonable care to protect third persons is unworkable because therapists cannot accurately predict whether or not a patient will resort to violence. In support of this argument amicus representing the American Psychiatric Association and other professional societies cites numerous articles which indicate that therapists, in the present state of the art, are unable reliably to predict violent acts; their forecasts, amicus claims, tend consistently to overpredict violence, and indeed are more often wrong than right. Since predictions of violence are often erroneous, amicus concludes, the courts should not render rulings that predicate the liability of therapists upon the validity of such predictions.

The role of the psychiatrist, who is indeed a practitioner of medicine, and that of the psychologist who performs an allied function, are like that of the physician who must conform to the standards of the profession and who must often make diagnoses and predictions based upon such evaluations. Thus the judgment of the therapist in diagnosing emotional disorders and in predicting whether a patient presents a serious danger of violence is comparable to the judgment which doctors and professionals must regularly render under accepted rules of responsibility.

We recognize the difficulty that a therapist encounters in attempting to forecast whether a patient presents a serious danger of violence. Obviously we do not require that the therapist, in making that determination, render a perfect performance; the therapist need only exercise "that reasonable degree of skill, knowledge, and care ordinarily possessed and exercised by members of [that professional specialty] under similar circumstances."

Within the broad range of reasonable practice and treatment in which professional opinion and judgment may differ, the therapist is free to exercise his or her own best judgment without liability; proof, aided by hindsight, that he or she judged wrongly is insufficient to establish negligence.

In the instant case, however, the pleadings do not raise any question as to failure of defendant therapists to predict that Poddar presented a serious danger of violence. On the contrary, the present complaints allege that defendant therapists did in fact predict that Poddar would kill, but were negligent in failing to warn.

The risk that unnecessary warnings may be given is a reasonable price to pay for the lives of possible victims that may be saved. We would hesitate to hold that the therapist who is aware that his patient expects to attempt to assassinate the President of the United States would not be obligated to warn the authorities because the therapist cannot predict with accuracy that his patient will commit the crime.

Defendants further argue that free and open communication is essential to psychotherapy; that "Unless a patient . . . is assured that . . . information [revealed by him] can and will be held in utmost confidence, he will be reluctant to make the full disclosure upon which diagnosis and treatment . . . depends." (Sen.Com. on Judiciary, comment on Evid.Code, § 1014.) The giving of a warning, defendants contend, constitutes a breach of trust which entails the revelation of confidential communications.

We recognize the public interest in supporting effective treatment of mental illness and in protecting the rights of patients to privacy, and the consequent public importance of safeguarding the confidential character of psychotherapeutic communication. Against this interest, however, we must weigh the public interest in safety from violent assault. The Legislature has undertaken the difficult task of balancing the countervailing concerns. In Evidence Code section 1014, it established a broad rule of privilege to protect confidential communications between patient and psychotherapist. In Evidence Code section 1024, the Legislature created specific and limited exception to the psychotherapist-patient privilege: "There is no privilege . . . if the psychotherapist has reasonable cause to believe that the patient is in such mental or emotional condition as to be dangerous to himself or to the person or property of another and that disclosure of the communication is necessary to prevent the threatened danger."

We realize that the open and confidential character of psychotherapeutic dialogue encourages patients to express threats of violence, few of which are ever executed. Certainly a therapist should not be encouraged routinely to reveal such threats; such disclosures could seriously disrupt the patient's relationship with his therapist and with the person threatened. To the contrary, the therapist's obligations to his patient require that he not disclose a confidence unless such disclosure is necessary to avert danger to others, and even then that he do so discreetly, and in a fashion that would preserve the privacy of his patient to the fullest extent compatible with the prevention of the threatened danger.

The revelation of a communication under the above circumstances is not a breach of trust or a violation of professional ethics; as stated in the Principles of Medical Ethics of the American Medical Association (1957), section 9: "A physician may not reveal the confidence entrusted to him in the course of medical attendance . . . *unless he is required to do so by law or unless it becomes necessary in order to protect the welfare of the individual or of the community."* (Emphasis added.) We conclude that the public policy favoring protection of the confidential character of patient-psychotherapist communications must yield to the extent to which disclosure is essential to avert danger to others. The protective privilege ends where the public peril begins.

Mosk, Justice (concurring and dissenting)

I concur in the result in this instance only because the complaints allege that defendant therapists did in fact predict Poddar would kill and were therefore negligent in failing to warn of that danger. Thus the issue here is very narrow: we are not concerned with whether the therapists, pursuant to the standards of their profession, "should have" predicted potential violence; they allegedly did so in actuality. Under these limited circumstances I agree that a cause of action can be stated.

Whether plaintiffs can ultimately prevail is problematical at best. As the complaints admit, the therapists *did* notify the police that Poddar was planning to kill a girl identifiable as Tatiana. While I doubt that more should be required, this issue may be raised in defense and its determination is a question of fact.

I cannot concur, however, in the majority's rule that a therapist may be held liable for failing to predict his patient's tendency to violence if other practitioners, pursuant to the "standards of the profession," would have done so. The question is, what standards? Defendants and a responsible amicus curiae, supported by an impressive body of literature discussed at length in our recent opinion in *People v. Burnick* (1975) 14 Cal.3d 306, 121 Cal. Rptr. 488, 535 P.2d 352, demonstrate that psychiatric predictions of violence are inherently unreliable.

I would restructure the rule designed by the majority to eliminate all reference to conformity to standards of the profession in predicting violence. If a psychiatrist does in fact predict violence, then a duty to warn arises. The majority's expansion of that rule will take us from the world of reality into the wonderland of clairvoyance.

Reprinted from Sup., 131 *California Reporter* 14, decided July 1, 1976.

4. IN THE MATTER OF KAREN QUINLAN, AN ALLEGED INCOMPETENT

Hughes, Chief Justice

The central figure in this tragic case is Karen Ann Quinlan, a New Jersey resident. At the age of 22, she lies in a debilitated and allegedly moribund state at Saint Clare's Hospital in Denville, New Jersey. The litigation has to do, in final analysis, with her life—its continuance or cessation—and the responsibilities, rights, and duties, with regard to any fateful decision concerning it, of her family, her guardian, her doctors, the hospital, the State through its law enforcement authorities, and finally the courts of justice. . . .

The matter is of transcendent importance, involving questions related to the definition and existence of death, the prolongation of life through artificial means developed by medical technology undreamed of in past generations of the practice of the healing arts; the impact of such durationally indeterminate and artificial life prolongation on the rights of the incompetent, her family and society in general; the bearing of constitutional right and the scope of judicial responsibility, as to the appropriate response of an equity court of justice to the extraordinary prayer for relief of the plaintiff. Involved as well is the right of the plaintiff, Joseph Quinlan, to guardianship of the person of his daughter.

On the night of April 15, 1975, for reasons still unclear, Karen Quinlan ceased breathing for at least two 15-minute periods. She received some ineffectual mouth-to-mouth resuscitation from friends. She was taken by ambulance to Newton Memorial Hospital. There she had a temperature of 100 degrees, her pupils were unreactive and she was unresponsive even to deep pain. The history at the time of her admission to that hospital was essentially incomplete and uninformative.

Three days later, Dr. Morse examined Karen at the request of the Newton admitting physician, Dr. McGee. He found her comatose with evidence of decortication, a condition relating to derangement of the cortex of the brain causing a physical posture in which the upper extremities are flexed and the lower extremities are extended. She required a respirator to assist her breathing. Dr. Morse was unable to obtain an adequate account of the circumstances and events leading up to Karen's admission to the Newton Hospital. Such initial history or etiology is crucial in neurological diagnosis. Relying as he did upon the Newton Memorial records and his own examination, he concluded that prolonged lack of oxygen in the bloodstream, anoxia, was identified with her condition as he saw it upon first observation. When she was later transferred to Saint Clare's Hospital she was still unconscious, still on a respirator and a tracheotomy had been performed. On her arrival Dr. Morse conducted extensive and detailed examinations. An electroencephalogram (EEG) measuring electrical rhythm of the brain was performed and Dr. Morse characterized the result as "abnormal but it showed some activity and was consistent with her clinical state." Other significant neurological tests, including a brain scan, an angiogram, and a lumbar puncture were normal in result. Dr. Morse testified that Karen has been in a state of coma, lack of consciousness, since he began treating her. He explained that there are basically two types of coma, sleep-like unresponsiveness and awake unresponsiveness. Karen was originally in a sleep-like unresponsive condition but soon developed "sleep-wake" cycles, apparently a normal improvement for comatose patients occurring within three to four weeks. In the awake cycle she blinks, cries out and does things of that sort but is still totally unaware of anyone or anything around her.

Dr. Morse and other expert physicians who examined her characterized Karen as being in a "chronic persistent vegetative state." Dr. Fred Plum, one of such expert witnesses, defined this as a "subject who remains with the capacity to maintain the vegetative parts of neurological function but who . . . no longer has any cognitive function."

Dr. Morse, as well as the several other medical and neurological experts who testified in this case, believed with certainty that Karen Quinlan is not "brain dead." They identified the Ad Hoc Committee of Harvard Medical School report . . . as the ordinary medical standard for determining brain death, and all of them were satisfied that Karen met none of the criteria specified in that report and was therefore not "brain dead" within its contemplation.

The experts believe that Karen cannot now survive without the assistance of the respirator; that exactly how long she would live without it is unknown; that the strong likelihood is that death would follow soon after its removal, and that removal would also risk further brain damage and would curtail the assistance the respirator presently provides in warding off infection.

It seemed to be the consensus not only of the treating physicians but also of the several qualified experts who testified in the case, that removal from the respirator would not conform to medical practices, standards and traditions.

The further medical consensus was that Karen in addition to being comatose is in a chronic and persistent "vegetative" state, having no awareness of anything or anyone around her and existing at a primitive reflex level. Although she does have some brain stem function (ineffective for respiration) and has other reactions one normally associates with being alive, such as moving, reacting to light, sound and noxious stimuli, blinking her eyes, and the like, the quality of her feeling impulses is unknown. She grimaces, makes stereotyped cries and sounds and has chewing motions. Her blood pressure is normal.

Karen remains in the intensive care unit at Saint Clare's Hospital, receiving 24-hour care by a team of four nurses characterized, as was the medical attention, as "excellent." She is nourished by feeding by way of a nasalgastro tube and is routinely examined for infection, which under these circumstances is a serious life threat. The result is that her condition is considered remarkable under the unhappy circumstances involved.

Karen is described as emaciated, having suffered a weight loss of at least 40 pounds, and undergoing a continuing deteriorative process. Her posture is described as fetal-like and grotesque; there is extreme flexion-rigidity of the arms, legs and related muscles and her joints are severely rigid and deformed.

From all of this evidence, and including the whole testimonial record, several basic findings in the physical area are mandated. Severe brain and associated damage, albeit of uncertain etiology, has left Karen in a chronic and persistent vegetative state. No form of treatment which can cure or improve that condition is known or available. As nearly as may be determined, considering the guarded area of remote uncertainties characteristic of most medical science predictions, she can *never* be restored to cognitive or sapient life. Even with regard to the vegetative level and improvement therein (if such it may be called) the prognosis is extremely poor and the extent unknown if it should in fact occur.

She is debilitated and moribund and although fairly stable at the time of argument before us (no new information having been filed in the meanwhile in expansion of the record), no physician risked the opinion that she could live more than a year and indeed she may die much earlier. Excellent medical and nursing care so far has been able to ward off the constant threat of infection, to which she is peculiarly susceptible because of the respirator, the tracheal tube and other incidents of care in her vulnerable condition. Her life accordingly is sustained by the respirator and tubal feeding, and removal from the respirator would cause her death soon, although the time cannot be stated with more precision. . . .

We have adverted to the "brain death" concept and Karen's disassociation with any of its criteria, to emphasize the basis of the medical decision made by Dr. Morse. When plaintiff and his family, finally reconciled to the certainty of Karen's impending death, requested the withdrawal of life support mechanisms, he demurred. His refusal was based upon his conception of medical standards, practice and ethics described in the medical testimony, such as in the evidence given by another neurologist, Dr. Sidney Diamond, a witness for the State.

Dr. Diamond asserted that no physician would have failed to provide respirator support at the outset, and none would interrupt its life-saving course thereafter, except in the case of cerebral death. In the latter case, he thought the respirator would in effect be disconnected from one already dead, entitling the physician under medical standards and, he thought, legal concepts, to terminate the supportive measures. We note Dr. Diamond's distinction of major surgical or transfusion procedures in a terminal case not involving cerebral death, such as here:

"The subject has lost human qualities. It would be incredible, and I think unlikely, that any physician would respond to a sudden hemorrhage, massive hemorrhage or a loss of all her defensive blood cells, by giving her large quantities of blood. I think that . . . major surgical procedures would be out of the question even if they were known to be essential for continued physical existence."

This distinction is adverted to also in the testimony of Dr. Julius Korein, a neurologist called by plaintiff. Dr. Korein described a medical practice concept of "judicious neglect" under which the physician will say: "Don't treat this patient any more, . . . it does not serve either the patient, the family, or society in any meaningful way to continue treatment with this patient."

Dr. Korein also told of the unwritten and unspoken standard of medical practice implied in the foreboding initials DNR (do not resuscitate), as applied to the extraordinary terminal case:

"Cancer, metastatic cancer, involving the lungs, the liver, the brain, multiple involvements, the physician may or may not write: Do not resuscitate. . . . [I]t could be said to the nurse: if this man stops breathing don't resuscitate him. . . . No physician that I know personally is going to try and resuscitate a man riddled with cancer and in agony and he stops breathing. They are not going to put him on a respirator. . . . I think that would be the height of misuse of technology."

While the thread of logic in such distinctions may be elusive to the non-medical lay mind, in relation to the supposed imperative to sustain life at all costs, they nevertheless relate to medical decisions, such as the decision of Dr. Morse in the present case. We agree with the trial court that that decision was in accord with Dr. Morse's conception of medical standards and practice. . . .

Constitutional and Legal Issues

The right of privacy. It is the issue of the constitutional right of privacy that has given us most concern, in the exceptional circumstances of this case. Here a loving parent, *qua* parent and raising the rights of his incompetent and profoundly damaged daughter, probably irreversibly doomed to no more than a biologically vegetative remnant of life, is before the court. He seeks authorization to abandon specialized technological procedures which can only maintain for a time a body having no potential for resumption or continuance of other than a "vegetative" existence.

We have no doubt, in these unhappy circumstances, that if Karen were herself miraculously lucid for an interval (not altering the existing prognosis of the condition to which she would soon return) and perceptive of her irreversible condition, she could effectively decide upon discontinuance of the life-support apparatus, even if it meant the prospect of natural death. To this extent we may distinguish [*John F. Kennedy Memorial Hosp. v. Heston*], . . .

which concerned a severely injured young woman (Delores Heston), whose life depended on surgery and blood transfusion; and who was in such extreme shock that she was unable to express an informed choice (although the Court apparently considered the case as if the patient's own religious decision to resist transfusion were at stake), but most importantly a patient apparently salvable to long life and vibrant health;—a situation not at all like the present case.

We have no hesitancy in deciding, in the instant diametrically opposite case, that no external compelling interest of the State could compel Karen to endure the unendurable, only to vegetate a few measurable months with no realistic possibility of returning to any semblance of cognitive or sapient life. We perceive no thread of logic distinguishing between such a choice on Karen's part and a similar choice which, under the evidence in this case, could be made by a competent patient terminally ill, riddled by cancer and suffering great pain; such a patient would not be resuscitated or put on a respirator in the example described by Dr. Korein, and *a fortiori* would not be kept *against his will* on a respirator. . . .

The claimed interests of the State in this case are essentially the preservation and sanctity of human life and defense of the right of the physician to administer medical treatment according to his best judgment. In this case the doctors say that removing Karen from the respirator will conflict with their professional judgment. The plaintiff answers that Karen's present treatment serves only a maintenance function; that the respirator cannot cure or improve her condition but at best can only prolong her inevitable slow deterioration and death; and that the interests of the patient, as seen by her surrogate, the guardian, must be evaluated by the court as predominant, even in the face of an opinion *contra* by the present attending physicians. Plaintiff's distinction is significant. The nature of Karen's care and the realistic chances of her recovery are quite unlike those of the patients discussed in many of the cases where treatments were ordered. In many of those cases the medical procedure required (usually a transfusion) constituted a minimal bodily invasion and the chances of recovery and return to functioning life were very good. We think that the State's interest *contra* weakens and the individual's right to privacy grows as the degree of bodily invasion increases and the prognosis dims. Ultimately there comes a point at which the individual's rights overcome the State interest. It is for that reason that we believe Karen's choice, if she were competent to make it, would be vindicated by the law. . . .

Our affirmation of Karen's independent right of choice, however, would ordinarily be based upon her competency to assert it. The sad truth, however, is that she is grossly incompetent and we cannot discern her supposed choice based on the testimony of her previous conversations with friends, where such testimony is without sufficient probative weight. 137 *N.J. Super.* at 260. Nevertheless we have concluded that Karen's right of privacy may be asserted on her behalf by her guardian under the peculiar circumstances here present.

If a putative decision by Karen to permit this non-cognitive, vegetative existence to terminate by natural forces is regarded as a valuable incident of her right of privacy, as we believe it to be, then it should not be discarded solely on the basis that her condition prevents her conscious exercise of the choice. The only practical way to prevent destruction of the right is to permit the guardian and family of Karen to render their best judgment, subject to the qualifications hereinafter stated, as to whether she would exercise it in these circumstances. If their conclusion is in the affirmative this decision should be accepted by a society the overwhelming majority of whose members would, we think, in similar circumstances, exercise such a choice in the same way for themselves or for those closest to them. It is for this reason that we determine that Karen's right of privacy may be asserted in her behalf, in this respect, by her guardian and family under the particular circumstances presented by this record. . . .

The medical factor. Having declared the substantive legal basis upon which plaintiff's rights as representative of Karen must be deemed predicated, we face and respond to the assertion on behalf of defendants that our premise unwarrantably offends prevailing medical standards. We thus turn to consideration of the medical decision supporting the determination made below, conscious of the paucity of pre-existing legislative and judicial guidance as to the rights and liabilities therein involved. . . .

The medical obligation is related to standards and practice prevailing in the profession. The physicians in charge of the case, as noted above, declined to withdraw the respirator. That decision was consistent with the proofs . . . [in the lower court] as to the then existing medical standards and practices. Under the law as it then stood, Judge Muir was correct in declining to authorize withdrawal of the respirator.

However, in relation to the matter of the declaratory relief sought by plaintiff as representative of Karen's interests, we are required to reevaluate the applicability of the medical standards projected in the court below. The question is whether there is such internal consistency and rationality in the application of such standards as should warrant their constituting an ineluctable bar to the effectuation of substantive relief for plaintiff at the hands of the court. We have concluded not.

In regard to the foregoing it is pertinent that we consider the impact on the standards both of the civil and criminal law as to medical liability and the new technological means of sustaining life irreversibly damaged.

The modern proliferation of substantial malpractice litigation and the less frequent but even more unnerving possibility of criminal sanctions would seem, for it is beyond human nature to suppose otherwise, to have bearing on the practice and standards as they exist. The brooding presence of such possible liability, it was testified here, had no part in the decision of the treating physicians. As did Judge Muir, we afford this testimony full credence. But we cannot believe that the stated factor has not had a strong influence on the standards, as the literature on the subject plainly reveals. Moreover our attention is drawn not so much to the recognition by Drs. Morse and Javed of the extant practice and standards but to the widening ambiguity of those standards themselves in their application to the medical problems we are discussing.

The agitation of the medical community in the face of modern life prolongation technology and its search for definitive policy are demonstrated in the large volume of relevant professional commentary.

The wide debate thus reflected contrasts with the relative paucity of legislative and judicial guides and standards in the same field. The medical profession has sought to devise guidelines such as the "brain death" concept of the Harvard Ad Hoc Committee mentioned above. But it is perfectly apparent from the testimony we have quoted of Dr. Korein, and indeed so clear as almost to be judicially noticeable, that humane decisions against resuscitative or maintenance therapy are frequently a recognized *de facto* response in the medical world to the irreversible, terminal, pain-ridden patient, especially with familial consent. And these cases, of course, are far short of "brain death."

We glean from the record here that physicians distinguish between curing the ill and comforting and easing the dying; that they refuse to treat the curable as if they were dying or ought to die, and that they have sometimes refused to treat the hopeless and dying as if they

were curable. In this sense, as we were reminded by the testimony of Drs. Korein and Diamond, many of them have refused to inflict an undesired prolongation of the process of dying
on a patient in irreversible condition when it is clear that such "therapy" offers neither human nor humane benefit. We think these attitudes represent a balanced implementation of a
profoundly realistic perspective on the meaning of life and death and that they respect the
whole Judeo-Christian tradition of regard for human life. No less would they seem consistent
with the moral matrix of medicine, "to heal," very much in the sense of the endless mission
of the law, "to do justice."

Yet this balance, we feel, is particularly difficult to perceive and apply in the context of
the development by advanced technology of sophisticated and artificial life-sustaining devices.
For those possibly curable, such devices are of great value, and, as ordinary medical procedures, are essential. Consequently, as pointed out by Dr. Diamond, they are necessary because
of the ethic of medical practice. But in light of the situation in the present case (while the
record here is somewhat hazy in distinguishing between "ordinary" and "extraordinary" measures), one would have to think that the use of the same respirator or like support could be
considered "ordinary" in the context of the possibly curable patient but "extraordinary" in
the context of the forced sustaining by cardio-respiratory processes of an irreversibly doomed
patient. And this dilemma is sharpened in the face of the malpractice and criminal action
threat which we have mentioned. . . .

There must be a way to free physicians, in the pursuit of their healing vocation, from possible contamination by self-interest or self-protection concerns which would inhibit their
independent medical judgments for the well-being of their dying patients. We would hope
that this opinion might be serviceable to some degree in ameliorating the professional problems under discussion.

A technique aimed at the underlying difficulty (though in a somewhat broader context)
is described by Dr. Karen Teel, a pediatrician and a director of Pediatric Education, who
writes in the *Baylor Law Review* under the title "The Physician's Dilemma: A Doctor's
View: What The Law Should Be." Dr. Teel recalls:

"Physicians, by virtue of their responsibility for medical judgments are, partly by choice
and partly by default, charged with the responsibility of making ethical judgments which
we are sometimes ill-equipped to make. We are not always morally and legally authorized to
make them. The physician is thereby assuming a civil and criminal liability that, as often
as not, he does not even realize as a factor in his decision. There is little or no dialogue in this
whole process. The physician assumes that his judgment is called for and, in good faith, he
acts. Someone must and it has been the physician who has assumed the responsibility and the
risk.

"I suggest that it would be more appropriate to provide a regular forum for more input and
dialogue in individual situations and to allow the responsibility of these judgments to be
shared. Many hospitals have established an Ethics Committee composed of physicians, social
workers, attorneys, and theologians, . . . which serves to review the individual circumstances
of ethical dilemma and which has provided much in the way of assistance and safeguards for
patients and their medical caretakers. Generally, the authority of these committees is primarily restricted to the hospital setting and their official status is more that of an advisory
body than of an enforcing body.

"The concept of an Ethics Committee which has this kind of organization and is readily
accessible to those persons rendering medical care to patients would be, I think, the most
promising direction for further study at this point. . . .

" [This would allow] some much needed dialogue regarding these issues and [force] the point of exploring all of the options for a particular patient. It diffuses the responsibility for making these judgments. Many physicians, in many circumstances, would welcome this sharing of responsibility. I believe that such an entity could lend itself well to an assumption of a legal status which would allow courses of action not now undertaken because of the concern for liability."

The most appealing factor in the technique suggested by Dr. Teel seems to us to be the diffusion of professional responsibility for decision, comparable in a way to the value of multi-judge courts in finally resolving on appeal difficult questions of law. Moreover, such a system would be protective to the hospital as well as the doctor in screening out, so to speak, a case which might be contaminated by less than worthy motivations of family or physician. In the real world and in relationship to the momentous decision contemplated, the value of additional views and diverse knowledge is apparent. . . .

And although the deliberations and decisions which we describe would be professional in nature they should obviously include at some stage the feelings of the family of an incompetent relative. Decision-making within health care if it is considered as an expression of a primary obligation of the physician, *primum non nocere,* should be controlled primarily within the patient-doctor-family relationship, as indeed was recognized by Judge Muir in his supplemental opinion of November 12, 1975.

If there could be created not necessarily this particular system but some reasonable counterpart, we would have no doubt that such decisions, thus determined to be in accordance with medical practice and prevailing standards, would be accepted by society and by the courts, at least in cases comparable to that of Karen Quinlan.

The evidence in this case convinces us that the focal point of decision should be the prognosis as to the reasonable possibility of return to cognitive and sapient life, as distinguished from the forced continuance of that biological vegetative existence to which Karen seems to be doomed.

In summary of the present Point of this opinion, we conclude that the state of the pertinent medical standards and practices which guided the attending physicians in this matter is not such as would justify this Court in deeming itself bound or controlled thereby in responding to the case for declaratory relief established by the parties on the record before us.

Alleged criminal liability. Having concluded that there is a right of privacy that might permit termination of treatment in the circumstances of this case, we turn to consider the relationship of the exercise of that right to the criminal law. We are aware that such termination of treatment would accelerate Karen's death. The County Prosecutor and the Attorney General stoutly maintain that there would be criminal liability for such acceleration. Under the statutes of this State, the unlawful killing of another human being is criminal homicide. We conclude that there would be no criminal homicide in the circumstances of this case. We believe, first, that the ensuing death would not be homicide but rather expiration from existing natural causes. Secondly, even if it were to be regarded as homicide, it would not be unlawful.

These conclusions rest upon definitional and constitutional bases. The termination of treatment pursuant to the right of privacy is, within the limitations of this case, *ipso facto* lawful. Thus, a death resulting from such an act would not come within the scope of the homicide statutes proscribing only the unlawful killing of another. There is a real and in this case determinative distinction between the unlawful taking of the life of another and the ending of artificial life-support systems as a matter of self-determination.

Declaratory Relief

We thus arrive at the formulation of the declaratory relief which we have concluded is appropriate to this case. Some time has passed since Karen's physical and mental condition was described to the Court. At that time her continuing deterioration was plainly projected. Since the record has not been expanded we assume that she is now even more fragile and nearer to death than she was then. Since her present treating physicians may give reconsideration to her present posture in the light of this opinion, and since we are transferring to the plaintiff as guardian the choice of the attending physician and therefore other physicians may be in charge of the case who may take a different view from that of the present attending physicians, we herewith declare the following affirmative relief on behalf of the plaintiff. Upon the concurrence of the guardian and family of Karen, should the responsible attending physicians conclude that there is no reasonable possibility of Karen's ever emerging from her present comatose condition to a cognitive, sapient state and that the life-support apparatus now being administered to Karen should be discontinued, they shall consult with the hospital "Ethics Committee" or like body of the institution in which Karen is then hospitalized. If that consultative body agrees that there is no reasonable possibility of Karen's ever emerging from her present comatose condition to a cognitive, sapient state, the present life-support system may be withdrawn and said action shall be without any civil or criminal liability therefor on the part of any participant, whether guardian, physician, hospital or others. We herewith specifically so hold.

Reprinted from 70 *New Jersey Reports* 10. Decided March 31, 1976.

5. SUPERINTENDENT OF BELCHERTOWN STATE SCHOOL V. SAIKEWICZ

Liacos, Justice

On April 26, 1976, William E. Jones, superintendent of the Belchertown State School (a facility of the Massachusetts Department of Mental Health), and Paul R. Rogers, a staff attorney at the school, petitioned the Probate Court for Hampshire County for the appointment of a guardian of Joseph Saikewicz, a resident of the State school. Simultaneously they filed a motion for the immediate appointment of a guardian ad litem, with authority to make the necessary decisions concerning the care and treatment of Saikewicz, who was suffering with acute myeloblastic monocytic leukemia. The petition alleged that Saikewicz was a retarded person in urgent need of medical treatment and that he was a person of disability incapable of giving informed consent for such treatment.

On May 5, 1976, the probate judge appointed a guardian ad litem. On May 6, 1976, the guardian ad litem filed a report with the court. The guardian ad litem's report indicated that Saikewicz's illness was an incurable one, and that although chemotherapy was the medically indicated course of treatment it would cause Saikewicz significant adverse side effects and discomfort. The guardian ad litem concluded that these factors, as well as the inability of the ward to understand the treatment to which he would be subjected and the fear and pain he would suffer as a result, outweighed the limited prospect of any benefit from such treatment, namely, the possibility of some uncertain but limited extension of life. He therefore recommended "that not treating Mr. Saikewicz would be in his best interests."

The judge below found that Joseph Saikewicz, at the time the matter arose, was sixty-seven years old, with an I.Q. of ten and a mental age of approximately two years and eight months. He was profoundly mentally retarded. He was physically strong and well built, nutritionally nourished, and ambulatory. He was not, however, able to communicate verbally—resorting to gestures and grunts to make his wishes known to others and responding only to gestures or physical contacts.

As a result of his condition, Saikewicz had lived in State institutions since 1923 and had resided at the Belchertown State School since 1928.

On April 19, 1976, Saikewicz was diagnosed as suffering from acute myeloblastic monocyctic leukemia. The disease is invariably fatal.

Chemotherapy involves the administration of drugs over several weeks, the purpose of which is to kill the leukemia cells. This treatment unfortunately affects normal cells as well. One expert testified that the end result, in effect, is to destroy the living vitality of the bone marrow. Because of this effect, the patient becomes very anemic and may bleed or suffer infections—a condition which requires a number of blood transfusions. Moreover, while most patients survive chemotherapy, remission of the leukemia is achieved in only thirty to fifty per cent of the cases. If remission does occur, it typically lasts for between two and thirteen months although longer periods of remission are possible. Estimates of the effectiveness of chemotherapy are complicated in cases, such as the one presented here, in which the patient's age becomes a factor. According to the medical testimony before the court below, persons over age sixty have more difficulty tolerating chemotherapy and the treatment is likely to be less successful than in younger patients. This prognosis may be compared with the doctors' estimates that, left untreated, a patient in Saikewicz's condition would live for a matter of weeks or, perhaps, several months. According to the testimony, a decision to allow the disease to run its natural course would not result in pain for the patient, and death would probably come without discomfort.

An important facet of the chemotherapy process, to which the judge below directed careful attention, is the problem of serious adverse side effects caused by the treating drugs. Among these side effects are severe nausea, bladder irritation, numbness and tingling of the extremities, and loss of hair. The bladder irritation can be avoided, however, if the patient drinks fluids, and the nausea can be treated by drugs. It was the opinion of the guardian ad litem, as well as the doctors who testified before the probate judge, that most people elect to suffer the side effects of chemotherapy rather than to allow their leukemia to run its natural course.

Drawing on the evidence before him including the testimony of the medical experts, and the report of the guardian ad litem, the probate judge issued detailed findings with regard to the costs and benefits of allowing Saikewicz to undergo chemotherapy. The judge concluded that the following considerations weighed *against* administering chemotherapy to Saikewicz: "(1) his age, (2) his inability to cooperate with the treatment, (3) probable adverse side effects of treatment, (4) low chance of producing remission, (5) the certainty that treatment will cause immediate suffering, and (6) the quality of life possible for him even if the treatment does bring about remission."

The following considerations were determined to weigh in *favor* of chemotherapy: "(1) the chance that his life may be lengthened thereby, and (2) the fact that most people in his situation when given a chance to do so elect to take the gamble of treatment."

Concluding that, in this case, the negative factors of treatment exceeded the benefits, the probate judge ordered on May 13, 1976, that no treatment be administered to Saikewicz for his condition of acute myeloblastic monocytic leukemia except by further order of the court. The judge further ordered that all reasonable and necessary supportive measures be taken, medical or otherwise, to safeguard the well-being of Saikewicz in all other respects and to reduce as far as possible any suffering or discomfort which he might experience.

It is within this factual context that we issued our order of July 9, 1976.

Saikewicz died on September 4, 1976, at the Belchertown State School hospital. Death was due to bronchial pneumonia, a complication of the leukemia. Saikewicz died without pain or discomfort.

We recognize at the outset that this case presents novel issues of fundamental importance that should not be resolved by mechanical reliance on legal doctrine. Our task of establishing a framework in the law on which the activities of health care personnel and other persons can find support is furthered by seeking the collective guidance of those in health care, moral ethics, philosophy, and other disciplines. The principal areas of determination are:

A. The nature of the right of any person, competent or incompetent, to decline potentially life-prolonging treatment.

B. The legal standards that control the course of decision whether or not potentially life-prolonging, but not life-saving, treatment should be administered to a person who is not competent to make the choice.

C. The procedures that must be followed in arriving at that decision.

We take the view that the substantive rights of the competent and the incompetent person are the same in regard to the right to decline potentially life-prolonging treatment. Factors which distinguish the two types of persons are found only in the area of how the State should approach the preservation and implementation of the rights of an incompetent person and in the procedures necessary to that process of preservation and implementation.

Advances in medical science have given doctors greater control over the time and nature of death. Chemotherapy is, as evident from our previous discussion, one of these advances. Prior to the development of such new techniques the physician perceived his duty as that of making every conceivable effort to prolong life. On the other hand, the context in which such an ethos prevailed did not provide the range of options available to the physician today in terms of taking steps to postpone death irrespective of the effect on the patient. With the development of the new techniques, serious questions as to what may constitute acting in the best interests of the patient have arisen.

The nature of the choice has become more difficult because physicians have begun to realize that in many cases the effect of using extraordinary measures to prolong life is to "only prolong suffering, isolate the family from their loved one at a time when they may be close at hand or result in economic ruin for the family."

The current state of medical ethics in this area is expressed by one commentator who states that: "we should not use *extraordinary* means of prolonging life or its semblance when, after careful consideration, consultation and the application of the most well conceived therapy it becomes apparent that there is no hope for the recovery of the patient. Recovery should not be defined simply as the ability to remain alive; it should mean life without intolerable suffering."

Our decision in this case is consistent with the current medical ethos in this area. There is implicit recognition in the law of the Commonwealth, as elsewhere, that a person has a strong interest in being free from nonconsensual invasion of his bodily integrity. One means by which the law has developed in a manner consistent with the protection of this interest is through the development of the doctrine of informed consent.

Of even broader import, but arising from the same regard for human dignity and self-determination, is the unwritten constitutional right of privacy found in the penumbra of specific guaranties of the Bill of Rights. In the case of a person incompetent to assert this constitutional right of privacy, it may be asserted by that person's guardian.

A survey of recent decisions involving the difficult question of the right of an individual to refuse medical intervention or treatment indicates that a relatively concise statement of countervailing State interests may be made. As distilled from the cases, the State has claimed interest in: (1) the preservation of life; (2) the protection of the interests of innocent third parties; (3) the prevention of suicide; and (4) maintaining the ethical integrity of the medical profession.

It is clear that the most significant of the asserted State interests is that of the preservation of human life. Recognition of such an interest, however, does not necessarily resolve the problem where the affliction or disease clearly indicates that life will soon, and inevitably, be extinguished. The interest of the State in prolonging a life must be reconciled with the interest of an individual to reject the traumatic cost of that prolongation. There is a substantial distinction in the State's insistence that human life be saved where the affliction is curable, as opposed to the State interest where, as here, the issue is not whether but when, for how long, and at what cost to the individual that life may be briefly extended. Even if we assume that the State has an additional interest in seeing to it that individual decisions on the prolongation of life do not in any way tend to "cheapen" the value which is placed in the concept of living (see *Roe v. Wade,* above), we believe it is not inconsistent to recognize a right to decline medical treatment in a situation of incurable illness. The constitutional right to privacy, as we conceive it, is an expression of the sanctity of individual free choice and self-determination as fundamental constituents of life. The value of life as so perceived is lessened not by a decision to refuse treatment, but by the failure to allow a competent human being the right of choice.

The last State interest requiring discussion is that of the maintenance of the ethical integrity of the medical profession as well as allowing hospitals the full opportunity to care for people under their control. Prevailing medical ethical practice does not, without exception, demand that all efforts toward life prolongation be made in all circumstances. Rather, as indicated in *Quinlan,* the prevailing ethical practice seems to be to recognize that the dying are more often in need of comfort than treatment. Recognition of the right to refuse necessary treatment in appropriate circumstances is consistent with existing medical mores; such a doctrine does not threaten either the integrity of the medical profession, the proper role of hospitals in caring for such patients or the State's interest in protecting the same.

Applying the considerations discussed in this subsection to the decision made by the probate judge in the circumstances of the case before us, we are satisfied that his decision was consistent with a proper balancing of applicable State and individual interests. Two of the four categories of State interests that we have identified, the protection of third parties and the prevention of suicide, are inapplicable to this case. The third, involving the protection of the ethical integrity of the medical profession, was satisfied on two grounds. The probate judge's decision was in accord with the testimony of the attending physicians of the patient. The decision is in accord with the generally accepted views of the medical profession, as set forth in this opinion. The fourth State interest—the preservation of life—has been viewed with proper regard for the heavy physical and emotional burdens on the patient if a vigorous regimen of drug therapy were to be imposed to effect a brief and uncertain delay in the natural process of death. To be balanced against these State interests was the individual's interest in the freedom to choose to reject, or refuse to consent to, intrusions of his bodily integrity and privacy. We cannot say that the facts of this case required a result contrary to that reached by the probate judge with regard to the right of any person, competent or incompetent, to be spared the deleterious consequences of life-prolonging treatment. We therefore turn to consider the unique considerations arising in this case by virtue of the patient's inability to appreciate his predicament and articulate his desires.

The question what legal standards govern the decision whether to administer potentially life-prolonging treatment to an incompetent person encompasses two distinct and important subissues. First, does a choice exist? That is, is it the unvarying responsibility of the State to order medical treatment in all circumstances involving the care of an incompetent person? Second, if a choice does exist under certain conditions, what considerations enter into the decision-making process?

We think that principles of equality and respect for all individuals require the conclusion that a choice exists. We recognize a general right in all persons to refuse medical treatment in appropriate circumstances. The recognition of that right must extend to the case of an incompetent, as well as a competent, patient because the value of human dignity extends to both.

This is not to deny that the State has a traditional power and responsibility, under the doctrine of parens patriae, to care for and protect the "best interests" of the incompetent person. The "best interests" of an incompetent person are not necessarily served by imposing on such persons results not mandated as to competent persons similarly situated. It does not advance the interest of the State or the ward to treat the ward as a person of lesser status or dignity than others.

To protect the incompetent person within its power, the State must recognize the dignity and worth of such a person and afford to that person the same panoply of rights and choices it recognizes in competent persons. If a competent person faced with death may choose to decline treatment which not only will not cure the person but which substantially may increase suffering in exchange for a possible yet brief prolongation of life, then it cannot be said that it is always in the "best interests" of the ward to require submission to such treatment. Nor do statistical factors indicating that a majority of competent persons similarly situated choose treatment resolve the issue. The significant decisions of life are more complex than statistical determinations. Individual choice is determined not by the vote of majority but by the complexities of the singular situation viewed from the unique perspective of the person called on to make the decision. To presume that the incompetent person must always be subjected to what many rational and intelligent persons may decline is to downgrade the status of the incompetent person by placing a lesser value on his intrinsic human worth and vitality.

We believe that both the guardian ad litem in his recommendation and the judge in his decision should have attempted (as they did) to ascertain the incompetent person's actual interests and preferences. In short, the decision in cases such as this should be that which would be made by the incompetent person, if that person were competent, but taking into account the present and future incompetency of the individual as one of the factors which would necessarily enter into the decision-making process of the competent person. Having recognized the right of a competent person to make for himself the same decision as the court made in this case, the question is, do the facts on the record support the proposition that Saikewicz himself would have made the decision under the standard set forth? We believe they do.

The two factors considered by the probate judge to weigh in favor of administering chemotherapy were: (1) the fact that most people elect chemotherapy and (2) the chance of a longer life. Both are appropriate indicators of what Saikewicz himself would have wanted, provided that due allowance is taken for this individual's present and future incompetency.

The probate judge identified six factors weighing against administration of chemotherapy. Four of these—Saikewicz's age, the probable side effects of treatment, the low chance of producing remission, and the certainty that treatment will cause immediate suffering—were clearly established by the medical testimony to be considerations that any individual would weigh carefully. A fifth factor—Saikewicz's inability to cooperate with the treatment—introduces those considerations that are unique to this individual and which therefore are essential to the proper exercise of substituted judgment. The judge heard testimony that Saikewicz would have no comprehension of the reasons for the severe disruption of his formerly secure and stable environment occasioned by the chemotherapy. He therefore would experience fear without the understanding from which other patients draw strength. The inability to anticipate and prepare for the severe side effects of the drugs leaves room only for confusion and disorientation. The possibility that such a naturally uncooperative patient would have to be physically restrained to allow the slow intravenous administration of drugs could only compound his pain and fear, as well as possibly jeopardize the ability of his body to withstand the toxic effects of the drugs.

The sixth factor identified by the judge as weighing against chemotherapy was "the quality of life possible for him even if the treatment does bring about remission." To the extent that this formulation equates the value of life with any measure of the quality of life, we firmly reject it. A reading of the entire record clearly reveals, however, the judge's concern that special care be taken to respect the dignity and worth of Saikewicz's life precisely because of his vulnerable position. The judge, as well as all the parties, were keenly aware that the supposed ability of Saikewicz, by virtue of his mental retardation, to appreciate or experience life had no place in the decision before them. Rather than reading the judge's formulation in a manner that demeans the value of the life of one who is mentally retarded, the vague, and perhaps ill-chosen, term "quality of life" should be understood as a reference to the continuing state of pain and disorientation precipitated by the chemotherapy treatment. Viewing the term in this manner, together with the other factors properly considered by the judge, we are satisfied that the decision to withhold treatment from Saikewicz was based on a regard for his actual interests and preferences and that the facts supported this decision.

Finding no State interest sufficient to counterbalance a patient's decision to decline life-prolonging medical treatment in the circumstances of this case, we conclude that the patient's right to privacy and self-determination is entitled to enforcement. Because of this conclusion, and in view of the position of equality of an incompetent person in Joseph Saikewicz's position, we conclude that the probate judge acted appropriately in this case. For these reasons we issued our order of July 9, 1976, and responded as we did to the questions of the probate judge.

Reprinted from Mass., 370 *North Eastern Reporter*, 2d Series 417, Decided November 28, 1977.

6. EICHNER V. DILLON

Mollen, Presiding Justice

This appeal concerns the right of a terminally ill patient in a comatose and essentially vegetative state to have extraordinary life-sustaining measures discontinued, and thereby to permit the process of death to run its natural course. The case raises issues which involve not only the life of the patient, but the interest of the State in maintaining that life. The issues are not difficult to frame, but their resolution will have a profound and far-reaching impact in a world where advances in medical technology sometimes blur the distinction between life and death. Ultimately, the question is whether the judicial system has the power to authorize termination of life-preserving measures and thereby, presumably, of life itself.

From the age of 16, Brother Joseph Charles Fox had lived a devout religious life in the Catholic Church. In 1970 he retired to the religious community of the Order of the Society of Mary living on the premises of the Chaminade High School. He had a close relationship with the president of the school, Rev. Philip Eichner, S.M., whom he had known since 1953 when Brother Fox was a prefect of novices during Father Eichner's novitiate. At the time of his retirement, Brother Fox was in excellent health suffering only from an eye condition which limited his vision. He remained both mentally and physically active, taking on duties as the high school's pastor and message coordinator.

In late August or early September, 1979, Brother Fox, then 83 years old, was working in the garden as was his usual practice. Apparently, in moving some large tubs of flowers, he sustained an inguinal hernia. His physician recommended that he undergo an operation, and corrective surgery was scheduled for October 2, 1979. Prior to the operation, Brother Fox was in good health and entered the hospital with all expectations of a successful recovery. The operation began and was proceeding in normal fashion when, near its conclusion, Brother Fox apparently suffered a cardiac arrest. Emergency procedures were applied in an attempt to revive him. Medication and heart massage were administered while an endotracheal tube was inserted between the tongue and teeth to permit air to flow into the lungs. These measures ultimately produced results in that Brother Fox's heart resumed beating. However, as a consequence of the interruption of the flow of oxygen caused by the cardiac arrest, Brother Fox suffered substantial brain damage. He was removed to the intensive care unit of the hospital and placed on a respirator, a mechanical breathing device used only for those who are extremely ill and in danger of dying. He slipped into a coma from which he was never to emerge and lost all comprehension of his surroundings. Moreover, with the passage of time, he showed little sign of ever regaining a state of sapience or consciousness.

When Father Eichner was informed of Brother Fox's dire condition, he arranged to have him examined by two neurosurgeons. Upon their negative prognosis, Father Eichner approached the hospital authorities and requested that Brother Fox be removed from the respirator. The authorities declined to comply with this request without a direction from the court and consequently Father Eichner, supported by Brother Fox's surviving relatives and members of the religious community, petitioned the court for relief pursuant to article 78 of the Mental Hygiene Law. Father Eichner asked to be appointed the Committee for Brother Fox and to be permitted to authorize discontinuance of the life-support system.

Supporting the verified petition were affidavits by, *inter alia,* the attending physician, Dr. Edward Kelly, and a neurosurgeon, Dr. Nicholas Poloukhine, detailing the extent of irreversible brain damage suffered by Brother Fox, as well as the overall gravity of his medical condition;

specifically, he had "suffered a cardio-respiratory arrest" resulting in "diffuse cerebral and brain stem anoxia"; he was terminally ill, remaining comatose "in a permanent vegetative state . . . and will not, in the future, come out of his permanent vegetative state."

With respect to Brother Fox's views on the use of "extraordinary" life-sustaining measures Father Eichner testified that in 1976, during the time that "the Karen Quinlan situation" was topical, the members of the Chaminade community engaged in extended discussions as to its significance, particularly in relation to the official position of the Catholic Church as expressed by the *allocutio* of Pope Pius XII and adopted by the New Jersey Church authorities. Father Eichner indicated that Brother Fox was an "active" participant in those discussions, agreeing with the position expressed by these religious authorities. In particular, Father Eichner recalled one incident when he heard Brother Fox expressly declare that he "would not want any of this extraordinary business . . . to be done for him."

Rev. Francis T. Keenan, S.M., the Provincial Superior of the Society of Mary, testified that he had been associated with Brother Fox since the witness' novitiate in 1951. With respect to the Chaminade community's discussions of the *Quinlan* case, Father Keenan testified that about two months prior to the hearing date Brother Fox had said to him, "Well, why don't they just let us go? I want to go." The witness also observed that "Brother Joseph would be a person who would revere the person of the Pope a great deal and the teaching of the church a great deal, and since Pius XII has been very clear on this issue, he would accept it."

Norbert Mechenbier, a nephew of Brother Fox, testified that he had discussed the petition of the nine other surviving blood relatives of Brother Fox. On October 16, 1979, after the operation, Mechenbier had visited Brother Fox in the hospital. Based on the statements of the medical staff, Mechenbier and his relatives favored withdrawal of the respirator unless there was a possibility of improvement beyond "a vegetative state."

In opposing the petition, the District Attorney sought to establish that Brother Fox was "improving" neurologically, or in the alternative that it was too early to determine his condition because he had yet to reach a state of neurological "stabilization." Toward this end the District Attorney presented two physicians who had conducted a neurological examination at his request. Dr. Eli Goldensohn, a neurologist, reviewed Brother Fox's records and noted "slight improvement" between October 12 and October 17. Brother Fox was in [a vegetative state], although Dr. Goldensohn was not certain whether this condition had stabilized. His prognosis was that the chances were "extremely remote" and that it was "entirely improbable" that Brother Fox would ever regain consciousness.

Dr. Richard Beresford, a neurologist, also examined Brother Fox, and his medical opinion was consistent with that of his colleagues. Specifically, he concluded that Brother Fox had entered into a vegetative state and it was "highly improbable" that he would ever regain cognitive function. While there was one case in the medical literature of a 43-year-old man who had fully recovered from a similar vegetative state after 17 months, this was an unexpected "deviation from the normal."

Finally, the guardian ad litem, Robert C. Minion, Esq., testified in favor of granting the relief sought by Father Eichner, including authorization to withdraw the respirator.

Turning our attention to the substantive legal problems, we begin by recognizing that, while the right of an *incompetent* patient to refuse medical treatment or to have it withdrawn may be subject to some controversy, by contrast, the right of a *competent* patient to do so is not. There exists a solid line of case authority recognizing the undeniable right of a terminally ill but competent individual to refuse medical care, even if it will inexorably result in his death. The underlying motive for the patient's decision is irrelevant. Its legal underpinnings have been carefully considered and variously described. The Court of Appeals has affirmed that " [e]very human being of adult years and sound mind has a right to determine what shall be done with his body."

Accordingly we conclude that, were Brother Fox competent, he could refuse medical treatment not only as an exercise of his common-law right to bodily self-determination, but also pursuant to his constitutional right to privacy. Although the two are quite clearly equivalent in effect since they compel the same result, the difference between them is something more than mere semantics. Common-law rights can be abrogated by statute in the exercise of the State's police powers subject only to due process requirements. It suffices for purposes of this analysis, however, that these two rights function in a complimentary manner, simultaneously affording the incurably ill the right to determine at what point aggressive therapy should cease.

We further conclude that by standards of logic, morality and medicine the terminally ill should be treated equally, whether competent or incompetent. Can it be doubted that the "value of human dignity extends to both?" What possible societal policy objective is vindicated or furthered by treating the two groups of terminally ill *differently?* What is gained by granting such a fundamental right only to those who, though terminally ill, have not suffered brain damage and coma in the last stages of the dying process? The very notion raises the spectre of constitutional infirmity when measured against the Supreme Court's recognition that incompetents must be afforded all their due process rights; indeed any State scheme which irrationally denies to the terminally ill incompetent that which it grants to the terminally ill competent patient is plainly subject to constitutional attack.

It is not enough, however, simply to declare that the terminally ill patient in a chronic coma is entitled to refuse further medical treatment: We are bound by *Roe v. Wade* to determine whether the exercise of that right contravenes some countervailing State interest, and we therefore measure the relief requested herein against the four major categories of relevant State interests.

(1) *Preservation and sanctity of life:* The principal State interest to be protected in this proceeding, as in *Roe v. Wade,* is the preservation of the sanctity of life. Yet, the patient in a permanent vegetative coma has no hope of recovery and merely lies, trapped in a technological limbo, awaiting the inevitable. As a matter of established fact, such a patient has *no* health and, in the true sense, no life, for the State to protect. Thus, the use of a respirator, or any other extraordinary means of life support, *under these circumstances,* does not serve to advance the State's interest in protecting health or life and, hence, that interest does not defeat the privacy right asserted here. Indeed, with *Roe v. Wade* in mind it is appropriate to note that the State's interest in preservation of the life of the fetus would appear to be *greater* than any possible interest the State may have in maintaining the continued life of a terminally ill comatose patient. The fetus is a potential person who, in the natural course, will develop into a whole functional human being; the terminally ill patient in a permanent vegetative coma, in striking contrast, has in most cases already enjoyed his life and now, at the last hour, depends for his continued existence upon an extraordinary life-sustaining technology. Such claim to personhood is certainly no greater than that of the fetus. Both the Quinlan and Saikewicz courts made similar determinations in this regard. The analysis of the Quinlan court was that " [t]he State's interest *contra* weakens and the in-

dividual's right to privacy grows as the degree of bodily invasion increases and the prognosis dims. Ultimately there comes a point at which the individual's rights overcome the State interest." Equally articulate, the Saikewicz court declared:

"The interest of the State in prolonging a life must be reconciled with the interest of an individual to reject the traumatic cost of that prolongation. There is a substantial distinction in the State's insistence that human life be saved where the affliction is curable, as opposed to the State interest where, as here, the issue is not whether but when, for how long, and at what cost to the individual that life may be briefly extended."

(2) *Protection of third parties:* This State interest turns on the facts of the particular controversy. It is incumbent upon Special Term to examine what potential harm may arise to dependents as a result of the patient's death and to consider such effect as one factor in the ultimate decision. In the case at bar, the 83-year-old Brother Fox had no dependents to "abandon"; accordingly, this State interest does not affect the outcome of this controversy.

(3) *Maintenance of the ethical integrity of the medical profession:* As previously alluded to, withdrawal of any extraordinary life-support systems for the terminally ill in an irreversible vegetative coma is consistent with and largely supported by the current state of medical ethics. The problem of potential liability to the hospital or medical staff can be obviated by protective provisions in the order ultimately issued.

(4) *Prevention of suicide:* Upon analysis, this protective State interest, under the circumstances at bar, is not compelling either. At common law, suicide required a *specific intent to die.* But withdrawal of the respirator evinces only an intent to forgo extraordinary measures and to allow the processes of nature to run their course. The legislative history of the criminal suicide statutes supports this analysis. Formerly, attempted suicide was a criminal offense which at common law worked a forfeiture of property. The common law was changed by statute to abolish the crime of attempted suicide and to recognize that suicide was merely "a grave public wrong." By 1890, suicide was no longer considered a crime in this State. The current Penal Law provides for criminal liability solely as to a third party who aids or promotes the suicide attempt; it does not impose liability against the *individual* himself. Hence, there seems to be no public policy against permitting a terminally ill patient to choose not to delay the inevitable and imminent termination of his life—at least insofar as public policy is reflected in the current Penal Law. Such decision, directed to terminating the artificial prolongation of life, cannot be deemed "irrational" in the sense generally connoted by the term "suicide."

We conclude, therefore, that there were no State interests sufficiently compelling in this proceeding to have precluded Brother Fox from exercising his right to discontinue life-prolonging medical treatment.

Accordingly, we hold that the following procedure shall be applicable to the proposed withdrawal of extraordinary life-sustaining measures from the terminally ill and comatose patient. The physicians attending the patient must first certify that he is terminally ill and in an irreversible, permanent or chronic vegetative coma, and that the prospects of his regaining cognitive brain function are extremely remote. Thereafter, the person to whom such certification is made, whether a member of the patient's family, someone having a close personal relationship with him, or an official of the hospital itself, may present the prognosis to an appropriate hospital committee. If the hospital has a standing committee for such purposes, composed of at least three physicians, then that committee shall either confirm or reject the prognosis. If the hospital has no such standing committee, then, upon the petition of the person seeking relief, the hospital's chief administrative officer shall appoint such a committee consisting of no fewer than three physicians with specialties relevant to the patient's case. Confirmation of the prognosis shall be a majority of the members of the committee, although lack of unanimity may later be considered by the court.

Upon confirmation of the prognosis, the person who secured it may commence a proceeding pursuant to article 78 of the Mental Hygiene Law for appointment as the Committee of the incompetent, and for permission to have the life-sustaining measures withdrawn. The Attorney-General and the appropriate District Attorney shall be given notice of the proceeding and, if they deem it necessary, shall be afforded an opportunity to have examinations conducted by physicians of their own choosing. Additionally, a guardian ad litem shall be appointed to assure that the interests of the patient are indeed protected by a neutral and detached party wholly free of self-interest.

Where this procedure is complied with, and where the court concludes, consistent with the principles announced herein, that the extraordinary life-sustaining measures should be discontinued, no participant—either medical or lay—shall be subject to criminal or civil liability as a result of the termination of such life-sustaining measures. Should death occur, its proximate cause shall be deemed to be whatever caused the patient to lapse into the coma in the first instance.

We recognize that, at first blush, the procedure we require may appear cumbersome and too time-consuming to accommodate the need for speedy determinations in cases where termination of treatment is proposed. We believe, however, that such procedure is both necessary for the protection of the rights of the incompetent and fully capable of expeditious completion through the co-operation of movants, physicians and judges all aware of the urgency which such situations present. Indeed, since we deal with profound issues of human life and of death with dignity, our society can tolerate no less thorough procedure and will expect nothing short of the best efforts of those involved to reach a decision with all possible speed.

As we have previously noted, the issues raised herein demand that a structural legal framework be created for future cases. We would consider it a veritable dereliction of our duty to decline to design a reasonable scheme at this time. In formulating this procedure, we are fully aware that the very nature of these issues will continue to provoke a wide-ranging disparity of views regarding the societal implications of the solution we have reached. Yet we are convinced that the framework we establish will serve both to protect the interests of the terminally ill and to ameliorate a difficult ethical problem facing the medical profession. Moreover, we firmly believe that by providing a procedure for the exercise of the right of the comatose and terminally ill to permit the immutable processes of nature to run their course, we ultimately affirm the dignity and worth of human life.

Reprinted from 426 New York Supplement 2nd Series 517, Decided March 27, 1980.

Author Index

Subject Index